2017

The Year Book of PEDIATRICS®

Editor

Michael D. Cabana, MD, MPH

Professor of Pediatrics, Epidemiology & Biostatistics and Chief, UCSF Division of General Pediatrics, University of California, San Francisco; Core Faculty, Philip R. Lee Institute for Health Policy Studies, San Francisco, California

Associate Editors

Allan M. Goldstein, MD

Marshall K. Bartlett Associate Professor of Surgery, Harvard Medical School; Chief of Pediatric Surgery, Massachusetts General Hospital; Surgeon-in-Chief, MassGeneral Hospital for Children, Boston, Massachusetts

Pascal Scemama de Gialluly, MD, MBA

Interim Director of Pediatric Pain, Assistant in Anesthesia, Department of Anesthesia, Critical Care and Pain Medicine, The Massachusetts General Hospital; Instructor, Harvard Medical School, Boston, Massachusetts

Alan R. Schroeder, MD

Director, PICU and Chief of Inpatient Pediatrics, Santa Clara Valley medicine Center, San Jose, CA; Associate Professor (affiliate) of Pediatrics, Stanford University School of Medicine, Stanford, California

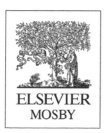

ELSEVIER
MOSBY

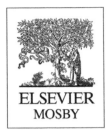

ELSEVIER
MOSBY

Vice President Global Content: Judith Fletcher
Acquisitions Editor: Kerry Holland
Developmental Editor: Casey Jackson
Production Supervisor, Electronic Year Books: Donna M. Skelton
Electronic Article Manager: Mahalakshmi Nithyanand
Illustrations and Permissions Coordinator: Dawn Vohsen

2017 EDITION

Printed in the United States of America
Composition by TNQ Books and Journals Pvt Ltd, India
Printing/binding by Sheridan Books, Inc.

Editorial Office:
Elsevier
Suite 1800
1600 John F. Kennedy Blvd.
Philadelphia, PA 19103-2899

International Standard Serial Number: 0084-3954
International Standard Book Number: 978-0-323-48035-2

Contributors

Jon S. Abramson, MD
Professor, Department of Pediatrics, Wake Forest Baptist Health Brenner Children's Hospital, Winston-Salem, NC

Janelle L. Aby, MD
Department of Pediatrics, Stanford University, Stanford Lucile Packard Children's Hospital, Palo Alto, CA

Michael J. Ackerman, MD, PhD
Windland Smith Rice Cardiovascular Genomics Research Professor, Professor of Medicine, Pediatrics, and Pharmacology, Director, Long QT Syndrome/ Genetic Heart Rhythm Clinic and Mayo Clinic Windland Smith Rice Sudden Death Genomics Laboratory, Mayo Clinic; President, Sudden Arrhythmia Death Syndromes (SADS) Foundation, Rochester, MN

Jeremy T. Aidlen, MD
Associate Professor of Surgery, Pediatrics and Urology, Department of Surgery, Division of Pediatric Surgery and Trauma, University of Massachusetts Medical School, Worcester, MA

Thomas B. Alexander, MD, MPH
Clinical Fellow, Hematology-Oncology, St. Jude's Children's Research Hospital, Memphis, TN

Elena Aragona, MD
Department of Pediatrics, Tufts Floating Hospital for Children, Boston, MA

Greg T. Armstrong, MD, MSCE
Associate Member, Department of Epidemiology and Cancer Control, Division of Neuro-Oncology, St. Jude's Research Hospital, Memphis, TN

John C. Arnold, MD
Chairman of Pediatrics, Pediatric Infectious Disease, and Head, Pediatric Clinic, Naval Medical San Diego, San Diego, CA

Paul L. Aronson, MD
Departments of Pediatrics and Emergency Medicine, Section of Pediatric Emergency Medicine, Yale School of Medicine, New Haven, CT

Judy Aschner, MD
Departments of Pediatrics, Obstetrics, Gynecology and Women's Health, Albert Einstein College of Medicine and the Children's Hospital of Montefiore, Bronx, NY

Peter F. Aziz, MD, FHRS
Assistant Professor, Pediatrics, Cleveland Clinic Lerner College of Medicine, Cleveland, OH

M. Douglas Baker, MD
Professor of Pediatrics, Johns Hopkins University School of Medicine, Vice Chair, Department of Pediatrics, Director, Division of Emergency Medicine, Charlotte R. Bloomberg Children's Center, Baltimore, MD

Sophie J. Balk, MD

Attending Pediatrician, Children's Hospital at Montefiore, Professor of Clinical Pediatrics, Albert Einstein College of Medicine, New York, NY

Naomi S. Bardach, MD, MAS

Department of Pediatrics, Philip R. Lee Institute for Health Policy Studies, University of California San Francisco, San Francisco, CA

John B. Bartholomew, PhD

Professor and Chair, Department of Kinesiology and Health Education, University of Texas at Austin, Austin, TX

Laurence S. Baskin, MD

Frank Hinman, Jr., MD, Distinguished Professorship in Pediatric Urology, UCSF Benioff Children's Hospital, Director KURe Training Program, Chief Pediatric Urology, Professor of Urology and Pediatrics, San Francisco, CA

Andrew J. Bauer, MD

Director, The Thyroid Center, Division of Endocrinology, The Children's Hospital of Philadelphia, Associate Professor, Department of Pediatrics, Perelman School of Medicine, The University of Pennsylvania, Philadelphia, PA

Michael W. Beets, MEd, MPH, PhD

Department of Exercise Science, Arnold School of Public Health, University of South Carolina, Columbia, SC

Carol D. Berkowitz, MD, FAAP, FACEP

Executive Vice Chair, Department of Pediatrics, Harbor-UCLA Medical Center, Distinguished Professor of Pediatrics, David Geffen School of Medicine at UCLA, Los Angeles, CA

Sarah N. Bernstein, MD

Massachusetts General Hospital, Department of Obstetrics and Gynecology, Division of Maternal Fetal Medicine, Boston, MA

Frank M. Biro, MD

Division of Adolescent Medicine, Cincinnati Children's Hospital Medical Center, Professor of Pediatrics, University of Cincinnati College of Medicine, Cincinnati, OH

Seth Bokser, MD, MPH

Associate Professor, Department of Pediatrics, University of California, San Francisco, San Francisco, CA

Jori F. Bogetz, MD

Assistant Clinical Professor of Pediatrics, Integrated Pain and Palliative Care Program (IP3), UCSF Benioff Children's Hospital, San Francisco, CA

J. Martijn Bos, MD, PhD

Assistant Professor of Pediatrics, Windland Smith Rice Sudden Death Genomics Laboratory, Mayo Clinic, Rochester, MN

Nelson Branco, MD, FAAP

Assistant Clinical Professor, Pediatrics, University of California San Francisco, San Francisco, CA; Tamalpais Pediatrics, Greenbrae, CA

Andreas Brunklaus, MD(Res)

Honorary Clinical Lecturer and Consultant Paediatric Neurologist, The Paediatric Neurosciences Research Group, Royal Hospital for Children, Glasgow, UK

Tyra Bryant-Stephens, MD
Director and Founder, The Community Asthma Prevention Program, Clinical Professor of Pediatrics, The Children's Hospital of Philadelphia, The Perelmann School of Medicine at the University of Pennsylvania, Philadelphia, PA

Supinda Bunyavanich, MD, MPH, MPhil
Assistant Professor, Department of Pediatrics- Allergy/Immunology, Department of Genetics and Genomic Sciences, Icahn School of Medicine at Mount Sinai, New York, NY

Elizabeth Bendig Burgener, MD
Pediatric Pulmonary Medicine, Lucile Packard Children's Hospital Stanford, Palo Alto, CA

Michael D. Cabana, MD, MPH
Professor of Pediatrics, Epidemiology & Biostatistics and Chief, UCSF Division of General Pediatrics, University of California, San Francisco; Core Faculty, Philip R. Lee Institute for Health Policy Studies, San Francisco, CA

Rashida T. Campwala, MD
Department of Pediatrics, Division of Emergency & Transport Medicine, Children's Hospital Los Angeles, Los Angeles, CA

Joseph A. Carcillo, MD
Professor, CCM and Pediatrics, Children's Hospital of Pittsburgh, Pittsburgh, PA

Alexandra N. Carey, MD
Instructor of Pediatrics, Harvard Medical School, Attending Physician, Division of Gastroenterology, Hepatology and Nutrition, Associate Medical Director, Center for Advanced Intestinal Rehabilitation Program, Boston Children's Hospital, Boston, MA

Donald H. Chace, PhD, MSFS, FACB
Pediatrix Analytical, Centers for Research, Education and Quality, Mednax Services, Inc, Sunrise, FL

Angela L. Chang, MD
Pediatric Fellow in the Division of Allergy, Immunology and Blood Marrow Transplantation, UCSF Benioff Children's Hospital, University of California San Francisco, San Francisco, CA

Christine S. Cho, MD, MPH, Med
Department of Pediatrics, Children's Hospital Los Angeles, USC Keck School of Medicine, Los Angeles, CA

Ian S. Chua, MD
Division of Hospital Medicine, Department of Pediatrics, Children's National Medical Center, George Washington School of Medicine, Washington, DC; Division of Pediatric Hospital Medicine, Department of Pediatrics, Lucile Packard Children's Hospital Stanford, Palo Alto, CA

Esther K. Chung, MD, MPH
Department of Pediatrics, The Sidney Kimmel Medical College, Thomas Jefferson University and Nemours, Philadelphia, PA

Michael J. Cisco, MD
Cardiac Intensive Care, Benioff Children's Hospital; Assistant Professor of Pediatrics, University of California San Francisco, San Francisco, CA

Reese H. Clark, MD
Director of Neonatal Research, MEDNAX Inc., Sunrise, FL

Taylor Clark, MD
Department of Pediatrics, Zuckerberg San Francisco General Hospital,
University of California San Francisco, San Francisco, CA

Stephen J. Cleland, BSc (Hons), PhD, FRCP (Glasg)
Emergency Care & Medical Services, Queen Elizabeth University Hospital,
Glasgow, Scotland

Ronald I. Clyman, MD
Professor of Pediatrics, University of California San Francisco,
San Francisco, CA

Sonja Colianni, MD, FAAP
Associate Chief, Department of Pediatrics, Hennepin County Medical Center,
Minneapolis, MN

Eric Coon, MD, MSCI
Assistant Professor of Pediatrics, Primary Children's Hospital, University of
Utah School of Medicine, Salt Lake City, UT

Kathleen Jo E. Corbin, MD, MHS
Department of Pediatrics, Division of Rheumatology, University of California
San Francisco, San Francisco, CA

Kelly M. Cordoro, MD
Associate Professor of Dermatology and Pediatrics, Assistant Chief, Pediatric
Dermatology, Director, Pediatric Dermatology Fellowship, University of
California San Francisco, San Francisco, CA

Kevin P. Coulter, MD
Professor and Interim Chair, Department of Pediatrics, University of California
Davis Children's Hospital, Sacramento, CA

Robert A. Cowles, MD
Associate Professor of Surgery, Program Director, Pediatric Surgery, Yale School
of Medicine, New Haven, CT

Edward S. Cruz, MD, MPH
Assistant Professor of Pediatrics, University of California San Francisco, San
Francisco General Hospital, San Francisco, CA

Megan Lea Curran, MD
Department of Pediatrics, Northwestern University Feinberg School or
Medicine, Ann & Robert H. Lurie Children's Hospital of Chicago, Chicago, IL

Peter A. Dargaville, MD
Staff Specialist and Professorial Research Fellow in Neonatology, Department of
Paediatrics, Royal Hobart Hospital and Menzies Research Institute, University
of Tasmania, Hobart, Australia

Augusto César Ferreira de Moraes, PhD
YCARE (Youth/Child and Cardiovascular Risk and Enviromental) Research
Group, School of Medicine, University of Sao Paulo/Brazil; GENUD (Growth,
Exercise, NUtrition and Development) Research Group, Faculty of Health
Services, University of Zaragoza, Zaragoza, Spain

Michael R. DeBaun, MD, MPH
Professor of Pediatrics and Medicine, Division of Pediatric Hematology/ Oncology, Monroe Carell Jr. Children's Hospital at Vanderbilt, Director, Vanderbilt-Meharry Center for Excellence in Sickle Cell Disease, Nashville, TN

Amanda Dempsey, MD, PhD, MPH
Department of Pediatrics, Division of General Pediatrics, Adult and Child Consortium for Outcomes Research and Dissemination Science, University of Colorado Denver, Denver, CO

Linda A. DiMeglio, MD, MPH
Professor of Pediatrics, Department of Pediatrics, Section of Endocrinology and Diabetology, Indiana University School of Medicine, Indianapolis, IN

Christopher Duggan, MD, MPH
Center for Nutrition at Boston Children's Hospital, Division of Gastroenterology, Hepatology and Nutrition, Department of Pediatrics, Harvard Medical School, Boston, MA

Marc A. Edwards, PhD, MS
Charles P. Lunsford Professor, Environmental and Water Resources Engineering, Virginia Tech, Blacksburg, VA

Jack S. Elder, MD, FACS
Chief, Division of Pediatric Urology, Massachusetts General Hospital, Harvard Medical School, Boston, MA

Elizabeth J. Elliott, AM, MD, MBBS, MPhil, FRACP, FRCPCH, FRCP
Professor of Paediatrics and Child Health, University of Sydney, Consultant Paediatrician, Sydney Children's Hospitals Network Westmead, National Health and Medical Research Council of Australia Practitioner Fellow, Westmead, Australia

Ayca Erkin-Cakmak, MD, MPH
Department of Pediatrics, UCSF Benioff Children's Hospital, San Francisco, CA

Jeffrey J. Fadrowski, MD, MHS
Associate Professor of Pediatrics, Division of Pediatric Nephrology, Johns Hopkins University School of Medicine, Baltimore, MD

Lauren E. Faricy, MD
Pediatric Pulmonary Medicine, Department of Pediatrics, UCSF Benioff Children's Hospital and University of California San Francisco, San Francisco, CA

Magali Fassiotto, PhD
Office of Faculty Development and Diversity, Stanford University School of Medicine, Stanford, CA

Joseph T. Flynn, MD, MS
Professor of Pediatrics, University of Washington, Chief, Division of Nephrology, Seattle Children's Hospital, Seattle, WA

Marc Foca, MD
Associate Professor of Pediatrics at Columbia University Medical Center, Department of Pediatrics, Division of Infectious Diseases, Children's Hospital of New York Presbyterian, New York, NY

Elizabeth E. Foglia, MD, MSCE
Department of Pediatrics, Division of Neonatology, University of Pennsylvania Perelman School of Medicine, Children's Hospital of Philadlephia, Philadelphia, PA

Mamta Fuloria, MD, FAAP
Assistant Professor, Department of Pediatrics, Albert Einstein College of Medicine and The Children's Hospital at Montefiore, Bronx, NY

Andrea K. Garber, PhD, RD
Associate Professor of Pediatrics, Division of Adolescent & Young Adult Medicine, UCSF Benioff Children's Hospital, University of California San Francisco, San Francisco, CA

Amy Gelfand, MD
Director of Pediatric Headache, UCSF Benioff Children's Hospital, San Francisco, CA

Elizabeth Gibb, MD
Department of Pediatrics, University of California San Francisco, San Francisco, CA

Shawn R. Gilbert, MD
Chief of Pediatric Orthopaedics, Orthopaedic Surgery, University of Alabama at Birmingham, Birmingham, AL

Robyn Gilden, PhD, RN
Director, Department of Family and Community Health Enviromental Health Certificate, University of Maryland School of Nursing, Baltimore, MD

Peter Girolami, PhD, BCBA-D
Program Director, Pediatric Feeding Disorders Program, Kennedy Krieger Institute, Assistant Professor, Department of Psychiatry and Behavioral Sciences, Johns Hopkins School of Medicine, Baltimore, MD

Christopher C. Giza, MD
Professor, Division of Pediatric Neurology, Department of Pediatrics; Department of Neurosurgery, Interdepartmental Programs for Neurosciences and Biomedical Engineering; Mattel Children's Hospital - UCLA & David Geffen School of Medicine at UCLA; Director, UCLA Steve Tisch BrainSPORT Program, Los Angeles, CA

Praveen S. Goday, MBBS
Professor, Pediatric Gastroenterology and Nutrition, Medical College of Wisconsin, Milwaukee, WI

Allan M. Goldstein, MD
Marshall K. Bartlett Associate Professor of Surgery, Harvard Medical School; Chief of Pediatric Surgery, Massachusetts General Hospital; Surgeon-in-Chief, MassGeneral Hospital for Children, Boston, MA

William V. Good, MD
Senior Scientist, Smith-Kettlewell Eye Research Institute, San Francisco, CA

Elizabeth Sinclair Goswami, PharmD, BCPS, BCPPS
Clinical Pharmacy Specialist, Pediatric Nephrology, Department of Pharmacy, The Johns Hopkins Hospital, Baltimore, MD

Eric Franklin Grabowski, MD, SCD
Associate Professor of Pediatrics, Director, Mass General Comprehensive Hemophilia Treatment Center, Co-Director, Pediatric Stroke Services, Director, Cardiovascular Thrombosis Laboratory, Massachusetts General Hospital, Harvard Medical School, Boston, MA

Donald E. Greydanus, MD, Dr. HC (ATHENS)
Professor and Founding Chair, Department of Pediatric and Adolescent Medicine, Western Michigan University Homer Stryker M.D. School of Medicine, Kalamazoo, MI

Jacqueline Grupp-Phelan, MD, MPH
Director of Research, Associate Director, Division of Pediatric Emergency Medicine, Ruddy Chair of Pediatric Emergency Medicine Research, Professor of Clinical Pediatrics, University of Cincinnati College of Medicine, Cincinnati, OH

Deepti Gupta, MD
Assistant Professor, Department of Pediatrics and Division of Dermatology, Seattle Children's Hospital, University of Washington School of Medicine, Seattle, WA

Philip J. Hashkes, MD, MSc, RhMSUS
Head, Pediatric Rheumatology Unit, Shaare Zedek Medical Center, Associate Professor of Pediatrics, Hebrew University, Jerusalem, Israel

Fern R. Hauck, MD, MS
Twenty-First Century Professor of Family Medicine and Public Health Sciences, Director, International Family Medicine Clinic, University of Virginia, Charlottesville, VA

William W. Hay Jr., MD
Professor of Pediatrics (Neonatology), Scientific Director, Perinatal Research Center, Co-Director for Child and Maternal Health, Colorado Clinical and Translational Sciences Institute, University of Colorado School of Medicine, Aurora, CO

Aimee Hersh, MD, MS
Department of Pediatrics, Division of Rheumatology, University of Utah, Salt Lake City, UT

William Hennrikus, MD
Professor, Penn State College of Medicine; Medical Director, Penn State Pediatric Bone and Joint Institute; Associate Dean of Education, Penn State College of Medicine, Hershey, PA

Merav Heshin-Bekenstein, MD
Fellow, Pediatric Rheumatology Division, University of California San Francisco, San Francisco, CA

Claus Højbjerg Gravholt, MD, PhD
Professor, Dr.Med.Sci., Department of Endocrinology and Internal Medicine MEA and Department of Molecular Medicine (MOMA), Aarhus University Hospital, Aarhus, Denmark

Peter F. Hoyer, Dr. med.
Department of Pediatrics II, Pediatric Nephrology, Gastroenterology, Endocrinology and Transplant Medicine, Children's Hospital Essen, University Duisburg-Essen, Essen, Germany

James Huang, MD
Department of Pediatrics, University of California San Francisco and UCSF Benioff Children's Hospital, San Francisco, CA

Abraham Jelin, MD
Associate Chairman of Pediatrics, Director of Pediatric Gastroenterology, The Brooklyn Hospital Center, Assistant Professor of Clinical Pediatrics, Icahn School of Medicine at Mount Sinai, New York, NY

Alan H. Jobe, MD, PhD
Cincinnati Children's Hospital, Division of Pulmonary Biology, University of Cincinnati, Cincinnati, OH

Christine L. Johnson, MD, FAAP
General Pediatrician, Naval Medical Center San Diego, San Diego, CA

Sebastian L. Johnston, MBBS, PhD, FERS, FRCP, FRSB, FMedSci
Airway Disease Infection Section, National Heart and Lung Institute, Imperial College London, London, United Kingdom

Ray Jurado, DDS
Division Head, Dentistry, Ann and Robert H. Lurie Children's Hospital of Chicago, Program Director, Pediatric Dentistry, Northwestern University Feinberg School of Medicine, Chicago, IL

Laura R. Kair, MD
Assistant Professor of Clinical Pediatrics, University of California Davis Medical Center, Sacramento, CA

Mitul Kapadia, MD, MSc
Assistant Clinical Professor of Physical Medicine and Rehabilitaion and Pediatrics, University of California San Francisco, Medical Director, Pediatric Rehabilitation Medicine, UCSF Benioff Children's Hospital, Co-Director of UCSF Sports Concussion Program, San Francisco, CA

Scarlett Karakash, MD
Director, Obstetrics, Maimonides Medical Center, Brooklyn, NY

Thomas K. Koch, MD
Chief, Division of Pediatric Neurology, Medical University of South Carolina, Charleston, SC

Prabhakar Kocherlakota, MD
Associate Professor of Pediatrics, Division of Neonatology, Department of Pediatrics, Maria Fareri Children's Hospital at Westchester Medical Center, New York Medical College, Valhalla, NY

Cassandra M. Kelleher, MD
Department of Pediatric Surgery, MassGeneral Hospital for Children, Harvard Medical School, Boston, MA

Kelly J. Kelleher, MD, MPH
Professor of Pediatrics and Public Health, Colleges of Medicine and Public Health, The Ohio State University; Vice President for Health Services Research, Director, Center for Innovation in Pediatric Practice, The Research Institute at Nationwide Children's Hospital, Columbus, OH

Roberta L. Keller, MD
Associate Professor of Pediatrics, Division of Neonatology, Director, Neonatal ECMO, Director of Neonatal Services, Fetal Treatment Center, University of California San Francisco, UCSF Benioff Children's Hospital, San Francisco, CA

Alex R. Kemper, MD, MPH, MS
Department of Pediatrics, Duke University, Durham, NC

Harry K.W. Kim, MD, MS
Director, Sara M. and Charles E. Seay Center for Muculoskeletal Research, Director, Center for Excellence in Hip Disorders, Texas Scottish Rite Hospital for Children, Professor, Orthopaedic Surgery, University of Texas Southwestern Medical Center, Dallas, TX

Walter K. Kraft, MD
Professor of Pharmacology, Medicine and Surgery, Department of Pharmcology and Experimental Therapeutics, Sidney Kimmel Medical College of Thomas Jefferson University, Philadelphia, PA

Scott D. Krugman, MD, MS, FAAP
Chairman, Department of Pediatrics, MedStar Franklin Square Medical Center, Professor, Pediatrics, Georgetown University School of Medicine, Associate Dean for Medical Education at MFSMC, Georgetown University School of Medicine, Washington, DC

Herwig Lackner, MD
Department of Pediatrics and Adolescent Medicine, Division of Pediatric Hematology/Oncology, Medical University of Graz, Graz, Austria

John D. Lantos, MD
Director, Children's Mercy Bioethics Center, Children's Mercy Hospital; and Professor of Pediatrics, University of Missouri, Kansas City, Kansas City, MO

Erica F. Lawson, MD
Department of Pediatrics, Division of Rheumatology, UCSF Benioff Children's Hospital, San Francisco, CA

Janet Y. Lee, MD, MPH
Clinical Fellow, Division of Endocrinology and Metabolism, Division of Pediatric Endocrinology and Diabetes, University of California San Francisco, San Francisco, CA

Harvey L. Leo, MD
Associate Research Scientist, Department of Health Behavior Health Education, University of Michigan School of Public Health, Washington Heights, Ann Arbor, MI

Melissa Liebowitz, MD
Department of Pediatrics, University of California San Francisco, San Francisco, CA

Nicole Ling, MD, MAS
Assistant Clinical Professor, Department of Pediatrics, Division of Pediatric Rheumatology, University of California San Francisco, Benioff Children's Hospitals, San Francisco, CA

Paul H. Lipkin, MD
Director, Interactive Autism Network, Kennedy Kreiger Institute, Associate Professor of Pediatrics, Johns Hopkins University School of Medicine, Baltimore, MD

Roger Long, MD
Department of Pediatrics, Benioff Children's Hospital San Francisco, University of California San Francisco School of Medicine, San Francisco, CA

Angela K. Lucas-Herald, MRCPCH, MBChC
Clinical Lecturer, Developmental Endocrinology Research Group, Royal Hospital for Children, University of Glasgow, Glasgow, United Kingdom

Robert Lustig, MD, MSL
Department of Pediatrics, UCSF Benioff Children's Hospital, and UCSF Institute for Health Policy Studies, San Francisco, CA

Ngoc P. Ly, MD, MPH
Pediatric Pulmonary Medicine, Department of Pediatrics, Benioff Children Hospital and University of California San Francisco, San Francisco, CA

Jeffrey M. Maisels, MB, BcH DSc
Chair Emeritus and Professor, Director, Academic Affairs, Department of Pediatrics, Oakland University William Beaumont School of Medicine, Beaumont Children's Hospital, Royal Oak, MI

Yvonne Maldonado, MD
Professor Pediatrics, Senior Associate Dean of Faculty Development and Diversity, Stanford University School of Medicine, Stanford, CA

Jyothi Marbin, MD
Department of Pediatrics, Pediatrics Leadership for the Undeserved Residency Program, University of California San Francisco, San Francisco General Hospital, San Francisco, CA

Jennifer R. Marin, MD, MSc
Division of Pediatric Emergency Medicine, Children's Hospital of Pittsburgh, Department of Pediatrics and Emergency Medicine, University of Pittsburgh School of Medicine, Pittsburgh, PA

Peter T. Masiakos, MD
Pediatric Surgery, MassGeneral Hospital for Children, Boston, MA

Jonathan M. Marron, MD
Department of Pediatric Oncology, Dana-Farber/Boston Children's Cancer and Blood Disorders Center, and Center for Bioethics, Harvard Medical School, Boston, MA

Elizabeth C. Matsui, MD, MHS
Department of Pediatrics, Division of Pediatric Allergy/Immunology, Johns Hopkins School of Medicine; Departments of Epidemiology and Environmental Health Sciences, Johns Hopkins Bloomberg School of Public Health, Baltimore, MD

Oliver F. Medzihradsky, MD, MPH, MSc
Division of Pediatric Infectious Diseases, Department of Pediatrics, University of California San Francisco, Malaria Elimination Initiative, Global Health Group, UCSF Global Health Sciences, San Francisco, CA

Dipika Menon, MD
Resident, Pediatrics, Cleveland Clinic Children's Hospital, Cleveland, OH

Daniel J. Merenstein, MD
Director of Research of Family Medicine, Associate Professor of Family Medicine, Georgetown University Medical Center, Washington, DC

Carol A. Miller, MD
HS Clinical Professor, Department of Pediatrics, University of California San Francisco, UCSF Benioff Children's Hospital, San Francisco, CA

Jennifer Miller, MD, FAAP
UCSF Benioff Children's Hospital, Oakland; East Bay Pediatrics Medical Group, Berkeley, CA

Mark D. Miller, MD, MPH
Assistant Clinical Professor Pediatrics and Co-Director, Western States Pediatric Environmental Health Specialty Unit at University of California San Francisco, San Francisco; Director, Children's Environmental Health Program, California Environmental Protection Agency, Sacramento, CA

Andrew F. Miller, MD
Boston Children's Hospital, Division of Emergency Medicine, Harvard Medical School, Boston, MA

Howard Minkoff, MD
Chairman, Department of Obstetrics and Gynecology, Maimonides Medical Center, Distinguished Professor of Obstetrics and Gynecology, SUNY Downstate Medical Center, Brooklyn, NY

Michael J. Morowitz, MD, FACS
Associate Professor of Surgery, University of Pittsburgh School of Medicine Attending Pediatric Surgeon, Division of Pediatric General and Thoracic Surgery, Children's Hospital of Pittsburgh of UPMC, Pittsburgh, PA

Thomas B. Newman, MD, MPH
Attending Pediatrician, UCSF Children's and Zuckerberg San Francisco General Hospitals, Professor of Epidemiology and Biostatistics and Pediatrics, University of California San Francisco San Francisco, CA

Josef Neu, MD
Professor of Pediatrics, Division of Neonatology; Director of Neonatology Fellowship Training Program, University of Florida Health, Gainesville, FL

Dennis W. Nielson, MD, PhD
Department of Pediatrics, University of California San Francisco, San Francisco, CA

Robin K. Ohls, MD
Professor of Pediatrics, Neonatology Division Chief, Neonatal Fellowship Program Director, Director, Neonatal Research, University of New Mexico, Albuquerque, NM

Sande Okelo, MD, PhD
Division of Pediatric Pulmonology, Department of Pediatrics, David Geffen School of Medicine at UCLA, Mattel Children's Hospital UCLA, Los Angeles, CA

Richard L. Oken, MD, FAAP
Clinical Professor of Pediatrics, University of California San Francisco, San Francisco, CA

Erica Pan, MD, MPH, FAAP
Director, Division of Communicable Disease Control and Prevention and Deputy Health Officer, Alameda County Public Health Department; Clinical Professor, Pediatric Infectious Diseases, University of California San Francisco, Benioff Children's Hospitals, San Francisco, CA

John Colin Partridge, MD, MPH
Division of Neonatology, UCSF Benioff Children's Hospital, San Francisco, CA

K.T. Park, MD, MS
Division of Gastroenterology, Hepatology and Nutrition, Department of Pediatrics, Standford University School of Medicine, Stanford, CA

Anisha Patel, MD, MSPH, MSHS
Department of Pediatrics and the Philip R. Lee Institute for Health Policy, University of California at San Francisco, San Francisco, CA

Ian M. Paul, MD, MSc
Professor of Pediatrics and Public Health Sciences, Chief, Division of Academic General Pediatrics, Vice Chair of Clinical Affairs, Department of Pediatrics, Penn State College of Medicine, Hershey, PA

Colin K.L. Phoon, MD
Department of Pediatrics, New York University School of Medicine, Hassenfield Children's Hospital of NYU Langone Medical Center, Bellevue Hospital Center, New York, NY

Frank S. Pidcock, MD
Director of Pediatric Rehabilitation, Associate Professor of Physical Medicine and Rehabilitation and Pediatrics, Department of Physical Medicine and Rehabilitation, Johns Hopkins University School of Medicine, Baltimore, MD

Janey Sue Pratt, MD
Division of General and Gastrointestinal Surgery, Department of Surgery, Massachusetts General Hospital, Assistant Professor of Surgery, Harvard Medical School, Boston, MA

Victoria E. Price, MBChB, MSc, FRCPC
Pediatric Hematologist/Oncologist, Associate Professor, Division Pediatric Hematology/Oncology, Deptartment of Pediatrics, Dalhousie University, IWK Health Centre, Halifax, Nova Scotia, Canada

Amanda Purington, MPS
Director of Evaluation and Research, ACT for Youth Center of Excellence, Bronfenbrenner Center for Translation Research, Cornell University, Doctoral Student, Department of Communication, Cornell University, Ithaca, NY

Ricardo A. Quinonez, MD, FAAP, FHM
Associate Professor of Pediatrics, Section Head and Service Chief, Pediatric Hospital Medicine, Baylor College of Medicine, Texas Children's Hospital, Houston, TX

Kacy A. Ramirez, MD
Department of Pediatric Infectious Disease, Wake Forest School of Medicine; Wake Forest Baptist Medial Center, Salem, NC

Danielle E. Ramo, PhD
Department of Psychiatry and Helen Diller Family Comprehensive Cancer Center, University of California San Francisco, San Francisco, CA

Matthew A. Rank, MD
Associate Professor of Medicine, Mayo Clinic Arizona, Phoenix, AZ

Kenneth B. Roberts, MD
Professor Emeritus of Pediatrics, University of North Carolina School of Medicine, Chapel Hill; Cone Health System, Greensboro, NC

Philip Rosenthal, MD
Professor of Pediatrics and Surgery, Director, Pediatric Clinical Research, Director, Pediatric Hepatology and Liver Transplant Research, Director, Pediatric Hepatology, University of California San Francisco, San Francisco, CA

Paul J. Rozance, MD
Perinatal Research Center, Department of Pediatrics, University of Colorado School of Medicine, Aurora, CO

Mark L. Rubinstein, MD
Professor, Fellowship Director, Division of Adolescent and Young Adult Medicine, UCSF Benioff Children's Hospital, University of California San Francisco, San Francisco, CA

George W. Rutherford, MD, AM
Department of Epidemiology and Biostatistics and Pediatrics, Program in Global Health Sciences, University of California San Francisco, San Francisco, CA

Loren D. Sacks, MD
Pediatric Cardiovascular Intensive Care Unit, Lucile Packard Children's Hospital Stanford, Palo Alto; Department of Pediatrics (Cardiology), Stanford University, Stanford, CA

Christy Sandborg, MD
Professor of Pediatrics, Stanford University School of Medicine, Stanford, CA

Georgiana M. Sanders, MD, MS
Clinical Associate Professor of Internal Medicine and Pediatrics, Division of Allergy and Clinical Immunology, Department of Internal Medicine and Department of Pediatrics and Communicable Diseases, Research Associate Professor, MH Weiser Food Allergy Research Center, University of Michigan Health System, Ann Arbor, MI

Mary Ellen Sanders, PhD
Dairy and Food Culture Technologies, Centennial, CO

Elisabeth Schainker, MD, MSc
Division of Pediatric Hospital Medicine, Tufts Floating Hospital for Children, Boston, MA

Adam Schickedanz, MD
Robert Wood Johnson Clinical Scholars Program, Department of Pediatrics, University of California Los Angeles, Los Angeles, CA

Alan R. Schroeder, MD
Director, PICU and Chief of Inpatient Pediatrics, Santa Clara Valley Medical Center, San Jose, CA; Associate Clinical Professor (affiliate) of Pediatrics, Stanford University School of Medicine, Stanford, CA

Melissa J. Schoelwer, MD
Department of Pediatrics, Section of Pediatric Endocrinology and Diabetology, Indiana University School of Medicine, Riley Hospital for Children, Indianapolis, IN

Deepa L. Sekhar, MD, MSc
Penn State College of Medicine, Department of Pediatrics, Division of Academic General Pediatrics, Hershey, PA

Marlene B. Schwartz, PhD
Director, Rudd Center for Food Policy and Obesity, Professor, Department of Human Development and Family Studies, University of Connecticut, Hartford, CT

Zachary Michael Sellers, MD, PhD
Division of Gastroenterology, Hepatology and Nutrition, Department of Pediatrics, Standford University School of Medicine, Stanford, CA

Erik S. Shank, MD
Division Chief, Pediatric Anesthesia, Department of Anesthesia, Critical Care and Pain Medicine, Massachusetts General Hospital and Harvard Medical School, Boston, MA

Nader Shaikh, MD
Associate Professor of Pediatrics, Children's Hospital of Pittsburgh of UPMC, University of Pittsburgh School of Medicine, Pittsburgh, PA

William J. Sheehan, MD
Division of Immunology, Boston Children's Hospital, Department of Pediatrics, Harvard Medical School, Boston, MA

Budd N. Shenkin, MD
President, Bayside Medical Group Inc, Clinical Instructor, Department of Pediatrics, University of California San Francisco, Affiliated Faculty Member, Philip R. Lee Institute for Health Policy Studies, University of California San Francisco, San Francisco, CA

Donald S. Shepard, PhD
Schneider Institutesfor Health Policy, Heller School for Social Policy and Management, Brandeis University, Waltham, MA

Jack P. Shonkoff, MD
Julius B. Richmond FAMRI Professor of Child Health and Development, Harvard T. H. Chan School of Public Health and Harvard Graduate School of Education, Professor of Pediatrics, Harvard Medical School and Boston Children's Hospital, Director, Center on the Developing Child at Harvard University, Cambridge, MA

Scott H. Sicherer, MD
Elliot and Roslyn Jaffe Professor of Pediatrics, Allergy and Immunology, Division Chief, Division of Pediatric Allergy and Immunology, Jaffe Food Allergy Institute, Icahn School of Medicine at Mount Sinai, New York, NY

Nanette Silverberg, MD
Chief, Pediatric Dermatology, Clinical Professor of Dermatology and Pediatrics, Icahn School of Medicine at Mount Sinai, New York, NY

Anne Slavotinek, MBBS, PhD
Professor of Clinical Pediatrics, Division of Genetics, Department of Pediatrics, University of California San Francisco, UCSF Benioff Children's Hospital, San Francisco, CA

Adam Spanier, MD, PhD, MPH, FAAP
Department of Pediatrics, University of Maryland School of Medicine, Baltimore, MD

Joseph W. St. Geme III, MD
Department of Pediatrics and Department of Microbiology, The Perelman School of Medicine at the University of Pennsylvania; Department of Pediatrics, The Children's Hospital of Philadelphia, Philadelphia, PA

Christopher C. Stewart, MD
Professor of Pediatrics, University of California San Francisco, San Francisco, CA

Sarah-Jo Stimpson, MD
Fellow, Division of Pediatric Hematology/Oncology, Monroe Carell Jr. Children's Hospital at Vanderbilt, Nashville, TN

Shannon S. Sullivan, MD
Clinical Assistant Professor, Division of Sleep Medicine, Department of Psychiatry, Stanford University School of Medicine, Stanford, CA

Sarah Tabbutt, MD, PhD
Department of Pediatrics, University of California San Francisco, UCSF Benioff Children's Hospital, San Francisco, CA

John I. Takayama, MD, MPH
Professor of Clinical Pediatrics, Department of Pediatrics, UCSF Benioff Children's Hospital, University of California San Francisco, San Francisco, CA

Phillip I. Tarr, MD
Melvin E. Carnahan Professor of Pediatrics, Professor of Molecular Microbiology, Director, Division of Gastroenterology, Hepatology, and Nutrition, Co-Leader, Pathobiology Research Unit, Washington University School of Medicine, St. Louis, MO

Kathleen Tebb, PhD
Department of Pediatrics, Division of Adolescent and Young Adult Medicine, UCSF Benioff Children's Hospital, University of California San Francisco, San Francisco, CA

Amit Thakral, MD, MBA
Department of Pediatrics, Northwestern University Feinberg School of Medicine, Ann and Robert H. Lurie Children's Hospital of Chicago, Chicago, IL

Darcy A. Thompson, MD, MPH
Department of Pediatrics, University of Colorado, Children's Hospital Colorado, Aurora, CO

Leonardo Trasande, MD, MPP
Departments of Pediatrics, Enviromental and Population Health, NYU School of Medicine, Health Policy, NYU Wagner School of Public Service, Public Health and Nutrition, NYU Steinhardt School of Culture, Education and Human Development, Public Health, NYU College of Public Health, New York, NY

Mary K. Tripp, PhD, MPH
Department of Behavioral Science, The University of Texas MD Anderson Cancer Center, Houston, TX

Angela Tsuang, MD, MSc
Fellow in Allergy/Immunology, Icahn School of Medicine at Mount Sinai, New York, NY

Kjell Tullus, MD, PhD, FRPCH
Nephrology Unit, Great Ormond Street Hospital for Children, London, UK

Michael P. Turmelle, MD
Melvin E. Carnahan Professor of Pediatrics, Professor of Molecular Microbiology, Director, Division of Gastroenterology, Hepatology, and Nutrition, Co-Leader, Pathobiology Research Unit, Department of Pediatrics, Washington University School of Medicine, St. Louis, MO

Eduardo A. Undurraga, PhD
Senior Research Associate, Schneider Institutes for Health Policy, Heller School, Brandeis University, Waltham, MA

Elliot P. Vichinsky, MD
Medical Director, Hematology/Oncology, UCSF Benioff Children's Hospital Oakland, Professor of Pediatrics, University of California San Francisco, San Francisco, CA

Karen Dineen Wagner, MD, PhD
Titus Harris Chair, Harry K. Davis Professor, Department of Psychiatry and Behavioral Sciences, University of Texas Medical Branch, Galveston, TX

Daniel Walmsley, DO
Department of Pediatrics, The Sidney Kimmel Medical College, Thomas Jefferson University and Nemours, Philadelphia, PA

Janis Whitlock, PhD, MPH
Director of the Cornell Research Program on Self-Injury Recovery, Bronfenbrenner Center for Translational Research, Cornell University, Ithaca, NY

R. Blake Windsor, MD
Hospice and Palliative Medicine, Hospitalist, Complementary and Integrative Medicine, Clinical Fellow in Pediatrics, Childrens Hospital Boston, Boston, MA

Janet M. Wojcicki, PhD, MPH
Associate Professor of Pediatrics, University of California San Francisco, UCSF Benioff Children's Hospital, San Francisco, CA

Charlene A. Wong, MD
Robert Wood Johnson Foundation Clinical Scholars Program, University of Pennsylvania; Division of Adolescent Medicine, The Children's Hospital of Philadelphia, Philadelphia, PA

Ernie H.C. Wong, MBBS, BSc, MRCP (UK)
Airway Disease Infection Section, National Heart and Lung Institute, Imperial College London, London, United Kingdom

Nicola A.M. Wright, MD, MSc, FRCPC
Division of Pediatric Hematology/Immunology, University of Calgary, Alberta Children's Hospital, Calgary, Alberta, Canada

Hsi-Yang Wu, MD
Associate Professor of Urology, Stanford University Medical Center, Pediatric Urology Fellowship Program Director, Lucile Packard Children's Hospital, Palo Alto, CA

H. Shonna Yin, MD, MS
Departments of Pediatrics and Population Health, New York University School of Medicine, New York, NY

William Qubty, MD
UCSF Benioff Children's Hospital, University of San Francisco, San Francisco, CA

Table of Contents

Journals Represented

Journals represented in this YEAR BOOK are listed below.

Academic Pediatrics
American Journal of Public Health
Annals of Surgery
Archives of Disease in Childhood
Blood
BMJ Quality and Safety
Clinical Pediatrics
Critical Care Medicine
Environmental Research
European Urology
Headache
Hospital Pediatrics
International Journal of Epidemiology
Journal of the Academy of Nutrition and Dietetics
Journal of Adolescent Health
Journal of Allergy and Clinical Immunology
Journal of Paediatrics and Child Health
Journal of Pediatric Gastroenterology and Nutrition
Journal of Pediatric Urology
Journal of Pediatrics
Journal of Rheumatology
Journal of the American Medical Association
Journal of the American Medical Association Dermatology
Journal of the American Medical Association Ophthalmology
Journal of the American Medical Association Pediatrics
Journal of the American Medical Association Surgery
Journal of the American Medical Informatics Association
Journal of Thoracic and Cardiovascular Surgery
Journal of Trauma and Acute Care Surgery
Lancet
New England Journal of Medicine
Pain
Pediatric Blood & Cancer
Pediatric Cardiology
Pediatric Infectious Disease Journal
Pediatric Nephrology
Pediatric Research
Pediatrics
Psychologie Medicale
Regional Anesthesia and Pain Medicine
Rheumatology International
The Journal of Clinical Endocrinology and Metabolism

STANDARD ABBREVIATIONS

The following terms are abbreviated in this edition: acquired immunodeficiency syndrome (AIDS), cardiopulmonary resuscitation (CPR), central nervous system

(CNS), cerebrospinal fluid (CSF), computed tomography (CT), deoxyribonucleic acid (DNA), electrocardiography (ECG), health maintenance organization (HMO), human immunodeficiency virus (HIV), intensive care unit (ICU), intramuscular (IM), intravenous (IV), magnetic resonance (MR) imaging (MRI), ribonucleic acid (RNA), ultrasound (US), and ultraviolet (UV).

NOTE

The YEAR BOOK OF PEDIATRICS® is a literature survey service providing abstracts of articles published in the professional literature. Every effort is made to assure the accuracy of the information presented in these pages. Neither the editors nor the publisher of the YEAR BOOK OF PEDIATRICS® can be responsible for errors in the original materials. The editors' comments are their own opinions. Mention of specific products within this publication does not constitute endorsement.

To facilitate the use of the YEAR BOOK OF PEDIATRICS® as a reference tool, all illustrations and tables included in this publication are now identified as they appear in the original article. This change is meant to help the reader recognize that any illustration or table appearing in the YEAR BOOK OF PEDIATRICS® may be only one of many in the original article. For this reason, figure and table numbers will often appear to be out of sequence within the YEAR BOOK OF PEDIATRICS.®

Introduction

Every new edition of the YEAR BOOK of Pediatrics is an opportunity to read the first remarks and impressions of some of the new discoveries, therapies or procedures from the last year. Through the years, the YEAR BOOK has commented on some of the most common and recognized advances in the field, when they were still considered novel, uncertain and unfamiliar. The novelty, uncertainty and unfamiliarity of these advances can be detected in the commentaries of the time.

The 1954-55 YEAR BOOK included a description of a "new method of evaluation of newborn infant," proposed by Dr. Virginia Apgar from Columbia University.[1] According to the description of the method, the score can be "used as a basis for discussion and comparison of results of obstetric practices, types of maternal pain relief and effects of resuscitation." The YEAR BOOK editor at the time, Dr. Sydney Gellis noted that it might be difficult for a single provider to accurately count a rapid newborn heart rate; however, "despite this drawback, the score sheet is a step in the right direction and should be used in the over-all evaluation of the newborn."[2]

A 1968 study published by Dr. Jerold Lucey and colleagues from the University of Vermont about a successful controlled trial of exposure to artificial light to prevent hyperbilirubinemia in premature infants was included in the 1970 YEAR BOOK.[3] The commentary described the method as, "simple, inexpensive and safe. It should reduce or eliminate the need for exchange transfusion in this condition, and phototherapy may be effective in reducing the incidence of brain damage in this group of infants." However, Dr. Gellis did voice concern about the dissemination of the 'light cradle' based on limited data. "As physicians we should view the light cradle as we would a new drug, requiring additional controlled studies, proper follow-up and a search for possible side effects such as injury to the eye or to normal growth and development. The rapid and widespread acceptance of this new and probably useful therapeutic tool is depressing in the face of the limited data available."[4] Dr. Gellis' comments are timeless and applicable to any new technology we would consider today. His concern was even prescient. Even today, 46 years later, we are still learning more about the slim but measurable risk in myeloid leukemia from phototherapy used to treat newborns with jaundice.[5]

The 1982 YEAR BOOK included an interesting case-control study published in 1980 by Dr. Karen M. Starko and colleagues from the Centers for Disease Control and Prevention, as well as the University of Arizona.[6] In an analysis of seven patients with Reye syndrome and 16 control classmates, the study noted that the use of salicylate-containing medications was significantly higher among cases. It was suggested that there may be a dose-dependent relationship between salicylate use and the risk of Reye syndrome. There was still some doubt in 1982. Dr. Frank Oski, who succeeded Dr. Gellis, commented, "Any suspicious-looking character is liable to be called in for questions, arrest and possible conviction.

Aspirin must be viewed as a suspect—but only as a suspect." However, he later admitted in the conclusion of his commentary that, "aspirin has been observed at the scene of the crime far more frequently than can be explained by coincidence. If you were on a Grand Jury, would you indict this drug? I would keep my children away from it until its name was cleared, while recognizing the danger of drawing conclusions based on guilt by association."[7]

In the 1987 YEAR BOOK, Dr. Oski commented on the first set of randomized double-blind clinical trials on the use of exogenous surfactant to prevent hyaline membrane disease. "Forms of therapy that offer to improve the survival rate and decrease long-term morbidity are most welcome...Not all studies are as conclusive, but preterm infants are not a homogenous group and not all surfactant that has been used in clinical trials is of the same composition." Additional studies were known to be in progress and the YEAR BOOK promised, "more next year."[8] And in 1988, as promised, a series of clinical trials on surfactant was discussed in the YEAR BOOK. Today, surfactant therapy has been credited with helping lower preterm mortality, as well as infant mortality in the developed world.

The 1996 YEAR BOOK included a 1995 analysis by Dr. Terence Dwyer and colleagues from the University of Tasmania on the incidence of deaths due to sudden infant death syndrome (SIDS) in Tasmania, Australia. After a number of public health interventions to encourage supine positioning of sleeping infants were introduced in Australia in 1991, there was a dramatic drop in SIDS cases. Based on a comprehensive analysis of an ongoing cohort study, the authors concluded that there was "evidence that the major contributing factor to the SIDS rate decline has been the reduction in the proportion of infants sleeping prone."[9] My immediate predecessor, Dr. James Stockman commented that, "this editor has previously expressed skepticism about the contribution of the recommendation against prone sleeping position and its benefits in preventing SIDS. It is possible that soon he may have to eat crow...whatever causes SIDS, be it sleep position or not, it is no longer having as major an impact on infant death. Thank goodness."[10]

This 2017 edition of the YEAR BOOK is no different from its predecessors. There is a promising report on the use of sirolimus for complicated vascular anomalies, as well as the publication of successful trial of sebelipase alfa for the treatment of lysosomal acid lipase deficiency (LALD). In addition, patients with hemolytic uremic syndrome (HUS) associated with Shiga toxin—producing *Escherichia coli* may benefit from early volume expansion. We also learn that spending time outdoors may have long-term beneficial effects on vision. There are warnings about the effects of phthalate and phenol exposure from personal care products, as well as crib bumpers and their association with SIDS. There is also a new clinical risk score reported for assessing persistent post-concussion symptoms in children. Who knows which one of these reports will turn out to be a new Apgar score or the next 'light cradle'?

If the commentaries suggest some caution, keep in mind the previous skepticism about supine sleep position or aspirin use. On the other hand, don't let too sanguine a commentary make you too credulous. Only time will tell. These commentaries are the best guesses from this year. They are only a 'first draft' in assessing and documenting our progress in improving the health and well-being of all infants, children and young adults.

Once again, this edition would not have been possible without all the expert colleagues who have contributed their commentaries to this edition. I am also in debt to the Associate Editors, Allan M. Goldstein, MD; Pascal H. Scemama de Gialluly, MD, MBA and Alan R. Schroeder, MD, who add great breadth and knowledge to this edition. Also, I am thankful for the team at Elsevier, including Ms. Casey Jackson and Ms. Kerry Holland, who kept our team on track and on time.

On behalf of our entire team, enjoy and read on!

Michael D. Cabana, MD, MPH

References

1. Apgar V. A proposal for a new method of evaluation of the newborn infant. *Curr Res Anesth Analg.* 1953;32:260-267.
2. Gellis SS. *Proposal for a new method of evaluation of newborn infant.* Chicago, IL: Year Book of Pediatrics. (The Year Book Publishers, Inc); 1954-1955:7.
3. Lucey J, Ferriero M, Hewitt J. Prevention of hyperbilirubinemia of prematurity by phototherapy. *Pediatrics.*. 1968;41:1047-1054.
4. Gellis SS. *Prevention of hyperbilirubinemia of prematurity by phototherapy.* Chicago, IL: Year Book of Pediatrics. (The Year Book Publishers, Inc); 1970:27-28.
5. Wickremasinghe AC, Kuzniewicz MW, Grimes BA, McCulloch CE, Newman TB. Neonatal phototherapy and infantile cancer. *Pediatrics.* 2016;137:e20151353.
6. Starko KM, Ray CG, Dominguez LB, Stromberg WL, Woodall DF. Reye's syndrome and salicylate use. *Pediatrics.* 1980;66:859-864.
7. Oski FA, Stockman JA. *Reye's syndrome and salicylate use.* Chicago, IL: Year Book of Pediatrics. (Year Book Medical Publishers, Inc); 1982:321-322.
8. Oski FA, Stockman JA. *Double-blind clinical trial of calf lung surfactant extract for the prevention of hyaline membrane disease in extremely premature infants. [commentary].* Chicago, IL: Year Book of Pediatrics. (Year Book Medical Publishers, Inc; 1987:43.
9. Dwyer T, Ponsonby AL, Blizzard L, Newman NM, Cochrane JA. The contribution of changes in the prevalence of prone sleeping position to the decline in sudden infant death syndrome in Tasmania. *JAMA.*. 1995;273:783-789.
10. Stockman JA. *The contributions of changes in the prevalence of prone sleeping position to the decline in sudden infant death syndrome in Tasmania [commentary].* Philadelphia, PA: Year Book of Pediatrics. (Mosby); 1996:254-256.

Dedication

AMG: *To the memory of my parents, Dr. Jacob and Rosa Goldstein, who were, and will always be, my greatest role models. Thank you for teaching me how to be a mensch.*

ARS: *To Lindsey, Owen and Dahlia.*

MDC: *To Cewin, Alexandra and Abigail.*

PHS: *To Marc, Paul, Benjamin and my wife Bettina. To Dr Padma Gulur for her mentorship.*

1 Adolescent Medicine

Secret Society 123: Understanding the Language of Self-Harm on Instagram

Moreno MA, Ton A, Selkie E, et al (Seattle Children's Res Inst, WA)

J Adolesc Health 58.78-84, 2016

Purpose.—Nonsuicidal self-injury (NSSI) content is present on social media and may influence adolescents. Instagram is a popular site among adolescents in which NSSI-related terms are user-generated as hashtags (words preceded by a #). These hashtags may be ambiguous and thus challenging for those outside the NSSI community to understand. The purpose of this study was to evaluate the meaning, popularity, and content advisory warnings related to ambiguous NSSI hashtags on Instagram.

Methods.—This study used the search term "#selfharmmm" to identify public Instagram posts. Hashtag terms co-listed with #selfharmmm on each post were evaluated for inclusion criteria; selected hashtags were then assessed using a structured evaluation for meaning and consistency. We also investigated the total number of Instagram search hits for each hashtag at two time points and determined whether the hashtag prompted a Content Advisory warning.

Results.—Our sample of 201 Instagram posts led to identification of 10 ambiguous NSSI hashtags. NSSI terms included #blithe, #cat, and #selfinjuryy. We discovered a popular image that described the broader community of NSSI and mental illness, called "#MySecretFamily." The term #MySecretFamily had approximately 900,000 search results at Time 1 and >1.5 million at Time 2. Only one-third of the relevant hashtags generated Content Advisory warnings.

Conclusions.—NSSI content is popular on Instagram and often veiled by ambiguous hashtags. Content Advisory warnings were not reliable; thus, parents and providers remain the cornerstone of prompting discussions about NSSI content on social media and providing resources for teens (Figs 1 and 2).

▶ Social media and youth are virtually synonymous in the contemporary era. The simple task of keeping up with the many mobile applications, platforms, Web sites, and other venues youth (and adults) use for social exchange and their shifting popularity can be a serious challenge for scholars, parents, youth-serving professionals, and even youth themselves. The subject of this report is a popular mobile and Web-based application (or app) called *Instagram*. This app allows its users to post images and text, which their followers

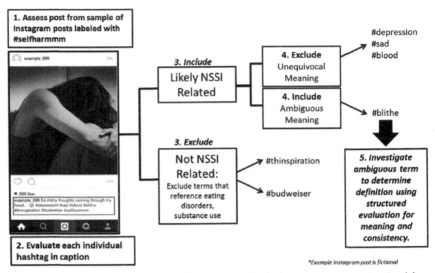

FIGURE 1.—Selection process to identify ambiguous NSSI hashtags on Instagram. (Reprinted from Moreno MA, Ton A, Selkie E, et al. Secret society 123: understanding the language of self-harm on instagram. *J Adolesc Health.* 2016;58:78-84, with permission from Society for Adolescent Health and Medicine.)

(which range from a mere few dozen to millions) can view through their own daily feeds. Images may be accompanied by a brief caption and any number of "hashtags" (#pony, #lovemydog). Clicking on any of the hashtags attached to a photo allows the viewer to see all other posts across Instagram with the same hashtag. In this way, Instagram users can create and find communities with shared interests (such as ponies or dog lovers in the above hashtags).

Because most Instagram users are adolescents, the authors of this report assume that most of the content on Instagram is created and consumed by teens. Because nonsuicidal self-injury (NSSI) is fairly common in adolescent populations, with a prevalence of between 7% and 24%, NSSI content on Instagram (and other online communities) is concerning because it may reinforce or trigger this behavior by posters and viewers. Research suggests that NSSI is contagious in peer systems and that normalization through repeated viewing may increase youth engagement in NSSI.

Because of these concerns, administrators of online communities often aim to prevent users from sharing potentially triggering content. Indeed, Instagram banned the hashtag "#selfharm" for this reason. But hashtags can convey multiple meanings to different individuals and communities, as the authors point out, not all of which are equally concerning. Instagram does have posting guidelines specifying what is and is not allowed (eg, no posts of self-injury, no pornography), and NSSI imagery deemed to promote self-injury can result in a deactivated account. NSSI imagery that may trigger but is not deemed to actively encourage NSSI may receive a Content Advisory warning, which alerts viewers to the graphic content of the posts. These warnings also contain a Learn More button that connects to more information and support about the topic.

Meaning

Step 1: What type of images accompany the hashtag ?

Are images consistent with NSSI?

Example: #Blithe as a search term on Instagram

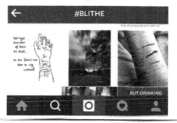

Consistency

Is the content related to the hashtag consistent across social media sites?

Step 2:
Use tagboard to search across social media sites using hashtag

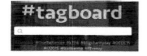

Step 3:
Use reverse Google image search to ensure images and text are consistent

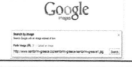

FIGURE 2.—Process for assessment of meaning and consistency of hashtags linked to the NSSI term #selfharmmm on Instagram. (Reprinted from Moreno MA, Ton A, Selkie E, et al. Secret society 123: understanding the language of self-harm on instagram. *J Adolesc Health*. 2016;58:78-84, with permission from Society for Adolescent Health and Medicine.)

The authors of this report set out to examine the extent and ways in which users circumnavigate Instagram rules to create NSSI communities using ambiguous hashtags such as #blithe or #cat or #secretsociety123. They conclude, not surprisingly, that circumnavigation using ambiguous hashtags referring to NSSI does occur and are accessed by what appear to be high volumes of Instagram users.

The methods used by the authors to conduct their study are straightforward, although results are not always easy to follow. Using a sample of content posted with the starting search "#selfharm" on Instagram between June 18, 2014 and June 30, 2014, the authors identified ambiguous hashtags associated with these posts that could be related to NSSI (Fig 1). The meaning and consistency for each of the identified hashtags was then determined by reviewing images that accompany the hashtag (meaning), the use of this hashtag across social media sites (consistency), and reverse Google image to ensure images and text align (consistency) (Fig 2). Frequency and growth of the hashtag were determined by the number of times the hashtag was used at 2 different time points 5 months apart. Finally, they recorded whether the hashtag activates a Content Advisory warning from Instagram.

The message of this report is that providers and parents need to be concerned about the way social media platforms, like Instagram, are used to share potentially harmful content and to create communities. This study fits in well with the small but growing body of descriptive research, which finds NSSI-focused communities and sharing to be widespread and users to be ceaselessly inventive in identifying and sharing content and connections. The capacity for continuous innovation in methods for circumventing social media administrator policies or guidelines (such as use of ambiguous hashtags) is an important element in building awareness about influences that may introduce or reinforce problematic (or unhealthy) youth behavior.

Such innovation is, however, also a central feature of adolescent and young adult identity development online. Descriptive studies such as this are exceptionally helpful in charting the general landscape of social media use, most of which is a fascinating fusion of human impulse and tendency coupled with the particularities of social media affordances. More often than not, however, the take-home messages for providers and parents can be boiled down to "be aware of how youth are using social media, foster opportunities for open conversation, and consult other available resources." In this case, the authors ultimately conclude that Instagram warnings are not sufficient to protect teens from exposure to NSSI content, and that clinicians should encourage parents to routinely check in with their teens about what they have viewed online and encourage parental monitoring and awareness of their children's online behavior.

While there is value in repeating this basic message, we encourage readers to understand that simple messages designed to alert parents to the dangers of what their teen may be doing online are not likely to be terribly helpful (although specific resources, such as Common Sense Media guides, can be). Unfortunately, until researchers successfully transcend the basic and descriptive approaches that currently characterize so many studies of this nature, we are ill prepared to understand or respond to the more complex relationship between human development and identity, on and offline behavior, and well-being. Assuming high homogeneity among users, motivations for use and effects of social media use on offline experiences and behavior will necessarily diminish effectiveness of clinician-imparted messages and assessments. This is particularly true, as many of these communities also include posts designed to convey hope, support, and encouragement for recovery goals. Assuming that use of social media tags and communities focused on self-injury (or other concerning behaviors) are likely to be more detrimental than helpful can limit generation of effective guidelines for assessing and responding to the inevitable and innovative ways young people do and will use virtual platforms for self-expression and coming together.

J. Whitlock, PhD, MPH
A. Purington, MPS

Adolescent depression, adult mental health and psychosocial outcomes at 30 and 35 years

McLeod GFH, Horwood LJ, Fergusson DM (Univ of Otago Christchurch, New Zealand)
Psychol Med 46:1401-1412, 2016

Background.—There is limited information on long-term outcomes of adolescent depression. This study examines the associations between severity of depression in adolescence and a broad array of adult functional outcomes.

Method.—Data were gathered as part of the Christchurch Health and Development Study, a 35-year longitudinal study of a birth cohort of 1265 children born in Christchurch, New Zealand in 1977. Severity of depression at age 14—16 years was classified into three levels according to DSM symptom criteria for major depression (no depression/sub-threshold symptoms/ major depression). This classification was related to adult functional outcomes assessed at ages 30 and 35 years using a generalized estimating equation modeling approach. Outcome measures spanned domains of mental disorder, education/economic circumstances, family circumstances and partner relationships.

Results.—There were modest but statistically significant bivariate associations between adolescent depression severity and most outcomes. After covariate adjustment there remained weak but significant ($p < 0.05$) associations with rates of major depression, anxiety disorder, illicit substance abuse/dependence, any mental health problem and intimate partner violence (IPV) victimization. Estimates of attributable risk for these outcomes ranged from 3.8% to 7.8%. For two outcomes there were significant ($p < 0.006$) gender interactions such that depression severity was significantly related to increased rates of unplanned pregnancy and IPV victimization for females but not for males.

Conclusions.—The findings reinforce the importance of the individual/ family context in which adolescent depression occurs. When contextual factors and probable maturational effects are taken into account the direct effects of adolescent depression on functioning in mature adulthood appear to be very modest.

▶ The destiny of human beings, as I see it,
 is to experience the world they inhabit—
 The universe inhabited by the immense
 scope of the human mind—and to construct
 That experience, that reality, in works of
 Uncompromised energy, unrestrained by FEAR
 —Lebbeus Woods (1940—2012)

Leonard Thompson was a 14-year-old boy admitted in January 1922 to the Toronto General Hospital with a then rapidly fatal disorder, diabetes mellitus. This was a disease puzzled over for thousands of years by clinicians that received the name "diabetes" from the 2nd century BC Greek physician Apollonius of Memphis, using the Greek words *dia* for "through" and *betes* for "to go"; later the word *siphon* for diabetes was taken from ancient Greek and also medieval Latin.[1,2] This disorder received its most elucidative ancient description from Areteus of Cappadocia (81–135 AD) of the late Hellenistic period; his comments about this deadly disease of disembogue and desinence rang out through the ages:

> "Diabetes is a remarkable affliction, not very frequent among men ... the patients never stop making water, but the flow is incessant, as if from the opening of aqueducts ... the nature of the disease, then, is chronic ... the patient is short-lived, ... the death speedy ... life is disgusting and painful.... Hence the disease appears to me to have got the name diabetes as if from the Greek word ... which signifies a siphon, because the fluid does not remain in the body, but uses the man's body as a ladder, whereby to leave it ... many parts of the flesh pass out along with the urine."[3,4]

The term *mellitus* is attributed by history to the great British (Oxford) physician and anatomist, Thomas Willis (1621–1675), who added it to diabetes in 1670 to separate out diabetes mellitus from other disorders causing polyuria.[5] It is unlikely that either Leonard Thompson or his parents knew about these medical terms nor their diaskeuastic derivations. However, both his parents and clinicians knew that this was an early death sentence, and management of the day consisted of futile treatments such as restrictive diets that sometimes killed the patient from starvation before the tabescence of diabetes did.

However, this fortunate young teenager was at the right time and the right place in history! A young orthopedic surgeon, Frederick Grant Banting (1891–1941), was involved with research on dogs (reported by the echoes of history to be border collies), and he had developed an extract from this research that could lower blood sugar. This pancreatic extract was developed by this hero from World War I by teaming up with other associates (Charles Herbert Best [1899–1978], John James Rickard [JJR] Macleod [1876–1935], and James Bertram Collip [1892–1965]). This fortunate young pediatric patient responded in a positive manner to this novel treatment, did not die in his adolescent years, and lived until age 27 years when he succumbed to pneumonia.[6–8]

Much progress has been made in purification and improvement in insulin since the early 1920s in Toronto, Canada, allowing millions of humans to live a life more closely related to their overall genetic potential based on having a more normal blood glucose milieu. As individuals lived longer, clinicians were able to more closely evaluate their quality of life. One important lesson that has been learned since that historic event in January 1922 in Toronto is that even though a diabetic person can use modern principles of medicine to avoid the early fate described by Areteus of Cappadocia, she or he may choose not to follow these rules of life and fugaciously die.

This quality-of-life concept has been raised by researchers such as Wibell et al, who published a study in 2001 that analyzed mortality in young adults (aged 15–34 years) after their diagnosis of diabetes mellitus had been made;

there was a mean follow-up of 5 years.[9] They reported an astonishing 3-fold increase in death in these persons and found that this rise in death was not from endocrine issues per se (ie, ketoacidosis or hypoglycemia) but from mental health issues that included substance abuse and drug overdose.[9] This work also raised the issue of how well do our youth with or without chronic illness transition to adulthood and what role should pediatricians and family physicians play in this transition? Why are some young adults not doing well in this regard?

Enter this salient study by McLeod and associates who provide some descriptive data on a timely topic that has not been well researched: what happens to adolescents with depression when they become adults? How well do they do in later life? Data were gathered from the Christchurch Health and Developmental Study, a 35-year longitudinal study of 1265 children born in Christchurch, New Zealand, in 1977. Individuals in this birth cohort with a diagnosis of depression between ages 14 and 16 years were assessed at ages 30 and 35 to evaluate any associations between their earlier depression and later outcomes.

Initially the criteria for depression and its severity was based on the American Psychiatric Association's third revised edition of the *Diagnostic and Statistical Manual of Mental Disorders* (DSM), which was published in 1987. Although new editions of the DSM were published in 1994, 2000, and 2013, it is not clear if these changes were accounted for in this study and if DSM criteria were used at follow-up. There is also no evidence of diversity of participants; no data are given with regard to socioeconomic status, ethnicity, race, cultural beliefs/practices, language, or religion.

These researchers write about classifying the level of depression dependent on scores on an assessment that was completed by both the adolescent and the parent. One potential problem some researchers would have with the way their level of depression (subthreshold and major depression) was classified was that instead of taking into account both results (parent and adolescent) as a whole to determine level of severity, they used either the parent or the individual's results. I assume that whichever assessment had higher scores yielded the recorded levels. What if this child did not endorse any levels but the parent rated them high? Who would be correct?

The study results appear to suggest that overall there is a mild or small relationship of adolescent depression and later adult mental health such as psychosocial outcomes. In this article, the authors do a good job explaining their conclusions by comparing results that were dependent only on the assessment outcomes to adding in covariates such as history as a contributing factor, reducing the relationship between depression and later outcomes. This stresses that environmental factors are extremely important in future outcomes, which also have generational implications. The study identifies 2 areas of increased risk due primarily to adolescent depression for females: unplanned pregnancy and intimate partner violence (IPV) victimization. This finding is an important consideration for early intervention for females.

Overall, this study by McLeod and associates provides some data showing that adolescent depression may continue into adulthood and/or contribute to negative psychosocial outcomes in adulthood. Although more studies are needed in this regard, we can learn some potential lessons about the importance of providing care to children and youth that involve both medical and mental health treatment. It reminds us of the importance of preventive services for children and adolescents to help mitigate the development of such negative outcomes in adulthood.

Mental health disorders are so common in adolescents that research notes that 25% of youth report a mental disorder during the past year in which they are surveyed and one-third will have a mental health disorder during their lifetimes.[10] Anxiety disorders are the most common but others occur, including behavioral disorders (eg, attention-deficit/hyperactivity disorder, among others), depression (mood) disorders, and substance use disorders.[11] The US National Institute of Mental Health statistics from 2014 concluded that 2.8 million youth (aged 12–17 years) had at least 1 major depressive episode, 10% to 15% had some depression symptoms at any 1 time, 5% had major depression at any 1 time, 8.3% had depression for at least 1 year at a time, and 2% of youth had a milder form of depression called dysthymia.[12]). Depression can last for months and may recur in many youth over the next year or two and before adulthood arrives.[12] The existence of depression in youth can have negative psychosocial outcomes in these youth and also, as noted by McLeod and associates, when they become young adults.[11]

There are many factors behind the development of depression and various complex factors that become comorbid with and in consequence of depression in youth. The neuroscience of depression is complex and undergoing intense research.[14] One factor to consider is that depression is common in youth with chronic illness, a phenomenon also lamentably prevalent in children and youth.[15,16] Approximately one-third of adolescents have a chronic illness or disability (with a duration of > 3 months), including 6% with a disability limiting daily activity. Nearly 75% of youth with a chronic illness have 1 disorder, 21% have 2 disorders, and 9% have 3 or more disorders.[14,15]

Studies have shown that youth with chronic illness have increased rates of depression and anxiety, as specifically seen with those having diabetes mellitus,[9,16] epilepsy,[17,18] asthma,[20,21] inflammatory bowel disease,[21] irritable bowel syndrome,[22] sickle cell disease,[23] chronic pain,[24] and others.[15] Depression in these youth may improve only to recur at various times later in adolescence or adulthood. Having medical and/or mental health problems can make this teen to young adult period even more difficult. Providing only a "medical" check-up in a patient with quasi-normal mental health status may miss underlying psychogenic problems—a missed ticking time bomb that goes off later in life.

Is this what happened to the adolescents and young adults with diabetes who had a 3 times mortality rate 5 or more years after their diagnosis of diabetes mellitus?[9] They died from suicide, drug overdose, and other negative psychosocial outcomes. The contribution of earlier depression is not known, but perhaps they were not able to develop a healthy self-esteem and were not able to survive their young adulthood with a longing to live. Pediatric patients with other chronic illnesses (eg, epilepsy, asthma) may have problems incorporating a normal self-esteem as well especially if there is comorbid depression or anxiety.

Such research suggests to me that caring for youth with chronic illness implies more than guilelessly applying pharmacologic principles in such complex situations. Providing the youth who has diabetes mellitus with information about the correct dose of insulin or how many calories to consume is not enough. If one does not assiduously assess patients' mental health status and, as a patient advocate or cicerone in life's dilemmas, help them incorporate their chronic illness into a healthy self-image during their juvenescence, this adumbrates a potential for low quality of life for many in their young adult years with Cimmerian consequences including depression and death. A Greek physician born in Turkey in the 6th century, Alexander Traillianus (525–605 AD), gave his peers in Rome and future clinicians of the world sage advice: "I like to use every possible means in treating my patients."

What is the purpose of the field of pediatrics? What is the role of the pediatrician? Is it to be a Laodicean clinician compendiously caring for as many patients as possible to maximize relative value units (RVUs), or is it to access each precious pediatric patient carefully with the goal of helping each one develop medical knowledge and psychosocial skills for a long and productive adult life?[15,25–27] Where is the balance between these 2 principles of modern health care? Are they inherently antipodal concepts of health care in the 21st century? If we ingenuously provide a pill prescription and not pay attention to our pediatric patients' overall well-being or quality of life, is this good enough? Do our patients deserve Icarian care that, much as Icarus with his poorly devised technology, leads to overall failure?

Whose responsibility is such a goal? Should contemporary comprehensive care of youth be an aleatory event dependent on finding a clinician who really cares for them and their future? Can we prevent the edacious, esurient RVU milieu of the 21st century health care industry from delivering a coup de grâce to competent clinical care? If we clinicians abjure or demit the real needs of our patients and do not address the depression or anxiety of our youth and allow them to die prematurely in young adulthood, have we done executed our professional responsibilities well enough?

Should the young adulthood period became a lamia or an oubliette for our youth much as war over the course of human history has done, or can we save our teens for a full and productive lifetime? Is ex post facto medical management (ie, in classic hysteron proteron logic, treat a suicidal 25-year-old versus initiating mental health screening and treatment in childhood or adolescence) a condign consequence for our children? Can we serve as a pharos to our hebetic patients in the often turbulent seas of life and guide them to a fulfilling adulthood? Generations now and yet unborn await our answer of Shakespearean fainéant ablution or acknowledgment befitting an Albert Schweitzer approach to health care. What is the leitmotiv of our clinical practice and indeed, our iatric lives in the 21st century?

> The purpose of human life is to serve
> and to show compassion
> and the will to help others.
>
> —Albert Schweitzer MD (1875–1965)

The field of pediatrics covers birth to age 21 years, and each phase of this life span has its complex, albeit cumbrous, challenges. This seminal study by McLeod and colleagues provides us with more dependable data in this regard and more challenges to what the specialty of pediatrics could be. Leonard Thompson's life was extended because of the discovery of insulin; however, it is a Cadmean victory if that is all we do for our young patients nearly a century after the remarkable démarche developed by the Toronto Team of Glory headed by Sir Frederick Grant Banting. The Leonard Thompsons' of the 21st century, we have learned, need much more than insulin to stay alive with discrete desideratum of a high quality of life throughout their adolescence and adulthood into this and the next century.

> There is a tide in the affairs of men.
> Which taken at the flood, leads on to fortune;
> Omitted, all the voyage of their life
> Is bound in shallows and in miseries.
> —William Shakespeare (*Julius Caesar*, Act IV, Scene III)

D. E. Greydanus, MD, Dr HC (ATHENS)

Contraceptive Provision to Adolescent Females Prescribed Teratogenic Medications
Stancil SL, Miller M, Briggs H, et al (Children's Mercy Hosp, Kansas City, MO; Kansas City Univ of Medicine and Biosciences, MO; et al)
Pediatrics 137:e20151454, 2016

Background and Objectives.—Rates of adult women receiving contraceptive provision when simultaneously prescribed a known teratogen are alarmingly low. The prevalence of this behavior among pediatric providers and their adolescent patients is unknown. The objective of this study was to describe pediatric provider behaviors for prescribing teratogens concurrently with counseling, referral, and/or prescribing of contraception (collectively called contraceptive provision) in the adolescent population.

Methods.—A retrospective review was conducted examining visits in 2008—2012 by adolescents aged 14 to 25 years in which a known teratogen (US Food and Drug Administration pregnancy risk category D or X) was prescribed. The electronic medical records were queried for demographic information, evidence of contraceptive provision, and menstrual and sexual histories. The data were analyzed using standard statistical methods.

Results.—Within 4172 clinic visits, 1694 females received 4506 prescriptions for teratogenic medications. The most commonly prescribed teratogens were topiramate, methotrexate, diazepam, isotretinoin, and enalapril. The subspecialties prescribing teratogens most frequently were neurology, hematology-oncology, and dermatology. Overall, contraceptive provision was documented in 28.6% of the visits. Whites versus nonwhites and older versus younger girls were more likely to receive contraceptive provision. The presence of a federal risk mitigation system for the teratogen also increased the likelihood of contraceptive provision.

Conclusions.—Our data demonstrate female adolescents prescribed teratogens receive inadequate contraception provision, which could increase their risk for negative pregnancy outcomes. Although the presence of a federal risk mitigation system appears to improve contraceptive provision, these systems are costly and, in some instances, difficult to implement. Efforts to improve provider practices are needed.

▶ Accurate characterization and assessment of adolescent sexual behavior in a clinical encounter is both an art and a challenge. For researchers, accurate description and quantification of clinician behavioral practices proves to be equally formidable. Clinical documentation in electronic health records and *International Classification of Diseases, Ninth Revision* (ICD-9) codes distill complex clinician-patient interactions and encounters into measurable morsels prime for statistical analysis.

Stancil et al describe valiant efforts to quantify clinician behavior surrounding contraceptive provision for adolescent females that have been prescribed teratogenic medications. Their definition of contraceptive provision includes documentation of counsel, prescription or referral for contraception through an ICD-9 and a novel key word search.

Overall, in their home institution, they found that contraceptive provision was documented in 28.6% of encounters. Their findings are similar to findings reported in the literature looking at adult women on teratogenic medications and stir up many follow-up questions. How accurately does documentation reflect actual conversation when it comes to sensitive and confidential information, such as contraception counseling? Knowing the somewhat fleeting attention span of some adolescents and their varying stages of development across the spectrum of ages 14 to 25 years, how much comprehension and understanding of teratogenic risk do our adolescent patients actually glean from our conversations?

Additionally, of the 1694 female patients on teratogenic medications that were seen over the course of 4172 clinical encounters, prescriptions for contraception were present in 11% of encounters. It is unclear what to make of this seemingly dismal prevalence, as the proportion of repeated visits of individuals on long-acting contraception can skew this number to be falsely inflated or underestimated. The importance of active contraception use is unequivocally imperative for sexually active, adolescent females who have sex with males. Without a denominator for this subpopulation in the study group, there is no context to interpret the value of this prevalence. Although the authors cite national data regarding prevalence of current sexual activity in adolescent females aged 14 to 18 years and their prevalence of contraceptive use, it is unclear whether study measurements are comparable, and even if they are, what the target benchmark should be.

For these patients who choose to use contraception, accurate measurement of provision is difficult, as access to contraceptive health care occurs across many organizations such as school based clinics and Planned Parenthood, that may or may not cross talk.

The authors postulate reasons for provider shortcomings in contraception provision in this vulnerable patient population including inadequate knowledge of teratogenic risk and adolescent reproductive health best practices, time constraints, and confidentiality issues. In a complex health care system that depends on multiple providers from different subspecialties and disciplines to provide comprehensive health care, who should be accountable for contraception provision, in all its varying degrees, for teenage girls taking teratogenic medications? For patients with complex medical issues requiring teratogenic medications, are their specialists responsible for discussing this risk and taking a sexual history at every visit if they are seen monthly, for example, and have been on the medication for years? Does the buck ultimately stop with the patient herself? If so, perhaps ensuring that she understands teratogenic risk and has access to contraception, should she choose to use it, is sufficient?

Taking a deeper dive into their data, Stancil et al identified the following characteristics associated with increased likelihood of contraceptive provision after attempts to control for confounding with multivariate regression analysis: white (vs nonwhite), older age (> 16 years vs < 16 years), more recent year of visit, noncommercial insurance coverage (vs Medicaid or no insurance) and presence of surveillance systems for a given teratogenic medication. The optimist inside of me would like to think that these issues are garnering more attention, which is reflected by more recent years being associated with increased likelihood of contraception provision. But the pessimist inside of me quickly resurfaces to wonder whether costly surveillance and risk mitigation systems such as REMS (Mycophenolate) and iPledge (Isotretinoin) actually improve quality and frequency of contraceptive provision affecting adolescent pregnancy outcomes or if they simply create a hard-stop framework that mandates improved clinician documentation of provision. Interestingly, for patients on teratogenic medications with established risk mitigation systems, providers were more likely to document contraception provision, but less likely to document sexual or menstrual histories.

The complexity of the issue expands further, as we have not even touched on the degree to which patients' families should or should not be involved. Still, Stancil et al should be lauded for their efforts to begin to characterize a gap in health care using a rigorous, quantitative approach, including sensitivity analysis of their development and use of novel key word electronic health record search. This work scratches the surface of a deep and complex issue and serves as a valuable launching point for further discussion, scholarly work, and a foundation for development of testable ways to improve clinical practice.

N. Ling, MD, MAS

Prevalence of HPV After Introduction of the Vaccination Program in the United States

Markowitz LE, Liu G, Hariri S, et al (Ctrs for Disease Control and Prevention, Atlanta, GA)
Pediatrics 137:e20151968, 2016

Background.—Since mid-2006, human papillomavirus (HPV) vaccination has been abstract recommended for females aged 11 to 12 years and through 26 years if not previously vaccinated.

Methods.—HPV DNA prevalence was analyzed in cervicovaginal specimens from females aged 14 to 34 years in NHANES in the prevaccine era (2003 2006) and 4 years of the vaccine era (2009–2012) according to age group. Prevalence of quadrivalent HPV vaccine (4vHPV) types (HPV-6, -11, -16, and -18) and other HPV type categories were compared between eras. Prevalence among sexually active females aged 14 to 24 years was also analyzed according to vaccination history.

Results.—Between the prevacccine and vaccine eras, 4vHPV type prevalence declined from 11.5% to 4.3% (adjusted prevalence ratio [aPR]: 0.36 [95% confidence interval (CI): 0.21–0.61]) among females aged 14 to 19 years and from 18.5% to 12.1% (aPR: 0.66 [95% CI: 0.47–0.93]) among females aged 20 to 24 years. There was no decrease in 4vHPV type prevalence in older age groups. Within the vaccine era, among sexually active females aged 14 to 24 years, 4vHPV type prevalence was lower in vaccinated (≥1 dose) compared with unvaccinated females: 2.1% vs 16.9% (aPR: 0.11 [95% CI: 0.05–0.24]). There were no statistically significant changes in other HPV type categories that indicate cross-protection.

Conclusions.—Within 6 years of vaccine introduction, there was a 64% decrease in 4vHPV type prevalence among females aged 14 to 19 years and a 34% decrease among those aged 20 to 24 years. This finding extends previous observations of population impact in the United States and demonstrates the first national evidence of impact among females in their 20s.

▶ In an age where pediatricians often feels like there is little they can do for common childhood problems such as obesity, exposure to violence, and toxic stress, it is so satisfying to be able to see measurable impacts of our interventions on health. In this follow-up study of female human papillomavirus (HPV) infection prevalence using National Health and Nutrition Examination Survey (NHANES) data, the authors show huge impacts on this outcome from HPV vaccination.

The drop in prevalence among 15- to 19-year-olds from 11.5% to 4.3% for the 4 most clinically relevant HPV types will no doubt result in huge cost savings related the to the prevention of future diseases such as abnormal Pap smears, genital warts and cervical cancer. This study shows that even with modest HPV vaccination rates, a lot is happening with the epidemiology of HPV in the population. However, it is important not to let these dramatic results obscure 4 equally important pieces of information about things that are not happening in this study.

First, the authors included in their analysis assessment of additional types of HPV not covered by the quadrivalent vaccine. This was done to address the ongoing question of whether this vaccine has any cross protection against related HPV types not included in the vaccine directly. The authors found no statistical differences in any of the additional HPV types assessed both when comparing vaccinated girls to those unvaccinated and when comparing the pre-vaccination era to the vaccination era. Unfortunately, the jury is still out on this question as data from this study somewhat contradict that of others. However, given the serial nature of the NHANES, systematically examining this issue over time is likely to eventually result in an answer.

A second thing that does not appear to be happening is HPV type replacement. That is, by lowering the prevalence of HPV 6, 11, 16, and 18 in the population, we are not seeing other strains simultaneously increasing in prevalence. When HPV vaccines first became available, some raised concerns about this possibility. However, this study adds to several others suggesting that type replacement is unlikely to occur.

Most clinicians at some time or another have heard parents raise concerns that giving the HPV vaccine to an adolescent might be misconstrued as also allowing permission to engage in sexual activity. Although this makes about as much sense as saying someone will drive recklessly because they put on a seatbelt, the issue is one with which clinicians must contend. Thus, a third important finding from this study is lack of difference in the number of lifetime sexual partners among 14- to 24-year-olds who were vaccinated compared with those who were not. Although this study was not designed to address the issue of sexual behavior specifically, the results support those of several others studies designed with this objective in mind that show, if anything, HPV vaccination is associated with a slightly lower chance of high-risk sexual behavior.

The fourth, and probably most important, thing that is not happening in this study is a lot of HPV vaccination! Only 1 out of 3 youth aged 14- to 19 years and 1 out of 5 of those aged 20 to 24 years had completed the 3-dose vaccination series as of 2012. Although these results are not surprising, they sure are depressing. Even as of 2014, the most recent year for which national adolescent vaccination data has been assessed, rates among females have not risen substantially from 2012.[1] The HPV vaccine has been recommended for routine use among girls in the United States now for a decade, yet our vaccination coverage can still be categorizes as "meh" at best.

So although it is exciting to see such declines in HPV infection prevalence, think about how much more we could achieve if HPV vaccination levels met that of other adolescent vaccines such as Tdap and meningococcal vaccines. Thus, an important take-home message from this study could be to continue to strongly and routinely recommend HPV vaccination for all adolescents in hopes that one day we can achieve the full health benefits this vaccine promises to provide.

A. F. Dempsey, MD, PhD, MPH

Reference

1. Elam-Evans LD, Yankey D, Jeyarajah J, et al. National, regional, state, and selected local area vaccination coverage among adolescents aged 13–17 years—United States, 2013. *MMWR Morb Mortal Wkly Rep.* 2014;63:625-633.

Adolescents' Self-Reported Recall of Anticipatory Guidance Provided During Well-Visits at Nine Medical Clinics in San Diego, California, 2009–2011

Peddecord KM, Wang W, Wang L, et al (San Diego State Univ, CA; Univ of California San Diego, La Jolla; et al)

J Adolesc Health 58:267-275, 2016

Purpose. Anticipatory guidance (AG) is recommended for adolescent well care. AG recall is important in the event sequence that might lead to behavioral change, reduced health risk, and improved health. We assessed factors influencing adolescents' self-reported recall of specific AG topics.

Methods.—Through convenience sampling of nine clinics in San Diego, California, 872 adolescents (429 aged 11–13 years; 443 aged 14–17 years) who had received well visits completed standardized surveys between 2009 and 2011. Adolescents were asked to report recall of either 17 or 23 age-appropriate AG topics that were analyzed in five categories (health maintenance; social/ emotional, safety/violence; smoking/substance abuse, and puberty/sexual health); a summary score for all categories was developed. Summary scores' associations with demographic variables, visit characteristics (including having time without parents present [private time]), clinic procedures, and lead physician attitudes were assessed.

Results.—AG recall was independently associated with adolescents having private time with clinicians, completing previsit questionnaires, reporting the well visit was helpful, and the well visit lasting at least 10 minutes. Higher summary recall scores were observed among adolescents who received care in clinics providing AG at both sick and well visits and having policies encouraging private time. Clinic electronic medical record use for AG prompts was associated with recall of fewer topics.

Conclusions.—To increase adolescents' AG recall and potentially foster behavior change, our results suggest medical providers should adopt procedures advocated by professional societies, including assuring adolescents receive private time during visits, increasing visit time during well visits, using patient-completed questionnaires, and providing AG during all visits.

▶ Anticipatory guidance is an essential part of our visits, regardless of the age of the patient. It is something we constantly strive to make time for. In the laundry list of material we should cover, the battle rages on, over which topic is most important. In the adolescent population, a group of patients who are developing, physically, educationally, and emotionally, this goal can be more daunting. For despite their thirst for knowledge, there is rarely an eagerness to receive a lecture from an authority figure of any generation.

This article attempts to highlight items that can make this experience, and our efforts, more successful, as we counsel young patients before they exit our care. In our opinion, this article provides some guidance, but its lack of focus confuses its conclusions.

In essence, the analysis includes too many variables in each category. Why evaluate adolescents from ages 11 to 13 and 14 to 17? One group would have simplified the study, as few practitioners provide private time to 11- and 12-year-olds.

Why have 17 to 23, age-appropriate topics analyzed in 5 categories? Is this number of topics a realistic expectation in a typical 30-minute well encounter, which already includes a physical exam, concluding remarks, a summary plan, and a separate meeting with the parents? This analysis doesn't even address the sick visit. How can we expect providers, in a focused 5 or 10 minutes, to get the history, do the exam, make the diagnosis, provide the treatment plan, and then provide adolescent anticipatory guidance on health maintenance issues, social emotional issues, substance abuse, sexual health, and/or safety?

In addition, the study surveyed 9 different clinical settings from 4 different strata. Such a diffuse group make the survey and its conclusions open to interpretation because of the wide range of settings and providers. Can a private practice setting with an average daily census of 20 to 25 patients, compete with a university setting or free clinic, where subsidy does not mandate volume?

What is most troubling however, is the statement that "chart data quality was so questionable that it could not be included in our analysis." One might take it a step further and suggest that, "if it's not recorded, it did not happen." How do we interpret the questionnaires if the "chart data quality was so variable in the sexual health category that it precluded validation of the topics discussed"?

Finally, this study suggests that the "clinical electronic record use was associated with recall of fewer items." One might say that the electronic health record inhibited anticipatory guidance! If a physician is just reading off a list from a computer screen, it seems like this might be less memorable to an adolescent patient than a physician efficiently going through a series of purposeful questions face-to-face in a meaningful way.

Despite these limitations, we took away several pearls from the authors' conclusions and modified some findings for future thought.

1. We need to provide private time to all adolescent encounters, with both sick and well patients.
2. Consider the use of an electronic questionnaire sent to the adolescent's smart phone, in advance, through an encrypted server.
3. Provide a broad range of anticipatory guidance in the well visit, and ask the patient what items to focus on during the more limited sick visit.
4. Focus the anticipatory guidance, as opposed to completing a checklist, because the adolescent will only remember what is helpful.

5. Remember to ask, "Are there any other issues to discuss, not related to your chief complaint?"

R. L. Oken, MD, FAAP

J. Miller, MD, FAAP

The feasibility of text reminders to improve medication adherence in adolescents with asthma

Johnson KB, Patterson BL, Ho Y-X, et al (Vanderbilt Univ School of Medicine, Nashville, TN)

J Am Med Inform Assoc 23:449-455, 2016

Objective.—Personal health applications have the potential to help patients with chronic disease by improving medication adherence, self-efficacy, and quality of life. The goal of this study was to assess the impact of MyMediHealth (MMH) — a website and a short messaging service (SMS)- based reminder system — on medication adherence and perceived self-efficacy in adolescents with asthma.

Methods.—We conducted a block-randomized controlled study in academic pediatric outpatient settings. There were 98 adolescents enrolled. Subjects who were randomized to use MMH were asked to create a medication schedule and receive SMS reminders at designated medication administration times for 3 weeks. Control subjects received action lists as a part of their usual care. Primary outcome measures included MMH usage patterns and self-reports of system usability, medication adherence, asthma control, self-efficacy, and quality of life.

Results.—Eighty-nine subjects completed the study, of whom 46 were randomized to the intervention arm. Compared to controls, we found improvements in self-reported medication adherence ($P = .011$), quality of life ($P = .037$), and self-efficacy ($P = .016$). Subjects reported high satisfaction with MMH; however, the level of system usage varied widely, with lower use among African American patients.

Conclusions.—MMH was associated with improved medication adherence, perceived quality of life, and self-efficacy.

Trial Registration.—This project was registered under http://clinicaltrials.gov/ identifier NCT01730235.

▶ Despite improvements in pharmacological regimens for asthma, the most recent data from the Centers for Disease Control and Prevention (CDC) show asthma prevalence at its highest in children under the age of 17 at 9.5%.[1] Data from the Youth Risk Behavior Survey (YRBS) have shown that up to 18.9% of high school students have been told by a doctor or nurse that they have asthma. Adolescents are at a higher risk of morbidity from asthma due to poor adherence to medication regimens, denial of symptoms, misreporting of symptoms, poor communication with parents, and engagement in risky behaviors. Medication adherence is one reason why adolescents have poor asthma control.[2]

Digital Health applications such as patient reminder systems using text-messaging, audiovisual reminder function, telephone messaging, Web-based messaging are ways that can potentially improve treatment adherence in chronic diseases such as asthma. One systematic review by Tran et al found that patient reminder systems do increase asthma medication adherence.[3] Although there is emerging literature on its use in asthma patients, there is a dearth of research on its use in adolescents with asthma.

Using a block randomized controlled design, Johnson et al. studied whether adolescents with asthma who used a personal health application called MyMediHealth (MMH) had increased medication adherence, self-efficacy, or quality of life (QOL). MMH is a web application that assists patients by managing their medications, establishing dosing schedules, providing a text-messaging–based reminder system, and recording medication adherence. The application reminds patients to take their medications by sending a text message reminder to their cell phone. The study's primary outcome measure was asthma controller medication adherence rate. Their secondary outcomes were self-perceived self-efficacy and QOL as measured using validated questionnaires. Johnson's study recruited adolescents aged 12 to 17 who had Internet access and who possessed a cell phone capable of receiving text reminders. They followed patients for 3 weeks and had a sample size of 98 patients between both intervention and control groups.

Johnson et al found that the adolescents in the intervention group had a statistically significant increase in self-reported 7-day controller adherence by an average of 1 day compared with the control group. Additionally, they found that the intervention group had a significant increase in perceived self-efficacy and QOL. Although they did not include asthma control as an outcome, they measured it and found no difference in pretrial and posttrial asthma control between both groups. The study investigators found large variability in usage of the MMH tool and they found no significant attitude differences about the tool between users and nonusers.

The authors noted that the results were innovative by showing that a digital health application could increase medication adherence, perceived self-efficacy, and QOL in adolescents with asthma. Nevertheless, it is difficult to generalize these results due to the short intervention period of 3 weeks. Future work should include larger and more diverse sample populations and measure long-term impact by increasing the time of the intervention. Both changes could show results that clinically correlate to improved asthma control and a reduction in disease morbidity.

Despite the positive results found in the study, usability of the tool varied widely especially in African American adolescents. The researchers noticed that 77% of MMH users who did not log in were African American. National asthma data shows that asthma prevalence disproportionately affects non-Hispanic blacks (11.2%) more than their white counterparts (7.7%). Research has also shown that minority adolescents have lower adherence than Caucasian adolescents. To reduce the asthma burden in all adolescents, especially those at higher risk, it is important to investigate the reasons for racial disparities.

The authors hypothesized that this could have been due to African American families having less web access than other groups. A study by MacDonell and colleagues measured the feasibility of text messaging in measuring asthma adherence in urban young adult African Americans.[4] They noted that most participants who did not take their asthma medication did it because of personal choice and dismissiveness. Past research has also suggested that high self-efficacy is associated with higher adherence.[5] If the goal is to use digital health tools to improve asthma control and reduce asthma morbidity in adolescents, we must study ways to make adolescents comfortable and confident in using these new tools, as well as ensuring that these tools are appealing, feasible, and accessible to all adolescents with asthma.

E. S. Cruz, MD, MPH

References

1. Centers for Disease Control and Prevention (CDC). Self-reported asthma among high school students—United States, 2003. *Morb Mortal Wkly Rep.* 2005;54: 765-767.
2. Eakin MN, Rand CS. Improving patient adherence with asthma self-management practices: what works? *Ann Allergy Asthma Immunol.* 2012;109:90-92.
3. Tran N, Coffman JM, Sumino K, Cabana MD. Patient reminder systems and asthma medication adherence: a systematic review. *J Asthma.* 2014;51:536-543.
4. MacDonell K, Gibson-Scipio W, Lam P, Naar-King S, Chen X. Text messaging to measure asthma medication use and symptoms in urban African American emerging adults: a feasibility study. *J Asthma.* 2012;49:1092-1096.
5. Riekert KA, Borrelli B, Bilderback A, Rand CS. The development of a motivational interviewing intervention to promote medication adherence among inner-city, African-American adolescents with asthma. *Patient Educ Couns.* 2011;82: 117-122.

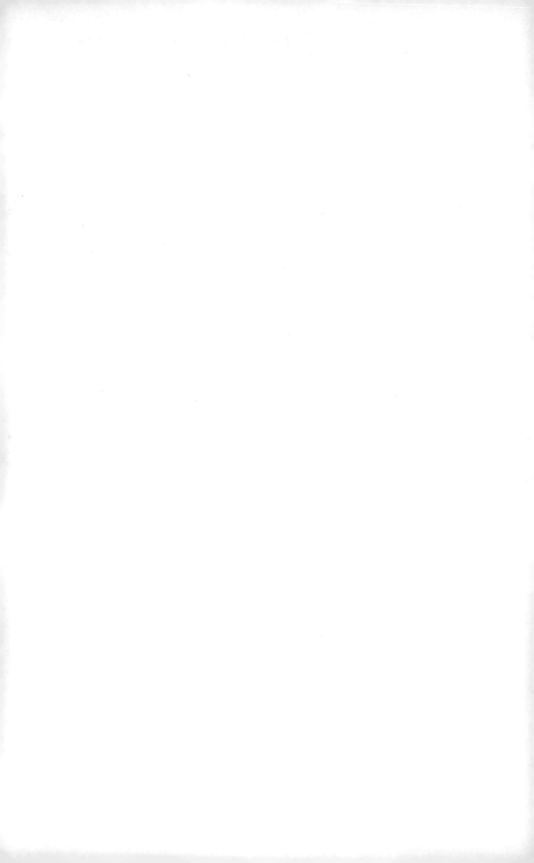

2 Allergy

Effect of Prenatal Supplementation With Vitamin D on Asthma or Recurrent Wheezing in Offspring by Age 3 Years: The VDAART Randomized Clinical Trial.
Litonjua AA, Carey VJ, Laranjo N, et al (Brigham and Women's Hosp, Boston, MA; et al)
JAMA 315:362-370, 2016

Importance.—Asthma and wheezing begin early in life, and prenatal vitamin D deficiency has been variably associated with these disorders in offspring.

Objective.—To determine whether prenatal vitamin D (cholecalciferol) supplementation can prevent asthma or recurrent wheeze in early childhood.

Design, Setting, and Participants.—The Vitamin D Antenatal Asthma Reduction Trialwas a randomized, double-blind, placebo-controlled trial conducted in 3 centers across the United States. Enrollment began in October 2009 and completed follow-up in January 2015. Eight hundred eighty-one pregnant women between the ages of 18 and 39 years at high risk of having children with asthma were randomized at 10 to 18 weeks' gestation. Five participants were deemed ineligible shortly after randomization and were discontinued.

Interventions.—Four hundred forty women were randomized to receive daily 4000 IU vitamin D plus a prenatal vitamin containing 400 IU vitamin D, and 436 women were randomized to receive a placebo plus a prenatal vitamin containing 400 IU vitamin D.

Main Outcomes and Measures.—Coprimary outcomes of (1) parental report of physician-diagnosed asthma or recurrent wheezing through 3 years of age and (2) third trimester maternal 25-hydroxyvitamin D levels.

Results.—Eight hundred ten infants were born in the study, and 806 were included in the analyses for the 3-year outcomes. Two hundred eighteen children developed asthma or recurrent wheeze: 98 of 405 (24.3%; 95% CI, 18.7%-28.5%) in the 4400-IU group vs 120 of 401 (30.4%, 95% CI, 25.7%-73.1%) in the 400-IU group (hazard ratio, 0.8; 95% CI, 0.6-1.0; P = .051). Of the women in the 4400-IU group whose blood levels were checked, 289 (74.9%) had 25-hydroxyvitamin D levels of 30 ng/mL or higher by the third trimester of pregnancy compared with 133 of 391 (34.0%) in the 400-IU group (difference, 40.9%; 95% CI, 34.2%-47.5%, P < .001).

Conclusions and Relevance.—In pregnant women at risk of having a child with asthma, supplementation with 4400 IU/d of vitamin D compared with 400 IU/d significantly increased vitamin D levels in the women. The incidence of asthma and recurrent wheezing in their children at age 3 years was lower by 6.1%, but this did not meet statistical significance; however, the study may have been underpowered. Longer follow-up of the children is ongoing to determine whether the difference is clinically important.

Trial Registration.—clinicaltrials.gov Identifier: NCT00920621.

▶ The primary source of vitamin D in the body is sun exposure, with dietary or supplemental intake playing a lesser role. Endogenous 7-dehydrocholesterol is converted to vitamin D3 in the skin after exposure to ultraviolet B radiation from the sun. Vitamin D3 is carried in the circulation by albumin or vitamin D—binding protein. In the liver, vitamin D3 is hydroxylated to its major circulating form, 25(OH)D3, which is the metabolite that can be measured in the serum and is generally accepted to reflect an individual's vitamin D status. Many tissues, including the respiratory epithelium, contain 1α-hydroxylase, which converts 25(OH)D3 to its biologically active form, 1,25(OH)2D3.

Vitamin D insufficiency (serum 25[OH]D3 of 20-30 ng/mL) or deficiency (serum 25[OH]D3 < 20 ng/mL) is widely prevalent across all age groups and is also notable in pregnant women. The prevalence of vitamin D deficiency and insufficiency is increasing over time. This trend has been attributed, at least in part, to deliberate sun avoidance and increasingly indoor lifestyles.

Levels greater than 30 ng/mL are required to avoid elevated parathyroid hormone and abnormal calcium transport. Cross-sectional studies of vitamin D insufficiency in children and adolescents in the United States note prevalence ranging from 48% to 61%.[1,2] People living at higher latitudes and those with dark skin pigmentation are disproportionately affected.

Interestingly, low levels of vitamin D have been associated with more severe asthma exacerbations, worse symptom control, and higher health care utilization. The understanding of how vitamin D deficiency modulates the pathophysiology of asthma is evolving. One plausible mechanism is that vitamin D reduces the inflammatory immune response. Many clinical trials are currently evaluating the effect of vitamin D supplementation on asthma outcomes in subjects of various ages and asthma phenotypes.

Pregnant women and their offspring have high rates of vitamin D deficiency despite supplementation with vitamin D—containing prenatal vitamins and high dietary intake.[3] Several prospective birth cohort studies suggest that higher maternal vitamin D intake is linked to decreased risk of wheezing in offspring during childhood,[4,5] whereas others have noted an increased risk of wheezing.[6,7] In animal models, maternal vitamin D deficiency results in increased airway reactivity in offspring.[8] Vitamin D supplementation to reduce asthma symptom severity and exacerbations would undoubtedly be a welcome therapy given the medication safety profile and low cost. What if this simple intervention could rewire a predisposition to asthma that has its roots in fetal development? Affecting prenatal development so that an at-risk infant never develops asthma would be the ultimate intervention for asthma prevention.

This study explores whether ensuring adequate maternal serum vitamin D levels during pregnancy may prevent early wheezing in infants and pre-school-age children who are at risk for wheezing based on family history. The study is rigorously designed and benefits from a high retention rate of subjects and close monitoring of medication adherence. Notably, the study population is racially diverse, and the study design used a randomization strategy that accounts for race.

The objective measurement of serum vitamin D levels in mothers and children is a strength of this study, as it avoids the pitfalls of the widely used dietary intake questionnaire in vitamin D studies. There was a trend toward a lower rate of asthma and recurrent wheezing at age 3 years in offspring of the intervention group, although the results did not reach statistical significance (Fig 2 in the original article). The findings suggest a possible protective effect of maternal vitamin D sufficiency, but follow-up of this birth cohort beyond the preschool years is important in clarify long-term protection. Longitudinal follow-up from this study is highly anticipated.

This study corroborates the wide prevalence of vitamin D insufficiency in adult women[9,10] but also interestingly highlights the failure of standard vitamin D–containing prenatal vitamins to achieve sufficiency. Infants born to mothers in the placebo group were vitamin D deficient at birth based on cord blood samples, and less than half of infants in the study received vitamin D supplementation in the first year of life. Regardless of study group, the children in the study were vitamin D insufficient at 1 and 3 years of age, indicating that hypovitaminosis D may be present very early in life.

Two recent randomized, controlled trials of maternal vitamin D supplementation similarly did not show a reduction in childhood wheezing. Goldring and colleagues[11] did not find a protective effect of prenatal vitamin D supplementation of 158 mother-child pairs, although the study was in a general population not one that was at high risk for asthma. In 2016, Chawes and colleagues[12] studied 581 mother-child pairs. A 4% reduction in persistent wheezing was noted by 3 years of age (which did not reach statistical significance) and a statistically significant reduction in troublesome pulmonary symptoms such as cough, wheeze, and dyspnea in the offspring of the intervention group. Both of these earlier trials supplemented only in the third trimester. This study began supplementation earlier in pregnancy (at 10-18 weeks of gestation). Women may need to achieve and maintain optimal vitamin D level prior to and throughout pregnancy to confer protection, as lung development begins at the fourth week of gestation. Finally, even with asthma protection from adequate prenatal vitamin D levels, children may need to maintain adequate levels in early childhood during a time of continued lung growth.

L. E. Faricy, MD

N. P. Ly, MD

References

1. Sullivan SS, Rosen CJ, Halteman WA, Chen TC, Holick MF. Adolescent girls in maine are at risk for vitamin D insufficiency. *J Am Diet Assoc.*. 2005;105: 971-974.
2. Kumar J, Muntner P, Kaskel FJ, Hailpern SM, Melamed ML. Prevalence and associations of 25-hydroxyvitamin D deficiency in US children: NHANES 2001–2004. *Pediatrics.* 2009;124:e362-e370.
3. Lee JM, Smith JR, Philipp BL, Chen TC, Mathieu J, Holick MF. Vitamin D deficiency in a healthy group of mothers and newborn infants. *Clin Pediatr (Phila).* 2007;46:42-44.
4. Camargo CA Jr, Rifas-Shiman SL, Litonjua AA, et al. Maternal intake of vitamin D during pregnancy and risk of recurrent wheeze in children at 3 y of age. *Am J Clin Nutr.* 2007;85:788-795.
5. Devereux G, Litonjua AA, Turner SW, et al. Maternal vitamin D intake during pregnancy and early childhood wheezing. *Am J Clin Nutr.* 2007;85:853-859.
6. Gale CR, Robinson SM, Harvey NC, et al. Maternal vitamin D status during pregnancy and child outcomes. *Eur J Clin Nutr.* 2008;62:68-77.
7. Hansen S, Maslova E, Strøm M, et al. The long-term programming effect of maternal 25-hydroxyvitamin D in pregnancy on allergic airway disease and lung function in offspring after 20 to 25 years of follow-up. *J Allergy Clin Immunol.* 2015;136:169-176.e2.
8. Yurt M, Liu J, Sakurai R, et al. Vitamin D supplementation blocks pulmonary structural and functional changes in a rat model of perinatal vitamin D deficiency. *Am J Physiol Lung Cell Mol Physiol.* 2014;307:L859-L867.
9. Ginde AA, Liu MC, Camargo CA. Demographic differences and trends of vitamin D insufficiency in the US population, 1988–2004. *Arch Intern Med.* 2009; 169:626-632.
10. Ginde AA, Sullivan AF, Mansbach JM, Camargo CA. Vitamin D insufficiency in pregnant and nonpregnant women of childbearing age in the united states. *Obstet Gynecol.* 2010;202:436.e1-e8.
11. Goldring ST, Griffiths CJ, Martineau AR, et al. Prenatal vitamin D supplementation and child respiratory health: a randomised controlled trial. *PLoS ONE.* 2013;8:e66627.
12. Chawes BL, Bønnelykke K, Stokholm J, et al. Effect of vitamin D3 supplementation during pregnancy on risk of persistent wheeze in the offspring: a randomized clinical trial. *JAMA.* 2016;315:353-361.

Allergy immunotherapy for allergic rhinitis effectively prevents asthma: Results from a large retrospective cohort study

Schmitt J, Schwarz K, Stadler E, et al (Med Faculty Carl Gustav Carus, TU Dresden, Germany)
J Allergy Clin Immunol 136:1511-1516, 2015

Background.—Allergic rhinitis (AR) is a main risk factor for the development of asthma. Two randomized open-label trials indicated that allergy immunotherapy (AIT) prevents the onset of asthma in patients with AR. However, these trials have methodological limitations, and it is unclear to what extent this experimental efficacy translates into clinical effectiveness.

Objectives.—We sought to investigate the effectiveness of AIT to prevent asthma in patients with AR.

Methods.—Using routine health care data from German National Health Insurance beneficiaries, we identified a consecutive cohort of 118,754 patients with AR but without asthma who had not received AIT in 2005. These patients were stratified into one group starting AIT in 2006 and one group receiving no AIT in 2006. Both groups were observed regarding the risk of incident asthma in 2007 to 2012. Risk ratios (RRs) were calculated with generalized linear models by using a Poisson link function with robust error variance and adjustment for age, sex, health care use because of AR, and use of antihistamines.

Results.—In a total of 2431 (2.0%) patients, AIT was started in 2006. Asthma was newly diagnosed from 2007-2012 in 1646 (1.4%) patients. The risk of incident asthma was significantly lower in patients exposed to AIT (RR, 0.60; 95% CI, 0.42-0.84) compared with patients receiving no AIT in 2006. Sensitivity analyses suggested significant preventive effects of subcutaneous immunotherapy (RR, 0.54; 95% CI, 0.38-0.84) and AIT including native (nonallergoid) allergens (RR, 0.22; 95% CI, 0.02-0.68). AIT for 3 or more years tended to have stronger preventive effects than AIT for less than 3 years.

Conclusion.—AIT effectively prevents asthma in patients with AR in a real-world setting. Confounding by indication cannot be excluded but would lead to an underestimation of the true preventive effects of AIT (Fig 1, Table 4).

▶ Allergy immunotherapy (AIT) has been established as an effective treatment for controlling allergic rhinitis symptoms. With AIT, an allergist administers incremental amounts of environmental allergen to an allergic individual over time until a maintenance dose is reached. The maintenance dose is then regularly administered, usually for at least 3 years. During and after this process, the individual becomes less symptomatic when exposed to the environmental allergen. AIT offers relief from bothersome nasal congestion, rhinorrhea, sneezing, itchy nose, and irritated eyes. AIT can be administered subcutaneously (subcutaneous immunotherapy [SCIT] or "allergy shots" colloquially) or sublingually (sublingual immunotherapy [SLIT]). SCIT has been available for decades, while SLIT has been more recently introduced.

Allergic rhinitis is a known risk factor for asthma, and studies have attempted to demonstrate that AIT can prevent the development of asthma. Schmitt and colleagues aimed to further investigate this theory through their analysis of a retrospective cohort of 118 754 patients within Saxony, Germany (Fig 1).

Schmitt et al's study differs from previous work in that it was a study of clinical effectiveness based on data derived from routine care rather than clinical trials. It provides further evidence that at least 3 years of AIT is associated with a decrease in development of asthma, particularly when AIT is targeted against native allergens (Table 4).

There were many limitations of the study because the data were from an administrative health database. Phenotyping was based on *International Classification of Diseases, 10th Revision* (ICD-10), codes, which can be notoriously inaccurate. The study was done in a primarily adult population with a

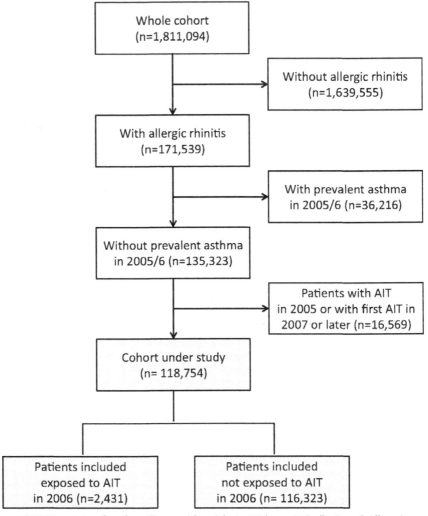

FIGURE 1.—Patient flow chart. (Reprinted from Schmitt J, Schwarz K, Stadler E, et al. Allergy immunotherapy for allergic rhinitis effectively prevents asthma: results from a large retrospective cohort study. *J Allergy Clin Immunol.* 2015;136:1511-1516, with permission from American Academy of Allergy, Asthma & Immunology.)

mean age of 37 years. In adults with possible new-onset asthma, further consideration needs to be given for other diagnoses or comorbidities including smoking history, occupational exposures, uncontrolled gastroesophageal reflux disease, and chronic obstructive pulmonary disease. The study would have also benefited from a stricter definition of "exposure" to AIT, as patients only needed at least 1 prescription of AIT to be considered in the exposed group, and there was no examination of type of environmental allergy (eg, tree pollen allergy vs dog allergy; single vs multiple allergen sensitizations).

TABLE 4.—Results of Multivariate Regression Analysis: RRs of Asthma in Patients with AR

Exposure Variable (Reference)	Multivariate Analysis (Adjusted for Age, Sex, Health Care Use Because of AR, and Prescribed Antihistamines)		
	RR	95% CI	P Value
Male sex (female)	1.09	0.99-1.20	.07
Age (per y)	0.98	0.97-0.98	$<10^{-17}$
Prescriptions of antihistamines (none)			
First quartile	2.85	2.43-3.34	$<10^{-17}$
Second quartile	1.99	1.74-2.28	$<10^{-17}$
Third quartile	2.21	1.92-2.55	$<10^{-17}$
Fourth quartile	2.26	1.95-2.63	$<10^{-17}$
Health care use because of AR (first quartile)			
Second quartile	1.31	1.12-1.54	.00088
Third quartile	1.77	1.53-2.04	$<10^{-17}$
Fourth quartile	1.83	1.57-2.15	$<10^{-17}$
Exposure to AIT in 2006 (not exposed)	0.60	0.42-0.84	.003
Route of administration of SIT (no AIT)			
SCIT	0.57	0.38-0.84	.005
SLIT drops	0.43	0.14-1.33	.14
Combinations	1.22	0.52-2.90	.65
Kind of allergen of AIT (no AIT)			
Seasonal	0.54	0.33-0.90	.02
Perennial	0.49	0.25-0.98	.04
Combinations	0.88	0.47-1.63	.68
Preparation of AIT (no AIT)			
Modified allergens (allergoids)	0.59	0.32-1.09	.09
Native allergens	0.22	0.02-0.68	.009
Combinations	0.90	0.48-1.66	.73
Not classified	0.73	0.39-1.35	.31
Duration of AIT (no AIT)			
<3 y	0.62	0.39-0.98	.04
≥3 y	0.57	0.34-0.94	.03

Reprinted from Schmitt J, Schwarz K, Stadler E, et al. Allergy immunotherapy for allergic rhinitis effectively prevents asthma: Results from a large retrospective cohort study. *J Allergy Clin Immunol.* 2015;136:1511-1516, with permission from American Academy of Allergy, Asthma & Immunology.

In comparing those who received AIT and those who did not, it is also important to make sure both groups are comparable in terms of asthma risk. It is not clear whether there is a subset of patients that may have been more atopic in terms of number of aeroallergen sensitizations, history of atopic dermatitis, history of bronchiolitis as a child, and family history of asthma. If there were more atopic patients in the group that did not receive AIT, this would skew the data to appear as if those who did not receive AIT were more likely to develop asthma.

Asthma was determined by an ICD-10 code noted twice in a patient's chart and at least 2 prescriptions of inhaled corticosteroids. Patients who met the database criteria for asthma at baseline were excluded, and this means there were some patients with 1 visit with an ICD-10 code of asthma and 1 prescription of inhaled steroids included in the cohort, and it is not apparent how these patients with possible asthma were distributed among the AIT versus non-AIT groups.

Furthermore, socioeconomic status should also be considered a confounding factor. Patients of higher status are more likely to be able to afford the time commitment of frequent AIT therapy and are also more likely to seek out treatment than those patients of lower socioeconomic standing. Asthma is more prevalent among lower socioeconomic classes in the United States according to most recent surveillance data from the Centers for Disease Control and Prevention.[1]

It is unclear whether these results would be generalizable to the population in the United States, where asthma is more prevalent in urban areas and among African Americans and Hispanics. Race or ethnicity and details of location (urban vs rural) are not mentioned in this study.

This cohort study adds to the limited literature in support of early AIT for prevention of asthma. An intervention such as AIT is attractive given the global burden of asthma on morbidity and mortality. The authors were aware of the limitations of their data and designed proxies for allergic rhinitis disease severity and for asthma diagnosis. However, further studies are still needed in the form of placebo-controlled, randomized clinical trials to provide stronger evidence of this association before influencing current practice.

A. Tsuang, MD, MSc
S. Bunyavanich, MD, MPH

Reference

1. Centers for Disease Control and Prevention. National Current Asthma Prevalence. 2014. http://www.cdc.gov/asthma/most_recent_data.htm. Accessed May 17, 2016

Preseasonal treatment with either omalizumab or an inhaled corticosteroid boost to prevent fall asthma exacerbations
Teach SJ, Gill MA, Togias A, et al (Children's Natl Health System, Washington, DC; Univ of Texas Southwestern Med Ctr, Dallas; The Natl Inst of Allergy and Infectious Diseases, Bethesda, MD; et al)
J Allergy Clin Immunol 136:1476-1485, 2015

Background.—Short-term targeted treatment can potentially prevent fall asthma exacerbations while limiting therapy exposure.

Objective.—We sought to compare (1) omalizumab with placebo and (2) omalizumab with an inhaled corticosteroid (ICS) boost with regard to fall exacerbation rates when initiated 4 to 6 weeks before return to school.

Methods.—A 3-arm, randomized, double-blind, double placebo-controlled, multicenter clinical trial was conducted among inner-city asthmatic children aged 6 to 17 years with 1 or more recent exacerbations (clincaltrials.gov #NCT01430403). Guidelines-based therapy was continued over a 4- to 9-month run-in phase and a 4-month intervention phase. In a subset the effects of omalizumab on IFN-α responses to rhinovirus in PBMCs were examined.

Results.—Before the falls of 2012 and 2013, 727 children were enrolled, 513 were randomized, and 478 were analyzed. The fall exacerbation rate was significantly lower in the omalizumab versus placebo arms (11.3% vs 21.0%; odds ratio [OR], 0.48; 95% CI, 0.25-0.92), but there was no significant difference between omalizumab and ICS boost (8.4% vs 11.1%; OR, 0.73; 95% CI, 0.33-1.64). In a prespecified subgroup analysis, among participants with an exacerbation during the run-in phase, omalizumab was significantly more efficacious than both placebo (6.4% vs 36.3%; OR, 0.12; 95% CI, 0.02-0.64) and ICS boost (2.0% vs 27.8%; OR, 0.05; 95% CI, 0.002-0.98). Omalizumab improved IFN-α responses to rhinovirus, and within the omalizumab group, greater IFN-α increases were associated with fewer exacerbations (OR, 0.14; 95% CI, 0.01-0.88). Adverse events were rare and similar among arms.

Conclusions.—Adding omalizumab before return to school to ongoing guidelines-based care among inner-city youth reduces fall asthma exacerbations, particularly among those with a recent exacerbation.

▶ Fall asthma exacerbations are a frustrating problem, especially among minority children living in low-income urban neighborhoods. Although I generally am opposed to the idea of a biologic, immune-modulator therapy as a solution to what is largely a public health problem, this particular population continues to have disproportionate asthma morbidity, so there is an urgent need to develop approaches, whatever they may be, that have real potential to work. This disparity in asthma exacerbations was the impetus behind this study, which was a multicenter randomized controlled arm comparing the effects of preseasonal treatment with omalizumab, inhaled corticosteroid (ICS) boost, and placebo on fall exacerbations.

Omalizumab is a monoclonal antibody against immunoglobulin (Ig)E that is injected in a clinical setting every 2 to 4 weeks, with dosing dependent on the patient's body mass index (BMI) and serum total IgE level. Estimated yearly costs of omalizumab range from $10 000 to $30 000 in the United States. Omalizumab is effective in reducing exacerbations in some populations and is approved for use in patients 12 years and older with moderate to severe asthma and skin test sensitivity to a perennial allergen. In a previous study, a post hoc analysis found that add-on treatment with omalizumab was associated with a marked reduction in fall exacerbations, and this current study formally tested this hypothesis.[1]

The researchers enrolled 6- to 17-year-olds living in inner-city neighborhoods who had had an exacerbation in the previous 19 months and were eligible to receive omalizumab (IgE sensitization to a perennial allergen and BMI and total IgE within the ranges required for omalizumab). The participants all received guidelines-based controller medication treatment and were randomized to receive 1 of the following starting 4 to 6 weeks before the first day of school: omalizumab, doubling of the ICS dose, or placebo. There were 2 primary analyses that lead to the following conclusions: (1) compared with placebo, omalizumab reduced fall exacerbation risk by about 50%, and (2) there was no difference between omalizumab and ICS boost in reduction of fall exacerbation risk.

There are a few wrinkles, though, that must be considered before thinking about how these findings might inform asthma management in this population. First, participants who were on high-dose ICS at baseline were not randomized to the ICS boost arm because they were already on maximal ICS therapy, so the lack of difference between omalizumab and ICS boost was only among participants who were on low to medium doses of ICS. Second, more than a third of potential participants were ineligible because they did not meet the prescribing criteria for omalizumab, suggesting that there is a substantial number of asthmatic children to whom these findings don't apply. Third, the researchers conducted a post hoc analysis examining the effect of these 3 treatment approaches among 2 groups: (1) those with an exacerbation during the 4-9 month run-in period and (2) those without an exacerbation in the run-in period. The researchers found that the omalizumab effect appeared to be restricted to those with an exacerbation in the run-in period and that ICS boost had no effect on reducing the risk of fall exacerbations in this subpopulation.

The study also addressed the mechanistic hypothesis that IgE inhibits the immune system s production of interferon-alpha in response to a rhinovirus infection, making atopic asthmatic children at higher risk of a rhinovirus-associated asthma exacerbation. To address this hypothesis, the researchers collected cells from study participants and measured the amount of interferon-alpha produced by cells in response to stimulation with rhinovirus. The researchers found that at baseline, participants' peripheral blood mononuclear cells had poor interferon-alpha responses to rhinovirus, but that treatment with omalizumab was associated with increased interferon alpha production in response to rhinovirus. These findings suggest that targeting the allergic, or IgE, component of asthma pathophysiology may enhance the immune system's ability to fend off rhinovirus, thereby reducing the risk of an asthma exacerbation. Although this finding has little immediate clinical relevance, the idea that it's the combination of allergy and respiratory viruses that is the major risk factor for fall exacerbations is intriguing and suggests that other approaches to targeting IgE, such as allergen exposure reduction, could also reduce the risk of viral-associated asthma exacerbations.

Should these findings alter clinical practice? For several reasons, it's not so clear. Although the findings suggest that similar children with an exacerbation in the 4- to 9-month period leading up to the start of school would benefit from the temporary, preseasonal addition of omalizumab but not an ICS boost, this approach would make the most sense for patients who have exacerbations that are largely restricted to the fall season. It's quite possible, for example, that those patients who might benefit from preseasonal treatment with omalizumab have exacerbations at different times of year and so should be treated yearround with omalizumab as would currently be done. In addition, among those randomized to placebo, 14% of those on low- to medium-dose maintenance ICS without a recent exacerbation went on to have a fall exacerbation, compared with 53% of those on high-dose ICS.

Adding an expensive biologic agent onto maintenance therapy before the fall may make sense for a group of patients with a high risk for fall exacerbation, such as those on high-dose ICS and who have had a recent exacerbation, but it is less clear that it makes sense for a group of patients who have a low risk of exacerbations, such as those on low- to medium-dose ICS without a recent exacerbation.

E. C. Matsui, MD, MHS

Reference

1. Busse WW, Morgan WJ, Gergen PJ, et al. Randomized trial of omalizumab (anti-IgE) for asthma in inner-city children. *N Engl J Med.* 2011;364:1005-1015.

Randomized Trial of Introduction of Allergenic Foods in Breast-Fed Infants
Perkin MR, for the LAI Study Team (Univ of London, UK; et al)
N Engl J Med 374:1733-1743, 2016

Background.—The age at which allergenic foods should be introduced into the diet of breast-fed infants is uncertain. We evaluated whether the early introduction of allergenic foods in the diet of breast-fed infants would protect against the development of food allergy.

Methods.—We recruited, from the general population, 1303 exclusively breast-fed infants who were 3 months of age and randomly assigned them to the early introduction of six allergenic foods (peanut, cooked egg, cow's milk, sesame, whitefish, and wheat; early-introduction group) or to the current practice recommended in the United Kingdom of exclusive breast-feeding to approximately 6 months of age (standard-introduction group). The primary outcome was food allergy to one or more of the six foods between 1 year and 3 years of age.

Results.—In the intention-to-treat analysis, food allergy to one or more of the six intervention foods developed in 7.1% of the participants in the standard-introduction group (42 of 595 participants) and in 5.6% of those in the early-introduction group (32 of 567) ($P = 0.32$). In the per-protocol analysis, the prevalence of any food allergy was significantly lower in the early-introduction group than in the standard-introduction group (2.4% vs. 7.3%, $P = 0.01$), as was the prevalence of peanut allergy (0% vs. 2.5%, $P = 0.003$) and egg allergy (1.4% vs. 5.5%, $P = 0.009$); there were no significant effects with respect to milk, sesame, fish, or wheat. The consumption of 2 g per week of peanut or egg-white protein was associated with a significantly lower prevalence of these respective allergies than was less consumption. The early introduction of all six foods was not easily achieved but was safe.

Conclusions.—The trial did not show the efficacy of early introduction of allergenic foods in an intention-to-treat analysis. Further analysis raised the question of whether the prevention of food allergy by means of early introduction of multiple allergenic foods was dose-dependent. (Funded by the Food Standards Agency and others; EAT Current Controlled Trials number, ISRCTN14254740.)

▶ With rates of food allergy apparently rising over the past 2 decades, there is strong motivation to find prevention strategies. About 15 years ago, the best recommendations for preventing food allergy were to delay introduction of dairy until 1 year, eggs until 2 years, and peanuts, tree nuts, and fish until 3 years of age in infants at risk for atopic conditions.[1] Eight years ago, these recommendations were rescinded because of a lack of supporting evidence and concern that delayed introduction may have contributed to increasing food allergy prevalence.[2-5]

The Learning Early about Peanut (LEAP) study, published in 2015, was the first prospective randomized trial that examined early introduction of a highly allergenic food. Highly atopic infants with severe atopic dermatitis and/or egg allergy but without large positive skin tests to peanut were randomized between 4 and 11 months of age to regularly ingest or to avoid peanut protein to age 5 years. The early introduction group had a significant reduction in the prevalence of peanut allergy at 5 years of age compared to those avoiding peanut (relative risk reduction of 86% in those with negative and 70% in those with positive peanut skin tests on enrollment).[6] However, the LEAP study did not address whether early introduction of peanut and other allergenic foods would be beneficial to infants in the general population.

The Enquiring about Tolerance (EAT) study is the first randomized study to examine the effect of early introduction of highly allergenic foods on food allergy prevalence in healthy breastfed infants (although participants self-selected toward an atopic disposition). Families in the early introduction group were instructed to give the infants prespecified amounts of 6 allergenic foods between 3 and 6 months of age. In the early introduction group, milk was introduced first and wheat was introduced last; in between, the order of peanut, egg, sesame, and whitefish was randomized.

The study aimed to have all foods introduced by 5 months of age, and infants were supposed to consume the allergenic foods until 1 year of age. After that, ongoing consumption was encouraged but not mandatory. In the standard introduction group, infants were breastfed exclusively until 6 months of age, and foods were introduced afterward per parental discretion. In the intention-to-treat analysis, the prevalence of food allergy to any food was not statistically significantly different between the early introduction and standard introduction groups, 7.1% in the standard-introduction group (42 of 595 participants) compared with 5.6% in the early-introduction group (32 of 567; $P = .32$).

Unfortunately, only 31.9% (208 of 652) of infants in the early introduction group adhered closely enough to the protocol to be included in the per-protocol analysis. Nonwhite race, parentally perceived symptoms in the child related to any of the early introduction foods, reduced maternal quality of life, and the presence of eczema at enrollment were associated with poor adherence. In a per-protocol analysis, the prevalence of food allergy at 1 to 3 years of age in the early introduction group was 67% lower than in the standard introduction group. Statistically significant decreases in peanut (0% vs 2.5%, $P = .003$)

and egg (1.4% vs 5.5%, $P = .009$) allergy were also found in the early versus standard introduction groups, respectively. The study found a dose-response relationship of increasing allergenic protein consumption, with decreasing allergy risk for egg and peanut (with prevention maximal for infants ingesting at least 2 g of peanut and 2 g of egg white protein weekly). The study also demonstrated that it is safe to introduce highly allergenic foods as early as 3 months, as no episode of anaphylaxis occurred during the initial introduction and there were no adverse effects on breastfeeding or growth.

In summary, the EAT study demonstrates that it is safe and may be beneficial to introduce highly allergenic foods starting at 3 to 6 months of age in the general population. However, the intention-to-treat analysis was negative, making the study inconclusive. The low adherence rate in the early introduction group also suggests that it may be difficult for parents to give highly allergenic foods on a regular basis. More studies are needed before definitive recommendations can be made regarding early introduction of highly allergenic foods for the general population, but the results are encouraging regarding a potential pathway toward prevention.

A. L. Chang, MD

S. H. Sicherer, MD

References

1. Committee on Nutrition. Hypoallergenic infant formulas. *Pediatrics*. 2000;106: 346-349.
2. Greer FR, Sicherer SH, Burks AW. Effects of early nutritional interventions on the development of atopic disease in infants and children: the role of maternal dietary restriction, breastfeeding, timing of introduction of complementary foods, and hydrolyzed formulas. *Pediatrics*. 2008;121:183-191.
3. Boyce JA, Assa'ad A, Burks AW, et al. Guidelines for the diagnosis and management of food allergy in the United States: report of the NIAID-sponsored expert panel. *J Allergy Clin Immunol*. 2010;126:S1-S58.
4. Fleischer DM, Spergel JM, Assa'ad AH, Pongracic JA. Primary prevention of allergic disease through nutritional interventions. *J Allergy Clin Immunol*. 2013;1: 29-36.
5. Du Toit G, Katz Y, Sasieni P, et al. Early consumption of peanuts in infancy is associated with a low prevalence of peanut allergy. *J Allergy Clin Immunol*. 2008;122: 984-991.
6. Du Toit G, Roberts G, Sayre PH, et al. Randomized trial of peanut consumption in infants at risk for peanut allergy. *N Engl J Med*. 2015;372:803-813.

Safety of live attenuated influenza vaccine in young people with egg allergy: multicentre prospective cohort study
Turner PJ, on behalf of the SNIFFLE-2 Study Investigators (Imperial College London, UK, et al)
BMJ 351:h6291, 2015

Study Question.—How safe is live attenuated influenza vaccine (LAIV), which contains egg protein, in young people with egg allergy?

Methods.—In this open label, phase IV intervention study, 779 young people (2-18 years) with egg allergy were recruited from 30 UK allergy centres and immunised with LAIV. The cohort included 270 (34.7%) young people with previous anaphylaxis to egg, of whom 157 (20.1%) had experienced respiratory and/or cardiovascular symptoms. 445 (57.1%) had doctor diagnosed asthma or recurrent wheeze. Participants were observed for at least 30 minutes after vaccination and followed-up by telephone 72 hours later. Participants with a history of recurrent wheeze or asthma underwent further follow-up four weeks later. The main outcome measure was incidence of an adverse event within two hours of vaccination in young people with egg allergy.

Study Answer and Limitations.—No systemic allergic reactions occurred (upper 95% confidence interval for population 0.47% and in participants with anaphylaxis to egg 1.36%). Nine participants (1.2%, 95% CI 0.5% to 2.2%) experienced mild symptoms, potentially consistent with a local, IgE mediated allergic reaction. Delayed events potentially related to the vaccine were reported in 221 participants. 62 participants (8.1%, 95% CI for population 6.3% to 10.3%) experienced lower respiratory tract symptoms within 72 hours, including 29 with parent reported wheeze. No participants were admitted to hospital. No increase in lower respiratory tract symptoms occurred in the four weeks after vaccination (assessed with asthma control test). The study cohort may represent young people with more severe allergy requiring specialist input, since they were recruited from secondary and tertiary allergy centres.

What This Study Adds.—LAIV is associated with a low risk of systemic allergic reactions in young people with egg allergy. The vaccine seems to be well tolerated in those with well controlled asthma or recurrent wheeze.

Funding, Competing Interests, Data Sharing.—This report is independent research commissioned and funded by a Department of Health policy research programme grant to the National Vaccine Evaluation Consortium. Additional funding was provided by the NIHR Clinical Research Networks, Health Protection Scotland (Edinburgh site), and Health & Social Care Services in Northern Ireland (Belfast site). PJT and MEL had support from the Department of Health for the submitted work; PJT has received research grants from the Medical Research Council and NIHR. No additional data available.

Study Registration.—ClinicalTrials.gov (NCT02111512) and the EU Clinical Trials Register EudraCT (2014-001537-92).

▶ Seasonal influenza is a significant global health problem, estimated to cause serious illness in 3 to 5 million people, and up to 500 000 deaths yearly.[1] From October 15, 2015, to April 29, 2016, there were 60 influenza-associated pediatric deaths in the United States.[2] To prevent spread of influenza, the Centers for Disease Control and Prevention (CDC) recommends immunization for all children > 6 months old, with either the inactivated influenza vaccine (IIV) or live attenuated influenza vaccine (LAIV) for those 2 years or older, whichever is available, with certain exclusions.[3] Both of these vaccines are grown on chick embryos, prompting concern for their use in children with egg allergy (estimated at 2%–3% of the population < 18 years old). Newer influenza vaccines that do not contain egg protein are not approved for children under 18 years old.

In the past 2 decades, numerous studies have evaluated the administration of IIV to children with egg allergy. Proof of safety is difficult due to the low reaction rate (estimated at 0.8–1.9 per million doses as reported in the Vaccine Adverse Event Reporting System). However, there are now at least 28 articles representing 4315 egg-allergic patients, including 656 with a history of egg-induced anaphylaxis, demonstrating that IIV administered as a single injection can be given safely to patients with egg allergy.[4]

Manufacturers of IIV indicate that these vaccines now contain less than 1 mcg of ovalbumin per dose, significantly below 30 to 130 mcg of egg protein, the amount required to induce a reaction in egg allergic patients. Currently, the CDC recommends that children with egg allergy, 6 months to 18 years old, be immunized with IIV, in a situation where the personnel are prepared to recognize and treat anaphylaxis, with a 30-minute observation after injection. LAIV is not recommended for egg-allergic children, due to lack of information on its use in this population. In addition, LAIV is not recommended for use in children 2 to 4 years old with a history of asthma or a significant wheezing episode in the previous 12 months.[3]

This open-label Phase IV study conducted in 30 UK specialty centers is the largest published study of LAIV in egg-allergic children and contributes greatly to our understanding of the safety of LAIV in this population. Turner et al evaluated 779 egg-allergic children aged 2 to 18 years, 57.1% who also had asthma or recurrent wheeze, and 34.7% with a history of egg-induced anaphylaxis, including respiratory and/or cardiovascular symptoms in 20.1%. Notably, they excluded children who previously required invasive ventilation for egg-induced anaphylaxis, had a diagnosis of severe asthma or other contraindications to LAIV. Evaluation at 3 time points allowed for assessment of early and delayed allergic reactions as well as any change in asthma symptoms in the month following immunization. There was excellent follow through with 98% of the children receiving a 72-hour assessment and 89% of the asthmatic children receiving a 4-week assessment.

The study participants had a total of 17 immediate adverse events, 11 of which were consistent with an immunoglobulin E—mediated allergic response. The reactions were mild and self-limiting, including rhinitis, urticaria, and oropharyngeal itch. All occurred in the first 30 minutes after immunization, and no predisposing factors could be identified. Importantly, there were no systemic reactions attributed to LAIV. As noted in the abstract, delayed reactions which occurred in 221 participants were primarily lower respiratory tract symptoms, including wheezing. There was a trend toward an increase in respiratory symptoms in younger children overall, and children < 5 years with asthma or recurrent wheeze were more likely to develop symptoms compared with older children, but only 1 child was seen in an emergency department, and none required hospital admission. Conversely, there was no effect on overall asthma control in the month after immunization, when comparing the asthma control test score 4 weeks after vaccination to baseline. In fact, there was a small improvement in overall asthma control for children 2 to 11 years old as well as the group younger than 5 years.

With this publication, there are now studies that include 955 children with egg allergy (338 with previous anaphylaxis) who have received LAIV without significant allergic reactions.[5] LAIV is unlikely to contain the amount of protein required to induce an allergic reaction; Flumist, the LAIV available in the United States, contains < 0.24 mcg ovalbumin/dose. This, combined with the larger numbers of egg-allergic children who have safely received IIV, suggests that LAIV should be well tolerated in egg-allergic children. In addition, this study adds to the evidence that LAIV will also be tolerated in children with a history of asthma or recurrent wheezing.

Pediatricians should be aware that there is still no information about use of LAIV in children with a history of anaphylaxis requiring invasive ventilation or severe or uncontrolled asthma, although history with IIV strongly suggests that LAIV should be tolerated in children with a history of egg anaphylaxis. Given the potentially fatal consequences of influenza infection and children's dislike of injections, the reactions seen with LAIV represent a reasonable risk in the studied population. It will be interesting to see whether there are changes to the upcoming recommendations from the CDC Advisory Committee on Immunization Practices.

G. M. Sanders, MD, MS

References

1. *Fact Sheet No 211.* 2014. World Health Organization; 2014, http://www.who.int/mediacentre/factsheets/fs211/en/. Accessed April 29, 2016.
2. MMWR. 2016. http://www.cdc.gov/mmwr/volumes/65/wr/mm6516md.htm?s_cid=mm6516md_w. Accessed April 29, 2016.
3. Grohskopf LA, Sokolow LZ, Olsen SJ, Bresee JS, Broder KR, Karron RA. Prevention and control of influenza with vaccines: recommendations of the Advisory Committee on Immunization Practices, United States, 2015-16 influenza season. *MMWR Morb Mortal Wkly Rep.* 2015;64:818-825.
4. Kelso J. Administering influenza vaccine to egg-allergic persons. *Expert Review in Vaccines.* 2014;13:1049-1057.
5. Des Roches A, Samaan K, Graham F, et al. Safe vaccination of patients with egg allergy by using live attenuated influenza vaccine. *J Allergy Clin Immunol Pract.* 2015;3:138-139.

Sensitization to cat and dog allergen molecules in childhood and prediction of symptoms of cat and dog allergy in adolescence: A BAMSE/MeDALL study
Asarnoj A, Hamsten C, Wadén K, et al (Karolinska Institutet and University Hospital, Stockholm, Sweden; et al)
J Allergy Clin Immunol 137:813-821, 2016

Background.—Sensitization to individual cat and dog allergen molecules can contribute differently to development of allergy to these animals.

Objective.—We sought to investigate the association between sensitization patterns to cat and dog allergen molecules during childhood and symptoms to these furry animals up to age 16 years.

Methods.—Data from 779 randomly collected children from the Barn/ Children Allergy/Asthma Milieu Stockholm Epidemiologic birth cohort at 4, 8, and 16 years were used. IgE levels to cat and dog were determined by using ImmunoCAP, and levels to allergen molecules were determined by using an allergen chip based on ISAC technology (Mechanisms for the Development of Allergy chip). Allergy was defined as reported rhinitis, conjunctivitis, or asthma at exposure to cat or dog.

Results.—Cross-sectionally, IgE to Fel d 1 and cat extract had similar positive predictive values for cat allergy. IgE to Can f 1 showed a higher positive predictive value for dog allergy than dog extract IgE. Sensitizations to Fel d 1 and Can f 1 in childhood were significantly associated with symptoms to cat or dog at age 16 years. Polysensitization to 3 or more allergen molecules from cat or dog was a better longitudinal predictor of cat or dog symptoms than results of IgE tests with cat or dog allergen extract, respectively. Cross-sectionally, cat/dogpolysensitized children had higher IgE levels and more frequent symptoms to cat and dog than monosensitized children.

Conclusions.—Sensitization to Fel d 1 and Can f 1 in childhood and polysensitization to either cat or dog allergen molecules predict cat and dog allergy cross-sectionally and longitudinally significantly better than IgE to cat or dog extract (Fig 4).

▶ There are very few things within the realm of allergic diseases that cause as much controversy as implicating a family pet as the cause of a child's atopic symptoms. Most families and clinicians would agree tobacco smoke exposure is an absolute detriment to an asthmatic or allergic child's health. Yet families seek out exotic treatments, "hypoallergenic" animals or aggressive allergy regimens to avoid removing a beloved pet from the home. Within this context, families often attempt to qualify the risks of allergic symptom development before bringing a furred animal into the home often with the guidance of their pediatrician or allergist.

Asarnoj et al provides guidance to clinicians attempting to counsel families on the overall risk of development of animal sensitization throughout a child's life. Utilizing a longitudinal birth cohort and microarray ImmunoCap screening methods, the investigators predict sensitization to the major allergenic proteins of domestic house cat and dog within this cohort by means of early life assessment of serum sensitization. Unlike previous studies in which other investigators used whole protein antigen ImmunoCap IgE response to determine sensitization to animals, the benefits of next generation microarray ImmunoCap serology testing can identify specific protein sensitization to specific epitopes, which improves accuracy of diagnosis of clinical sensitization. In addition, the authors were able to identify stages of sensitization from early childhood, elementary school age, and into adolescence by means of sensitization response to multiple allergenic epitopes.

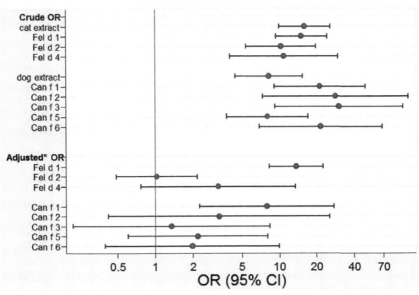

FIGURE 4.—Longitudinal logistic regression. Crude and adjusted ORs for IgE sensitizations to cat and dog allergen (ISU-E ≥ 0.3) at 4 and 8 years of age in relation to reported cat/dog allergy at 16 years of age (n = 779). *Adjusted for concomitant sensitization to the other cat or dog components, respectively. For sensitization matrix, see Table E5. *Editor's Note*: Please refer to original journal article for full references. (Reprinted from Asarnoj A, Hamsten C, Wadén K, et al. Sensitization to cat and dog allergen molecules in childhood and prediction of symptoms of cat and dog allergy in adolescence: A BAMSE/MeDALL study. *J Allergy Clin Immunol.* 2016;137:813-821, with permission from American Academy of Allergy, Asthma & Immunology.)

No matter what families hope for, both cat and dogs shed major and minor allergens, which can affect human health. There is no truly "hypo-allergenic furred pet" despite the claims of breeders, the Internet, and avid pet owners. For purposes of the investigation, the major and minor cat (Fel d 1-5) allergens and dog (Can f 1-5) allergens were measured throughout the cohort at different intervals. The continued sensitization to major allergens (ie, Fel d 1 and Can f 1) could predict which child would carry clinical sensitization later in adolescence (Fig 4). Asarnoj et al further note that specific sensitization to the major allergens Fel d 1 and Can f 1 play a roll in the development of clinical symptoms in vulnerable individuals and moreover, poly-sensitization to multiple allergenic epitopes in early childhood was an accurate predictive marker for clinical sensitization in adolescence.

There are several minor weaknesses of this study due to the sample population, limited genetic variability of the birth cohort, and the method of determining sensitization (questionnaires vs challenges). Although some would also note the variability of animal breed playing a roll, it is unlikely this would affect the outcome of this study. Despite these issues, the authors have provided clinicians a useful means of assessing the risk of pet allergy development throughout a child's life, which in its own way, has almost limitless benefits considering the heartbreak of asking a family to give up a pet.

H. L. Leo, MD

3 Anesthesia Pain

Epidural Steroid Injections for Radiculopathy and/or Back Pain in Children and Adolescents: A Retrospective Cohort Study With a Prospective Follow-Up

Kurgansky KE, Rodriguez ST, Kralj MS, et al (Boston Children's Hosp and Harvard Med School, Boston, MA)
Reg Anesth Pain Med 41:86-92, 2016

Background and Objectives.—Epidural steroid injections (ESIs) are commonly performed for adults with spinal pain and/or radiculopathy. Previous pediatric ESI case series were not identified by literature review. The primary aim of this study was to examine the safety and provisional outcomes of pediatric ESIs.

Methods.—With institutional review board approval, medical records were reviewed for patients aged 9 to 20 years receiving a first ESI at Boston Children's Hospital from 2003 through 2013. A subset of patients completed a Web-based follow-up questionnaire. Descriptive statistics included frequencies, medians, interquartile ranges, and Kaplan-Meier methods. Statistical comparisons were made using Wilcoxon rank sum, χ^2, Fisher exact, and Cox proportional hazards regression analyses.

Results.—A total of 224 patients aged 9 to 20 years underwent 428 ESIs. One hundred seventyfour (76.0%) patients had a lumbar disc herniation with radiculopathy; the others had a spectrum of other spinal disorders. There were no serious adverse events, hospitalizations, dural punctures, or nerve injuries. During follow-up, 69 (41.6%) of 166 previously nonoperated lumbar disc plus radiculopathy patients underwent discectomy at a median time of 128 days (interquartile range, 76–235 days) after first injection. Degrees of straight-leg raising at presentation was significantly associated with subsequent discectomy. On followup, patients who did and did not undergo discectomy had low pain scores and high function scores.

Conclusions.—Children and adolescents can receive ESIs under conscious sedation with good safety. Further prospective studies may better define the role for these injections in the comprehensive management of pediatric spinal pain disorders.

▶ Epidural steroid injection for axial back pain due to disc herniations with and without radiculopathy is common practice in adults. Current estimates approximate a 20% to 40% prevalence of back pain among adults and that 1% to 5% of these patients have lumbar radiculopathy from disc herniations.[1,2]

The factors associated with this risk are many, including obesity, older age, occupation, sedentary lifestyle, degenerative changes, family history, and psychological stress.[2] Approximately one-quarter to one-half of cases spontaneously resolve, and between 5% and 15% go on to need surgery.[2,3] Epidural steroid injections are currently part of the conservative, nonsurgical approach to treating persistently painful disc herniations, especially with radiculopathy, although the evidence to support this approach is mixed.[4]

The literature regarding disc herniations in the pediatric population is largely centered on the various surgical treatments for patients who fail conservative therapy. Conservative therapy typically includes physical therapy, bracing, and anti-inflammatory medications.[5] Operative treatments include discectomy, laminectomy, and/or spinal fusion.[5] The current data suggest a surgical rate of 55% to 80%, which is significantly higher than the rate for adults.[6,7] These data suggest that children and adolescents with painful disc herniations are a different subset of patients than their adult counterparts. They also have significantly better outcomes after surgery than the adult population. The hypothesis is that young people are more likely to have traumatic (as opposed to degenerative) disc herniations, be physically active, have a nucleus pulposus that is less likely to resorb, and that the inciting trauma may rupture the vertebral epiphyseal ring forming an additional mass in addition to the herniated disc.[5]

In this important, first of its kind, retrospective cohort study, Kurgansky et al showed that epidural steroid injections should be further evaluated as part of the conservative approach to disc herniations with and without radiculopathy. Although limited by its retrospective nature, the results are promising. In the study, they showed that 41.6% of their previously nonoperated patients underwent discectomy within a year after first injection. This is significantly less than the neurosurgical literature suggesting a rate of 55% to 80% of patients failing conservative treatment and proceeding to surgery. The single most predictive factor of discectomy in this study was the degree of straight leg raise positivity on initial presentation. A positive SLR of 30 degrees or less was associated with an increased need for surgical intervention. There were no serious adverse events reported from ESI, and no significant difference in outcomes between patients who did and did not proceed to surgery.

Limitations to the study included its retrospective design, single center with interventional techniques varying throughout the 10 years of review, and significant referral biases. The practice patterns at the study site included referrals to Sports Medicine and Orthopedic Spine Clinics for conservative management followed by neurosurgery evaluation for refractory patients. Because this refractory population was then referred to the Pain Treatment Clinic for epidural steroid injection, the studied patients likely were a preselected population.

Overall, this well-conducted retrospective study made 3 well-supported conclusions. First, epidural steroid injections can be performed safely on children and adolescents under conscious sedation using currently accepted techniques with fluoroscopic guidance. Second, these initial data suggest a need to further validate this approach through prospective, randomized studies. Finally, inclusion of epidural steroid injections into the treatment algorithm for pediatric patients may reduce the need for operative treatment.

R. Blake Windsor, MD

References

1. Konstantinou K, Dunn KM. Sciatica: review of epidemiological studies and prevalence estimates. *Spine (Phila Pa 1976)*. 2008;33:2464-2472.
2. Hoy D, Brooks P, Blyth F, Buchbinder R. The epidemiology of low back pain. *Best Pract Res Clin Rheumatol*. 2010;24:769-781.
3. Gaskin DJ, Richard P. The economic costs of pain in the United States. *J Pain*. 2012;13:715-724.
4. Manchikanti L, Knezevic NN, Boswell MV, Kaye AD, Hirsch JA. Epidural injections for lumbar radiculopathy and spinal stenosis: a comparative systematic review and meta-analysis. *Pain Physician*. 2016;19:E365-E410.
5. Dang L, Liu Z. A review of current treatment for lumbar disc herniation in children and adolescents. *Eur Spine J*. 2010;19:205-214.
6. Kurth AA, Rau S, Wang C, Schmitt E. Treatment of lumbar disc herniation in the second decade of life. *Eur Spine J*. 1996;5:220-224.
7. DeLuca PF, Mason DE, Weiand R, Howard R, Bassett GS. Excision of herniated nucleus pulposus in children and adolescents. *J Pediatr Orthop*. 1994;14:318-322.

Pediatric Pain Screening Tool: rapid identification of risk in youth with pain complaints

Simons LF, Smith A, Ibagon C, et al (Boston Children's Hosp, MA; et al)
Pain 156:1511-1518, 2015

Moderate to severe chronic pain is a problem for 1.7 million children, costing $19.5 billion dollars annually in the United States alone. Risk-stratified care is known to improve outcomes in adults with chronic pain. However, no tool exists to stratify youth who present with pain complaints to appropriate interventions. The Pediatric Pain Screening Tool (PPST) presented here assesses prognostic factors associated with adverse outcomes among youth and defines risk groups to inform efficient treatment decision making. Youth (n = 321, ages 8-18, 90.0% Caucasian, 74.8% female) presenting for multidisciplinary pain clinic evaluation at a tertiary care center participated. Of these, 195 (61.1%) participated at 4-month follow-up. Participants completed the 9-item PPST in addition to measures of functional disability, pain catastrophizing, fear of pain, anxiety, and depressive symptoms. Sensitivity and specificity for the PPST ranged from adequate to excellent, with regard to significant disability (78%, 68%) and high emotional distress (81%, 63%). Participants were classified into low- (11%), medium-(32%), and high-(57%) risk groups. Risk groups did not significantly differ by pain diagnosis, location, or duration. Only 2% to 7% of patients who met reference standard case status for disability and emotional distress at 4-month follow-up were classified as low risk at baseline, whereas 71% to 79% of patients who met reference standard case status at follow-up were classified as high risk at baseline. A 9-item screening tool identifying factors associated with adverse outcomes among youth who present with pain complaints seems valid and provides risk stratification that can potentially guide effective pain treatment recommendations in the clinic setting.

▶ Pain complaints in children and adolescents are common. Chronic pain is defined as pain lasting longer than 3 to 5 months, or longer than anticipated.[1] It is often associated with complex biopsychosocial dynamics, including persistent pain from unexplained causes, emotional distress, catastrophizing behaviors, fear of pain, and development of functional disability.[2-5] Current estimates are that 5% of children and adolescents have chronic pain that result in functional disability.[6]

Rates of chronic pain in pediatrics appear to be increasing. Coffelt, Bauer, and Carroll showed that the rate of inpatient hospitalization for children with chronic pain increased 831% between 2004 and 2010 and that their stays were 3 days longer than expected for the complaint.[7] A retrospective cost analysis from a multidisciplinary, academic pediatric pain center demonstrated that the mean economic cost of their patients was $11 787 in the year before referral. Extrapolated across the estimated prevalence of pediatric pain with disability, Groenwald et al estimated a national economic burden of $19.5 billion annually— comparable to disorders such as ADHD.[8] A multidisciplinary team approach to treatment, including physicians, psychologists, physical and/or occupational therapists, nurses, and social workers have been shown to be the most effective treatment strategy for this challenging population.[9] Unfortunately, few medical centers currently have multidisciplinary treatment teams in place.

Simons et al aimed to address this issue with the creation of a brief, validated, 9-question screening survey to stratify the risk of persistent pain symptoms and disability in this population. The study took place at the initial visit, and at 2-week and 4-month follow-up of patients referred to a large, academic multidisciplinary pain clinic. The study recruited 321 patients (71% of eligible patients) with multiple pain complaints, including musculoskeletal pain (43.2%), complex regional pain syndrome (18.6%), neuropathic pain (7.3%), functional abdominal pain (6.6%), headache (6.0%), endometriosis (3.5%), and other diseases (14.8%). The mean age was 13.2 years, and duration of pain ranged from less than 1 month to longer than 15 years (median 13 months).

The screening survey, named the Pediatric Pain Screening Tool (PPST), is modified from an adult screening instrument used for a similar purpose, the Keele STaRT Back Screening Tool (SBST).[10] The scale consists of 2 subscales, physical and psychosocial metrics. Physical subscale questions identify widespread pain, impaired ability to walk long distances or attend school, and sleep disturbance due to pain. Psychosocial questions identify feelings of worry, hopelessness, and lack of enjoyment in activities due to pain. This prospective study compared screening scores against validated instruments, including the Numeric Rating Scale of pain intensity (NRS), Functional Disability Inventory (FDI),[4,5] Fear of Pain Questionnaire (FOPQ) for children,[11] Pain Catastrophizing Scale-Child report (PSC-C),[2] Children's Depression Inventory (CDI-2), and the Revised Children's Manifest Anxiety Scale.

The study found 2 statistically significant cutoff scores. A PPST total score greater than 5, or a psychosocial subset score greater than or equal to 3 was associated with persistent pain, disability, and emotional distress. At follow-up, 71% to 79% of patients who met the reference standard for high disability, catastrophizing, fear, anxiety, and depression at 4-month follow-up were initially scored as high risk. Only 2% to 7% of children with who met this reference standard were initially scored as low risk. Overall, only 11% of studied patients were identified as low risk, which is much less than the adult primary care data of 40% to 47%. This was likely due to the severe impairment of the preselected and complex patient population that was ultimately referred to a large academic medical center.

The PPST is an important concept to help quickly stratify the risk of persistent pain, disability, and emotional distress in children and predict which patients are likely to be refractory to typical care. Because of the limited availability of multi-disciplinary pain treatment centers, the PPST may help guide the appropriate and efficient referral of high-risk patients.

This is a first-time study that evaluated patients referred to a single, multidisciplinary pain clinic and is limited by its preselected, complex population. Through an attempt to keep the screening test rapid (1—2 minutes), the PPST may not include all facets associated with an increased risk. The authors' stated goal is to test implementation in primary and specialty clinics (ie, gastroenterology), in an attempt to guide escalation of services. Early identification of high-risk patients may ultimately improve recovery rates and intervene on maladaptive long-term trajectories.

R. Blake Windsor, MD

References

1. McGrath PJ, Stevens BJ, Walker SM, Zempsky WT. *Oxford Textbook of Pediatric Pain*. 1st edition. Oxford: Oxford University Press; 2013.
2. Crombez G, Bijttebier P, Eccleston C, et al. The child version of the pain catastrophizing scale (PCS-C): a preliminary validation. *Pain*. 2003;104: 639-646.
3. Eccleston C, Crombez G, Scotford A, Clinch J, Connell H. Adolescent chronic pain: patterns and predictors of emotional distress in adolescents with chronic pain and their parents. *Pain*. 2004;108:221-229.
4. Walker LS, Greene JW. The functional disability inventory: measuring a neglected dimension of child health status. *J Pediatr Psychol*. 1991;16:39-58.
5. Kashikar-Zuck S, Flowers SR, Claar RL, et al. Clinical utility and validity of the functional disability inventory among a multicenter sample of youth with chronic pain. *Pain*. 2011;152:1600-1607.
6. Huguet A, Miro J. The severity of chronic pediatric pain: an epidemiological study. *J Pain*. 2008;9:226-236.
7. Coffelt TA, Bauer BD, Carroll AE. Inpatient characteristics of the child admitted with chronic pain. *Pediatrics*. 2013;132:e422-e429.
8. Groenewald CB, Essner BS, Wright D, Fesinmeyer MD, Palermo TM. The economic costs of chronic pain among a cohort of treatment-seeking adolescents in the United States. *J Pain*. 2014;15:925-933.
9. Gatchel RJ, McGeary DD, McGeary CA, Lippe B. Interdisciplinary chronic pain management: past, present, and future. *Am Psychol*. 2014;69:119-130.

10. Hay EM, Dunn KM, Hill JC, et al. A randomised clinical trial of subgrouping and targeted treatment for low back pain compared with best current care. The STarT Back Trial Study Protocol. *BMC Musculoskelet Disord.* 2008;9:58.
11. Simons LE, Sieberg CB, Carpino E, Logan D, Berde C. The Fear of Pain Questionnaire (FOPQ): assessment of pain-related fear among children and adolescents with chronic pain. *J Pain.* 2011;12:677-686.

Surgery and Neurodevelopmental Outcome of Very Low-Birth-Weight Infants

Morriss FH Jr, for the Eunice Kennedy Shriver National Institute of Child Health and Human Development Neonatal Research Network (Univ of Iowa; et al)
JAMA Pediatr 168:746-754, 2014

Importance.—Reduced death and neurodevelopmental impairment among infants is a goal of perinatal medicine.

Objective.—To assess the association between surgery during the initial hospitalization and death or neurodevelopmental impairment of very low-birth-weight infants.

Design, Setting, and Participants.—A retrospective cohort analysiswas conducted of patients enrolled in the National Institute of Child Health and Human Development Neonatal Research Network Generic Database from 1998 through 2009 and evaluated at 18 to 22 months' corrected age. Twenty-two academic neonatal intensive care units participated. Inclusion criteria were birth weight 401 to 1500 g, survival to 12 hours, and availability for follow-up. A total of 12 111 infants were included in analyses.

Exposures.—Surgical procedures; surgery also was classified by expected anesthesia type as major (general anesthesia) or minor (nongeneral anesthesia).

Main Outcomes and Measures.—Multivariable logistic regression analyses planned a priori were performed for the primary outcome of death or neurodevelopmental impairment and for the secondary outcome of neurodevelopmental impairment among survivors. Multivariable linear regression analyses were performed as planned for the adjusted mean scores of the Mental Developmental Index and Psychomotor Developmental Index of the Bayley Scales of Infant Development, Second Edition, for patients born before 2006.

Results.—A total of 2186 infants underwent major surgery, 784 had minor surgery, and 9141 infants did not undergo surgery. The risk-adjusted odds ratio of death or neurodevelopmental impairment for all surgery patients compared with those who had no surgery was 1.29 (95% CI, 1.08-1.55). For patients who had major surgery compared with those who had no surgery, the risk-adjusted odds ratio of death or neurodevelopmental impairment was 1.52 (95% CI, 1.24-1.87). Patients classified as having minor surgery had no increased adjusted risk. Among survivors who had major surgery compared with those who had no surgery, the adjusted risk of neurodevelopmental impairment was greater and the adjusted mean Bayley scores were lower.

Conclusions and Relevance.—Major surgery in very low-birth-weight infants is independently associated with a greater than 50% increased risk of death or neurodevelopmental impairment and of neurodevelopmental impairment at 18 to 22 months' corrected age. The role of general anesthesia is implicated but remains unproven.

▶ The clinical question of neurotoxicity and potential harm from general anesthesia in pediatric patients is of significant concern to physicians, scientists, and, of course, parents. Recent publications in both the lay press (the *New York Times*[1]) and highly cited medical journals[2] have made this a subject of worry and, sometimes, fear for caregivers and lay people alike. The recognition that general anesthetics appear to promote apoptosis of brain cells not only in laboratory animals but also in human children has prompted further clinical and basic science investigations trying to determine which specific agents are most dangerous and what periods of development the child may be most vulnerable to these agents.[3]

The current study by Morris et al is an attempt to investigate 1 such period of vulnerability to anesthetics—that is, the infant with very low birth weight having surgery, as a surrogate for clinical exposure to anesthetics in the earliest postnatal stages of development. This study is a multicenter retrospective cohort analysis of 12 111 infants born weighing between 401 and 1 500 g. Primary end points were death or neurodevelopmental impairment (NDI). They further classified the infants into 3 groups: major surgery, minor surgery, and no surgery. "Major surgery" was defined as surgery in which the expected anesthesia would have been general anesthesia, and "minor surgery" was defined as surgery where the expected anesthetic technique would have been nongeneral anesthesia (local or central neuraxial [spinal], for example).

The author's analysis demonstrated that the risk adjusted odds ratio of death or NDI for all the surgery patients versus the no surgery group, was 1.29 (95% confidence interval, 1.08—1.55). This result was more dramatic for the major surgery group alone, compared with no surgery group, where the odds ratio was 1.52 (95% confidence interval, 1.24—1.87) of death or NDI. Patients classified as minor surgery (ie, likely had surgery without general anesthesia) had no additional risk of death or NDI versus the no surgery group.

The glaring flaw of this study is the use of 2 subgroups (major surgery and minor surgery) as proxies for general anesthesia versus nongeneral anesthesia. They justify this because the database that they employed (Neonatal Research Network Generic Database) provides data on specific surgeries but not specific anesthetics. They make no efforts to drill-down on their data to identify specific anesthetic agents or even whether general anesthesia or nongeneral was used. For instance, the authors state that gastrostomy procedures where defined as "minor surgery" because it "could have been performed under neuraxial, regional, or local." It could also have been performed under general anesthesia. Other variables of their "major surgery" group could include greater physiological stress, hypoxia, postoperative analgesics, for example.

Regarding specific general anesthetics, many laboratory investigations have suggested tremendous variability in apoptosis levels based on anesthetic chosen.

For example, GABA-ergic agonists (eg, midazolam), and N-methyl-D-aspartate receptor antagonists (NMDA blockers) such as ketamine, appear much more dangerous than other agents (eg, alpha-2 agonists such as dexmedetomidine).[4]

The authors cite a study by Blakely et al, which prospectively evaluated neonates with necrotizing enterocolitis undergoing laparotomy (under general anesthesia) compared with those having a peritoneal drain placement (without general anesthesia). This study demonstrated no difference in adjusted odds ratio for death or NDI between these groups suggesting the need to look at other factors than anesthetic versus no anesthesia.

Finally, it may be that neither death nor NDI are the correct end points to study in this age group. Severely premature and extremely small neonates have many different causes of NDIs and/or death. Factors such as physiological stress, hyperoxia, hypoxia, hypothermia, caffeine use, prenatal insults (eg, maternal opioid use), and surgical volume shifts may all be more significant determinants of these endpoints than general anesthesia.[5]

The retrospective nature of this study, using type of surgery as a surrogate for presumed type of anesthesia, and the lack of anesthetic type—specific data make this study's conclusions less applicable to the important questions of safety and neurotoxicity of anesthesia in low birth weight infants, and more applicable to the dangers of extensive surgery in these tiny, usually premature, infants. The authors' statement that "this analysis supports the concern that surgery with general anesthesia during a vulnerable period of infancy has an adverse effect on neurodevelopmental outcome" is not adequately supported by this study.

E. S. Shank, MD

References

1. Grady D. Researchers call for more study of anesthesia's risks to brains of young children. *New York Times.* 2015:A20.
2. Rappaport BA, Suresh S, Hertz S, et al. Anesthetic neurotoxicity - clinical implications of animal models. *N Engl J Med.* 2015;372:796-797.
3. Shafer SL. Neurotoxicity of anesthetic agents in children. *Anesth Analg.* 2007;105: 882-883.
4. Lin EP, Soriano SG, Loepke AW. Anesthetic neurotoxicity. *Anesthesiol Clin.* 2014; 32:133-155.
5. Blakely ML, Tyson JE, Lally KP, et al. NICHD Neonatal Research Network. Laparotomy versus peritoneal drainage for necrotizing enterocolitis or isolated intestinal perforation in extremely low birth weight infants. *Pediatrics.* 2006;117:e680-e687.

Sedatives and Analgesics Given to Infants in Neonatal Intensive Care Units at the End of Life

Zimmerman KO, Hornik CP, Ku L, et al (Duke Univ School of Medicine, Durham, NC; et al)
J Pediatr 167:299-304, 2015

Objective.—To describe the administration of sedatives and analgesics at the end of life in a large cohort of infants in North American neonatal intensive care units.

Study Design.—Data on mortality and sedative and analgesic administration were from infants who died from 1997-2012 in 348 neonatal intensive care units managed by the Pediatrix Medical Group. Sedatives and analgesics of interest included opioids (fentanyl, methadone, morphine), benzodiazepines (clonazepam, diazepam, lorazepam, midazolam), central alpha-2 agonists (clonidine, dexmedetomidine), ketamine, and pentobarbital. We used multivariable logistic regression to evaluate the association between administration of these drugs on the day of death and infant demographics and illness severity.

Results.—We identified 19 726 infants who died. Of these, 6188 (31%) received a sedative or analgesic on the day of death; opioids were most frequently administered, 5366/19 726 (27%). Administration of opioids and benzodiazepines increased during the study period, from 16/283 (6%) for both in 1997 to 523/1465 (36%) and 295/1465 (20%) in 2012, respectively. Increasing gestational age, increasing postnatal age, invasive procedure within 2 days of death, more recent year of death, mechanical ventilation, inotropic support, and antibiotics on the day of death were associated with exposure to sedatives or analgesics.

Conclusions.—Administration of sedatives and analgesics increased over time. Infants of older gestational age and those more critically ill were more likely to receive these drugs on the day of death. These findings suggest that drug administration may be driven by severity of illness. (Figs 1 and 2)

▶ No one wants to die in pain.

Prior retrospective studies from a single tertiary level neonatal intensive care unit (NICU) in 1997 and again in 2015 in 4 university centers in 3 countries show that a significant proportion of dying newborns do not receive analgesics or sedatives during end-of-life care.[1,2] In the large multicenter study by Zimmerman and colleagues, only 31% of the infants received a sedative or analgesic on the day of death, 41% within the last 2 days of life, and 48% at any point during their hospitalization.

This is the largest study of end-of-life care for newborns to date, including 19 726 infants who died in 348 NICUs in North America. In this study, sedative and analgesic use among ranged from 0 to 60% (Fig 1). Prior studies in 1 to 4 centers have shown higher rates of administration (79%–97%) in the 48 hours before death.[1-4] Studies of withdrawal or withholding of life-sustaining interventions in the NICU have shown similarly high rates of analgesic administration.[2] The NICUs in this study may differ from other tertiary NICUs in that they are part of the Pediatrix Medical Group; this potential bias in not addressed by the authors. On the other hand, a particular strength of this North American study is its breadth. Zimmerman and coworkers were able to demonstrate large center-to-center variations across North America, with an analgesic or sedative administered to 18% (median, interquartile range 0–34) of dying infants. The infrequent use of these medications in end-of-life care is striking.

Multivariate analysis of sedative or analgesic use on the day of death showed associations with increasing gestational age, increasing postnatal age, invasive

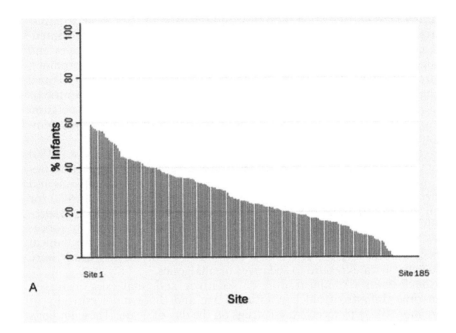

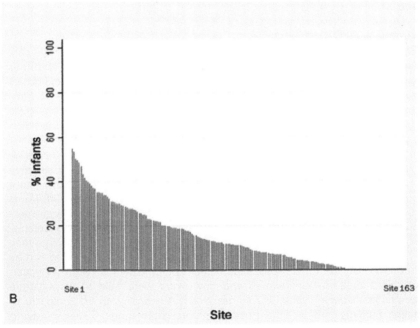

FIGURE 1.—Use of **A,** opioids and **B,** benzodiazepines on day of death among all sites with >10 deaths. (Reprinted from Zimmerman KO, Hornik CP, Ku L, et al. Sedatives and analgesics given to infants in neonatal intensive care units at the end of life. *J Pediatr.* 2015;167:299-304, with permission Elsevier Inc.)

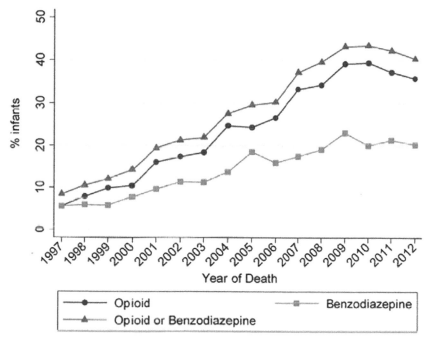

FIGURE 2.—Exposure to opioids and benzodiazepines by year of death (exposure on the day of death). (Reprinted from Zimmerman KO, Hornik CP, Ku L, et al. Sedatives and analgesics given to infants in neonatal intensive care units at the end of life. *J Pediatr.* 2015;167:299-304, with permission Elsevier Inc.)

procedures within 2 days of death, and measures of critical illness (mechanical ventilation, inotropic support, and antibiotics) on the day of death.

However controversial, it is clear that most, if not all, neonates admitted to the NICU are mature enough to have the capacity to perceive pain.[5,6] Although not all infants experience significant pain during an NICU admission, most undergo a series of uncomfortable or outright painful procedures as part of their lives in the NICU.[7] Pain has significant short- and long-term deleterious effects among survivors of the NICU.[8] Unfortunately, so may opioids.[9] Physicians' reluctance to medicate infants in the NICU is understandable given the potential for side effects, such as respiratory depression or hypotension. But for those infants who cannot survive the delivery room or the NICU, there are few, if any, valid contraindications to administering either benzodiazepines or opioid during end-of-life care. Dying infants will not become addicted to opioids. Fear of litigation should not render health care providers unresponsive to their pain and suffering.

Fear of hastening their death also acts as a barrier to administering analgesics and sedatives in end-of-life care. However, the ethical doctrine of double effect permits actions that might cause serious harm or death as a side effect if the intent of the actions is to promote a larger good, such as the prevention of pain and suffering.[10] Thus, in the context of withdrawal or withholding of life-sustaining interventions, the intent is the prevention of pain and suffering as the infant dies, not shortening the course. In fact, there is growing evidence that opiates do not affect the time of death after compassionate extubation.[2]

There are, of course, situations in which analgesics or sedatives are either inappropriate or not feasible, such as sudden unexpected death, death during a code, or conditions in which perception of pain may be severely diminished or absent (profound brain injury or, rarely, brain death). The authors did not measure the extent to which this might have affected sedative or analgesic use; however, they justified this with the assumption that their results would resemble prior reports that up to 73% of infants die after withdrawal or withholding of life support, and that < 10% of NICU deaths occur because of physiologic instability or requirement for cardiopulmonary resuscitation (CPR) outside the delivery room.[1,11]

The authors suggest improvements to end-of-life care for neonates that may not be completely novel but that, at the same time, have not been widely adopted. These include guidelines for end-of-life care, pediatric palliative care teams, and improved methods for recognizing pain in all infants and especially in those most difficult to assess, such as in infants who are extremely premature, neurologically compromised, or born with life-threatening congenital anomalies. Health care providers can do better.

There is hope, though. The authors demonstrate an increasing use of both sedatives and analgesics on the day of death during the study period (1997–2012), from 6% to 36% for opioids and from 6% to 20% for benzodiazepines (Fig 2). Further studies of physician intent, and dosing regimens could help clarify remaining obstacles to preventing pain and suffering among infants destined to die.

We all die at some point. Do unto others as you would have them do unto you.

J. C. Partridge, MD, MPH

References

1. Wall SN, Partridge JC. Death in the intensive care nursery: physician practice of withdrawing and withholding life support. *Pediatrics*. 1997;99:64-70.
2. Partridge JC, Wall SN. Analgesia for dying infants whose life support is withdrawn or withheld. *Pediatrics*. 1997;99:76-79.
3. Janvier A, Meadow W, Leuthner SR, et al. Whom are we comforting? An analysis of comfort medications delivered to dying neonates. *J Pediatr*. 2011;159: 206-210.
4. Provoost V, Colls F, Bilsen J, et al. The use of drugs with a life-shortening effect in end-of-life care in neonates and infants. *Intensive Care Med*. 2006;32:133-139.
5. Lee SJ, Ralston HJ, Drey EA, Partridge JC, Rosen MA. Fetal pain: a systematic multidisciplinary review of the evidence. *JAMA*. 2005;294:947-954.
6. Anand KJ, Hall RW. Controversies in neonatal pain: an introduction. *Semin Perinatol*. 2007;31:273-274.
7. Carbajal R, Rousset A, Danan C, et al. Epidemiology and treatment of painful procedures in neonates in intensive care units. *JAMA*. 2008;300:60-70.
8. Ranger M, Zwicker JG, Chau CM, et al. Neonatal pain and infection relate to smaller cerebellum in very preterm children at school age. *J Pediatr*. 2015;167: 292-298.e1.

9. Zwicker JG, Miller SP, Grunau RE, et al. Smaller cerebellar growth and poorer neurodevelopmental outcomes in very preterm infants exposed to neonatal morphine. *J Pediatr.* 2016;172:81-87.e2.
10. Wilkinson D. Three myths in end-of-life care. *J Med Ethics.* 2013;39:389-390.
11. Fontana MS, Farrell C, Gauvin F, Lacroix J, Janvier A. Modes of death in pediatrics: differences in the ethical approach in neonatal and pediatric patients. *J Pediatr.* 2013;162:1107-1111.

4 Blood

Effect of Transfusion of Red Blood Cells With Longer vs Shorter Storage Duration on Elevated Blood Lactate Levels in Children With Severe Anemia: The TOTAL Randomized Clinical Trial

Dhabangi A, Ainomugisha B, Cserti Gazdewich C, et al (Makerere Univ, Kampala, Uganda; Mulago Hosp, Kampala, Uganda; Univ of Toronto, Canada; et al)

JAMA 314.2514-2523, 2015

Importance.—Although millions of transfusions are given annually worldwide, the effect of red blood cell (RBC) unit storage duration on oxygen delivery is uncertain.

Objective.—To determine if longer-storage RBC units are not inferior to shorter-storage RBC units for tissue oxygenation as measured by reduction in blood lactate levels and improvement in cerebral tissue oxygen saturation among children with severe anemia.

Design, Setting, and Participants.—Randomized noninferiority trial of 290 children (aged 6-60 months), most with malaria or sickle cell disease, presenting February 2013 through May 2015 to a university-affiliated national referral hospital in Kampala, Uganda, with a hemoglobin level of 5 g/dL or lower and a lactate level of 5 mmol/L or higher.

Interventions.—Patients were randomly assigned to receive RBC units stored 25 to 35 days (longer-storage group; n = 145) vs 1 to 10 days (shorter-storage group; n = 145). All units were leukoreduced prior to storage. All patients received 10 mL/kg of RBCs during hours 0 through 2 and, if indicated per protocol, an additional 10 mL/kg during hours 4 through 6.

Main Outcomes and Measures.—The primary outcome was the proportion of patients with a lactate level of 3 mmol/L or lower at 8 hours using a margin of noninferiority equal to an absolute difference of 25%. Secondary measures included noninvasive cerebral tissue oxygen saturation during the first transfusion, clinical and laboratory changes up to 24 hours, and survival and health at 30 days after transfusion. Adverse events were monitored up to 24 hours.

Results.—In the total population of 290 children, the mean (SD) presenting hemoglobin level was 3.7 g/dL (1.3) and mean lactate level was 9.3 mmol/L (3.4). Median (interquartile range) RBC unit storage was 8 days (7-9) for shorter storage vs 32 days (30-34) for longer storage without overlap. The proportion achieving the primary end point was 0.61 (95% CI, 0.52 to 0.69) in the longer-storage group vs 0.58 (95% CI, 0.49 to 0.66) in the shorter-storage group (between-group difference, 0.03 [95% CI, −0.07 to ∞], $P < .001$), meeting the prespecified margin of noninferiority. Mean lactate levels were not statistically different between the 2 groups at 0, 2, 4, 6, 8, or 24 hours. Kaplan-Meier analysis and global nonlinear regression revealed no statistical difference in lactate reduction between the 2 groups. Clinical assessment, cerebral oxygen saturation, electrolyte abnormalities, adverse events, survival, and 30-day recovery were also not significantly different between the groups.

Conclusions and Relevance.—Among children with lactic acidosis due to severe anemia, transfusion of longer-storage compared with shorter-storage RBC units did not result in inferior reduction of elevated blood lactate levels. These findings have relevance regarding the efficacy of stored RBC transfusion for patients with critical tissue hypoxia and lactic acidosis due to anemia.

Trial Registration.—clinicaltrials.gov Identifier: NCT01586923.

▶ Red blood cells (RBCs) have long been known to undergo biochemical and morphological changes during storage. However, whether these changes (termed the "red cell storage lesion") impact clinical outcomes remains an open question.[1] In the past 10 years, the potentially deleterious clinical consequences of transfusing RBCs that have been stored for prolonged periods has gained prominence.

Among the first and most influential studies is a single institution observational study in adult patients undergoing cardiothoracic surgery published in the *New England Journal of Medicine* in 2008. In that report, Koch and colleagues at the Cleveland Clinic examined data from patients given RBC transfusions during coronary-artery bypass grafting, heart-valve surgery, or both between 1998 and 2006. They compared the outcomes for 2872 patients who received blood that had been stored for 14 days or less (median 11 days) with that for 3130 patients who received blood that had been stored for more than 14 days (median 20 days) and found that patients who were given older units had higher rates of in-hospital mortality, complications, and long-term (1 year) mortality.[2]

However, the data on the clinical impact of the red cell storage lesion remains far from clear. Observational studies in both adult and pediatric patients, and meta-analyses based on these studies, have given contradictory answers, and, in general, have been limited by sample size and methodological concerns.[3-5] This contrasts with data from preclinical animal models that have shown clearer associations between transfusion of longer-stored RBCs and increased mortality or morbidity, or decreased efficacy. Notably, the animal models point to the possibility that storage lesion elements which impact endothelial function, iron load, and oxidative damage may affect outcome specifically in recipients with underlying infections or inflammatory states.[3,5,6]

In an attempt to clarify this question, several randomized clinical trials (RCT) in both pediatric and adult patients have been conducted to determine the effect of RBC age at transfusion on morbidity and mortality. To date, these have found no significant differences in adverse outcomes between patients receiving longer versus shorter-stored RBCs.[6]

This study by Dhabangi and colleagues is now the first to examine whether RBC age affects the efficacy of oxygen delivery in children presenting with severe anemia and lactic acidosis. They found that longer-stored RBCs reduce blood lactate levels and improve cerebral tissue oxygen saturation in a comparable fashion to shorter-stored RBCs in children with severe anemia. This study is notable in several respects. It provides an example of how a carefully designed and executed randomized clinical trial (RCT) can be conducted in the developing world and may be better able to be done there because of the patient population. In fact, compared with the RCTs done to date, this study achieved better separation of the duration of storage between the 2 study cohorts. Previous RCTs examining the red cell storage lesion question, such as the Age of Red Blood Cells in Premature Infants (ARIPI) trial, have been criticized for comparing "fresh" with "fresher" cells.[5]

Furthermore, the high prevalence of malaria in Uganda (~80% of the patients on the study) provided a cohort of severely anemic patients that is not as readily available in North America or Europe. As the authors point out, previous RCTs done in North America and Europe have not been able to assess tissue oxygenation because patients are generally transfused earlier. Finally, together with the results of the other RCTs, this study provides reassurance that for the populations studied to date, which includes some of the sickest patients in neonatal intensive and critical care units, there is no significant benefit to be gained by changing RBC storage age requirements in current transfusion practice. It is therefore likely that the impact of the red cell storage lesion will only become clear with further elucidation of the role that donor- and recipient-specific characteristics play in transfusion outcomes.

J. Huang, MD

References

1. Hess JR. Red cell changes during storage. *Transfus Apher Sci..* 2010;43:51-59.
2. Koch CG, Li L, Sessler DI, et al. Duration of red-cell storage and complications after cardiac surgery. *N Engl J Med.* 2008;358:1229-1239.
3. Cohen B, Matot I. Aged erythrocytes: a fine wine or sour grapes? *Br J Anaesth.* 2013;111:i62-i70.
4. Qu L, Triulzi DJ. Clinical effects of red blood cell storage. *Cancer Control.* 2015;22:26-37.
5. Remy KE, Natanson C, Klein HG. The influence of the storage lesion(s) on pediatric red cell transfusion. *Curr Opin Pediatr.* 2015;27:277-285.
6. Glynn SA, Klein HG, Ness PM. The red blood cell storage lesion: the end of the beginning. *Transfusion.* 2016;56:1462-1468.

A multicenter randomized controlled trial of intravenous magnesium for sickle cell pain crisis in children

Brousseau DC, for the Pediatric Emergency Care Applied Research Network (PECARN) (Children's Res Inst, Milwaukee, WI; et al)
Blood 126:1651-1657, 2015

Magnesium, a vasodilator, anti-inflammatory, and pain reliever, could alter the pathophysiology of sickle cellpain crises. We hypothesized that intravenous magnesium would shorten length of stay, decrease opioid use, and improve health-related quality of life (HRQL) for pediatric patients hospitalized with sickle cell pain crises. The Magnesium for Children in Crisis (MAGiC) study was a randomized, double-blind, placebo-controlled trial of intravenous magnesium vs normal saline placebo conducted at 8 sites within the Pediatric Emergency Care Applied Research Network (PECARN). Children 4 to 21 years old with hemoglobin SS or Sβ^0 thalassemia requiring hospitalization for pain were eligible. Children received 40 mg/kg of magnesium or placebo every 8 hours for up to 6 doses plus standard therapy. The primary outcome was length of stay in hours from the time of first study drug infusion, compared using a Van Elteren test. Secondary outcomes included opioid use and HRQL. Of 208 children enrolled, 204 received the study drug (101 magnesium, 103 placebo). Between-group demographics and prerandomization treatment were similar. The median interquartile range (IQR) length of stay was 56.0 (27.0-109.0) hours for magnesium vs 47.0 (24.0-99.0) hours for placebo ($P = .24$). Magnesium patients received 1.46 mg/kg morphine equivalents vs 1.28 mg/kg for placebo ($P = .12$). Changes in HRQL before discharge and 1 week after discharge were similar ($P > .05$ for all comparisons). The addition of intravenous magnesium did not shorten length of stay, reduce opioid use, or improve quality of life in children hospitalized for sickle cell pain crisis. This trial was registered at www.clinicaltrials.gov as #NCT01197417.

▶ Despite the ongoing improvements in childhood survival from sickle cell disease (SCD), the vast majority will still experience vaso-occlusive pain episodes, the leading cause of hospitalization for individuals with SCD. The primary therapy of acutely severe vaso-occlusive pain includes intravenous (IV) opioids, hydration, supportive care, and hospital admission. We applaud the multidisciplinary team of emergency medicine physicians, pediatric hematologists, and other staff members for completing a randomized controlled trial (RCT) to address the efficacy of treating vaso-occlusive pain upon admission with IV magnesium in conjunction with standard therapy.

The foundation for the Magnesium for Children in Crisis (MAGiC) trial, which is the phase III RCT described in this article, was the completion of a single center, prospective, nonrandomized and nonblinded pilot study. The pilot study aimed to determine the feasibility and safety of IV magnesium for acute vaso-occlusive pain episodes. Magnesium was selected as the intervention based on its biological effects of vasodilation and ability to alter inflammation.

Given these biological interactions, the investigators elected to test the hypothesis that the addition of IV magnesium would decrease the length of stay (LOS) for vaso-occlusive pain compared with standard therapy alone. In 2004, Brousseau et al investigated LOS for 19 children with hemoglobin SS (HbSS) and hemoglobin Sβ thalassemia zero (HbSβ0), aged 4 to 18 years, admitted with vaso-occlusive pain and treated with magnesium infusions in addition to standard therapy. The LOS was shorter during the magnesium admission (median 3.0 days, compared with 5.0 and 4.0 days for the previous 2 admissions; $P = .006$).[1] These results from the initial pilot study suggested that IV magnesium might shorten hospitalization for children admitted for vaso-occlusive pain, which prompted further investigation in MAGiC.

MAGiC was a multicenter, randomized, parallel, double-blinded, placebo-controlled trial designed to assess the benefits of IV magnesium vs normal saline in addition to standard supportive therapy for pediatric vaso-occlusive pain management. The primary hypothesis was that adding IV magnesium to standard therapy for vaso-occlusive pain would shorten LOS by at least 20 hours. LOS was the time between the first opioid infusion to 12 hours after the last opioid infusion or time of discharge (whichever came first). The power calculation based on the primary outcome revealed that 91 participants were needed to detect a 20-hour difference in LOS. Accounting for both 5% noncompliance and interim monitoring limitations, the sample size was increased to 104 per group. The secondary outcomes were decreased opioid use, improved health related quality of life (HRQL), and changes in inflammatory markers.

A total of 204 participants were randomly allocated (101 in the magnesium and 103 in the placebo groups). For the primary outcome, the intention-to-treat results revealed median interquartile range LOS for the magnesium group compared with the placebo group were 56.0 (27.0—109.0) and 47.0 (24.0—99.0) hours, respectively ($P = 0.24$). The morphine equivalents between the magnesium treatment and placebo groups were 1.46 mg/kg and 1.28 mg/kg, respectively ($P = 0.12$). HRQL outcomes were measured predischarge and emergency department to 1-week follow-up in both trial participants and their parents using the PedsQL Generic Core Scale, PedsQL Multidimensional Fatigue Scale, and the PedsQL SCD Module, which is the only validated quality of life measure specific to SCD. Regardless of the scale and time administered, there were no statistical differences between the magnesium and placebo groups for all HRQL measures, both for trial participants and parents. Additionally, there were no statistically significant differences in markers of inflammation, hemolysis, and endothelial activation after 25 hours between the magnesium and placebo groups. After the completion of the trial, the investigators concluded that IV magnesium does not reduce LOS, decrease opioid use, or improve quality of life for children admitted for a vaso-occlusive pain crisis.

When comparing the conflicting results between the pilot study and MAGiC, the results are consistent with what would be expected. Typically, single-center trials exhibit a higher treatment effect than when the similar study question is investigated as a multicenter trial.[2] The multicenter MAGiC trial effectively addressed the limitations and inherent biases associated with a single-center, single-arm trial and demonstrates the importance of not overinterpreting results from pilot studies and single-center trials.

Despite the negative results of MAGiC, there are several key points that can be learned from this trial. First, MAGiC demonstrated that overcoming enrollment challenges through collaborations between pediatric hematology and emergency medicine physicians within the Pediatric Emergency Care Applied Research Network (PECARN) was possible. Second, the strategic design of MAGiC explains why a RCT can effectively answer the clinical question: What is the impact of IV magnesium on hospital LOS for children with sickle cell anemia admitted for vaso-occlusive pain? This was achieved with well-matched magnesium and placebo groups in baseline characteristics. In addition to similar ages and gender, both groups previously experienced similar complications from their SCD such as acute chest syndrome and asthma, were taking hydroxyurea within the last 3 months, and had similar baseline laboratory values, including median hemoglobin and white blood cell levels.

Additionally, there are a few limitations of MAGiC. MAGiC focused on children with HbSS and HbSβ0 and did not include other SCD phenotypes. The strongest limitation is that children with SCD often come to the emergency department at different states of pain, including early vs late vaso-occlusive pain that has failed both long- and short-acting opioid administration. Without standardizing the intervention for the same magnitude of pain, heterogeneity in the intervention may exceed any successful intervention.

In summary, MAGiC was a well-conducted RCT, which effectively answered the question that there is no benefit for using IV magnesium in the management of vaso-occlusive pain for children with sickle cell anemia. Given that there have not been many improvements in standard therapies for management of acute vaso-occlusive pain, the trial offers promise for future trials focused on attenuating the most common cause of hospital admission for children with sickle cell anemia.

S.-J. Stimpson, MD
M. R. DeBaun, MD, MPH

References

1. Brousseau DC, Scott JP, Hillery CA, Panepinto JA. The effect of magnesium on LOS for pediatric sickle cell pain crisis. *Acad Emerg Med.* 2004;11:968-972.
2. Unverzagt S, Prondzinsky R, Peinemann F. Single-center trials tend to provide larger treatment effects than multicenter trials: a systematic review. *J Clin Epidemiol.* 2013;66:1271-1280.

A Multinational Trial of Prasugrel for Sickle Cell Vaso-Occlusive Events
Heeney MM, for the DOVE Investigators (Dana—Farber/Boston Children's Cancer and Blood Disorders Ctr, MA; et al)
N Engl J Med 374:625-635, 2016

Background.—Sickle cell anemia is an inherited blood disorder that is characterized by painful vaso-occlusive crises, for which there are few treatment options. Platelets mediate intercellular adhesion and thrombosis during vaso-occlusion in sickle cell anemia, which suggests a role for anti-platelet agents in modifying disease events.

Methods.—Children and adolescents 2 through 17 years of age with sickle cell anemia were randomly assigned to receive oral prasugrel or placebo for 9 to 24 months. The primary end point was the rate of vaso-occlusive crisis, a composite of painful crisis or acute chest syndrome. The secondary end points were the rate of sickle cell—related pain and the intensity of pain, which were assessed daily with the use of pain diaries.

Results.—A total of 341 patients underwent randomization at 51 sites in 13 countries across the Americas, Europe, Asia, and Africa. The rate of vaso-occlusive crisis events per person-year was 2.30 in the prasugrel group and 2.77 in the placebo group (rate ratio, 0.83; 95% confidence interval, 0.66 to 1.05; $P = 0.12$). There were no significant differences between the groups in the secondary end points of diary-reported events. The safety end points, including the frequency of bleeding events requiring medical intervention, of hemorrhagic and nonhemorrhagic adverse events that occurred while patients were taking prasugrel or placebo, and of discontinuations due to prasugrel or placebo, did not differ significantly between the groups.

Conclusions.—Among children and adolescents with sickle cell anemia, the rate of vaso-occlusive crisis was not significantly lower among those who received prasugrel than among those who received placebo. There were no significant between-group differences in the safety findings. (Funded by Daiichi Sankyo and Eli Lilly; ClinicalTrials.gov number, NCT01794000.)

▶ Sickle cell disease is one of the most common severe genetic disorders worldwide with more than 300 000 children born annually with sickle cell anemia.[1] Despite dramatic advances in understanding its complex pathophysiology, little has changed in therapy.[2] Whereas 35 new treatments have been approved by the US Food and Drug Administration for human immunodeficiency virus, only hydroxyurea approved in 1995 is available for therapy for sickle cell disease.

The multifactorial factors affecting the pathophysiology and the lack of large prospective well-designed studies are the 2 most important factors for this lack of progress. Many new targeted therapies are being evolving including coagulation modifying drugs, such as prasugrel.[3,4] This study demonstrates that multinational well-designed and monitored studies can be performed and answer critical therapeutic questions. This study included 51 sites in 13 countries and successfully accomplished dose escalation adjustments, excellent compliance, and answered the primary end point, which was the rate of vaso-occlusive events. This study provides a foundation for the evolving new trials to be successful (hemoglobin F inducers, antioxidants, antiadhesive agents, antiinflammatory agents, antisickling agents, anticoagulants, and antiplatelet agents).

This study, like majority of drug trials, targets acute painful events as the primary clinical end point. Pain is only 1 manifestation of the disease and does not reflect the chronic progressive organ failure or many of the other complications, such as pulmonary hypertension, avascular necrosis, priapism, stroke, and leg ulcers. Furthermore, this study, like others, defines a painful event as requiring medical management with the treatment of prescribed analgesics. Most painful events occur at home and are underreported.

Unfortunately, diaries have not been validated as outcome tools. The clinical and laboratory endpoints for drug therapy trials need to be expanded. Health-related quality of life, patient outcomes, 6-minute walk tests, elevated tricuspid regurgitant jet, and aggregate complication models need to be considered as primary end points. Validated surrogate markers of disease severity such as hemoglobin F need to be accepted. Most importantly, long-term studies are necessary to assess therapeutic effects on chronic organ failure, the most serious morbidity afflicting this population.

The subgroup analysis of this study found prasugrel, an inhibitor of adenosine diphosphate (ADP) platelet activation, almost reaching clinical significance in the older childhood population. Prasugrel may have therapeutic benefit particularly in older patients. This study was appropriately concerned about hemorrhage and patient safety.[5] Therefore, platelet inhibition goals were modest and lower than other studies in non—sickle cell patients. Further research evaluating dose response and safety is warranted.

E. Vichinsky, MD

References

1. Piel F, Hay SI, Gupta S, et al. Global burden of SCA in children under five 2010—2050: modeling based on demographics, excess mortality, and interventions. *PLoS Med.* 2013;10:e1001484.
2. Ataga K, Stocker J. The trials and hopes for drug development in sickle cell disease. *Brit J Haematol.* 2015;170:768.
3. Vichinsky E, ed. *Emerging therapies targeting the pathophysiology of sickle cell disease. Hematology/Oncology Clinics of North America.* 2014;Vol 28. Philadelphia, PA: Elsevier Inc; 2014.
4. Villagra J, Shiva S, Hunter LA, et al. Platelet activation in patients with sickle disease, hemolysis-associated pulmonary hypertension, and nitric oxide scavenging by cell-free hemoglobin. *Blood.* 2007;110:2166.
5. Wun T, Soulieres D, Frelinger AL, et al. A double-blind, randomized, multi-center phase 2 study of prasugrel versus placebo in adult patients with sickle cell disease. *J Hem Oncol.* 2016;6:17.

Sirolimus is effective in relapsed/refractory autoimmune cytopenias: results of a prospective multi-institutional trial
Bride KL, Vincent T, Smith-Whitley K, et al (The Children's Hosp of Philadelphia, PA; Perelman School of Medicine at the Univ of Pennsylvania, Philadelphia; et al)
Blood 127:17-28, 2016

Patients with autoimmune multilineage cytopenias are often refractory to standard therapies requiring chronic immunosuppression with medications with limited efficacy and high toxicity. We present data on 30 patients treated on a multicenter prospective clinical trial using sirolimus as monotherapy. All children (N = 12) with autoimmune lymphoproliferative syndrome (ALPS) achieved a durable complete response (CR), including rapid improvement in autoimmune disease, lymphadenopathy, and splenomegaly within 1 to 3 months of starting sirolimus. Double-negative T cells were no longer detectable in most, yet other lymphocyte populations were spared, suggesting a targeted effect of sirolimus. We also treated 12 patients with multilineage cytopenias secondary to common variable immunodeficiency (CVID), Evans syndrome (ES), or systemic lupus erythematosus (SLE), and most achieved a CR (N = 8), although the time to CR was often slower than was seen in ALPS. Six children with single-lineage autoimmune cytopenias were treated and only 2 responded. Sirolimus was well tolerated with very few side effects. All of the responding patients have remained on therapy for over 1 year (median, 2 years; range, 1 to 4.5 years). In summary, sirolimus led to CR and durable responses in a majority of children with refractory multilineage autoimmune cytopenias. The responses seen in ALPS patients were profound, suggesting that sirolimus should be considered as a first-line, steroid-sparing treatment of patients needing chronic therapy. The results in other multilineage autoimmune cytopenia cohorts were encouraging, and sirolimus should be considered in children with SLE, ES, and CVID. This trial was registered at www.clinicaltrials.gov as #NCT00392951.

▶ Autoimmune cytopenias are characterized by the production of antibodies against blood cells and include autoimmune hemolytic anemia (AIHA), autoimmune neutropenia (AIN), and immune thrombocytopenic purpura (ITP). The association of AIHA and ITP is referred to as Evans syndrome. However, the term *autoimmune multilineage cytopenias* is more inclusive, referring to the occurrence of 2 or more autoimmune cytopenias in a patient, either concurrently or sequentially. The presence of more than 1 autoimmune cytopenia in a patient is often a symptom of a significant underlying disturbance in their immune regulatory system. Autoimmune multilineage cytopenias may be idiopathic or associated with underlying immunodeficiency such as autoimmune lymphoproliferative syndrome (ALPS), common variable immunodeficiency, or autoimmune disease such as systemic lupus erythematosus. With the advent of improved genetic diagnostics, the discovery of defects in immune regulatory genes such as *CLTA-4*, *LRBA*, and *PI3 K* has led to an improved understanding of the pathophysiology that can result in an immune set-up for autoimmune multilineage cytopenias in some of these patients.

This study by Bride et al is the first prospective study of single drug therapy in this patient population. There is very little existing literature on pediatric patients with autoimmune multilineage cytopenias, and treatment varies significantly with no consensus on management. These patients are notoriously difficult to manage, with poor responses to standard therapies such as corticosteroids or intravenous immunoglobulin. Many require trials of multiple drugs, and in our review of this patient population, 78% required more than 2 therapies, and only

13% of patients were able to achieve a complete remission.[1] Bride et al illustrate the value of studying a therapy directed at the underlying pathophysiology of the disease.

In this study, all 12 patients with ALPS achieved a durable complete response (CR) with resolution of their autoimmune multilineage cytopenias and rapid improvement in their lymphadenopathy and splenomegaly; 11 of 12 achieved CR within 3 months of starting sirolimus. This response rate is notable, considering that a median of 3 other therapies failed in these patients prior to the sirolimus trial. Response was durable, with a median follow-up of 3.5 years (range, 1.5–8 years). Sirolimus was also trialed in other populations, with responses in 4 of 8 Evans syndrome patients, 2 of 2 common variable immunodeficiency patients, and 2 of 2 patients with systemic lupus erythematosus; overall 8 of 12 of these patients achieved CR by 12 months on therapy and another 2 attained a partial response (PR). Again, this outcome is remarkable, as a median of 3 other therapies failed in these patients prior to sirolimus.

A surprising result was the significant improvement in neutrophil count seen in patients with AIN. Immune suppression is rarely used to treat AIN because of poor response rates and the benign nature of AIN; however, the patients in this study showed resolution of their AIN with the use of sirolimus. A retrospective study by Miano et al[2] supports a demonstrated improved response to sirolimus in non-ALPS patients with chronic/refractory autoimmune cytopenias.

The response rate was lower in 6 patients with single autoimmune cytopenias, with PR in only 1 of 4 ITP patients, CR in 1 AIHA patient, and PR in another AIHA patient. This finding likely speaks to a different underlying pathophysiology in patients with single autoimmune cytopenias compared with those with multilineage cytopenias (Fig 2A, B in the original article).

Sirolimus was well tolerated, with the most common side effects being transient mild mucositis in one- third of patients and elevated triglycerides and cholesterol in 2 patients that responded to fish oil or atorvastatin. Only 1 patient discontinued sirolimus use because of headache; however, the etiology of the headache was eventually determined to be caused by to underlying disease-associated vasculitis. Immune function, as measured by absolute lymphocyte count, T-cell numbers, IgG level, and mitogen stimulation response, was not affected in a subset of ALPS patients; although some non-ALPS patients did show reductions. Numbers and severity of infection while on sirolimus were not discussed in this report.

Sirolimus is a mammalian target of rapamycin inhibitor, the principle mechanism of action of which is to inhibit cell proliferation via proteins involved in cell cycle control. It also inhibits interleukin-2 production, blocking T- and B-cell activation. It is, therefore, not surprising that response rate with sirolimus is superior in ALPS patients; ALPS results from a defect in apoptosis (mammalian target of rapamycin pathway), resulting in uncontrolled lymphoproliferation. It would, therefore, make sense that a drug targeting proliferation through the cell cycle would be more effective than drugs that target lymphocyte cell signaling and activation pathways, such as cyclosporin, a calcineurin inhibitor that affects inerleukin-2 production and T-cell activation, and mycophenolate mofetil, that does not induce lymphocyte death or have any effect on lymphoproliferation. Sirolimus has also been found to be more effective in treating autoimmunity in some primary immunodeficiencies that mimic ALPS, such as PI3K deficiency and CTLA-4 deficiency.[3]

Treatment of patients with chronic, refractory and multilineage cytopenias has traditionally been empirical with a lack of evidence-based approaches. This study is one of the first prospective studies using a pathophysiology-based treatment for autoimmune multilineage cytopenias. Autoimmune multilineage cytopenias can be a common presentation of several underlying disorders with different pathophysiologies, such as lymphoproliferation in ALPS, immune dysregulation in primary immunodeficiencies, and autoimmunity in rheumatologic disease. We cannot emphasize enough the importance of investigating patients with autoimmune multilineage cytopenias for these various underlying pathologies.

A suggested algorithm for screening can be found in Al Ghaithi et al.[1] Understanding what caused the cytopenias in a patient may significantly affect the approach to therapy, response rates, and other complications for which the patient may be at risk. An excellent example is one of the patients in the Bride et al study who initially presented as Evans syndrome and was eventually diagnosed with an underlying T cell primary immunodeficiency requiring hematopoietic stem cell transplantation.

Based on the results of this study, we recommend using sirolimus early in the therapy of patients with ALPS and considering its use early in therapy of other patients with autoimmune multilineage cytopenias. Further research is required in these patient populations, including prospective, multicenter studies assessing response to therapies and bench research to gain a better understanding of the underlying cause of autoimmunity.

N. A. M. Wright, MD, MSc, FRCPC

V. Price, MBChB, MSc, FRCPC

References

1. Al Ghaithi I, Wright NAM, Breakey VR, et al. Combined autoimmune cytopenias presenting in childhood. *Pediatr Blood Cancer.* 2016;63:292-298.
2. Miano M, Scalzone M, Perri K, et al. Mycophenolate mofetil and sirolimus as second or further line treatment in children with chronic refractory primitive or secondary autoimmune cytopenias: a single centre experience. *Br J Haematol.* 2015; 171:247-253.
3. Lucas CL, Kuehn HS, Zhao F, et al. Dominant activating germline mutations in the gene encoding the PI(3)K catalytic subunit p110δ result in T cell senescence and human immunodeficiency. *Nat Immunol.* 2014;15:88-97.

5 Child Development/ Behavior

Impact of the Great East Japan Earthquake on Child's IQ
Tatsuta N, Nakai K, Satoh H, et al (Tohoku Univ Graduate School of Medicine, Sendai, Japan; et al)
J Pediatr 167:745-751, 2015

Objective.—To assess the neurodevelopmental effects of the Great East Japan Earthquake in resident children.

Study Design.—The disaster on March 11, 2011, caused severe damage to the Sanriku coastal area, where we had been conducting a birth cohort study since 2003. It occurred in the middle of our 7-year-old examination. Approximately 500 mother-child pairs were compulsorily divided into 2 groups: 123 children finished the examination in the predisaster period, and 289 did in the postdisaster period. The remainder died or moved from that area. At the time of 7-year-old examination, we administered the Wechsler Intelligence Scale for Children-Third Edition and electrocardiography to assess autonomic function. According to the Child Behavior Checklist for ages 2-3 years and the Kaufman Assessment Battery for Children that had been administered at 30 months and 42 months of age, respectively, there were no significant differences in them between the 2 groups.

Results.—Verbal IQ, including information, arithmetic, and vocabulary subscores of the Wechsler Intelligence Scale for Children-Third Edition, at 7 years of age was significantly lower in the postdisaster group than in the predisaster group. However, there were no significant differences in performance IQ, full-scale IQ, or autonomic nervous indicators between the 2 groups.

Conclusions.—Since many schools were utilized as primary refuges after the disaster, the deficits in verbal IQ of 7-year-old children may have been due to the interrupted schooling. Further follow-up and more specific posttraumatic stress disorder testing will be required to determine the cause and long-term implications (Fig 1).

▶ On March 11, 2011, a massive earthquake, followed by a devastating tsunami and associated nuclear plant disaster, struck northeastern Japan (Fig 1). In this article, Tatsuta et al analyzed data from an ongoing prospective birth cohort study to determine whether neurological functioning in 7-year-olds

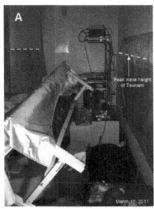 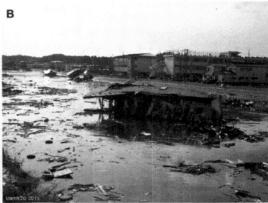

FIGURE 1.—The ravages of the Great East Japan Earthquake. **A,** The tsunamis following the earthquake destroyed the electromyograph that we used for measurements of brainstem auditory and visual evoked potentials in our electrophysiological laboratory, and the device for assessing autonomic nervous function was barely saved. **B,** An elementary school (the 2 three-story buildings in the photo) located near our laboratory in the Sanriku coastal area was destroyed. For this reason, the pupils had no school to go for a month and transferred to another elementary school. (Reprinted from Tatsuta N, Nakai K, Satoh H, et al. Impact of the Great East Japan Earthquake on child's IQ. *J Pediatr.* 2015;167:745-751, with permission from Elsevier.)

were affected by the disasters. The Tohoku Study of Child Development was started in the period 2003–2006 to determine whether prenatal exposure to neurotoxins, such as lead and mercury, affects child development.

The current analysis was limited to participants from the Sanriku coastal region, Miyagi Prefecture, which suffered much destruction from the tsunami. Among 498 children originally registered in the study, 160 completed their 7-year assessment before the disaster; 338 not until approximately 6 months after the disaster. The assessment included the Wechsler Intelligence Scale for Children—Third Edition (WISC-III), an ECG (to assess heart rate variability) and the ICCE (Index of Child Care Environment),[1] a modified version of the Home Observation for Measurement of Environment, completed by mothers.

Tatsuta et al compared the results of the baseline assessment, conducted earlier in the study, and the 7-year assessment between 123 children in the predisaster and 289 children in the postdisaster groups whose data were complete. Maternal alcohol consumption during pregnancy was greater in the predisaster (23.4%) than postdisaster group (13.1%); no differences were identified in other baseline characteristics, including gestational age, birth weight, maternal age, birth order, delivery type, cigarette smoking during pregnancy, exposure biomarkers for environmental toxins (ie, lead, mercury), parent education or parent income between the 2 groups. There were also no differences in EES (Evaluation of Environmental Stimulation - assesses interaction between child and caregiver) scores at 18 months, CBCL (Child Behavior Check List) scores at 30 months and K-ABC (Kaufman Assessment Battery for Children) scores at 42 months of age.

Given the association between prenatal exposure to alcohol and postnatal intellectual quotient (IQ), the authors adjusted the WISC-III scores for alcohol consumption. Verbal IQ (WISC-III) was significantly lower for the postdisaster

(100.0 11.9) compared with the predisaster group (103.5 14.0, $P = .020$). Performance IQ did not differ (101.6 11.7 vs 100.4 11.7, $P = .383$). Within Verbal IQ, scores were lower in the postdisaster group for information ($P = .011$), arithmetic ($P = .011$), vocabulary ($P = .041$) and digit span ($P = .078$). Within Performance IQ, there were no differences in subscale scores. Further adjustment for 2 K-ABC subset scores did not affect the results. Autonomic nervous function, as measured using the ECG; and the ICCE scores did not differ between the 2 groups.

In their discussion, the authors attempt to answer 2 questions, why differences between the pre- and postdisaster groups were so subtle, and why the subtle but significant differences were limited to the verbal IQ and did not include the performance IQ scores. First and foremost, not all mother-child pairs completed the assessment; according to the authors, they may have "died or moved from that area." Those most seriously affected may not have participated in the study. As part of data collection, the researchers asked "each mother whether she heard from a health specialist that her child had trouble related to post-traumatic stress disorder (PTSD), but all of them answered no." This, along with lack of differences in the ICCE scores, is interpreted as "no history of PTSD or poor parenting" (presumably from PTSD). The researchers appear not to have asked specific questions about exposure to disaster trauma. To their credit, they recognize that the post-disaster group may not be representative and "more specific PTSD testing may be required." In fact, collecting additional data could have yielded more accurate information.[2]

On the other hand, the authors could have been more forthcoming with available information. They mention that the "research field" included the "Sanriku coastal area." Sanriku is in northern Miyagi Prefecture and part stretches 12 to 18 miles inland; it consists of 4 townships with a total population of nearly 250 000 people. The degree of direct and indirect impact of the earthquake and subsequent tsunami may have varied widely. In fact, the authors attribute verbal IQ differences to potentially interrupted education from the routine use of school buildings for refuge for at least some children.

Why were pre- and postdisaster group differences limited to verbal IQ? Interestingly, one past study compared the WISC-III scores of traumatized youth with PTSD to those of trauma-exposed and nonexposed comparison groups without PTSD and found that the PTSD group scored significantly lower than the comparison groups on Verbal but not Performance IQ.[3] Lower Verbal IQ may be a marker for PTSD. A disaster of this magnitude may have also affected the administration of the WISC-III. Would testers have been more likely to adhere to procedures more loosely and score responses more generously? Although no published studies have examined this question, several have described variations in administration of the WISC-III.[4,5]

Natural disasters of this magnitude affect entire communities. The authors should be lauded for their resiliency in resuming their research so quickly and their resourcefulness in adapting an ongoing cohort study to determine the effect of the disaster on child IQ; the limitations of such analyses notwithstanding, this effort raises several new and intriguing lines of query. What is the impact of large-scale disasters on ongoing studies and how should the integrity of the original study be maintained? More specifically, when measurements may be measurer dependent, as in the administration of scales such as the WISC-III, how do we adjust or interpret? Finally, if such measures are found to provide indirect evidence of conditions such as PTSD, what is the responsibility of researchers to advocate for appropriate care?

J. I. Takayama, MD, MPH

References

1. Sugisawa Y, Shinohara R, Tong L, et al. The trajectory patterns of parenting and the social competence of toddlers: a longitudinal perspective. *J Epidemiol.* 2010; 20:S459-S465.
2. Fujiwara T, Yagi J, Homma H, et al. Clinically significant behavior problems among young children 2 years after the Great East Japan Earthquake. *PLoS One.* 2014;9:e109342.
3. Saigh PA, Yasik AE, Oberfield RA, Halamandaris PV, Bremner JD. The intellectual performance of traumatized children and adolescents with or without posttraumatic stress disorder. *J Abnorm Psych.* 2006;115:332-340.
4. Platt TL, Zachar P, Ray GE, Lobello SG, Underhill AT. Does Wechsler Intelligence Scale administration and scoring proficiency improve during assessment training? *Psychol Rep.* 2007;100:547-555.
5. Belk MS, Lobello SG, Ray GE, Zachar P. WISC-III administration, clerical, and scoring errors made by student examiners. *J Psychoed Assess.* 2002;20:290-300.

Physically Active Math and Language Lessons Improve Academic Achievement: A Cluster Randomized Controlled Trial

Mullender-Wijnsma MJ, Hartman E, de Greeff JW, et al (Univ Med Ctr Groningen, Netherlands; et al)
Pediatrics 137:e20152743, 2016

Objectives.—Using physical activity in the teaching of academic lessons is a new way of learning. The aim of this study was to investigate the effects of an innovative physically active academic intervention ("Fit & Vaardig op School" [F&V]) on academic achievement of children.

Methods.—Using physical activity to teach math and spelling lessons was studied in a cluster-randomized controlled trial. Participants were 499 children (mean age 8.1 years) from second- and third-grade classes of 12 elementary schools. At each school, a second- and third-grade class were randomly assigned to the intervention or control group. The intervention group participated in F&V lessons for 2 years, 22 weeks per year, 3 times a week. The control group participated in regular classroom lessons. Children's academic achievement was measured before the intervention started and after the first and second intervention years. Academic achievement was measured by 2 mathematics tests (speed and general math skills) and 2 language tests (reading and spelling).

Results.—After 2 years, multilevel analysis showed that children in the intervention group had significantly greater gains in mathematics speed test ($P < .001$; effect size [ES] 0.51), general mathematics ($P < .001$; ES 0.42), and spelling ($P < .001$; ES 0.45) scores. This equates to 4 months more learning gains in comparison with the control group. No differences were found on the reading test.

Conclusions.—Physically active academic lessons significantly improved mathematics and spelling performance of elementary school children and are therefore a promising new way of teaching.

▶ Children spend more time in school than in any other setting outside the home.[1] As a result, if children are going to meet the recommended guidelines for daily physical activity, schools must be a setting where they can spend significant time moving. Unfortunately, of the approximately 35 hours spent at school, 92% of students spend the majority of that time sedentary.[2] Moreover, with the increased emphasis on standardized testing, time in physical education is being reduced.[3] This shifts the burden for physical activity from the physical education teacher to the classroom teacher and begs the question: Why would a classroom teacher have an interest in sacrificing classroom time for physical activity?

Mullender-Wijnsma and colleagues provide an answer. To improve math and spelling performance, they argue that teachers need not make a choice between physical activity and academics but can employ physical activity as a strategy to improve academic performance. This is an important shift in the discussion. Rather than argue for the health benefit of physical activity, the emphasis is on the academic benefits. This is an argument that is likely to resonate. Although teachers care deeply about the health of their students, their job is to improve learning. Thus, this shift in the discussion from health to academics—and data to support this shift—is critical if we are to motivate teachers and school administrators to adopt physical activity in the classroom.[4]

To pursue this goal, Mullender-Wijnsma and colleagues test a series of lessons that teach math and spelling in combination with physical activity (eg, executing a series of jumping jacks whose number corresponds to the answer of a math problem). These lessons were carried out 3 times per week, 22 weeks per year, for 2 years, in second- and third-grade classes. Although there have been a number of studies that have integrated physical activity into the regular education classroom, few have done so as a randomized control trial, for this duration, and with the explicit intent to improve academic performance. Thus, this study represents a clear movement forward for the literature.

The results are moderate, with minimal effects after 1 year, and 2-year effects averaging between 0.4 and 0.5 standard deviations between the intervention and control classrooms. That said, these findings nicely extend the growing body of literature that have shown relationships among physical fitness, cognitive function, and test performance. The present study extends this from a cross-sectional factor (ie, fitness) to a behavior factor (ie, physical activity) and provides a model to place this into practice through a series of physically active lessons that can be easily disseminated.

On the basis of these results, can we positively respond to teachers who question whether they should work to integrate physical activity into their lessons? Yes, we can. If teachers implement this or similar programs elementary-age students are likely to respond with some improvement in math and spelling.

Is the expected improvement in scores over the course of 2 years enough to motivate teachers to implement this intervention? This answer is less certain. Behavioral science tells us that motivation will flow from strong rewards that closely follow a behavior. Thus, if teachers experience an immediate, positive reward in conjunction with these lessons, they will be likely to consistently implement the intervention. Unfortunately, it is difficult to expect teachers to continue an intervention for more than a year with little sign of impact. Thus, if this approach to instruction is to be widely adopted, it must be refined to bring about larger and more immediate results.

How might this be achieved? Refinement of the intervention depends on our knowledge of the underlying mechanism for the effect. The authors offer numerous suggestions for why the combination of physical activity combined with academic instruction benefits learning. However, mechanisms for change were not tested as a part of this study, nor have they been tested in other school-based research. As a result, it is not clear whether the present findings require the combination of activity and academic content or if they are simply due to the added 20 to 30 minutes of physical activity per day (10–15 minutes for spelling and 10–15 minutes for math). Is it the physical activity or the active lessons? This is the central question for the research to come. That said, a potential mechanism is drawn from evidence that students respond to these interventions with improved attention and behavior control for the subsequent 20 to 30 minutes,[5] which is likely to result in more efficient learning.

There are few things teachers value more in the short term than a well-behaved classroom. Thus, the improved attention and behavior control might both support student learning and serve as a motivating factor for teachers. In addition, the present study tested the intervention 3 times per week, across only 22 weeks and in one classroom per school. I would expect larger effects from daily implementation throughout the school, for the full academic year. An active school is likely to achieve much higher implementation fidelity than a single, active classroom.

In summary, physically active academic lessons hold great promise and the present study adds to this conclusion. These lessons result in increased physical activity, attention control, and academic performance. Like any intervention, its effectiveness lies in the willingness of teachers to implement the lessons.[6] Targeting teacher motivation will represent an important, next phase of this research.

J. B. Bartholomew, PhD

References

1. Story M, Nanney MS, Schwartz MB. Schools and obesity prevention: creating school environments and policies to promote healthy eating and physical activity. *Milbank Q.* 2009;87:71-100.
2. Burns RD, Brusseau TA, Fang Y, Myrer RS, Fu Y, Hannon JC. Predictors and grade level trends of school day physical activity achievement in low-income children from the U.S. *Prev Med Rep.* 2015;2:868-873.
3. Trost SG, van der Mars H. Why we should not cut P.E. *Educ Leadersh.* 2009;67:60-65.

4. Department of Kinesiology and Health Education at the University of Texas at Austin, Austin, TX, Bartholomew JB. Environments change child behavior, but who changes environments? *Kinesiol Rev.* 2015;4:71-76.

5. Grieco L, Jowers E, Bartholomew J. Physically active academic lessons and time on task: the moderating effect of body mass index. *Med Sci Sports Exerc.* 2009;41: 1921-1926.

6. Donnelly J, Greene J, Gibson C, et al. Physical activity across the curriculum (PAAC): a randomized controlled trial to promote physical activity and diminish overweight and obesity in elementary school children. *Prev Med.* 2009;49: 336-341.

Two-Year Outcomes of a Population-Based Intervention for Preschool Language Delay: An RCT

Wake M, Levickis P, Tobin S, et al (Royal Children's Hosp, Parkville, Melbourne, Australia; et al)
Pediatrics 130.e838-e847, 2015

Objective.—We have previously shown short-term benefits to phonology, letter knowledge, and possibly expressive language from systematically ascertaining language delay at age 4 years followed by the Language for Learning intervention. Here, we report the trial's definitive 6-year outcomes.

Methods.—Randomized trial nested in a population-based ascertainment. Children with language scores >1.25 SD below the mean at age 4 were randomized, with intervention children receiving 18 1-hour home-based therapy sessions. Primary outcome was receptive/expressive language. Secondary outcomes were phonological, receptive vocabulary, literacy, and narrative skills; parent-reported pragmatic language, behavior, and health-related quality of life; costs of intervention; and health service use. For intention-to-treat analyses, trial arms were compared using linear regression models.

Results.—Of 1464 children assessed at age 4, 266 were eligible and 200 randomized; 90% and 82% of intervention and control children were retained respectively. By age 6, mean language scores had normalized, but there was little evidence of a treatment effect for receptive (adjusted mean difference 2.3; 95% confidence interval [CI] −1.2 to 5.7; P = .20) or expressive (0.8; 95% CI −1.6 to 3.2; P = .49) language. Of the secondary outcomes, only phonological awareness skills (effect size 0.36; 95% CI 0.08−0.65; P = .01) showed benefit. Costs were higher for intervention families (mean difference AU $4276; 95% CI: $3424 to $5128).

Conclusions.—Population-based intervention targeting 4-year-old language delay was feasible but did not have lasting impacts on language, possibly reflecting resolution in both groups. Long-term literacy benefits remain possible but must be weighed against its cost.

▶ One in 6 US children have a developmental disability.[1] This number is increasing, most notably among autism and attention deficit hyperactivity disorder diagnoses, which have increased by 290% and 33%, respectively.[1] Presumably, contributions to this trend include increased awareness and screening for developmental disabilities. The American Academy of Pediatrics recommends standardized developmental screening for all children at 9, 18, 24, and 30 months of age, including the use of an autism-specific instrument at 18 and 24 months. In the setting of profoundly increasing rates of disease detection, it is important to ask if the increasing amount of diagnosis is translating into patient benefit.

The accurate detection of an abnormality or a disease from which patients do not experience net benefit is termed *overdiagnosis,* and much of what we have learned about overdiagnosis comes from studies of cancer screening. For example, widespread screening for thyroid cancer in South Korea was accompanied by a 15-fold increase in the incidence of thyroid cancer between 1993 and 2011, triggering an investigation of disease characteristics and patient benefit from diagnosis.[2] Notably, the entire increase can be attributed to smaller, more benign forms of the cancer. Most importantly, increased detection of these cancers has not been accompanied by a measurable change in thyroid cancer mortality rates; more disease has been discovered, with no apparent benefit to patients. The screen-detected thyroid cancers did not need to be found in the first place.

Examples of overdiagnosis extend well beyond cancer screening and likely include developmental disabilities in children.[3] To investigate this hypothesis, we need a better understanding of the natural history of diagnoses and the impact of ensuing interventions. Wake et al's well-done randomized trial comparing a home-based language therapy intervention with usual care among children screened for language delay adds meaningful data to our understanding of the impact of screening and interventions. It also provides evidence suggesting the possibility of overdiagnosis. Four-year-old children with expressive or receptive language scores greater than 1.25 standard deviations below the normative mean were enrolled. Although the study's principal finding was that the language therapy intervention did not appear to impact expressive or receptive language scores, an intriguing discovery was that expressive and receptive language scores normalized at the 2-year follow-up among children randomly assigned to usual care. Likely, children assigned to the usual care arm received some kind of intervention for their diagnosis. The extent and success of these interventions are unknown. An additional explanation for the normalization in scores observed among the usual care group may be that the diagnosed language delays largely represented variants of normal language development and that their natural, unadulterated progression is normalization with time. If most young children with screen-detected language delays experience symptom resolution without significant intervention, is detection warranted? Could the harms of detection outweigh the benefits?

To truly evaluate the possibility that language delay and other developmental disabilities are being overdiagnosed by screening, a comprehensive evaluation of harms and benefits experienced by children as a result of diagnosis is needed. While a portion of symptomatic children undoubtedly benefit from diagnosis of developmental disabilities, it is unclear if screening for these conditions benefits children. The US Preventive Services Task Force found inadequate evidence that screening for autism and speech-language delays improve outcomes and found no studies that addressed the harms of screening for these conditions.[4,5] Potential harms resulting from a screen-detected developmental disability include stigma, costly treatments, medication side effects, and lowered parent and teacher expectations for academic, behavioral, or social success. As widespread testing and screening programs become entrenched, and increasing numbers of children are told they have a developmental disability, it is imperative that future research is directed toward evaluating the balance between harm and benefit to children as a result of such policies.

E. Coon, MD, MSCI

References

1. Boyle CA, Boulet S, Schieve LA, et al. Trends in the prevalence of developmental disabilities in US children, 1997–2008. *Pediatrics.* 2011;127:1034-1042.
2. Ahn HS, Kim HJ, Welch HG. Korea's thyroid-cancer "epidemic"—screening and overdiagnosis. *N Engl J Med.* 2014;371:1765-1767.
3. Coon ER, Quinonez RA, Moyer VA, Schroeder AR. Overdiagnosis: how our compulsion for diagnosis may be harming children. *Pediatrics.* 2014;134:1013-1023.
4. McPheeters M, Weitlauf A, Vehorn A, et al. *Screening for Autism Spectrum Disorder in Young Children: A Systematic Evidence Review for the U.S. Preventive Services Task Force.* Rockville (MD): AHRQ Publication; 2015.
5. Wallace IF, Berkman ND, Watson LR, et al. Screening for speech and language delay in children 5 years old and younger: a systematic review. *Pediatrics.* 2015; 136:e448-e462.

Primary Care Providers' Initial Evaluation of Children with Global Developmental Delay: A Clinical Vignette Study

Tarini BA, Zikmund-Fisher BJ, Saal HM, et al (Univ of Michigan, Ann Arbor; Cincinnati Children's Hosp Med Ctr, OH)
J Pediatr 167:1404-1408, 2015

Objective.—To examine the decisions of pediatric primary care physicians about their diagnostic evaluation for a child with suspected global developmental delay (GDD).

Study Design.—A survey was mailed to a sample of pediatricians (n = 600) and family physicians (n = 600) randomly selected from the American Medical Association Physician Masterfile. The survey contained a clinical vignette describing a 9-month-old nondysmorphic boy with GDD. Participants were asked their initial evaluation steps (test, refer, or both test and refer) and what types of referral and/or testing they would pursue. We examined bivariate associations between physician/clinical practice characteristics and participants' evaluation decision.

Results.—More pediatricians than family physicians completed the survey (response rates: 55% vs 38%). Almost three-quarters of the respondents (74%) reported that their first step in a diagnostic evaluation would be to refer the child without testing, 22% would test only, and 4% would both test and refer. As their initial step, most physicians referred to a developmental pediatrician (58%), and only 5% would refer to a geneticist. The most commonly ordered test was general biochemical testing (64%). The most commonly ordered genetic test was a karyotype (39%).

Conclusions.—When evaluating a child with GDD, few primary care physicians would order genetic testing or refer to a genetics specialist as a first evaluation step. Future studies should examine both barriers to and utilization of a genetic evaluation for children with GDD (Fig 3).

▶ In this study, Tarini and colleagues surveyed pediatricians and family physicians on their initial management decisions in the case of a 9-month-old male child with global developmental delay (GDD). Their finding, that most primary care physicians (PCP) would refer this child, was not surprising. What was surprising and "most concerning" to the authors was that "despite a child with GDD being at increased risk for having a genetic disorder, accessing genetics services from a genetics provider were not at the forefront of pediatric PCPs' considerations." The authors cite the American Academy of Pediatrics clinical report "Comprehensive Evaluation of the Child With Intellectual Disability (ID) or Global Developmental Delays,"[1] where the purpose of a comprehensive genetics evaluation are laid out, including clarifying etiology and providing information about prognosis and treatment options, parental support, and access to research projects.

The authors provide some potential explanations for their findings, all of which are reasonable but deserve explanation from the perspective of the PCP. The first explanation presented is that PCPs may refer initially to developmental pediatricians or neurologists rather than a geneticist because of a desire to have a specialist offer a therapeutic intervention as well as a diagnostic evaluation (Fig 3). This is a key point and is not to be overlooked: PCPs who have a longitudinal relationship with parents and children with GDD are more concerned with initiating therapy than documenting etiology. If there were any surprises for me in this study, it was the low number of PCPs who referred to early intervention services as a first step. I suspect that if the survey allowed for

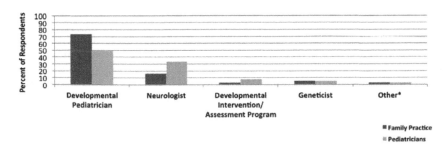

* other included pediatrician, regional/tertiary care medical center, Occupational Therapy/Physical Therapy

FIGURE 3.—Specialist referral for children with GDD: FPs vs pediatricians. (Reprinted from Tarini BA, Zikmund-Fisher BJ, Saal HM, et al. Primary care providers' initial evaluation of children with global developmental delay: a clinical vignette study. *J Pediatr.* 2015;167:1404-1408, with permission from Elsevier.)

multiple choices that could be ranked in chronological order of completion, closer to 100% of PCPs would seek out early intervention or therapy services and genetic referral or testing.

The authors also point out that the most frequent testing ordered was general biochemical testing, despite the fact that the yield of metabolic testing is low. I would argue that this is another example of the pragmatism of the pediatric PCP. Although a relatively small number of children will have a metabolic condition leading to GDD, finding that condition and initiating appropriate therapy early may significantly alter the course of disease, and the testing is familiar and (relative to genetic testing) inexpensive. The authors also felt that the lack of history or physical exam findings that would influence referral or suggest a diagnosis may have led to a more cautionary first step. I would agree that in the absence of a clearly defined phenotype, the first impulse will be to refer for more evaluation and close monitoring while investigating proper referrals and workup.

I was somewhat surprised that 11% of the respondents would order a genetic test instead of or prior to referral to a geneticist and, like the authors, was glad the number was not higher.

As has often been said, half of what is learned in medical school will be wrong or out of date within 10 years of graduation; the trouble is knowing which half is wrong or out of date. Given advances in the fields of genetics, metabolism, genomics, molecular medicine, and laboratory testing, I suspect that many PCPs should be concerned that they may do an incomplete or ineffective genetic workup. Knowing when to order karyotype, chromosomal microarray, specific testing for a genetic disorder, or whole exome sequencing can be confusing.

The authors have some good suggestions for future areas of study. To these I will add my own suggestions—not for study, but for improving access to and the relevance of genetic services. To help PCPs understand and initiate an appropriate workup, geneticists should avail themselves of new technology platforms that provide access for PCPs and patients. A workup and evaluation could begin with a telemedicine discussion between the geneticist and PCP, including a review of documents and images or videos, followed by a visit to the genetics clinic. I would also advocate for geneticists to be involved with regional early intervention programs. A multidisciplinary approach to early intervention would achieve the goal of initiation of therapy with a concurrent genetics evaluation when appropriate. Geneticists can provide an important perspective on prognosis and advice around symptoms and comorbidities to families, PCPs, and the early intervention team.

This is an interesting and relevant article; appropriate workup and referral of these children can have long-lasting implications for them and their families. Genetic evaluation is important not only for the affected child but also for their parents, who may be interested in assessing risk of recurrence in future children. The challenge is not only in making genetic services available but also demonstrating the importance and value to pediatric PCPs and the affected families.

N. Branco, MD

Reference

1. Moeschler JB, Shevell M. Comprehensive evaluation of the child with intellectual disability or global developmental delay. *Pediatrics*. 2014;134:e903-e918.

Screening for Autism Spectrum Disorder in Young Children US Preventive Services Task Force Recommendation Statement
Siu AL, the US Preventive Services Task Force (USPSTF) (Mount Sinai School of Medicine, NY)
JAMA 315:691-696, 2016

Description.—New US Preventive Services Task Force (USPSTF) recommendation on screening for autism spectrum disorder (ASD) in young children.

Methods.—The USPSTF reviewed the evidence on the accuracy, benefits, and potential harms of brief, formal screening instruments for ASD administered during routine primary care visits and the benefits and potential harms of early behavioral treatment for young children identified with ASD through screening.

Population.—This recommendation applies to children aged 18 to 30 months who have not been diagnosed with ASD or developmental delay and for whom no concerns of ASD have been raised by parents, other caregivers, or health care professionals.

Recommendation.—The USPSTF concludes that the current evidence is insufficient to assess the balance of benefits and harms of screening for ASD in young children for whom no concerns of ASD have been raised by their parents or a clinician. (I statement) (Fig 1).

▶ It is fundamental to the optimism embedded in pediatric thought and practice that the earliest identification of a health condition will ultimately lead to improved health and well-being of a child. Such thinking has led to successful population screening efforts for various treatable pediatric conditions, including newborn metabolic testing, early hearing detection, and anemia screening. It is this same line of reasoning that has energized both health care providers specializing in the care of children with developmental disorders as well as parents of affected children.

Now, after a decade of specific efforts on the part of the pediatric and public health communities directed at improved screening for the developmental disorders, including autism, in the pediatric office setting,[1-4] evidence is growing suggesting increased developmental and autism screening in primary care pediatrics.[5] In autism, these efforts also appear to be resulting in a lowering of the age of identification of children with autism spectrum disorders (ASD), with earlier diagnosis and treatment being put in place.[6] Families have promoted and lauded these efforts as they strive to maximize their child's opportunities in education, socialization, and community integration.

What the USPSTF Grades Mean and Suggestions for Practice

Grade	Definition	Suggestions for Practice
A	The USPSTF recommends the service. There is high certainty that the net benefit is substantial.	Offer or provide this service.
B	The USPSTF recommends the service. There is high certainty that the net benefit is moderate, or there is moderate certainty that the net benefit is moderate to substantial.	Offer or provide this service.
C	The USPSTF recommends selectively offering or providing this service to individual patients based on professional judgment and patient preferences. There is at least moderate certainty that the net benefit is small.	Offer or provide this service for selected patients depending on individual circumstances.
D	The USPSTF recommends against the service. There is moderate or high certainty that the service has no net benefit or that the harms outweigh the benefits.	Discourage the use of this service.
I statement	The USPSTF concludes that the current evidence is insufficient to assess the balance of benefits and harms of the service. Evidence is lacking, of poor quality, or conflicting, and the balance of benefits and harms cannot be determined.	Read the Clinical Considerations section of the USPSTF Recommendation Statement. If the service is offered, patients should understand the uncertainty about the balance of benefits and harms.

USPSTF Levels of Certainty Regarding Net Benefit

Level of Certainty	Description
High	The available evidence usually includes consistent results from well-designed, well-conducted studies in representative primary care populations. These studies assess the effects of the preventive service on health outcomes. This conclusion is therefore unlikely to be strongly affected by the results of future studies.
Moderate	The available evidence is sufficient to determine the effects of the preventive service on health outcomes, but confidence in the estimate is constrained by such factors as the number, size, or quality of individual studies. inconsistency of findings across individual studies. limited generalizability of findings to routine primary care practice. lack of coherence in the chain of evidence. As more information becomes available, the magnitude or direction of the observed effect could change, and this change may be large enough to alter the conclusion.
Low	The available evidence is insufficient to assess effects on health outcomes. Evidence is insufficient because of the limited number or size of studies. important flaws in study design or methods. inconsistency of findings across individual studies. gaps in the chain of evidence. findings not generalizable to routine primary care practice. lack of information on important health outcomes. More information may allow estimation of effects on health outcomes.

The USPSTF defines certainty as "likelihood that the USPSTF assessment of the net benefit of a preventive service is correct." The net benefit is defined as benefit minus harm of the preventive service as implemented in a general, primary care population. The USPSTF assigns a certainty level based on the nature of the overall evidence available to assess the net benefit of a preventive service.

FIGURE 1.—US preventive services task force grades and levels of certainty. (Reprinted from Siu AL, the US Preventive Services Task Force (USPSTF). Screening for autism spectrum disorder in young children US preventive services task force recommendation statement. *JAMA.* 2016;315:691-696, wit permission from American Medical Association.)

On the heels of these success stories, the US Preventive Services Task Force (USPSTF) has entered into a review of screening for autism spectrum disorders in young children.[7] Having worked in the halls of the US government on health policy, I highly respect the Task Force and the difficult decisions with which it is tasked. It is with deep seriousness that it strives to find effective evidence-based health screening and preventive care for the American public.

In recent years, the USPSTF has been met with both respect as well as disdain for controversial recommendations on breast cancer and prostate cancer screening. The USPSTF has now entered into the world of early childhood development and disabilities and, in doing so, has again walked into a minefield, populated by a passionate public striving to improve the lives of children and adults with ASD. This public has seen a rapid rise in interest and empathy for those with this condition, along with accompanying support and funding for the specialized health and service needs of the children and adults. They have also witnessed the improvements and expansion of treatments available to children and adults, even at the youngest ages, even before age 2 years.

The takeaway for the pediatrician and other early childhood professionals on their recommendations on ASD screening is summed up by a single letter, "I," indicating "Insufficient" evidence "to assess the balance of benefits and harms of screening" for ASD in young children for whom specifically there are no concerns raised by parents or a clinician. Pediatric clinicians, early childhood professionals, as well as those in public health, public education, and the health insurance industry, should take it no further! The USPSTF has not said that screening should not be done but are instead suggesting that more research be done on the benefits and risks of such screening. They specifically recommend that the clinician exercise judgment on screening at this time for the child without overt signs or concerns (Fig 1).

They have posed specific research questions to be answered and methods to use for gaining the necessary knowledge around the benefits of early screening for ASD. Although they are currently agnostic on the benefits of ASD screening, they support the Modified Checklist for Autism in Toddlers, with Follow-Up (M-CHAT/F) and the Modified Checklist for Autism in Toddlers, Revised with Follow-Up (M-CHAT-R/F) as autism screening tools. They also support the treatment of children with ASD with early intensive behavioral and developmental interventions, based on evidence of improved cognition and language outcomes.

This "I" recommendation is interestingly a significant contrast to recommendations in the United Kingdom, where developmental and ASD screening are not recommended,[8] and in Canada where a recommendation against screening was made for developmental delay in young children.[9] In the United States, the American Academy of Pediatrics continues to promote ASD screening at 18 and 24 months,[1,2,10] while the American Academy of Family Physicians has echoed the conclusions of the USPSTF.

So where does that leave the practicing pediatrician and the families with young children? With increased developmental and autism screening, we now have evidence of earlier identification of children with ASD, with the median age of diagnosis decreasing from 35 months of age in children born in 2002 to 32 months of age in those children born in 2006 in a Centers for Disease Control and Prevention (CDC) cohort.[6] At the same time, there is continuing evidence regarding the benefits of early intervention and autism specific interventions.

We have a highly educated and empowered parent community who are telling physicians that they want to take charge of their personal health and decision making as well as their children's. Perfect should not be the enemy of the good when it comes to the early identification and intervention for children with ASD or other neurodevelopmental, genetic, or behavior disorders. ASD screening of all children should continue as recommended at 18 and 24 months of age,[1,2,10] alongside general developmental screening at 9, 18, 30, and 48 months of age, while researchers in health screening, early child health and development, and autism continue to strengthen the body of evidence around such practice.

It is the responsibility of the pediatrician and other professionals to advocate for the optimal health and well-being of each child. Although the benefits of autism screening for all are uncertain, there is little argument about the need for early identification and treating those affected. Such practice should continue.

P. H. Lipkin, MD

References

1. Council on Children With Disabilities, Section on Developmental Behavioral Pediatrics, Bright Futures Steering Committee, and Medical Home Initiatives for Children With Special Needs Project Advisory Committee. Identifying infants and young children with developmental disorders in the medical home: an algorithm for developmental surveillance and screening. *Pediatrics.* 2006;118: 405-420.
2. Johnson CP, Myers SM.American Academy of Pediatrics Council on Children with Disabilities. Identification and evaluation of children with autism spectrum disorders. *Pediatrics.* 2007;120:1183-1215.
3. King TM, Tandon SD, Macias MM, et al. Implementing developmental screening and referrals: lessons learned from a national project. *Pediatrics.* 2010;125: 350-360.
4. Guevara JP, Gerdes M, Localio R, et al. Effectiveness of developmental screening in an urban setting. *Pediatrics.* 2013;131:30-37.
5. Radecki L, Sand-Loud N, O'Connor KG, Sharp S, Olson LM. Trends in the use of standardized tools for developmental screening in early childhood: 2002–2009. *Pediatrics.* 2011;128:14-19.
6. Christensen DL, Bilder DA, Zahorodny W, et al. Prevalence and characteristics of autism spectrum disorder among 4-year-old children in the autism and developmental disabilities monitoring network. *J Dev Behav Pediatr.* 2016;37:1-8.
7. The UK NSC recommendation on Autism screening in children. http://legacy. screening.nhs.uk/autism. Accessed April 4, 2016.
8. Tonelli M, Parkin P, Leduc D, et al. Canadian Task Force on Preventive Health Care. Recommendations on screening for developmental delay. *CMAJ.* 2016; 188:579-587.
9. AAP Statement on U.S. Preventive Services Task Force Final Recommendation Statement on Autism Screening. https://www.aap.org/en-us/about-the-aap/aap-press-room/Pages/AAP-Statement-on-US-Preventive-Services-Task-Force-Final-Recommendation-Statement-on-Autism-Screening.aspx. Accessed April 4, 2016.
10. Clinical Preventive Service Recommendation- Autism Spectrum: Children (Aged 18 to 30 Months). http://www.aafp.org/patient-care/clinical-recommendations/all/autism-children.html. Accessed April 4, 2016.

Psychological and Psychosocial Impairment in Preschoolers With Selective Eating

Zucker N, Copeland W, Franz L, et al (Duke Univ School of Medicine, Durham, NC)
Pediatrics 136:e582-e590, 2015

Objective.—We examined the clinical significance of moderate and severe selective eating (SE). Two levels of SE were examined in relation to concurrent psychiatric symptoms and as a risk factor for the emergence of later psychiatric symptoms. Findings are intended to guide healthcare providers to recognize when SE is a problem worthy of intervention.

Methods.—A population cohort sample of 917 children aged 24 to 71 months and designated caregivers were recruited via primary care practices at a major medical center in the Southeast as part of an epidemiologic study of preschool anxiety. Caregivers were administered structured diagnostic interviews (the Preschool Age Psychiatric Assessment) regarding the child's eating and related self-regulatory capacities, psychiatric symptoms, functioning, and home environment variables. A subset of 188 dyads were assessed a second time ~24.7 months from the initial assessment.

Results.—Both moderate and severe levels of SE were associated with psychopathological symptoms (anxiety, depression, attention-deficit/hyperactivity disorder) both concurrently and prospectively. However, the severity of psychopathological symptoms worsened as SE became more severe. Impairment in family functioning was reported at both levels of SE, as was sensory sensitivity in domains outside of food and the experience of food aversion.

Conclusions.—Findings suggest that health care providers should intervene at even moderate levels of SE. SE associated with impairment in function should now be diagnosed as avoidant/restrictive food intake disorder, an eating disorder that encapsulates maladaptive food restriction, which is new to the *Diagnostic and Statistical Manual of Mental Disorders, Fifth Edition.*

▶ Upon initiating services for the treatment of a feeding/eating problem, parents often report that they were told (maybe by a pediatrician or family member) that the eating problem would fade over time, that it's normal, and/or not to worry about it. Zucker and colleagues take these viewpoints to task and challenge the health care community to (1) recognize that a significant number of families are reporting problems that warrant attention and (2) be more prepared to identify and refer for appropriate treatment. This study is particularly relevant to the field because it highlights and provides empirical support to long-standing anecdotal reports provided by clinicians based on their own experiences with this population.

Downplaying or dismissing (even inadvertently) mealtime problems that will not remediate without intervention may end up exacerbating the problem, leading to added stress for family members and disruption of the family dynamic. Parents are increasingly aware of the importance of a varied diet and are under pressure to make sure their child is meeting their required intake of fruits and vegetables. This message is then contrasted with advice that tells them not to worry if their child refuses to eat certain foods.

If we accept the rates of moderate and severe selective eating and comorbid conditions are representative of preschoolers, then a large number or families are in need of additional support. In defense of front-line health care providers, it is correct that some children do improve their intake. However, even with the information presented in the results of this study, it's not clear which children or families will most require intervention and to what extent. As we learn more about this population, there needs to be further development of appropriate guidelines for referrals or recommendations.

Although a reasonable starting point, the reliance on parent report is a potential concern and actual behavioral observations of food intake across settings and contexts should be used to support findings. Despite scoring high on parent-generated sensory profiles indicating hypersensitivity to stimuli (food or other), a number of children seem very comfortable with certain tastes, textures, and smells after only a few exposures. Detailed observational data would add more information about the pervasiveness of the perceived sensitivity and the extent that experience or learned behavior serves to maintain the selective eating.

More research is still needed to confirm whether the numbers reported are representative to other potential demographic groups.[1] There are also questions as to the relationships between selective eating and anxiety, depressive symptoms, and other conditions. For example, what comes first, the selective eating or the anxiety? If one condition is improved, does the other also improve? Selective eating is also associated with a number of variables not mentioned in the study, including history of parent-child interaction, previous medical conditions, exposure to tastes/smells, and genetic influences.[2,3]

Although the authors mention the need to develop interventions or provide further guidance to caregivers about selective eating, there is little mention of the treatment approaches that have been demonstrated to be effective with the avoidant/restrictive food intake disorder (AFRID) population. This is especially important when we consider (as the authors note) the "variability in the range of clinical presentations." Multi- or interdisciplinary feeding teams have experience with children diagnosed with ARFID including those reported to be hypersensitive (as described in the article) and unwilling to try new foods. The complexity of the problem requires a comprehensive individualized assessment to ensure that all the variables associated with onset or maintenance of selective eating are identified. A wide range of behavioral strategies have been shown to be effective to help restructure the mealtime environment and enable children to participate meals both in and out of the home.

Overall, I'm not sure we're at the point yet to render the term "picky eating" obsolete until we get a greater consensus on what constitutes developmentally appropriate, nutritionally sufficient, and socially productive (or at least tolerable) mealtime interactions. The creation and description of 3 categories of normal, moderate, and severe selective eating provided a helpful framework to differentiate eating behavior, but we're still left without a definition of picky eating or specificity of adequate "ranges" of consumption.

Hopefully after reading this study, health care providers will be more apt to look a little deeper into reports of eating problems. Familiarity with the ARFID criteria may help identify families that would benefit from referrals to clinicians with experience with feeding/eating problems in this population.

P. Girolami, PhD, BCBA-D

References

1. Zucker NL, Copeland W, Egger H. Authors' response. *Pediatrics*. 2016;137.
2. Mennella JA, Jagnow CP, Beauchamp GK. Prenatal and postnatal flavor learning by human infants. *Pediatrics*. 2001;107:E88.
3. Bartoshuk LM, Duffy VB, Miller IJ. PTC/PROP tasting: anatomy, psychophysics, and sex effects. *Physiol Behav*. 1994;56:1165-1171.

6 Dentistry Otolaryngology

After-Hours Versus Office-Hours Dental Injuries in Children: Does Timing Influence Outcome?

Vukovic A, Vukovic R, Markovic D, et al (Univ of Belgrade, Serbia; Mother and Child Health Care Inst of Serbia "Dr Vukan Cupic," Belgrade; et al)
Clin Pediatr 55:29-35, 2016

Aim.—The aim of this study was to analyze the outcomes and factors associated with after-hours dental trauma.

Methods.—Study sample consisted of 1762 permanent teeth injuries in children, gender and age matched with office-hours injuries. Epidemiological and clinical data were collected from 4 university dental trauma centers.

Results.—During median follow-up time of 4.3 years, complications have occurred in 14.5% of injured teeth. Age, type, and degree of tissue injury and after-hours time of injury were significantly associated with complications. Unfavorable outcomes were 34% more likely in the after-hours group compared with office-hours. Urgent treatment was significantly delayed in after-hours group with a delay of more than 3 hours in 90.5% versus 38.9% in the office-hours group. Multivariate regression model showed that after-hours time of injury was significant predictor of complications.

Conclusion.—Delayed urgent treatment was one of the main factors associated with unfavorable outcome of after-hours injuries.

▶ Dental trauma during office hours is by its very nature is "inconvenient" for the family, dentist, and physician. Not discounting the child's traumatic experience, it is an unscheduled time expense for the parent who must leave work, leading to lost hours, and risk the appearance of being unreliable. This financial concern is compounded by the fact that a visit to the dentist or hospital can be costly.

For the busy dentist, a trauma visit during office hours is invariably a "fit-in" appointment. Virtually all dentists know that trauma must be immediately managed, therefore fitting in these visits leads to backed-up schedules, dissatisfied parents, and increased stress.

The study presented factors leading to increased traumatic dental injuries (TDI) complications when treated after hours. I agree that delayed presentation and management is a major determinant of prognosis. Parents may wait until they feel that the trauma must be treated, which is usually after work or even dinner. Financial concerns often lead to biased judgment in severity and delayed presentation.

Experienced community dentists may not be available after hours, only because treatment without support staff may not be worth their time and aggravation. A referral to the local hospital is often the protocol, leading to possible delayed ED triage and wait times. If the hospital finds it is unequipped to handle the dental emergency, referral to a children's hospital usually takes place, further delaying crucial attention to the injury.

Finally, in the treatment chair, the child is at times managed by less experienced, but willing and available, dentists. Many times, dental residents with limited experience are managing complicated situations requiring technique sensitive treatment. Long- and short-term complications are likely to increase in this scenario.

Lastly, children who may be cooperative in the dental chair often times find it difficult to cope in such an extreme, emotional situation. Management of uncooperative behavior while simultaneously treating the dental issue often leads to limitation of procedures and lower success rates. Furthermore, if after -hours sedation is necessary, lack of NPO status can be a factor increasing treatment delay.

This study, although retrospective, reinforces the trend that treatment of TDI after hours is likely to increase complications. It is paramount for the urgent and primary care physician to provide timely assessment, referral, and possibly an urgent phone call to the dentist to help mitigate the delay in treatment of the child with TDI.

R. Jurado, DDS

Exclusive Breastfeeding and Risk of Dental Malocclusion

Peres KG, Cascaes AM, Peres MA, et al (Univ of Adelaide, Australia; Federal Univ of Pelotas, RS, Brazil; et al)
Pediatrics 136:e60-e67, 2015

Objectives.—The distinct effect of exclusive and predominant breastfeeding on primary dentition malocclusions is still unclear. We hypothesized that exclusive breastfeeding presents a higher protective effect against malocclusions than predominant breastfeeding and that the use of a pacifier modifies the association between breastfeeding and primary dentition malocclusions.

Methods.—An oral health study nested in a birth cohort study was conducted at age 5 years ($N = 1303$). The type of breastfeeding was recorded at birth and at 3, 12, and 24 months of age. Open bite (OB), crossbite, overjet (OJ), and moderate/severe malocclusion (MSM) were assessed. Poisson regression analyses were conducted by controlling for sociodemographic and anthropometric characteristics, sucking habits along the life course, dental caries, and dental treatment.

Results.—Predominant breastfeeding was associated with a lower prevalence of OB, OJ, and MSM, but pacifier use modified these associations. The same findings were noted between exclusive breastfeeding and OJ and between exclusive breastfeeding and crossbite. A lower prevalence of OB was found among children exposed to exclusive breastfeeding from 3 to 5.9 months (33%) and up to 6 months (44%) of age. Those who were exclusively breastfed from 3 to 5.9 months and up to 6 months of age exhibited 41% and 72% lower prevalence of MSM, respectively, than those who were never breastfed.

Conclusions.—A common risk approach, promoting exclusive breastfeeding up to 6 months of age to prevent childhood diseases and disorders, should be an effective population strategy to prevent malocclusion.

▶ Exclusive breastfeeding for the first 6 months is associated with a decreased risk of childhood infectious and allergic diseases as well as multiple chronic health conditions across the lifecourse.[1] In addition to the benefits of breast milk, breastfeeding, versus bottle feeding, has been shown to contribute positively to orofacial development.[2] Pacifier use, although common, is controversial both because of its association with dental malocclusions as well as concerns that it may interfere with breastfeeding.

In this article, Perez et al provide evidence that breastfeeding for more than 6 months helps protect against dental malocclusions. The new knowledge that this study adds to the existing literature is subtle yet important to consider: exclusive breastfeeding for 6 months is associated with a lower risk of dental malocclusions regardless of pacifier use, but duration of pacifier use of 48 months nullifies the association between predominant breastfeeding for 6 months and dental malocclusions. This new evidence provides support in favor of the World Health Organization (WHO) recommendation that infants should be exclusively breastfed for the first 6 months.

Overall the design and conduct of the study were exceptional. It was a study of 5-year-old children nested in a prospective birth cohort study, so information on infant feeding mode and pacifier use were collected when participants were 3, 12, 24, and 48 months of age, greatly reducing the risk of recall bias. The study benefitted from a robust sample size and adequate power. The fieldwork was performed by 8 trained and calibrated dentists, and there was good inter-examiner reliability.

One limitation of the study is the lack of information about overall breastfeeding duration. The authors do not show whether there is a strong correlation between pacifier use for 48 months and duration of any breastfeeding. It is possible that the duration of any breastfeeding could be a confounding variable and may explain the reason that the inverse association between predominant breastfeeding for 6 months and dental malocclusion was nullified when pacifier use for 48 months was added to the model. Additionally, the possibility of reverse causality is not discussed by the study authors, but it seems to me that infants with craniofacial structural differences that predispose them to the development of dental malocclusions may be more likely to discontinue breastfeeding earlier due to latching difficulties.

I also caution that the authors of this study present only 1 side of the evidence about the impact of pacifier use on breastfeeding duration. Although it is true that a well-designed randomized controlled trial (RCT) published by Howard et al in 2003 found that early pacifier exposure led to shortened exclusive breastfeeding duration,[3] this is in contrast to the results of 3 other RCTs, and 2 recent systematic reviews have concluded that the available evidence does not conclusively demonstrate an adverse relationship between pacifier use and breastfeeding duration or breastfeeding exclusivity.[4,5] Couple this lack of consensus with the known association between pacifier use and reduced risk of sudden infant death syndrome (SIDS),[6] and the decision of whether to recommend pacifier use during infancy becomes much more complex. This article does; however, call into question how long is too long for children to use pacifiers. The study population boasted 40.1% of children using a pacifier daily through 4 years of age—definitely past the window of any SIDS-reducing benefit!

In reading this article, I also could not help but wonder what effect the duration of partial breastfeeding and the duration of exclusive breastfeeding but with some of the feeds given as expressed breast milk by bottle would have on the risk of dental malocclusions. It is possible that some of the infants in the exclusive breastfeeding and predominant breastfeeding categories in this study were receiving expressed breast milk by bottle, but that was not entirely clear in the methods. In societies where infants enter day care as early as 6 to 12 weeks of age, many exclusively breastfed infants feed at breast by night and drink breast milk from the bottle by day. It would stand to reason that bottle feeding breast milk for a portion of the day might attenuate the relationship between exclusive breastfeeding and malocclusion.[7] As a next step, comparing the risks of dental malocclusion among exclusively breastfed infants with varied proportions of feedings at the breast would help to elucidate what proportion of feeds at breast are needed to minimize the risk of dental malocclusion. This information would help inform on-site day care and maternity leave policy in middle and high-income countries.

Perez et al's findings evoke the easily overlooked fact that infants benefit not only from breast milk but also from breastfeeding. This well-designed study offers additional support to the WHO recommendation that infants should be exclusively breastfed for the first 6 months and also highlights important areas where further research and advocacy are needed in the fields of breastfeeding promotion and oral health promotion.

L. R. Kair, MD

References

1. Section on Breastfeeding. Breastfeeding and the use of human milk. *Pediatrics.* 2012;129:e827-841.
2. Sanchez-Molins M, Grau Carbo J, Lischeid Gaig C, Ustrell Torrent JM. Comparative study of the craniofacial growth depending on the type of lactation received. *Eur J Paediatr Dent.* 2010;11:87-92.

3. Howard CR, Howard FM, Lanphear B, et al. Randomized clinical trial of pacifier use and bottle-feeding or cupfeeding and their effect on breastfeeding. *Pediatrics.* 2003;111:511-518.
4. Jaafar SH, Jahanfar S, Angolkar M, Ho JJ. Effect of restricted pacifier use in breastfeeding term infants for increasing duration of breastfeeding. *Cochrane Database Syst Rev.* 2012;(7). CD007202.
5. O'Connor NR, Tanabe KO, Siadaty MS, Hauck FR. Pacifiers and breastfeeding: a systematic review. *Arch Pediatr Adolesc Med.* 2009;163:378 382.
6. Task Force on Sudden Infant Death Syndrome, Moon RY. SIDS and other sleep-related infant deaths: expansion of recommendations for a safe infant sleeping environment. *Pediatrics.* 2011;128:1030-1039.
7. Diouf JS, Ngom PI, Badiane A, et al. Influence of the mode of nutritive and non-nutritive sucking on the dimensions of primary dental arches. *Int Orthod.* 2010;8: 372-385.

No Visible Dental Staining In Children Treated with Doxycycline for Suspected Rocky Mountain Spotted Fever

Todd SR, Dahlgren FS, Traeger MS, et al (Ctrs for Disease Control and Prevention, Atlanta, GA; Indian Health Service, Whiteriver, AZ; et al)
J Pediatr 166:1246-1251, 2015

Objective.—To evaluate whether cosmetically relevant dental effects occurred among children who had received doxycycline for treatment of suspected Rocky Mountain spotted fever (RMSF).

Study Design.—Children who lived on an American Indian reservation with high incidence of RMSF were classified as exposed or unexposed to doxycycline, based on medical and pharmacy record abstraction. Licensed, trained dentists examined each child's teeth and evaluated visible staining patterns and enamel hypoplasia. Objective tooth color was evaluated with a spectrophotometer.

Results.—Fifty-eight children who received an average of 1.8 courses of doxycycline before 8 years of age and who now had exposed permanent teeth erupted were compared with 213 children who had never received doxycycline. No tetracycline-like staining was observed in any of the exposed children's teeth (0/58, 95% CI 0%-5%), and no significant difference in tooth shade ($P = .20$) or hypoplasia ($P = 1.0$) was found between the 2 groups.

Conclusions.—This study failed to demonstrate dental staining, enamel hypoplasia, or tooth color differences among children who received short-term courses of doxycycline at <8 years of age. Healthcare provider confidence in use of doxycycline for suspected RMSF in children may be improved by modifying the drug's label (Fig 1, Table 2).

▶ Doxycycline, a tetracycline derivative, is first-line therapy for treatment of life-threatening infections caused by pathogens in the *Rickettsia/Ehrlichia/Anaplasma* group including Rocky Mountain spotted fever (RMSF).[1] Early empiric treatment, often done on an outpatient basis, is recommended in suspected cases before presentation of classic symptoms (eg, petechiae, if present)

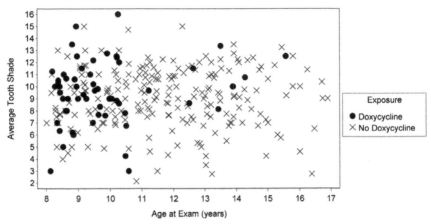

FIGURE 1.—A scatterplot of average tooth shade by age at examination, stratified by doxycycline exposure. (Reprinted from Todd SR, Dahlgren FS, Traeger MS, et al. No visible dental staining in children treated with doxycycline for suspected rocky mountain spotted fever. *J Pediatr.* 2015;166:1246-1251, with permission from Elsevier Inc.)

or laboratory confirmation because (1) delay in therapy beyond the fifth day of illness could lead to increased morbidity and death and (2) results of current diagnostic testing modalities including blood or tissue DNA polymerase chain reaction (PCR) and convalescent serology could take several days for the results to be reported or up to 7 to 10 days for the antibody result to become positive, respectively, for definitive diagnosis.[1-3]

There is a paucity of evidence supporting dental staining effects of doxycycline compared with older tetracyclines. In addition, administration of the drug can prevent fatal outcomes if given early as recommended by the American Academy of Pediatrics (AAP) and the Centers for Disease Control (CDC).[1] Despite these points, pediatricians continue to exhibit hesitancy when prescribing doxycycline to children younger than 8 years of age. This practice has resulted in unfavorable outcomes, evidenced by mortality rates that are 5 times higher in children less than 10 years of age compared with older children with RMSF.

Tetracycline use has been limited in pediatric patients younger than 8 years.[4] Incorporated into enamel during odontogenesis, their colored degradation products can cause permanent dental discoloration and enamel hypoplasia in 23% to 92% of developing teeth. Doxycycline, a newer tetracycline derivative, binds less readily to calcium. Several studies, although small and possibly subject to interpretation bias, have failed to demonstrate evidence of dental effects even after repeated courses of administration.[5-7] Chloramphenicol is considered second-line therapy for RMSF given its inferiority at preventing fatal outcomes compared with tetracyclines.[1] Additionally, its side effect profile includes aplastic anemia, and oral formulations are no longer available in the United States.[1] The use of chloramphenicol was favored by the AAP for children younger than 9 years of age until 2000,[8,9] when all hesitancy to utilize doxycycline was removed in 2003 and it became the drug of choice for pathogens in the *Rickettsia/Ehrlichia/Anaplasma* group.[10,11]

TABLE 2.—The Prevalence of Enamel Hypoplasia, the Prevalence of Fluorosis, and Dental Hygiene Habits by Whether Exposed to Doxycycline

	Doxycycline <8 y, N (%)	No Doxycycline, N (%)	Crude PR (95% CI)	Crude PR, P Value	Breslow-Day, P Value	Age-Adjusted PR (95% CI)	Age-Adjusted PR, P Value
Enamel hypoplasia	2 (4)	8 (4)	0.92 (0.2-4.2)	1.00	.79	1.6 (0.2-13.5)	.65
Fluorosis	5 (9)	28 (13)	0.66 (0.3-1.6)	.35	.54	0.86 (0.4-2.0)	.72
Brushes ≥2 times daily	40 (75)	148 (71)	1.1 (0.9-1.3)	.50	.32	1.1 (0.9-1.4)	.34
Any dark drinks	41 (71)	163 (77)	0.9 (0.77-1.1)	.36	.32	0.93 (0.8-1.1)	.48
Tobacco use	2 (4)	21 (10)	0.4 (0.1-1.4)	.18	.64	0.75 (0.2-3.1)	.68

PR, prevalence ratio.
The crude PR and its 95% CI are presented, as well as the age-adjusted PR.
Results of the Breslow-Day test for the homogeneity of the associations are stratified by age as a whole number.
Reprinted from Todd SR, Dahlgren FS, Traeger MS, et al. No visible dental staining in children treated with doxycycline for suspected rocky mountain spotted fever. *J Pediatr.* 2015;166:1246-1251, with permission from Elsevier Inc.

Provider apprehension to prescribe doxycycline despite current AAP and CDC recommendations is potentially fueled by the current US Food and Drug Administration (FDA) drug label warning against its use in children younger than 8 years of age and the dental-staining stigma of the older tetracyclines. In the recently published article by Todd et al, treatment courses (averaging 7 days duration) of doxycycline given to 58 children younger than 8 years of age failed to demonstrate subsequent dental staining, enamel hypoplasia, or tooth color differences, providing further evidence to potentially modify the FDA drug label and improve clinical outcomes.

RMSF has contributed to significant morbidity and mortality on several American Indian reservations in Arizona since 2002, possibly linked to an unexpected vector, *Rhipicephalus sanguineus* (the brown dog tick) and large populations of free-roaming dogs.[12] Compared with other US regions, clinical presentations, more notably in younger children (median age, 11 years), were often nonspecific, variable, and difficult to differentiate from other illnesses.[12] A large population (n = 58) of children received 1 or more empiric doxycycline courses (average 1.8 per child, and sometimes up to 3) regardless of age due to intensive education on these tribal lands.

Todd et al decided to objectively measure the potential adverse effects on teeth for those treated with doxycycline on the Indian reservations. This study is the largest retrospective study to date of children treated with doxycycline, and also the first to apply objective cross-sectional dental examinations utilizing trained dentists and a spectrophotometer to assess dental shade and enamel hypoplasia. Overall, the results from this study support the findings in smaller studies[5-7] that doxycycline does not cause dental staining after short and even repeated treatment courses for RMSF in children younger than eight 8 of age (Table 2).

Several study limitations include recall bias in regards to children's ability to relay dental behaviors and an inability to confirm completion of total duration of prescribed doxycycline. A range of tooth shade differences are appreciable among exposed and unexposed children, but average tooth shade among groups is alternatively assessed to minimize individual variability (Fig 1). Inter-rater variability always exist in both visual assessments and spectrophotometer results although efforts are made to make the most objective measurements through training dentists using a single identification standard.

Doxycycline is the single oral antibiotic available in the United States capable of reducing fatal outcomes if initiated early in children with RMSF.[2,3] Limited evidence exists to support dental staining effects of its routine use in children less than 8 years of age compared with the older tetracyclines, although the FDA maintains a cautionary warning label against its use in this age group. Hesitancy among pediatricians to prescribe doxycycline despite AAP and CDC recommendations is problematic, given increased mortality rates seen in young children with RMSF. Results from the study by Todd et al further support the lack of association between routine doxycycline use and dental staining in children less than eight years of age. Modifications of the current FDA warning labels against doxycycline should be considered.

K. A. Ramirez, MD
J. S. Abramson, MD

References

1. American Academy of Pediatrics. Rocky mountain spotted fever. In: Kimberlin DW, Brady MT, Jackson MA, Long SS, eds. *Red Book: 2015 Report of the Committee on Infectious Diseases.* 30th ed. Elk Grove Village, IL: American Academy of Pediatrics; 2015:682-684.
2. Regan JJ, Traeger MS, Humpherys D, et al. Risk factors for fatal outcome from rocky mountain spotted fever in a highly endemic area—Arizona, 2002–2011. *Clin Infect Dis.* 2015;60:1659-1666.
3. Holman RC, Paddock CD, Curns AT, Krebs JW, McQuiston JH, Childs JE. Analysis of risk factors for fatal Rocky Mountain Spotted Fever: evidence for superiority of tetracyclines for therapy. *J Infect Dis.* 2001;184:1437-1444.
4. American Academy of Pediatrics. Tetracyclines. In: Kimberlin DW, Brady MT, Jackson MA, Long SS, eds. *Red Book: Report of the Committee on Infectious Diseases.* 30th ed. Elk Grove Village, IL: American Academy of Pediatrics; 2015:873.
5. Volovitz B, Shkap R, Amir J, Calderon S, Varsano I, Nussinovitch M. Absence of tooth staining with doxycycline treatment in young children. *Clin Pediatr (Phila).* 2007;46:121-126.
6. Forti G, Benincori C. Doxycycline and the teeth. *Lancet.* 1969;1:782.
7. Lochary ME, Lockhart PB, Williams WT Jr. Doxycycline and staining of permanent teeth. *Pediatr Infect Dis J.* 1998;17:429-431.
8. American Academy of Pediatrics. Rocky mountain spotted fever. In: Peter G, Lepow ML, McCracken GH, Philips CF, eds. *Red Book: Report on the Committee on Infectious Diseases.* 22nd ed. Elk Grove Village, IL: American Academy of Pediatrics; 1991:405-407.
9. American Academy of Pediatrics. Rocky mountain spotted fever. In: Pickering LK, Peter G, Baker C, et al., eds. *Red Book: Report of the Committee on Infectious Diseases.* Elk Grove Village, IL: American Academy of Pediatrics; 2000:491-493.
10. Abramson JS, Givner LB. Should tetracycline be contraindicated for therapy of presumed Rocky Mountain spotted fever in children less than 9 years of age? *Pediatrics.* 1990;86:123-124.
11. American Academy of Pediatrics. Rocky mountain spotted fever. In: Abramson JS, Pickering LK, et al., eds. *Red Book: Committee on Infectious Diseases 2001–2003.* Elk Grove Village, IL: American Academy of Pediatrics; 2003:532-534.
12. Traeger MS, Regan JJ, Humpherys D, et al. Rocky mountain spotted fever characterization and comparison to similar illnesses in a highly endemic area—Arizona, 2002–2011. *Clin Infect Dis.* 2015;60:1650-1658.

Risk of Sensorineural Hearing Loss and Bilirubin Exchange Transfusion Thresholds

Wickremasinghe AC, Risley RJ, Kuzniewicz MW, et al (Kaiser Permanente Northern California, Santa Clara; Hearing Health Ctr, Oak Brook, IL; Kaiser Permanente Northern California, Oakland; et al)

Pediatrics 136:505-512, 2015

Background and Objectives.—High bilirubin levels are associated with sensorineural hearing loss (SNHL). However, few large studies of relative and excess risk exist. We sought to quantify the risk of SNHL in newborns who had bilirubin levels at or above American Academy of Pediatrics exchange transfusion thresholds (ETT).

Methods.—Infants born at ≥35 weeks gestation in 15 Kaiser Perma-nente Northern California hospitals from 1995-2011 were eligible ($N = 525\,409$). We used a nested double cohort design. The exposed cohort included subjects with ≥1 bilirubin level at or above ETT. The unexposed cohort was a 3.6% random sample of subjects with all biliru-bin levels below ETT (10 unexposed per exposed). An audiologist, blinded to bilirubin levels, reviewed the charts of children in whom SNHL had been diagnosed before age 8 years to confirm the diagnosis. We calculated Cox proportional hazard ratios for time to diagnosis of SNHL.

Results.—SNHL was confirmed in 11 (0.60%) of the 1834 exposed sub-jects and in 43 (0.23%) of the 19 004 unexposed. Only bilirubin levels ≥10 mg/dL above ETT were associated with a statistically significant increased risk of SNHL (hazard ratio: 36 [95% confidence interval (CI): 13 to 101]). Likewise, only bilirubin levels ≥35 mg/dL were associated with a statistically significant increased risk of SNHL (hazard ratio: 91 [95% CI: 32 to 255]). For subjects with total serum bilirubin levels 0 to 4.9 mg/dL above ETT, the upper limit of the 95% CI for excess risk was 0.5%.

Conclusions.—Only bilirubin levels well above ETT were associated with SNHL. At lower bilirubin levels, the excess risk of SNHL was low.

▶ Hyperbilirubinemia affects 60% of newborns in the United States and is a common problem encountered by both general pediatricians and neonatolo-gists.[1] In 1994, the American Academy of Pediatrics (AAP) published its first guidelines on management of hyperbilirubinemia, and this statement was sub-sequently updated in 2004.[1,2] The 2004 practice parameter included additional criteria for exchange transfusion by stratifying infants based on gestational age, hours of life, and relevant risk factors.[2]

Wickremasinghe et al's well-designed retrospective cohort study attempts to better quantify the risk of sensorineural hearing loss (SNHL) with bilirubin levels at or above the exchange transfusion threshold (ETT). Only subjects with extremely elevated total serum bilirubin (TSB) levels (> 10 mg/dL above the AAP ETT or > 35 mg/dL) were more likely to have SNHL compared with those with lower TSB levels. The authors conclude that for TSB levels just exceeding ETT, exchange transfusions may not be needed to prevent SNHL and may pose additional risks.

Yet for most physicians managing newborn hyperbilirubinemia and contem-plating an exchange transfusion, the primary concern is not SNHL but bilirubin-related encephalopathy and kernicterus.[2,3] Kernicterus is defined as the chronic and permanent clinical sequelae of bilirubin toxicity, which includes damage to the brain. Survivors may demonstrate severe athetoid cerebral palsy, paralysis of upward gaze, developmental delay, and hearing loss.[2,3] Because the threshold at which hyperbilirubinemia causes kernicterus is complicated by a variety of neonatal factors,[2] it would be more relevant to determine the risk of kernicterus in relation to the ETT.

Wickremasinghe worked with Wu et al[4] to present these data in a March 2015 *JAMA Pediatrics* publication using the same cohort of infants. The authors found that cerebral palsy with kernicterus occurred in 3 infants, all with TSB levels > 5.0 mg/dL above the ETT and 2 neurotoxicity risk factors. Two of the 3 infants with kernicterus also experienced SNHL.[4] The current article would have benefitted greatly from additional consideration of the cerebral palsy and kernicterus data in combination with the SNHL data. The tables presented in the 2 articles on the 7 infants with cerebral palsy and the 11 with SNHL cannot be easily compared by the reader. However, the results suggest significant risk of SNHL occurs at higher bilirubin levels (> 10 mg/dL above the ETT) than cerebral palsy with kernicterus (> 5.0 mg/dL above the ETT with two neurotoxicity risk factors).[4]

Wickremasinghe et al state that a greater proportion of subjects exposed to bilirubin levels above the ETT who developed SNHL underwent exchange transfusion (18.2% vs 2.2%, $P = .03$). These subjects also demonstrated significantly higher peak serum bilirubin levels (mean SD: 30.1 11.7 vs 23.4 3.1; $P < .001$). Although the auditory system is particularly sensitive to the toxic effects of bilirubin, SNHL has also been linked to anemia and ischemia, which may be exacerbated in an exchange transfusion.[5] The authors comment on the additional risks of exchange transfusion (morbidity of 5% and mortality risks of 0.3%–1.9%). Considering how this treatment may affect the development of SNHL, especially if complicated by hypotension or arrhythmias, would be of interest. This may in part explain why SNHL seems to occur at higher bilirubin levels than cerebral palsy with kernicterus. Perhaps infants with higher TSB were more likely to undergo exchange transfusion and experience complications such as SNHL.

The impact of the study results is limited by the significant decline in the number of exchange transfusions performed in the United States. As Hansen[3] notes in an editorial, even multiregional referral centers report performing as few as 0 to 2 exchange transfusions annually. The finding that intravenous immunoglobulin can be given to slow the rate of rise of hyperbilirubinemia has further reduced the use of exchange transfusions.[6] The use of intravenous immunoglobulin was not reported in this study, but the article similarly finds that those infants with bilirubin levels exceeding the ETT were more likely to have been born in the early years of the study. The information on cerebral palsy, kernicterus, and SNHL is certainly valuable for the limited cases of exchange transfusion performed in the United States.

In summary, Wickremasinghe et al present a well-designed retrospective cohort study to quantify the risk of SNHL at TSB exceeding the AAP ETT. The results would have been greatly enhanced by further discussion of these data in combination with their analysis on the risk of cerebral palsy and kernicterus in the same cohort. As SNHL seemed to occur at higher TSB than cerebral palsy and kernicterus, additional consideration of the complications of treatment with exchange transfusion would have been a worthwhile addition to the article. Overall the data suggest risks of cerebral palsy, kernicterus, and SNHL are low at < 5 mg/dL above the AAP ETT (note 1 case of kernicterus occurred at 5.5 mg/dL above the ETT). This information is valuable for clinicians in speaking with families and making the decision to proceed to exchange transfusion. However, it is hoped close adherence to the AAP clinical practice recommendations for management of newborn hyperbilirubinemia will continue to make the need for exchange transfusion in the United States increasingly rare.

D. L. Sekhar, MD, MSc

References

1. American Academy of Pediatrics. Practice parameter: management of hyperbilirubinemia in the healthy term newborn. *Pediatrics*. 1994;94:558-565.
2. American Academy of Pediatrics. Management of hyperbilirubinemia in the newborn infant 35 or more weeks of gestation. *Pediatrics*. 2004;114:297-316.
3. Hansen TWR. Kernicterus in neonatal jaundice — finding the needle in the haystack. *PCCM*. 2016;17:266-267.
4. Wu YW, Kuzniewicz MW, Wickremasinghe AC, et al. Risk for cerebral palsy in infants with total serum bilirubin levels at or above the exchange transfusion threshold: a population-based study. *JAMA Pediatr*. 2015;169:239-246.
5. Chung SD, Chen PY, Lin HC, Hung SH. Sudden sensorineural hearing loss associated with iron-deficiency anemia: a population-based study. *JAMA Otolaryngol Head Neck Surg*. 2014;140:417-422.
6. Steiner LA, Bizzarro MJ, Ehrenkranz RA, Gallagher PG. A decline in the frequency of neonatal exchange transfusions and its effect on exchange-related morbidity and mortality. *Pediatrics*. 2007;120:27-32.

Clinical Features, Virus Identification, and Sinusitis as a Complication of Upper Respiratory Tract Illness in Children Ages 4-7 Years

DeMuri GP, Gern JE, Moyer SC, et al (Univ of Wisconsin School of Medicine and Public Health, Madison; et al)
J Pediatr 171:133-139, 2016

Objective.—To determine the rate of sinusitis complicating upper respiratory tract illnesses (URIs) in children. We prospectively identified the clinical, virologic, and epidemiologic characteristics of URIs in a population of 4- to 7-year-old children followed for 1 year.

Study Design.—This was an observational cohort study in 2 primary care pediatric practices in Madison, Wisconsin. Nasal samples were obtained during 4 asymptomatic surveillance visits and during symptomatic URIs. A polymerase chain reaction-based assay for 9 respiratory viruses was performed on nasal samples. A diagnosis of sinusitis was based on published criteria.

Results.—Two hundred thirty-six children ages 48-96 months were enrolled. A total of 327 URIs were characterized. The mean number of URIs per child was 1.3 (range 0-9) per year. Viruses were detected in 81% of URIs; rhinovirus (RV) was most common. Seventy-two percent of URIs were resolved clinically by the 10th day. RV-A and RV-C were detected more frequently at URI visits; RV-B was detected at the same rate for both asymptomatic surveillance visits and URI visits. Sinusitis was diagnosed in 8.8% of symptomatic URIs. Viruses were detected frequently (33%) in samples from asymptomatic children.

Conclusions.—Sinusitis occurred in 8.8% of symptomatic URIs in our study. The virus most frequently detected with URIs in children was RV;

RV-A and RV-C detection but not RV-B detection were associated with illness. Viruses, especially RV, are detected frequently in asymptomatic children. Most URIs have improved or resolved by the 10th day after onset. Children experienced a mean of 1.3 URIs per year, which was lower than expected (Figs 1-4).

▶ This prospective cohort study describing the virology and complications of upper respiratory infections (URIs) in children 4 to 7 years old fills in a surprising gap in our knowledge about an incredibly common medical occurrence (Figs 1 and 2). The application of polymerase chain reaction (PCR)-based viral detection provides an opportunity for better identification of viruses during URIs and, coupled with detailed clinical data, provides a new look at the epidemiology of URIs in this age group (Fig 3). The study is important because it informs the clinical differentiation of self-limited URI and sinusitis, which has implications for appropriate use of antibiotics in children.

The key strength of the study is its prospective design, which allowed for preplanned collection of key clinical and virological data. Having a clear definition of sinusitis that would be accepted by most practicing pediatricians helped to determine the rate of sinusitis complications (8.8%). Application of the multiplex PCR technology allowed for the best ability to characterize viral detection, leading to a rate of 81% for viral detection during symptomatic URIs. Another novel feature of the study design was the collection of nasal mucous during asymptomatic periods, which led to the observation that specific viral strains may be just as likely to be detected during asymptomatic or symptomatic sampling frames (which was the case for human rhinovirus-B) (Fig 4).

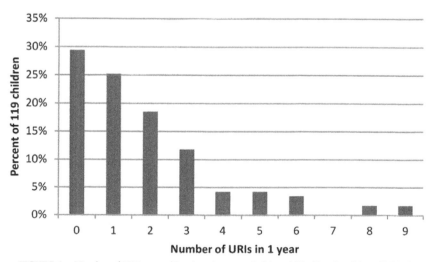

FIGURE 1.—Number of URIs per subject in a 1-year period ($n = 119$). (Reprinted from DeMuri GP, Gern JE, Moyer SC, et al. Clinical features, virus identification, and sinusitis as a complication of upper respiratory tract illness in children ages 4-7 years. *J Pediatr.* 2016;171:133-139, with permission from Elsevier.)

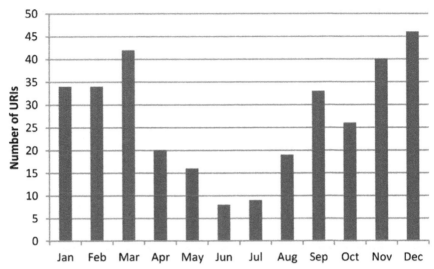

FIGURE 2.—Number of URIs (n = 327) by month in 236 children. (Reprinted from DeMuri GP, Gern JE, Moyer SC, et al. Clinical features, virus identification, and sinusitis as a complication of upper respiratory tract illness in children ages 4-7 years. *J Pediatr.* 2016;171:133-139, with permission from Elsevier.)

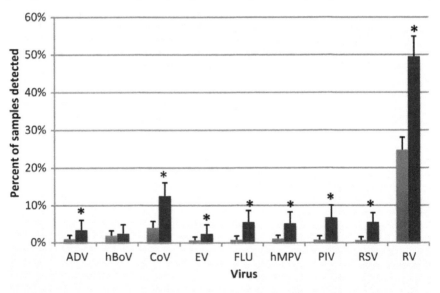

■ Surveillance (n = 725)   ■ URI (n = 327)

FIGURE 3.—Respiratory viruses detected in nasal specimens from 725 asymptomatic surveillance visits and 327 URI visits from 236 study subjects. The detection rates shown include samples with both single and multiple viruses detected. ORs and 95% CIs (shown in parentheses) for the difference in detection of each virus between URI and surveillance specimens: ADV 3.6 (1.4-9.3), hBoV 1.3 (0.5-3.1), CoV 3.4 (2.1-5.7), EV 3.6 (1.2-11.1), FLU 7.0 (2.8-17.8), hMPV 4.9 (2.1-11.5), PIV 8.7 (3.5-21.5), RSV 8.4 (3.1-22.8), and RV 3.0 (2.3-3.9). There were 242 viruses detected in surveillance visits and 266 viruses in URI visits. *P < .001 for an OR different than 1. (Reprinted from DeMuri GP, Gern JE, Moyer SC, et al. Clinical features, virus identification, and sinusitis as a complication of upper respiratory tract illness in children ages 4-7 years. *J Pediatr.* 2016;171:133-139, with permission from Elsevier.)

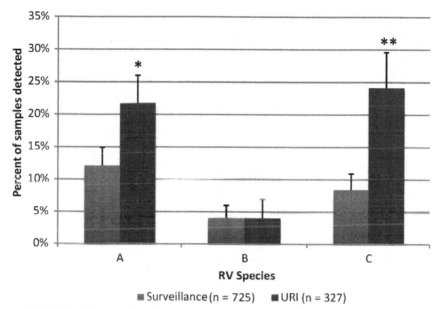

■ Surveillance (n = 725)   ■ URI (n = 327)

FIGURE 4.—RV species detected in nasal specimens (n = 179) in 725 surveillance (n = 725) vs 327 URI visits (n = 327). ORs for the comparison between surveillance and URI visits for each species: RV-A 2.0 (1.4-2.8,*P < .001), RV-B 0.9 (0.5-1.7, P = Not Significant), RV-C 3.5 (2.3-5.1, **P < .001). (Reprinted from DeMuri GP, Gern JE, Moyer SC, et al. Clinical features, virus identification, and sinusitis as a complication of upper respiratory tract illness in children ages 4-7 years. *J Pediatr.* 2016;171:133-139, with permission from Elsevier.)

The main limitation of this study is that only 29 sinusitis episodes occurred in 24 children, which limited the ability of the authors to identify key epidemiologic or viral factors that are more likely to result in sinusitis. Similarly, few otitis media episodes were captured, also limiting statistical analyses. Therefore, it was not determined whether specific virus strains were more likely to result in sinusitis or otitis. In addition, the overall somewhat lower rate of URIs in this 1-year study makes one wonder if they captured all of the URIs in the cohort. Although study coordinator contact monthly likely captured most severe episodes, it is possible that milder URIs were not fully characterized in this cohort. Finally, measurement of immunologic responses to URIs (eg, interleukin-6) was not reported. Linking specific immunologic responses, virus type/strain, and likelihood of sinusitis would have implications for diagnosis and treatment of URIs.

The clinical implication of this study is that most URIs are uncomplicated, with only 8.8% associated with sinusitis and 5.8% associated with otitis media. The observation that most URI symptoms had resolved by 10 days supports the current guidelines for differentiating self-limited URI and sinusitis. The research implication of this study is that not all viruses appear to cause similar clinical disease, paving the way for hypothesis-driven studies that can explain this observation.

M. A. Rank, MD

7 Dermatology

Antibiotic Exposure, Infection, and the Development of Pediatric Psoriasis: A Nested Case-Control Study
Horton DB, Scott Fl, Haynes K, et al (Univ of Pennsylvania, Philadelphia; et al)
JAMA Dermatol 152.191 199, 2016

Importance.—Antibiotics disrupt human microbiota and have been associated with several pediatric autoimmune diseases. Psoriasis activity has been linked to group A streptococcal and viral infections.

Objective.—To determine whether antibiotic exposure and infections are independently associated with incident psoriasis in children.

Design, Setting, and Participants.—This nested case-control study used data from the Health Improvement Network database, a population-representative electronic health records database from the United Kingdom, from June 27, 1994, through January 15, 2013. Data were analyzed from September 17, 2014, through August 12, 2015. Children aged 1 to 15 years with newly diagnosed psoriasis (n = 845) were compared with age- and sex-matched controls (n = 8450) randomly chosen at the time of psoriasis diagnosis from general practices with at least one case, excluding children with immunodeficiency, inflammatory bowel disease, and juvenile arthritis.

Exposures.—Systemic antibacterial prescriptions and infections of the skin and other sites within 2 years before psoriasis diagnosis.

Main Outcomes and Measures.—Incident psoriasis as determined by validated diagnostic codes. The association of antibiotic exposure and infections with incident psoriasis was determined by conditional logistic regression, adjusting for confounders.

Results.—After adjusting for matching, country, socioeconomic deprivation, outpatient visits, and infections within the past 2 years, antibiotic exposure in the last 2 years was weakly associated with incident psoriasis (adjusted odds ratio [aOR], 1.2; 95%CI, 1.0-1.5). The associations for infections of skin (aOR, 1.5; 95% CI, 1.2-1.7) and other sites (aOR, 1.3; 95% CI, 1.1-1.6) were similar. Untreated nonskin infections (aOR, 1.5; 95% CI, 1.3-1.8) but not antibiotic-treated nonskin infections (aOR, 1.1; 95% CI, 0.9-1.4) were associated with psoriasis. Results were similar when using a lifetime exposure window. Different classes of antibiotics and age of first antibiotic exposure were also not associated with psoriasis. The findings did not substantively change when excluding periods of varying length before diagnosis.

Conclusions and Relevance.—Infections are associated with the development of pediatric psoriasis, but antibiotics do not appear to contribute substantially to that risk.

▶ Psoriasis has recently been identified as a chronic, multisystem inflammatory disease with predominantly skin and joint manifestations.[1] For decades, the association of group A beta hemolytic streptococcal infections have been known to be a potential trigger of pediatric psoriasis and guttate disease.[2] The mechanism through which this occurs is believed to be via streptococcal superantigens and is associated with HLA CW* 0602 and CLA + T-cell-dependent epidermal cell activation which triggers TH17 response in guttate psoriasis.[3,4]

The story has largely in the past suggested that the infection is a trigger of psoriatic disease in childhood. First, we know that psoriasis is considered one of the many recognized autoimmune diseases, that is, psoriatic inflammation is triggered by recognition of self and inflammatory attack triggered by such recognition by the immune system.[5] It has been demonstrable that there is a homology between some epidermal antigens (eg, streptococcal M surface antigen) and beta hemolytic *Streptococcus*, such that streptococcal infections could be trigger an accidental recognition of self.[6] Tonsillectomy has been demonstrated to improve both psoriasis and circulating T cells that recognize streptococcal determinants.[7] Recently 6 of 7 adult patients with guttate psoriasis have been found to have streptococcal ribosomal DNA circulating in their blood.[8]

Despite the basic data that exist in the literature, in fact, the question has not been previously answered as to whether the psoriatic trigger in childhood is the antibiotic usage to treat strep or the strep infections which the antibiotics are treating, that is, is the trigger the chicken or the egg?

Antibiotic usage, likely via microbiome alteration, has also been variably linked, although not fully proven and somewhat controversial, to autoimmune disease such as inflammatory bowel disease and autoimmune hepatitis.[9,10] Therefore, the question about the antibiotic linkage to psoriatic triggering is one that should be answered.

On the other hand, we know that the usage of antibiotics in childhood has independent risks that may be linked to psoriasis. First, chronic antibiotic exposure may be independently linked to obesity.[11] Obesity as measured by large waist circumference has been linked to psoriasis of childhood. Obesity with features of metabolic syndrome including inflammatory markers and lipid abnormalities have been linked to pediatric psoriasis. In adults, obesity, metabolic syndrome, hypertension and lipid metabolism abnormalities are linked to the diagnosis of psoriasis.[12]

Horton et al, using a nested case-controlled cohort of children from the Health Improvement Network database of the United Kingdom, addressed the relationship of psoriasis to infections and to antibiotics. The database was screened from 1994 through 2013, and 845 children with psoriasis aged 1 to 15 years were assessed and compared with 8450 age- and sex-matched controls without psoriasis.

Infections and antibiotics exposure in the past 2 years were studied as they relate to psoriasis. Infections were associated with psoriasis, including infections of the skin and nonskin (eg, upper respiratory infections) and untreated nonskin infections, but not antibiotic treated nonskin infections. Antibiotic usage was only weakly associated with psoriatic disease in children.

In addition, children were compared with their mothers. Maternal psoriasis and autoimmune diseases were associated with pediatric psoriasis.

Horton et al provide the first strong evidence that infections, but not the use of antibiotics, trigger what is likely a genetic tendency to the disease.[3] The study is the first to address a large pediatric cohort and is the first credible evidence that pediatric psoriasis onset is linked to infections. Interestingly, infections with strep pyogenes were not the only infections linked to pediatric disease. Clearly, the story on how psoriasis is triggered by infections is yet to be fully delineated. This study provides a new overview of the infectious players in pediatric psoriatic disease.

N. Silverberg, MD

References

1. Menter A, Gottlieb A, Feldman SR, et al. Guidelines of care for the management of psoriasis and psoriatic arthritis: Section 1. Overview of psoriasis and guidelines of care for the treatment of psoriasis with biologics. *J Am Acad Dermatol.* 2008; 58:826-850.
2. Leung DY, Travers JB, Giorno R, et al. Evidence for a streptococcal superantigen-driven process in acute guttate psoriasis. *J Clin Invest.* 1995;96:2106-2112.
3. Ferran M, Galván AB, Rincón C, et al. Streptococcus induces circulating CLA(+) memory T-cell-dependent epidermal cell activation in psoriasis. *J Invest Dermatol.* 2013;133:999-1007.
4. Ruiz-Romeu E, Ferran M, Sagristà M, et al. Streptococcus pyogenes-induced cutaneous lymphocyte antigen-positive T cell-dependent epidermal cell activation triggers T_H17 responses in patients with guttate psoriasis. *J Allergy Clin Immunol.* 2016;138:491-499.e6.
5. http://www.niaid.nih.gov/topics/autoimmune/Pages/diseases.aspx#. Accessed May 21, 2016.
6. Sigmundsdottir H, Sigurgeirsson B, Troye-Blomberg M, Good MF, Valdimarsson H, Jonsdottir I. Circulating T cells of patients with active psoriasis respond to streptococcal M-peptides sharing sequences with human epidermal keratins. *Scand J Immunol.* 1997;45:688-697.
7. Thorleifsdottir RH, Sigurdardottir SL, Sigurgeirsson B, et al. Improvement of psoriasis after tonsillectomy is associated with a decrease in the frequency of circulating T cells that recognize streptococcal determinants and homologous skin determinants. *J Immunol.* 2012;188:5160-5165.
8. Munz OH, Sela S, Baker BS, Griffiths CE, Powles AV, Fry L. Evidence for the presence of bacteria in the blood of psoriasis patients. *Arch Dermatol Res.* 2010;302:495-498.
9. Dubeau MF, Iacucci M, Beck PL, et al. Drug-induced inflammatory bowel disease and IBD-like conditions. *Inflamm Bowel Dis.* 2013;19:445-456.
10. Healy J, Alexander B, Eapen C, Roberts-Thomson IC. Minocycline-induced autoimmune hepatitis. *Intern Med J.* 2009;39:487-488.
11. Turta O, Rautava S. Antibiotics, obesity and the link to microbes—what are we doing to our children? *BMC Med.* 2016;14:57.
12. Gutmark-Little I, Shah KN. Obesity and the metabolic syndrome in pediatric psoriasis. *Clin Dermatol.* 2015;33:305-315.

Effectiveness of a Multicomponent Sun Protection Program for Young Children: A Randomized Clinical Trial

Ho BK, Reidy K, Huerta I, et al (Northwestern Univ Feinberg School of Medicine, Chicago, IL; Advocate Children's Hosp, Park Ridge and Oak Lawn, IL; et al)

JAMA Pediatr 170:334-342, 2016

Importance.—Emphasizing sun protection behaviors among young children may minimize sun damage and foster lifelong sun protection behaviors that will reduce the likelihood of developing skin cancer, especially melanoma.

Objective.—To determine whether a multicomponent sun protection program delivered in pediatric clinics during the summer could increase summertime sun protection among young children.

Design, Setting, and Participants.—Randomized controlled clinical trial with 4-week follow-up that included 300 parents or relatives (hereafter simply referred to as caregivers [mean age, 36.0 years]) who brought the child (2-6 years of age) in their care to an Advocate Medical Group clinic during the period from May 15 to August 14, 2015. Of the 300 caregiver-child pairs, 153 (51.0%) were randomly assigned to receive a read-along book, swim shirt, and weekly text-message reminders related to sun protection behaviors (intervention group) and 147 (49.0%) were randomly assigned to receive the information usually provided at a well-child visit (control group). Data analysis was performed from August 20 to 30, 2015.

Intervention.—Multicomponent sun protection program composed of a read-along book, swim shirt, and weekly text-message reminders related to sun protection behaviors.

Main Outcomes and Measures.—Outcomes were caregiver-reported use of sun protection by the child (seeking shade and wearing sun-protective clothing and sunscreen) using a 5-point Likert scale, duration of outdoor activities, and number of children who had sunburn or skin irritation. The biologic measurement of the skin pigment of a child s arm was performed with a spectrophotometer at baseline and 4 weeks later.

Results.—Of the 300 caregiver-child pairs, the 153 children in the intervention group had significantly higher scores related to sun protection behaviors on both sunny (mean [SE], 15.748 [0.267] for the intervention group; mean [SE], 14.780 [0.282] for the control group; mean difference, 0.968) and cloudy days (mean [SE], 14.286 [0.282] for the intervention group; mean [SE], 12.850 [0.297] for the control group; mean difference, 1.436). Examination of pigmentary changes by spectrophotometry revealed that the children in the control group significantly increased their melanin levels, whereas the children in the intervention group did not have a significant change in melanin level on their protected upper arms ($P < .001$ for skin type 1, $P = .008$ for skin type 2, and $P < .001$ for skin types 4-6).

Conclusions and Relevance.—A multicomponent intervention using text-message reminders and distribution of read-along books and swim shirts was associated with increased sun protection behaviors among young children. This was corroborated by a smaller change in skin pigment among children receiving the intervention. This implementable program can help augment anticipatory sun protection guidance in pediatric clinics and decrease children's future skin cancer risk.

Trial Registration.—clinicaltrials.gov Identifier: NCT02376517.

▶ This study is important and timely, considering that the US Surgeon General published a Call to Action to Prevent Skin Cancer[1] in July 2014 to highlight the significant public health burden of skin cancer, the most common cancer in the United States. Annually, almost 5 million patients receive treatment for skin cancer.[2] The incidence rate of melanoma, the most commonly fatal skin cancer, continues to increase.[3] However, most skin cancer cases are potentially preventable by minimizing sun exposure and avoiding indoor tanning. Sunburn during childhood is a recognized risk factor.[4] The Call to Action emphasizes sun protection interventions in children, to reduce their lifetime risk of skin cancer. This need is urgent because research indicates that children are not adequately protected and sunburns are prevalent.[5,6]

There are relatively few investigations of sun protection interventions delivered in the pediatric setting. The American Academy of Pediatrics (AAP) acknowledges the importance of the pediatrician's role in skin cancer prevention and recommends that clinicians incorporate prevention advice into at least 1 well-child visit per year.[7] An engaging and feasible intervention for children and their parents/caregivers that reinforces pediatricians' efforts may potentially be effective in increasing children's sun protection.

A strength of this study conducted by Ho and colleagues is that it evaluated an innovative intervention that leveraged technology (4 weekly text message reminders to caregivers about sun protection) and ongoing pediatrician efforts to improve literacy (distributing a read-along book about sun protection) while providing a sun-protective swim shirt to address the potential barrier of lack of protective clothing. Results show that this multicomponent intervention significantly increased sun protection, although not sunburn rates, in children. The mean differences across sun protection outcomes between intervention and control groups were small, but these positive changes in the desired direction across the population may translate into public health significance, which is important to determine. Further research is critical to examine whether these behavior changes may be sustained past this study's short-term follow-up period.

Although the results are encouraging, the study design did not enable researchers to evaluate the effectiveness of individual intervention components (text messages, read-along book, or swim shirt) or determine which were responsible for the observed behavior changes. The study also would have benefitted from collecting follow-up data to characterize use of the read-along book and swim shirt, rather than relying solely on caregivers' yes/no responses to related questions posed in the weekly text messages, which provided limited information. Authors did not report response rates for text message questions, but described that 62% of caregivers reported reading the book with their child during the first week of intervention and 57.5% reported that their child wore the swim shirt during the third week. Details on frequency of use throughout the intervention period would have enabled analysis of the association between intervention exposure and outcomes. It is critical to better understand how intervention components may have accounted for the observed behavior change, especially if researchers aim to scale up dissemination.

Researchers also did not evaluate the effect of pediatrician counseling on outcomes because pediatricians in the study did not provide verbal sun protection counseling. In 2012, the US Preventive Services Task Force (USPSTF) an independent group of experts in prevention, primary care and evidence-based medicine who evaluate the effectiveness of clinical preventive services, recommended that clinicians counsel children, adolescents, and young adults aged 10 to 24 years who have fair skin about minimizing their ultraviolet (UV) radiation exposure to reduce skin cancer risk.[8] Too few studies were available to determine the effectiveness of counseling parents/guardians to prevent UV exposure in children younger than 10 years; therefore, the USPSTF did not address the effectiveness of counseling parents of young children. In the current study, it is unclear why pediatricians did not provide verbal sun protection counseling.

Researchers reported that some pediatricians gave caregivers Bright Futures handouts containing sun protection information, but they did not describe whether the proportion of pediatricians doing so was balanced across study groups, which may affect results interpretation. Given AAP's recommendation that clinicians provide skin cancer prevention advice during well-child visits, it would have been appropriate for pediatricians to provide verbal sun protection counseling in the context of this study. It is possible that pediatrician counseling could have reinforced the other interventions, leading to improved results.

A noteworthy aspect of this study was the inclusion of reflectance spectrophotometry to assess any changes in melanin levels over the intervention period. Melanin is produced by melanocytes in the skin in response to UV exposure, indicating overexposure to the sun.[1] The study's control group significantly increased their melanin levels on the upper arm compared to the intervention group. Authors discussed that these findings provided biological support for self-report results that showed children in the intervention group were significantly more likely to wear sleeved shirts. However, the exploratory nature of these analyses, which authors acknowledged, and the lack of information on sunscreen or shade coverage of the upper arm, makes it challenging to confirm whether the spectrophotometry findings corroborate self-report in this study. Future research on biologic endpoints, including melanin levels, is warranted.

The study also reminds pediatricians that wearing clothing is an important sun protection strategy. Sunscreen is the most commonly used sun protection method, including by adults for their children.[9] Sunscreen, however, often is not applied in large enough amounts to provide adequate protection and needs to be reapplied frequently. Clothing made of fabrics with a tight weave and wide-brimmed hats offer sun protection without the application issues posed by sunscreen. Wearing clothing and hats, seeking shade, and applying sunscreen are part of an overall program of sun protection advised by many organizations including the AAP.[7]

Overall, this is an interesting study to inform interventions that pediatricians may disseminate to their patients and caregivers, to reinforce sun protection messaging received during the well-child visit. Appealing interventions such as the one evaluated in this study may facilitate the adoption of sun protection behaviors and, importantly, motivate continued practice to develop lifelong habits to reduce skin cancer risk.

M. K. Tripp, PhD, MPH

S. J. Balk, MD

References

1. U.S. Department of Health and Human Services. *The Surgeon General's Call to Action to Prevent Skin Cancer.* Washington, DC: U.S. Department of Health and Human Services, Office of the Surgeon General; 2014, www.surgeongeneral.gov/library/calls/prevent-skin-cancer/call-to-action-prevent-skin-cancer.pdf.
2. Guy GP Jr, Machlin SR, Ekwueme DU, Yabroff KR. Prevalence and costs of skin cancer treatment in the U.S., 2002–2006 and 2007–2011. *Am J Prev Med.* 2015; 48:183-187.
3. Siegel RL, Miller KD, Jemal A. Cancer statistics, 2016. *CA Cancer J Clin.* 2016; 66:7-30.
4. Dennis LK, Vanbeek MJ, Beane Freeman LE, Smith BJ, Dawson DV, Coughlin JA. Sunburns and risk of cutaneous melanoma: does age matter? A comprehensive meta-analysis. *Ann Epidemiol.* 2008;18:614-627.
5. Cokkinides V, Weinstock M, Glanz K, Albano J, Ward E, Thun M. Trends in sunburns, sun protection practices, and attitudes toward sun exposure protection and tanning among US adolescents, 1998–2004. *Pediatrics.* 2006;118:853-864.
6. Dusza SW, Halpern AC, Satagopan JM, et al. Prospective study of sunburn and sun behavior patterns during adolescence. *Pediatrics.* 2012;129:309-317.
7. American Academy of Pediatrics Council on Environmental Health and Section on Dermatology. Policy Statement. Ultraviolet radiation: a hazard to children and adolescents. *Pediatrics.* 2011;127:588-597.
8. Moyer VA, on behalf of the U.S. Preventive Services Task Force. Behavioral counseling to prevent skin cancer: U.S. Preventive Services Task Force recommendation statement. *Ann Intern Med.* 2012;157:59-65.
9. Robinson JK, Rigel DS, Amonette RA. Summertime sun protection used by adults for their children. *J Am Acad Dermatol.* 2000;42:746-753.

Efficacy and Safety of Sirolimus in the Treatment of Complicated Vascular Anomalies

Adams DM, Trenor CC, Hammill AM, et al (Cincinnati Children's Hosp Med Ctr, OH; Boston Children's Hosp and Harvard Med School, MA; et al)
Pediatrics 137:e20153257, 2016

Background and Objectives.—Complicated vascular anomalies have limited therapeutic options and cause significant morbidity and mortality. This Phase II trial enrolled patients with complicated vascular anomalies to determine the efficacy and safety of treatment with sirolimus for 12 courses; each course was defined as 28 days.

Methods.—Treatment consisted of a continuous dosing schedule of oral sirolimus starting at 0.8 mg/m^2 per dose twice daily, with pharmacokinetic-guided target serum trough levels of 10 to 15 ng/mL. The primary outcomes were responsiveness to sirolimus by the end of course 6 (evaluated according to functional impairment score, quality of life, and radiologic assessment) and the incidence of toxicities and/or infection-related deaths.

Results.—Sixty-one patients were enrolled; 57 patients were evaluable for efficacy at the end of course 6, and 53 were evaluable at the end of course 12. No patient had a complete response at the end of course 6 or 12 as anticipated. At the end of course 6, a total of 47 patients had a partial response, 3 patients had stable disease, and 7 patients had progressive disease. Two patients were taken off of study medicine secondary to persistent adverse effects. Grade 3 and higher toxicities attributable to sirolimus included blood/bone marrow toxicity in 27% of patients, gastrointestinal toxicity in 3%, and metabolic/laboratory toxicity in 3%. No toxicity-related deaths occurred.

Conclusions.—Sirolimus was efficacious and well tolerated in these study patients with complicated vascular anomalies. Clinical activity was reported in the majority of the disorders.

▶ Adams et al report the results of a phase II trial to evaluate the efficacy and safety of sirolimus in the treatment of patients with complicated vascular anomalies.[1] Fifty-seven patients between 0 and 31 years of age received oral sirolimus targeted at blood levels between 5 and 15 ng/mL. Most of the underlying diseases were lymphatic (n = 22), venous (n = 13), and mixed malformations (n = 3) and Kaposiform hemangioendotheliomas (KHE) (n = 13). The authors observed a partial response in 47 patients, stable disease in 3 patients, and progressive disease in 7 patients (Fig 1 in the original article). Toxicity seemed to be acceptable; bone marrow toxicity was seen in 27%, gastrointestinal toxicity in 3% and metabolic toxicity was seen in 3% of patients.

The mammalian target of rapamycin (mTOR) is a serine-threonine kinase that regulates cell growth, cell proliferation, and angiogenesis by activation of the vascular endothelial growth factor (VEGF), a known key regulator of angiogenesis and lymphangiogenesis. The anti-angiogenic potential of sirolimus, an inhibitor of mTOR, offers fascinating new treatment options for patients with complicated vascular lesions. For the first time, an effective and well-tolerated systemic treatment option has become available for children with lymphatic and venous malformations. In addition, sirolimus has shown to be effective also in patients with locally aggressive vascular tumors such as KHE and tufted angiomas; thus, avoiding some of the negatives of the cytotoxic first-line therapy (eg, vincristine) in these patients.

Only sporadic case reports or small case series describing the use of sirolimus in vascular anomalies have been published so far.[2,3] This article reports on the largest number of treated patients up to now and suggests considerable clinical importance for the future management of patients with vascular anomalies. In patients with locally aggressive vascular tumors, a paradigm shift might occur from cytotoxic chemotherapy to anti-angiogenic mTOR inhibition. In patients with lymphatic or venous malformations, sirolimus might represent some kind of neoadjuvant therapy preceding and/or enabling further local treatment.

However, a randomized study regarding the efficacy of sirolimus in comparison with the currently used standard of care (eg, vincristine) is lacking in this article. Second, the heterogeneity of patients makes it difficult to draw general conclusions. Finally, the criteria of response in this article could have been defined more precisely. Several questions remain to be answered: What is the optimal dose of sirolimus, and which serum levels should be achieved? What is the optimal duration of treatment with sirolimus? Is there a place of combination therapy with sirolimus and other treatment options (eg, local therapy, cytotoxic drugs)? What is the future role of other mTOR inhibitors (eg, everolimus, temsirolimus, deforolimus) in the management of vascular anomalies? What are the long-term side effects of sirolimus?

Nevertheless, anti-angiogenic therapy with mTOR inhibition might represent a new era in the management of vascular anomalies. However, it must be emphasized that treatment with sirolimus always should be planned within a multidisciplinary approach, and possible side effects of sirolimus should be monitored closely, including infectious and/or metabolic complications.

H. Lackner, MD

References

1. Adams DM, Trenor CC III, Hammill AM, et al. Efficacy and safety of sirolimus in the treatment of complicated vascular anomalies. *Pediatrics*. 2016;137: e20153257.
2. Nadal M, Giraudeau B, Tavernier E, et al. Efficacy and safety of mammalian target of rapamycin inhibitors in vascular anomalies: a systematic review. *Acta Derm Venereol*. 2015;96:448-452.
3. Lackner H, Karastaneva A, Schwinger W, et al. Sirolimus for the treatment of children with various complicated vascular anomalies. *Eur J Pediatr*. 2015;174: 1579-1584.

The Genetic Evolution of Melanoma from Precursor Lesions

Shain AH, Yeh I, Kovalyshyn I, et al (Univ of California, San Francisco (UCSF); Cleveland Clinic, OH; et al)
N Engl J Med 373:1926-1936, 2015

Background.—The pathogenic mutations in melanoma have been largely catalogued; however, the order of their occurrence is not known.

Methods.—We sequenced 293 cancer-relevant genes in 150 areas of 37 primary melanomas and their adjacent precursor lesions. The histopathological spectrum of these areas included unequivocally benign lesions, intermediate lesions, and intraepidermal or invasive melanomas.

Results.—Precursor lesions were initiated by mutations of genes that are known to activate the mitogen-activated protein kinase pathway. Unequivocally benign lesions harbored BRAF V600E mutations exclusively, whereas those categorized as intermediate were enriched for NRAS mutations and additional driver mutations. A total of 77% of areas of intermediate lesions and melanomas in situ harbored TERT promoter mutations, a finding that indicates that these mutations are selected at an unexpectedly early stage of the neoplastic progression. Biallelic inactivation of CDKN2A emerged exclusively in invasive melanomas. PTEN and TP53 mutations were found only in advanced primary melanomas. The point-mutation burden increased from benign through intermediate lesions to melanoma, with a strong signature of the effects of ultraviolet radiation detectable at all evolutionary stages. Copy-number alterations became prevalent only in invasive melanomas. Tumor heterogeneity became apparent in the form of genetically distinct subpopulations as melanomas progressed.

Conclusions.—Our study defined the succession of genetic alterations during melanoma progression, showing distinct evolutionary trajectories for different melanoma subtypes. It identified an intermediate category of melanocytic neoplasia, characterized by the presence of more than one pathogenic genetic alteration and distinctive histopathological features. Finally, our study implicated ultraviolet radiation as a major factor in both the initiation and progression of melanoma. (Funded by the National Institutes of Health and others.)

▶ The bad news? Melanoma in children and adults is often fatal when detected late in the invasive stage.

The good news? Many melanomas are preventable. Most melanomas, if caught early, can be successfully treated and cured. The importance of primary prevention and early detection of melanoma is underscored by Shain et al's article, which elegantly and clearly demonstrates the evolutionary trajectory of benign nevi to invasive melanoma. This group sequenced genes from 150 micro-dissections of benign precursor, intermediate and malignant areas of 37 primary melanomas.

They identified a "progression cascade" of genetic changes from early activation of cell proliferation pathways at initiation to later disruption of critical cell cycle "check-point" genes. The researchers found that the number of mutations at each stage of progression from benign to malignant rose significantly. As the mutational burden increased, so did the heterogeneity of the tumor, with genetically distinct subpopulations within each tumor becoming more apparent at each stage of progression. Importantly, the genetic signature of the effects of UV radiation (UVR) was detectable at every evolutionary stage. In summary, this study defined the succession of genetic alterations during melanoma progression and implicated ultraviolet (UV) radiation as a dominant factor in both the initiation and progression of melanoma. The authors state, "In aggregate, these findings indicate that sun protection should reduce melanoma risk, especially among persons with a high nevus count."

So what does it all mean? How do we tie these laboratory bench findings to how we counsel patients and screen for and diagnose melanoma at the bedside? Although many important messages derive from this research, the clinical bottom line is that the main preventive strategy against melanoma is protection from ultraviolet (UV) light. Pediatric patients accumulate an enormous amount of UV exposure from everyday outdoor activities to beach vacations to the frustratingly popular indoor tanning industry.[1] The known association between UV radiation, in any form, and skin cancer including melanoma, represents a tremendous opportunity for early educational intervention by primary care physicians. There are a few caveats, however. The conventional clinical construct of melanoma, largely derived from adult presentations, may not hold up clinically for children. Although melanoma accounts for very few overall cancers in children, it can be fatal. Early recognition will save lives.

A recent study by Cordoro, et al[2] underscored the notion that pediatric melanoma is not just adult melanoma in arising in kids. It may present clinically, appear histologically, and behave biologically different from its adult counterparts. Patients younger than 20 years old account for 2% and prepubertal patients only 0.4% of all reported melanomas.[3] Although rare, the incidence of childhood melanoma is increasing and may be fatal.[4] Pediatric melanoma can often go undiagnosed due to lack of "classic" presentation, mimicking benign diagnoses (ie, warts, pyogenic granulomas, etc) and a low index of suspicion by the practitioner. This can delay the time to diagnosis, sometimes greater than 1 year.

"ABCDE" is an acronym that represents widely adopted criteria for the visual detection of melanoma and stands for Asymmetry, Border irregularity, Color variegation, Diameter > 6 mm, and Evolution. These criteria often do not apply to the pediatric population, especially to melanomas found in prepubertal children. Thus, a modified ABCDE criteria for children has been proposed to facilitate earlier recognition of melanoma in children and is as follows[2]:

A: Amelanotic

B: Bleeding, Bump

C: Color uniformity

D: De Novo, any Diameter

E: Evolution

In this study, the majority of melanomas, especially in prepubertal children, presented with amelanosis, regular borders, uniform color, and variable diameter and arose de novo without the presence of a precursor lesion. This is very different from the clinical presentation that is classically taught and recalled by the conventional ABCDs. Critically important at the bedside is the awareness of the possibility of amelanotic (lacking pigment) melanoma, a common presentation in prepubertal children.

Practitioners should also be aware of lesional evolution—defined as a change in appearance or symptoms such as itching, scabbing, or bleeding—as a key characteristic of pediatric melanoma. Recent evolution of a lesion was reported and observed in almost 100% of pediatric melanomas in this study. The use of modified criteria in conjunction with the conventional ABCD criteria may facilitate earlier recognition of melanoma in the pediatric population. Early recognition is important because pediatric melanomas often present at more advanced stages. Despite this, the prognosis of pediatric melanoma overall tends to be more favorable than for adult melanomas at similar stages.

Histologically, pediatric melanomas also tended to differ compared with adult counterparts. Pediatric melanoma did not follow the classic adult subtypes of melanoma and were more often found to be Spitzoid, nodular, or unclassifiable variants. These pathologic differences seem to parallel the non-ABCD morphology that is observed clinically. Given the differences in histologic features and that pediatric melanoma cases can arise de novo (in the absence of a precursor lesion), it remains to be determined if the genetic progression cascade identified in Shain et al's study will also apply to pediatric melanoma.

In summary, melanoma occurs in kids and can have a fatal outcome. Melanoma in younger children may not look like "typical" melanoma at all, resulting in delayed diagnosis and potentially poorer outcomes. There is a clear succession of genetic alterations that occur during progression from benign nevi to invasive melanoma. UV radiation is a major factor in all stages of this progression.

So what can you do? Most important, remember that melanoma can and does occur in children and may present with clinical features that are different from conventional adult melanomas. Incorporate the modified ABCDs for children into your examination of individual lesions on the skin. Maintain a high index of suspicion for melanoma when observing a persistent, otherwise unexplained lesion, especially one that has recently evolved in size, appearance, or symptomatology. Be relentless in your educational messaging to patients and families that UV light of any kind—natural or synthetic—is the greatest preventable risk factor for melanoma. Advise strict photoprotection and annual skin examinations, especially for children with risk factors for melanoma such as a family history of melanoma, fair skin, and lots of nevi. Although the chance of a skin lesion on a child being melanoma is small, it is always better to have it checked out. Refer any patient with a suspicious lesion to a dermatologist immediately.

K. M. Cordoro, MD

D. Gupta, MD

References

1. Wehner MR, Chren MM, Nameth D, et al. International prevalence of indoor tanning: a systematic review and meta-analysis. *JAMA Dermatol.* 2014;150:390-400.
2. Cordoro KC, Gupta D, Frieden IJ, Mccalmont T, Kashani-Sabet M. Pediatric melanoma: results of a large cohort study and proposal for modified ABCD criteria for children. *J Am Acad Derm.* 2013;68:913-925.
3. Pappo AS. Melanoma in children and adolescents. *Eur J Cancer.* 2003;39: 2651-2661.
4. Strouse JJ, Fears TR, Tucker MA, Wayne AS. Pediatric melanoma: risk factor and survival analysis of the Surveillance, Epidemiology, and End Results database. *J Clin Oncol.* 2005;23:4735-4741.

8 Emergency Medicine

A Validation Study of the PAWPER (Pediatric Advanced Weight Prediction Tool in the Emergency Room) Tape—A New Weight Estimation Tool

Garcia CM, Meltzer JA, Chan KN, et al (Albert Einstein College of Medicine, Bronx, NY)

J Pediatr 167:173-177, 2015

Objective.—To evaluate the performance of the PAWPER (Pediatric Advanced Weight Prediction in the Emergency Room) tape, a new weight-estimation tool with a modifier for body habitus, in our increasingly obese population.

Study Design.—A convenience sample of children presenting to the pediatric emergency department of an urban public hospital was enrolled. A nurse or doctor assigned the patient a body habitus score and used the PAWPER tape to estimate the weight. The true weight was then recorded for comparison. The estimated weight was considered accurate if it was within 10% of the true weight.

Results. We enrolled 1698 patients; 579 (34%) were overweight or obese. Overall, the estimated weight was accurate for 64% of patients (95% CI 61%-65%). For children with an above-average body habitus, the tape was accurate 50% of the time (95%CI 46%-55%). There was no significant difference in the accuracy of the PAWPER tape for children assessed during medical and trauma resuscitations.

Conclusion.—Although the PAWPER tape may ultimately be useful, its initial performance was not replicated in our population. A simple, accurate method of weight estimation remains elusive (Fig 1).

▶ During a resuscitation, when a critically ill child's weight is unknown and measurement by scale is not possible, accurate weight estimation is crucial. The weight is used to calculate drug dosages, equipment sizes, fluid replacement rates, and defibrillator joules, which are essential components of care in the emergent treatment of a pediatric patient.

Many weight estimation methods can be used, from parental recall or health care provider estimations, to age-based formulas and length-based weight estimation tapes. Of these resuscitation aids, perhaps the most widely used tool, and arguably the gold standard, is a length-based measuring tool called the Broselow Tape.[1] However, studies have shown that with the growing prevalence of obesity in the United States, the Broselow Tape tends to underestimate weight.[2,3] Thus, Wells et al developed the Pediatric Advanced Weight Prediction Tool in the Emergency Room (PAWPER) tape, which takes into account body habitus.

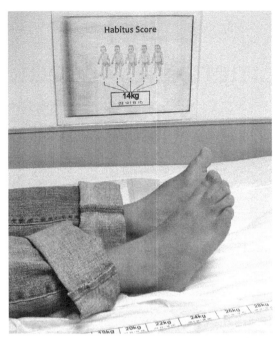

FIGURE 1.—The PAWPER tape in use at the bedside with the HS diagram hanging on the wall. Note the tape has been encased in hard plastic. With permission from Wells et al.[19] *Editor's Note*: Please refer to original journal article for full references. (Reprinted from Garcia CM, Meltzer JA, Chan KN, et al. A validation study of the PAWPER (pediatric advanced weight prediction tool in the emergency room) tape—a new weight estimation tool. *J Pediatr.* 2015;167:173-177, with permission from Elsevier Inc.)

Now, what is the PAWPER tape and how exactly does it work? To give some detail not found in the study: the tape, similar to Broselow, first requires a baseline weight estimation from a supine length. This weight corresponds to the 50th percentile on the World Health Organization weight-for-length growth chart. This baseline weight is then modified according to the body habitus of the child. The habitus score (HS) is chosen by the health care provider by a general visual impression of the child's habitus. This is a 5-point scale that then approximates the weight to the 5th, 25th, 50th, 75th, and 95th percentiles, respectively, for that length (Fig 1).

The authors of this study had a relatively straightforward aim: to validate the PAWPER tape in their population. The methodology and analysis were similar to the original study by Wells et al in order to easily compare results. Population characteristics and indicators of bias and precision were evaluated in the measured weight categories (all patients, ≤12 kg, 12.1–20 kg, >20 kg) and assigned habitus score categories (ie, HS < 3, HS = 3, HS > 3).

Overall, the current version of the PAWPER tape did not perform well, particularly for obese children. For children with an above-average body habitus, the tape was accurate approximately 50% of the time (95% confidence interval 46%–55%).

Of note, it is interesting that the authors of both the original paper[4] and this one grouped patients into categories based on their actual weight in order to examine the tape's ability to estimate a true weight, irrespective of their age or length. By doing so, they evaluated all children in their study who are 10 kg, for example, regardless of whether they are underweight, normal, overweight, or obese for their length, and looked to see how well the tape performed for that weight category. Additionally, they categorized patients by the assigned HS, which is a subjective measure inherent to the tape itself. Instead, perhaps a better alternative might have been to assign groups based on length categories, examine estimated weight versus actual weight within those length categories, and calculate the actual BMI in order to evaluate how the PAWPER tape performed in weight estimation.

An interesting observation was made in this article regarding the assignment of a habitus score. They found that a lower habitus score was often given when in fact the patient was overweight or obese, making a score or 4 or 5 more appropriate. The article suggests that this may be due to effects of living in an overweight society, which alters our perception of what is "normal."

Per current Centers for Disease Control and Prevention reports from 2011–2012, more than one-third of adults, and 17% (12.7 million) of children and adolescents aged 2 to 19 in the United States are not just overweight but obese. In some communities, the prevalence of obesity is even higher.[5] This epidemic clearly presents a challenge in weight estimation. To add one more layer of complexity, some drugs are better dosed using ideal body weight and others using actual body weight. Whether it's a formula, a length-based weight estimation tape, or another tool, the hope is that an accurate method for weight estimation is developed to help us care for critically ill patients presenting to the emergency department. Perhaps with some fine-tuning, the PAWPER tape could be that tool!

Rashida T. Campwala, MD

C. S. Cho, MD, MPH, MEd

References

1. Leten RC, Wears RL, Broselow J, et al. Length-based endotracheal tube and emergency equipment in pediatrics. *Ann Emerg Med.* 1992;21:900-904.
2. Nieman CT, Manacci CF, Super DM, Mancuso C, Fallon WF Jr. Use of the Broselow tape may result in the underresuscitation of children. *Acad Emerg Med.* 2006; 13:1011-1019.
3. Hofer CK, Ganter M, Tucci M, Klaghofer R, Zollinger A. How reliable is length-based determination of body weight and tracheal tube size in the paediatric age group? The Broselow tape reconsidered. *Br J Anaesth.* 2002;88:283-285.
4. Hofer CK, Ganter M, Tucci M, Klaghofer R, Zollinger A. How reliable is length-based determination of body weight and tracheal tube size in the paediatric age group? The Broselow tape reconsidered. *Br J Anaesth.* 2002;88:283-285.
5. Division of Nutrition, Physical Activity, and Obesity, National Center for Chronic Disease Prevention and Health Promotion. Version 2015/06/19. http://www.cdc.gov/obesity/data/childhood.html. Accessed April 11, 2016.

Point-of-Care Ultrasonography for the Diagnosis of Pediatric Soft Tissue Infection

Adams CM, Neuman MI, Levy JA (Boston Childrens Hosp, MA; et al)
J Pediatr 169:122-127.e1, 2016

Objectives.—To determine the test characteristics of point-of-care ultrasonography for the identification of a drainable abscess and to compare the test characteristics of ultrasonography with physical examination. In addition, we sought to measure the extent to which ultrasonography impacts clinical management of children with skin and soft tissue infections (SSTIs).

Study Design.—We performed a prospective study of children with SSTIs evaluated in a pediatric emergency department. Treating physicians recorded their initial impression of whether a drainable abscess was present based on physical examination. Another physician, blinded to the treating physician's assessment, performed an ultrasound study and conveyed their interpretation and recommendations to the treating physician. Any management change was recorded. An abscess was defined as a lesion from which purulent fluid was expressed during a drainage procedure in the emergency department or during the 2- to 5-day follow-up period. We defined a change in management as correct when the ultrasound diagnosis was discordant from physical examination and matched the ultimate lesion classification.

Results.—Of 151 SSTIs evaluated among 148 patients, the sensitivity and specificity of point-of-care ultrasonography for the presence of abscess were 96% (95% CI 90%-99%) and 87% (74%-95%), respectively. The sensitivity and specificity of physical examination for the presence of abscess were 84% (75%-90%) and 60% (44%-73%), respectively. For every 4 ultrasound examinations performed, there was 1 correct change in management.

Conclusions.—Point-of-care ultrasonography demonstrates excellent test characteristics for the identification of skin abscess and has superior test characteristics compared with physical examination alone (Fig 3, Table 2).

▶ Soft tissue infections account for more than 14 million outpatient visits per year in the United States.[1] These lesions fall somewhere on a diagnostic spectrum. At one end there is an abscess, a pus-filled lesion that requires drainage as the primary management. At the other end is a cellulitis, a lesion that will improve with systemic antibiotics alone.

Although we'd like to believe our clinical acumen is such that we can easily and reliably diagnose the lesions that fall along this spectrum based solely on our clinical examination, it's often not that easy.[2] Accuracy is key and misdiagnosis of a cellulitis as an abscess results in an unnecessary (usually painful) drainage procedure; conversely, misdiagnosing an abscess as a cellulitis leads to delays in definitive management and the associated progression of disease. The study by Adams et al adds to the literature regarding an objective, increasingly adopted,

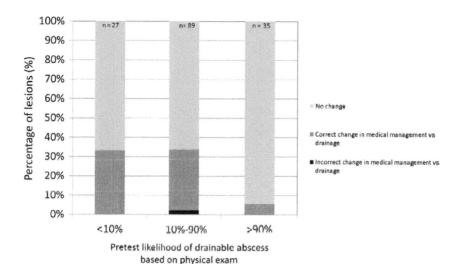

FIGURE 3.—Change in management based on pretest likelihood of abscess. (Reprinted from Adams CM, Neuman MI, Levy JA. Point-of-care ultrasonography for the diagnosis of pediatric soft tissue infection. *J Pediatr.* 2016;169:122-7.e1, with permission from Elsevier Inc.)

metric by which we can evaluate these lesions: point-of-care ultrasound (POCUS).

POCUS use in children, until recently, has been extrapolated from studies and use in adult patients, and POCUS has been part of the general emergency physician's armamentarium for decades. Studies of adults with soft tissue infections show a clear benefit of POCUS over clinical examination alone.[3,4] However, the benefit to pediatric patients has been less apparent.[5-7] The study by Adams et al highlights the higher accuracy of POCUS compared with clinical examination alone (Table 2). In addition, the study compellingly demonstrates that for 1 in every 4 patients with a soft tissue infection, the initial management strategy based on clinical examination alone was changed (appropriately) as a result of the POCUS findings, sparing painful drainage procedures (and often procedural sedations, and the risks associated with them) and leading to a drainage procedure that might not otherwise have been performed (Fig 3).

Only recently, POCUS has become integrated into pediatric emergency medicine (PEM) practice,[8] and most PEM physicians practicing today did not receive POCUS education as part of their training. But we are learning. More pediatric emergency departments are hiring POCUS directors, developing curriculums, and integrating POCUS into clinical care. A POCUS curriculum is part of PEM fellowship training, and POCUS is part of the American Board of Pediatrics subspecialty content for PEM. There are even 1-year PEM POCUS fellowships for those seeking more intensive training.

What about general pediatricians, though? They are often the first to assess soft tissue infections and, based on their examination, have to decide in some cases whether a patient should be referred to a busy emergency department to have a drainage procedure. We cannot necessarily generalize the findings

TABLE 2.—Test Characteristics of Physical Examination and Point-of-Care Ultrasonography Stratified by Pretest Likelihood of a Drainable Abscess

	Sensitivity, % (95% CI)	Specificity, % (95% CI)	PPV (95% CI)	NPV (95% CI)	LR+ (95% CI)	LR− (95% CI)
All lesions (n = 151)						
Physical examination	84 (75-90)	60 (44-73)	82 (73-89)	62 (47-76)	2.1 (1.5-3.0)	0.3 (0.2-0.5)
Point-of-care ultrasonography	96 (90-99)	87 (74-95)	94 (88-98)	91 (79-97)	7.5 (3.6-15.9)	0.04 (0.02-0.1)
High certainty lesions (n = 62)						
Physical examination	84 (69-94)	88 (68-97)	91 (77-98)	78 (58-91)	6.7 (2.3-19.6)	0.2 (0.1-0.4)
Point-of-care ultrasonography	97 (86-100)	96 (79-99)	97 (86-99)	96 (79-99)	23.4 (3.4-159.3)	0.03 (0-0.2)
Equivocal lesions (n = 89)						
Physical examination	83 (72-91)	30 (13-53)	77 (66-87)	39 (17-64)	1.2 (0.9-1.6)	0.6 (0.2-1.2)
Point-of-care ultrasonography	95 (87-99)	78 (56-92)	93 (84-98)	86 (64-97)	4.4 (2.0-9.6)	0.06 (0.02-0.2)

LR−, negative likelihood ratio; LR+, positive likelihood ratio; NPV, negative predictive value; PPV, positive predictive value.
Reprinted from Adams CM, Neuman MI, Levy JA. Point-of-care ultrasonography for the diagnosis of pediatric soft tissue infection. J Pediatr. 2016;169:122-7.e1, with permission from Elsevier Inc.

of Adams et al's to outpatient pediatric practices. Anyone who performs POCUS will tell you: learning POCUS takes time and a lot of practice. Furthermore, the sonologists in Adams et al's study all had significant experience with soft tissue ultrasound. However, it should be asked whether POCUS would be appropriate in the office setting. The use of POCUS in this manner could potentially have a significant impact on resource utilization and alter referral patterns for these patients. It is an area that is certainly ripe for investigation. Nevertheless, we are at a point where we can at least embrace the evidence-based use of POCUS in the emergency department evaluation of pediatric soft tissue infections to improve clinical care.

J. R. Marin, MD, MSc

References

1. Hersh AL, Chambers HF, Maselli JH, Gonzales R. National trends in ambulatory visits and antibiotic prescribing for skin and soft tissue infections. *Arch Intern Med.* 2008;168:1585-1591.
2. Marin JR, Bilker W, Lautenbach E, Alpern ER. Reliability of clinical examinations for pediatric skin and soft-tissue infections. *Pediatrics.* 2010;126:925-930.
3. Tayal VS, Hasan N, Norton HJ, Tomaszewski CA. The effect of soft-tissue ultrasound on the management of cellulitis in the emergency department. *Acad Emerg Med.* 2006;13:384-388.
4. Squire BT, Fox JC, Anderson C. ABSCESS: applied bedside sonography for convenient evaluation of superficial soft tissue infections. *Acad Emerg Med.* 2005; 12:601-606.
5. Iverson K, Haritos D, Thomas R, Kannikeswaran N. The effect of bedside ultrasound on diagnosis and management of soft tissue infections in a pediatric ED. *Am J Emerg Med.* 2012;30:1347-1351.
6. Sivitz AB, Lam SHF, Ramirez-Schrempp D, Valente JH, Nagdev AD. Effect of bedside ultrasound on management of pediatric soft-tissue infection. *J Emerg Med.* 2010;39:637-643.
7. Marin JR, Dean AJ, Bilker WB, Panebianco NL, Brown NJ, Alpern ER. Emergency ultrasound-assisted examination of skin and soft tissue infections in the pediatric emergency department. *Acad Emerg Med.* 2013;20:545-553.
8. American Academy of Pediatrics, Committee on Pediatric Emergency Medicine, Society for Academic Emergency Medicine, Academy of Emergency Ultrasound, American College of Emergency Physicians, Pediatric Emergency Medicine Committee, World Interactive Network Focused on Critical Ultrasound. Policy statement: point-of-care ultrasonography by Pediatric Emergency Medicine Physicians. *Pediatrics.* 2015;135:e1097-e1104.

Effect of Oxygen Desaturations on Subsequent Medical Visits in Infants Discharged From the Emergency Department With Bronchiolitis
Principi T, Coates AL, Parkin PC, et al (The Hosp for Sick Children, Toronto, Ontario, Canada)
JAMA Pediatr 170:602-608, 2016

Importance.—Reliance on pulse oximetry has been associated with increased hospitalizations, prolonged hospital stay, and escalation of care.

Objective.—To examine whether there is a difference in the proportion of unscheduled medical visits within 72 hours of emergency department discharge in infants with bronchiolitis who have oxygen desaturations to lower than 90% for at least 1 minute during home oximetry monitoring vs those without desaturations.

Design, Setting, and Participants.—Prospective cohort study conducted from February 6, 2008, to April 30, 2013, at a tertiary care pediatric emergency department in Toronto, Ontario, Canada, among 118 otherwise healthy infants aged 6 weeks to 12 months discharged home from the emergency department with a diagnosis of acute bronchiolitis.

Main Outcomes and Measures.—The primary outcome was unscheduled medical visits for bronchiolitis, including a visit to any health care professional due to concerns about respiratory symptoms, within 72 hours of discharge in infants with and without desaturations. Secondary outcomes included examination of the severity and duration of the desaturations, delayed hospitalizations within 72 hours of discharge, and the effect of activity on desaturations.

Results.—A total of 118 infants were included (mean [SD] age, 4.5 [2.1] months; 69 male [58%]). During a mean (SD) monitoring period of 19 hours 57 minutes (10 hours 37 minutes), 75 of 118 infants (64%) had at least 1 desaturation event (median continuous duration, 3 minutes 22 seconds; interquartile range, 1 minute 54 seconds to 8 minutes 50 seconds). Among the 118 infants, 59 (50%) had at least 3 desaturations, 12 (10%) had desaturation for more than 10% of the monitored time, and 51 (43%) had desaturations lasting 3 or more minutes continuously. Of the 75 infants who had desaturations, 59 (79%) had desaturation to 80% or less for at least 1 minute and 29 (39%) had desaturation to 70%or less for at least 1 minute. Of the 75 infants with desaturations, 18 (24%) had an unscheduled visit for bronchiolitis as compared with 11 of the 43 infants without desaturation (26%) (difference, −1.6%; 95% CI, −0.15 to ∞; $P = .66$). One of the 75 infants with desaturations (1%) and 2 of the 43 infants without desaturations (5%) were hospitalized within 72 hours (difference, −3.3%; 95% CI, −0.04 to 0.10; $P = .27$). Among the 62 infants with desaturations who had diary information, 48 (77%) experienced them during sleep or while feeding.

Conclusions and Relevance.—The majority of infants with mild bronchiolitis experienced recurrent or sustained desaturations after discharge home. Children with and without desaturations had comparable rates of return for care, with no difference in unscheduled return medical visits and delayed hospitalizations.

▶ Bronchiolitis is common and frustrating for providers and for families. Although much has been tried, such as bronchodilators, hypertonic saline, and corticosteroids, there is really no treatment or strategy to make these miserable infants better faster. Symptomatic care is what we are left with; if they are dehydrated give fluids, if they are hypoxemic give oxygen, and teach all parents to bulb suction. And even with these interventions, there are lingering uncertainties, especially concerning supplemental oxygen. How hypoxemic is too hypoxemic?

As Principi points out, after the introduction of routine pulse oximetry in the 1980s the hospitalization rate for bronchiolitis more than doubled, yet the mortality rate did not change, which is suggestive of overdiagnosis of hypoxemia. Now 30 years later, we still do not have evidence to rationalize this increase in hospitalization; although we know we are still admitting patients based on pulse oximetry.[1] Some feel that oximetry is a proxy for illness severity or risk of decompensation, but where are the data to support this?

The American Academy of Pediatrics has stated in the most recent bronchiolitis guidelines in 2013 that "clinicians may choose not to use continuous pulse oximetry" as a level C recommendation, indicating there are single or few observational studies, or multiple studies but with inconsistent findings.[2] The Choosing Wisely Campaign's 2013 Five Opportunities for Improved Health Care Value in Pediatric Hospital Medicine stated it more forcefully, "Do not use continuous pulse oximetry... unless they are on supplemental oxygen."[3] The evidence cited for these recommendations focused on prolonged hospitalization caused by perceived need for oxygen, avoiding the risks involved in a longer hospitalization, and the lack of evidence that transient desaturation has any adverse outcomes.

In this study, Principi describes a well-designed prospective study in which infants with bronchiolitis were discharged from the emergency room with home oximetry monitoring. Both families and providers were blinded to the oxygen saturation. The aim of the study was to assess whether well-appearing infants with bronchiolitis who experience brief desaturations have worse outcomes than those who do not. The magnitude of desaturations noted is worth highlighting: 65% of the infants enrolled had desaturations (defined as lasting >1 minute) of less than 90%, which may not be a surprise to many pediatricians. However, half of the patients enrolled had desaturations to less than 80%, and 25% had desaturations less than 70%! However, the investigators found no difference in the primary outcome (unscheduled medical visits) or in the secondary outcome (hospitalizations) between children with desaturation and those with no desaturation. Therefore, there is no evidence that well-appearing children with bronchiolitis and intermittent hypoxemia are at risk for adverse events in the short term.

There are still further questions: are these transient episodes of hypoxemia similarly inconsequential in hospitalized infants? Are there any long-term adverse effects of brief periods of hypoxemia? Although we do not yet have all the answers, we now have additional data from a prospective, blinded study to support the recommendations to avoid continuous pulse oximetry in infants with bronchiolitis who have otherwise reassuring examinations, and, more importantly, to reassure providers that transient desaturations in the emergency room or clinic do not always have to trigger hospitalization. Avoidance of unnecessary hospitalization has many potential advantages: reduced costs, reduced risk of nosocomial infections and medication errors, and perhaps most relevant to this study ... less noise from alarming pulse oximeters!

E. B. Burgener, MD

References

1. Mallory MD, Shay DK, Garrett J, Bordley WC. Bronchiolitis management preferences and the influence of pulse oximetry and respiratory rate on the decision to admit. *Pediatrics.* 2003;111:e45-e51.
2. Quinonez RA, Garber MD, Schroeder AR, et al. Choosing wisely in pediatric hospital medicine: Five opportunities for improved healthcare value. *J Hosp Med.* 2013;8:479-485.
3. Ralston SL, Lieberthal AS, Meissner HC, et al. Clinical practice guideline: the diagnosis, management, and prevention of bronchiolitis. *Pediatrics.* 2014;134: e1474-e1502.

Hazards Associated with Sitting and Carrying Devices for Children Two Years and Younger

Batra EK, Midgett JD, Moon RY (Penn State College of Medicine, Hershey, PA; US Consumer Product Safety Commission, Bethesda, MD; Children's Natl Med Ctr, Washington, DC)
J Pediatr 167:183-187, 2015

Objective.—To analyze reported mechanisms of injury and characterize risk factors for infants and young children ≤2 years of age who died in sitting and carrying devices.

Study Design.—A retrospective review of deaths involving sitting and carrying devices (car seats, bouncers, swings, strollers, and slings) reported to the US Consumer Product Safety Commission between 2004 and 2008.

Results.—Of the 47 deaths analyzed, 31 occurred in car seats, 5 in slings, 4 each in swings and bouncers, and 3 in strollers. The reported elapsed time between the last time a child was seen by a caregiver and found deceased varied greatly, with a mean of 26 minutes in slings; 32 minutes in strollers; 140 minutes in car seats; 150 minutes in bouncers; and 300 minutes in swings. The cause of death was asphyxiation in all cases except one. Fifty-two percent of deaths in car seats were attributed to strangulation from straps; the others were attributed to positional asphyxia.

Conclusion.—Infants and children 2 years of age and younger should be properly restrained and not be left unsupervised in sitting and carrying devices. Car seats should not be used as sleeping areas outside of the vehicle, and children should never be in a car seat with unbuckled or partially buckled straps. Infants in slings should have their faces visible and above the edge of the sling, should not have their faces covered by fabric, and their chins should not be compressed into their chests (Tables 1 and 2).

▶ Every year in the United States, approximately 3500 infants under the age of 1 year die from a sleep-related cause, including sudden infant death syndrome (SIDS), suffocation, strangulation, and entrapment.[1] The Back to Sleep Campaign was launched in 1994 to focus attention on the risk of SIDS associated with infants sleeping supine. As a result of widespread educational outreach,

TABLE 1.—Hazards of Sitting and Carrying Devices for Children 2 Years and Younger (Gender and Age Ranges for Each Device)

Device	No.	Male	Female	Unknown	% of Total in Study	Mean Age at Death, mo	Median Age at Death, mo	Age Range
Car seats	31	14	16	1	66	9.7	9	1-24 mo
Slings	5	3	2	0	11	2	1	10 d to 5 mo
Swings	4	3	1	0	9	3.6	2.9	18 d to 8 mo
Bouncers	4	3	1	0	9	2.5	2.5	2-3 mo
Strollers	3	2	1	0	6	5.7	7	2-8 mo
Total	47	25	21	1		7.5	7	

Reprinted from Batra EK, Midgett JD, Moon RY. Hazards associated with sitting and carrying devices for children two years and younger. *J Pediatr.* 2015;167:183-187, with permission from Elsevier.

TABLE 2.—Hazards of Sitting and Carrying Devices for Children 2 Years and Younger (Mean and Median Elapsed Time)

Device	No. Cases with Elapsed Time	Mean Elapsed Time	Median Elapsed Time	Range
Car seats	10	2.3 h	55 min	4 min-11 h
Slings	4	26 min	18 min	10-60 min
Swings	4	5 h	5 h	1-9 h
Bouncers	3	2.5 h	2 h	1.5-4 h
Strollers	3	32 min	30 min	5-60 min

Reprinted from Batra EK, Midgett JD, Moon RY. Hazards associated with sitting and carrying devices for children two years and younger. *J Pediatr.* 2015;167:183-187, with permission from Elsevier.

between 1994 and 1999, there was a greater than 50% reduction in the rate of SIDS concomitant with a doubling in infants being placed supine for sleep.[2] However, after 1999, rates of SIDS remained relatively unchanged, with small declines likely due to a "diagnostic shift" in categorizing the cause of death.[3] Deaths once attributed to SIDS were being attributed to other causes of death such as accidental suffocation or ill-defined or unspecified cause. As a result of this shift, the campaign, now known as Safe to Sleep, expanded its focus to include guidelines for a safe sleep environment to reduce all sleep-related infant deaths.

The American Academy of Pediatrics Task Force on SIDS, in its most recent 2011 policy statement, "SIDS and Other Sleep-related Infant Death: Expansion of Recommendations for a Safe Infant Sleeping Environment," explicitly identified the need to include all sleep-related sudden unexpected infant deaths including suffocation, asphyxia, or entrapment, in addition to SIDS, in its recommendations.[4] The guidelines for a safe sleeping location include the following: (1) using a firm, flat mattress; (2) using a crib, bassinet, portable crib, or play yard that conforms to the safety standards of the Consumer Product Safety Commission (CPSC) and ASTM International (formerly the American Society for Testing and Materials); (3) soft materials or objects such as pillows, quilts, comforters, or sheepskins, even if covered by a sheet, should not be placed under a sleeping infant; and (4) sitting devices, such as car seats, strollers, swings, infant carriers, and infant slings, are not recommended for routine sleep in the hospital or at home. Infants who are younger than 4 months are particularly at risk because they may assume positions that can create risk for suffocation or airway obstruction. When infant slings are used for carrying, it is important to ensure that the infant's head is up and above the fabric, the face is visible, and that the nose and mouth are clear of obstructions.

Despite these clear guidelines, parents continue to place infants in devices that are not intended for sleeping. As described in the publication by Batra et al, 47 deaths of children 2 years of age and younger that occurred in sitting and carrying devices (car seats, swings, bouncers, strollers, and slings) were reported to the US Consumer Product Safety Commission (CPSC) from April 2004 to December 2008.5 As a voluntary reporting system, this number likely represents an underestimation of the true number of deaths that occurred in these devices, but the analysis provides useful information to help understand the circumstances of these events and to illustrate potential mechanisms of injury.

Of the 47 deaths, 66% occurred in car seats. The remainder occurred in slings (11%), swings (9%), bouncers (9%), and strollers (6%) (Table 1). The time between when the infant was last seen alive and discovered ranged from 4 minutes to 11 hours (Table 2), demonstrating that a death from asphyxiation in these devices can occur in just minutes while some infants may be left unattended for dangerously long periods of time. Twenty-seven of the cases had information about why the child had been placed in the device. Seventeen of these indicated that the intention was for the child to fall asleep, 5 were placed in car seats for travel, 4 were to contain the child, and 1 child died after crawling into a car seat that subsequently flipped over.

The cause of death for 46 of the 47 cases was asphyxiation, either from positional asphyxia or strangulation. Of note, 52% of the car-seat deaths were attributed to strangulation from straps and 48% to positional asphyxia. Of the 42 cases found in devices that had restraints or straps (car seats, swings, bouncers, and strollers), 15 had information about whether they were present and used properly. Improper use of the restraints or straps was reported in 10 car-seat cases and 3 stroller cases.

The authors conclude that "most, if not all, of these deaths might have been prevented had the device been used properly and/or had there been adequate supervision." One excellent suggestion made by the authors to help prevent deaths was to encourage manufacturers in designing these devices to make suffocation or strangulation less likely when supervision is not optimal, such as in the design of restraints. Ideally, restraints that are built in and require less parental adjustment would be more effective because caregivers may ignore warnings to from ASTM about the risk of strangulation from improperly buckled straps on certain devices and the need to always use them correctly. The proper use of slings is particularly difficult because it is easy for the infant's airway to become compromised in a short period of time without constant supervision. It is important for caregivers to only use slings that allow them to see the infant's face.

Unfortunately, in those cases studied where the device was used for sleep, the authors were unable to assess the reasons for parents choosing these locations due to lack of data available for such analysis. Given the widespread dissemination of the Safe to Sleep guidelines, clearly there are gaps—parents not receiving the advice about recommended sleep locations for their infants and the hazards of being placed in sitting and carrying devices for sleep (or awake but unattended) or despite knowledge of these recommendations and warnings on products, choosing to use these devices for reasons such as perceived comfort of the infant or nonacceptance that they pose risk. As we continue to expand the recommendations to prevent all sleep-related infant deaths, health professionals who counsel parents and campaigns that promote the guidelines need to include a thorough explanation of the hazards of these devices and ensure that parents have alternatives for safe infant sleep. This article provides powerful examples of these hazards that can be used to strengthen the impact of such educational activities.

F. R. Hauck, MD, MS

References

1. Centers for Disease Control and Prevention. Sudden Unexpected Infant Death and Sudden Infant Death Syndrome. Data and Statistics. http://www.cdc.gov/sids/data.htm. Accessed August 25, 2015.
2. Eunice Kennedy Shriver National Institute of Child Health and Human Development. Safe to Sleep Public Education Campaign. Progress in Reducing SIDS. http://www.nichd.nih.gov/sts/about/SIDS/Pages/progress.aspx. Accessed August 25, 2015.
3. Moon RY. American Academy of Pediatrics Task Force on Sudden Infant Death Syndrome, Technical Report. SIDS and other sleep-related infant deaths: Expansion of recommendations for a safe infant sleeping environment. *Pediatrics.* 2011;128:e1341-e1349.
4. Moon RY. American Academy of Pediatrics Task Force on Sudden Infant Death Syndrome, Policy Statement. SIDS and other sleep-related infant deaths: Expansion of recommendations for a safe infant sleeping environment. *Pediatrics.* 2011;128:1030-1039.

US Poison Control Center Calls for Infants 6 Months of Age and Younger

Kang AM, Brooks DE (Banner—Univ Med Ctr Phoenix, AZ; et al)
Pediatrics 137:e20151865, 2016

Background.—Anticipatory guidance and prevention efforts to decrease poisonings in young children have historically focused on restricting access to minimize exploratory ingestions. Because infants through 6 months of age have limited mobility, such exposures are expected to be less frequent and therapeutic (or dosing) errors should be more frequent. Although recent prevention efforts target some types of therapeutic errors, the epidemiology of these exposures is not well characterized in this age group. This could have important implications for the effectiveness of current prevention efforts.

Methods.—A 10-year (2004–2013) retrospective review of exposure calls for infants through 6 months of age was conducted on National Poison Data System files.

Results.—A total of 271 513 exposures were reported, of which 96.7% were unintentional. Of these, the most common reasons were general unintentional (50.7%), which includes exploratory exposures, and therapeutic error (36.7%). Among the latter, 47.0% involved quantitative dosing errors (a different amount than intended) and 42.8% involved nonquantitative dosing errors (a medication given twice or too soon, the wrong medication, or wrong route). Most exposures (97.5%) occurred in the home but only 85.2% of calls came from the home; 80.4% of self-referrals to a healthcare facility were not admitted.

Conclusions.—General unintentional (including exploratory) exposures and therapeutic errors both comprise a large proportion of calls in this age group. Among therapeutic errors, quantitative and nonquantitative dosing errors are equally concerning. There are appreciable numbers of patients presenting to healthcare prior to poison center consultation. These data can help target future anticipatory guidance and prevention measures.

▶ Anticipatory guidance related to poison prevention typically begins at well-child visits in the second half of the first year of life, once children become more mobile, with poison prevention efforts focused on keeping medications and other potentially harmful substances out of the reach of young children. This article is unique in its focus on children in the first 6 months of life. Using data from the National Poison Data Systems files, which contains information on US Poison Control Center calls, the authors conducted a 10-year retrospective review (covering 2004–2013 and more than 270 000 exposures), to characterize the epidemiology of exposure in this age group and guide future poison prevention efforts.

Prior studies have grouped together findings for all infants < 1 year of age, or have involved a smaller sample size. In infants younger than 6 months of age, one might hypothesize that there would be more therapeutic errors, such as parent errors in dosing a medication, compared with problems related to the exploratory behavior of children, such as unintentional ingestions.

Interestingly, the authors found that "general intentional" errors were most common, representing a little over half of all cases, whereas therapeutic errors accounted for a little more than a third of cases. It is important to point out, however, that the category of "general intentional" errors served as the "default coding" for all poison control center calls and was quite broad, including exploratory ingestions of any product, plant, or object, as well as scenarios in which access was involved (eg, an infant given a medication container to play with; sibling providing a substance to an infant). Exploratory ingestions were not specifically coded for within this category. The authors do note this as a limitation.

Therapeutic errors, on the hand, focused specifically on medication dosing errors. Nearly half of those were noted to be "quantitative" in nature, defined as giving a different dose than intended, while a little more than 40% were considered "nonquantitative," such as when a medication was given too frequently, the wrong medication was administered, or a medication was given via an incorrect route.

The article provides valuable data that enhances our understanding of the epidemiology of poisonings in the United States, which is helpful for both providers and policy makers. The majority of exposures was acute (89%) and involved a single product (98%). Diaper care and rash products were the most common substances involved in unintentional exposures; acetaminophen alone was most commonly involved in therapeutic errors. Of note, ibuprofen exposure frequency increased during the study period, even though it is generally not recommended for infants less than 6 months of age, and over-the-counter packaging does not include dosing information for this age group.

Of particular interest, the authors describe cases in which exposures played a significant role in deaths. Understanding what led to these scenarios is important in the development of strategies to prevent those cases that can lead to the greatest harm. In total, there were 73 infant deaths. Ethanol contributed to the most serious outcomes for unintentional exposures. Combination cough/cold medications and gastrointestinal products contributed to the most major clinical effects with therapeutic errors, followed by acetaminophen, methadone, and systemic antibiotics. The authors provide limited detail about these deaths, however; it would have been helpful to know more. Only a dozen of these cases were described as out-of-hospital general unintentional exposures or therapeutic errors, with the remainder of fatalities including a range of scenarios such as in-hospital therapeutic errors, dog bites, carbon monoxide, and 3 cases of 1-day-old neonates where methamphetamine or phencyclidine were involved.

Luckily, the vast majority of exposures (88%) were not serious and did not require referral to a health care facility. Among the < 10% of patients who were "self-referred" and taken by their caregiver to a health care facility, only about 1 in 10 were admitted. Only approximately 1% of all calls in the sample led to what was considered a "moderate" or "severe" effect or death. These findings suggest that many cases of self-triage to a health care facility were unnecessary and could have been prevented with earlier involvement of the Poison Control Center or another health care provider. The findings support expansion of current anticipatory guidance to include poison prevention counseling earlier in life, potentially beginning at discharge from the nursery. The availability of the Poison Control Center as a resource could be mentioned at that time and reinforced at subsequent well-child visits.

Therapeutic errors due to quantitative errors might be prevented by provision of oral syringes of appropriate size (eg, smallest syringe size to accommodate dose, but not requiring measurement of multiple syringes or instruments), as well as through simplification of dosing instructions such that only 1 unit of measurement is consistently used, with avoidance of vague terms such as teaspoon and tablespoon (using only milliliter is recommended in an American Academy of Pediatrics Policy statement released in 2015). It is less clear, however, what strategies should be employed to address "nonquantitative" dosing errors, such as giving a medication too frequently, although provision of medication "logs" with prescribed medications might be helpful.

In looking at the study findings, it is important to remember some of the limitations of the study. These data come only from Poison Control Center data. As such, the data may be biased toward representing cases of unintentional ingestions, where a parent might feel an urgency to contact their local Poison Control Center. In a situation with a therapeutic error, parents may be more likely to reach out to their health care provider rather than the Poison Control Center, and such data would likely not be captured in this data set. The data hinge on the reliability of the caller. In addition, coding errors by Poison Control Center staff may occur. For example, included in the sample are implausible scenarios of "suspected suicide" and "abuse" that the authors deemed likely to be misclassified. Ultimately, however, this study provides important data to guide poison prevention efforts in families with children less than 6 months of age.

H. S. Yin, MD, MSc

9 Endocrinology

Effect of Metformin Added to Insulin on Glycemic Control Among Overweight/Obese Adolescents with Type 1 Diabetes: A Randomized Clinical Trial

Libman IM, for the T1D Exchange Clinic Network Metformin RCT Study Group (Children's Hosp of Pittsburgh of UPMC, PA; et al)
JAMA 314:2241-2250, 2015

Importance. — Previous studies assessing the effect of metformin on glycemic control in adolescents with type 1 diabetes have produced inconclusive results.

Objective. — To assess the efficacy and safety of metformin as an adjunct to insulin in treating overweight adolescents with type 1 diabetes.

Design, Setting, and Participants. — Multicenter (26 pediatric endocrinology clinics), double-blind, placebo-controlled randomized clinical trial involving 140 adolescents aged 12.1 to 19.6 years (mean [SD] 15.3 [1.7] years) with mean type 1 diabetes duration 7.0 (3.3) years, mean body mass index (BMI) 94th (4) percentile, mean total daily insulin 1.1 (0.2) U/kg, and mean HbA_{1c} 8.8% (0.7%).

Interventions. — Randomization to receive metformin (n = 71) (≤2000 mg/d) or placebo (n = 69).

Main Outcomes and Measures. — Primary outcome was change in HbA_{1c} from baseline to 26 weeks adjusted for baseline HbA_{1c}. Secondary outcomes included change in blinded continuous glucose monitor indices, total daily insulin, BMI, waist circumference, body composition, blood pressure, and lipids.

Results. — Between October 2013 and February 2014, 140 participants were enrolled. Baseline HbA_{1c} was 8.8% in each group. At 13-week follow-up, reduction in HbA_{1c} was greater with metformin (−0.2%) than placebo (0.1%; mean difference, −0.3% [95% CI, −0.6% to 0.0%]; $P = .02$). However, this differential effect was not sustained at 26-week follow up when mean change in HbA_{1c} from baseline was 0.2% in each group (mean difference, 0% [95% CI, −0.3% to 0.3%]; $P = .92$). At 26-week follow-up, total daily insulin per kg of body weight was reduced by at least 25% from baseline among 23% (16) of participants in the metformin group vs 1% (1) of participants in the placebo group (mean difference, 21% [95% CI, 11% to 32%]; $P = .003$), and 24% (17) of participants in the metformin group and 7% (5) of participants in the placebo group had a reduction in BMI z score of 10% or greater from baseline to 26 weeks (mean difference, 17% [95% CI, 5%

to 29%]; $P = .01$). Gastrointestinal adverse events were reported by more participants in the metformin group than in the placebo group (mean difference, 36% [95% CI, 19% to 51%]; $P < .001$).

Conclusions and Relevance.—Among overweight adolescents with type 1 diabetes, the addition of metformin to insulin did not improve glycemic control after 6 months. Of multiple secondary end points, findings favored metformin only for insulin dose and measures of adiposity; conversely, use of metformin resulted in an increased risk for gastrointestinal adverse events. These results do not support prescribing metformin to overweight adolescents with type 1 diabetes to improve glycemic control.

Trial Registration.—clinicaltrials.org Identifier: NCT01881828

▶ For several years, physicians (both adult and pediatric) have been experimenting with the use of metformin as an adjunct therapy in type 1 Diabetes (T1D). We tend to use this in patients who have poor glycemic control despite relatively high insulin doses in whom there is fear of promotion of weight gain if insulin doses are pushed up further. In some patients who try metformin, there is stabilization of weight with some reduction in insulin requirement, and occasionally a small drop in hemoglobin A1c (HbA_{1c}).

This pattern has been replicated in previous small studies of metformin in T1D. The current 26-week randomized controlled trial by Libman et al was well powered to show $> 0.5\%$ change in HbA_{1c} in a group of 140 adolescents (mean age 15 years). The study participants were predominantly white females with baseline HbA_{1c} 8.8%, body mass index z score 1.6, and total daily insulin dose 1.1 units/kg. Although there was absolutely no effect on HbA_{1c}, there was a significant reduction in total daily insulin dose (around 10%), with weight maintenance in the metformin group compared with a 2-kg weight increase in the placebo group. Secondary outcomes included measures of blood pressure (BP), lipids, and inflammatory markers, none of which changed significantly over the course of the study.

The authors concluded that "these results do not support prescribing metformin to adolescents to improve glycemic control." However, there remains a bigger question: whether insulin-sensitizing strategies (healthy lifestyle and/or drugs) can influence longer term outcomes in T1D.

There is increasing epidemiological evidence to suggest that patients with TID who gain excess fat, have raised markers of insulin resistance, and have features of the metabolic syndrome including relatively lower high-density lipoprotein (HDL) cholesterol and higher BP, are at increased risk of a cardiovascular event, in particular, a coronary event. Where insulin resistance has been directly measured in T1D patients using the clamp technique, there is a strong correlation with coronary artery calcification load, a surrogate for ischemic heart disease. When "survivors" of T1D are studied (patients with T1D > 50 years), the phenotype is consistently insulin sensitive.

All of this circumstantial evidence would support the idea that cardiovascular risk in T1D is augmented by a concurrent insulin-resistant phenotype and, therefore, that it might be a good thing for T1D at all age groups to remain as insulin sensitive as possible. The primary approach should be promotion of healthy eating and physical activity, but there may well be a role for drugs such as metformin. Potential target patients for this approach might have (1) central obesity, (2) sedentary lifestyle, (3) relatively high total insulin requirement, (4) relatively low HDL cholesterol, or (5) positive family history of type 2 diabetes in first-degree relatives.

A long-term randomized controlled trial of metformin in T1D patients looking at cardiovascular event outcomes will never be done; the sample size and duration of follow-up would be impractical. However, we may get some useful information from the REMOVAl study (REducing with MetfOrmin Vascular Adverse Lesions in Type 1 Diabetes; clinicaltrials.gov identifier: NCT01483560). This study has recruited adults with T1D > 40 years who have 3 or more cardiovascular risk factors, randomized to metformin or placebo for 3 years. The primary outcome measure is progression of carotid intima-media thickness (a surrogate for atherosclerosis). The results are anticipated in 2017. Although this study may seem far from the minds of pediatric diabetologists, it may help support the belief that insulin-sensitizing strategies may confer long-term benefit in adolescents with T1D, even if there are no obvious short-term benefits in glycemic control.

S. Cleland, MB,ChB, PhD, MRCP, FRCP

The effect of early, comprehensive genomic testing on clinical care in neonatal diabetes: an international cohort study
De Franco E, Flanagan SE, Houghton JA, et al (Univ of Exeter Med School, UK; et al)
Lancet 386:957-963, 2015

Background.—Traditional genetic testing focusses on analysis of one or a few genes according to clinical features; this approach is changing as improved sequencing methods enable simultaneous analysis of several genes. Neonatal diabetes is the presenting feature of many discrete clinical phenotypes defined by different genetic causes. Genetic subtype defines treatment, with improved glycaemic control on sulfonylurea treatment for most patients with potassium channel mutations. We investigated the effect of early, comprehensive testing of all known genetic causes of neonatal diabetes.

Methods.—In this large, international, cohort study, we studied patients with neonatal diabetes diagnosed with diabetes before 6 months of age who were referred from 79 countries. We identified mutations by comprehensive genetic testing including Sanger sequencing, 6q24 methylation analysis, and targeted next-generation sequencing of all known neonatal diabetes genes.

Findings.—Between January, 2000, and August, 2013, genetic testing was done in 1020 patients (571 boys, 449 girls). Mutations in the potassium channel genes were the most common cause (n = 390) of neonatal diabetes, but were identified less frequently in consanguineous families (12% in consanguineous families vs 46% in non-consanguineous families; $p < 0.0001$). Median duration of diabetes at the time of genetic testing decreased from more than 4 years before 2005 to less than 3 months after 2012. Earlier referral for genetic testing affected the clinical phenotype. In patients with genetically diagnosed Wolcott-Rallison syndrome, 23 (88%) of 26 patients tested within 3 months from diagnosis had isolated diabetes, compared with three (17%) of 18 patients referred later (>4 years; $p < 0.0001$), in whom skeletal and liver involvement was common. Similarly, for patients with genetically diagnosed transient neonatal diabetes, the diabetes had remitted in only ten (10%) of 101 patients tested early (<3 months) compared with 60 (100%) of the 60 later referrals ($p < 0.0001$).

Interpretation.—Patients are now referred for genetic testing closer to their presentation with neonatal diabetes. Comprehensive testing of all causes identified causal mutations in more than 80% of cases. The genetic result predicts the best diabetes treatment and development of related features. This model represents a new framework for clinical care with genetic diagnosis preceding development of clinical features and guiding clinical management.

Funding.—Wellcome Trust and Diabetes UK (Fig 1).

▶ She had been dreading the impending meeting with Genetics. Her third child, a son, had just been diagnosed with high sugars and diabetes at 1 month of age, just like her first son 4 years earlier. She hadn't forgotten the Genetics visit with her oldest child. There had been a lot of chatter she hadn't understood, and no one had been able to give them an answer as to why it had happened, although they had taken lots of blood. This time she expected the same. Instead, they talked about a new test. She agreed resignedly that they could do it but didn't hold out hope until she answered a phone call several weeks later. They had the result, and could they also test her older boy? At first she didn't believe them.

In contrast to Sanger sequencing, next-generation sequencing (NGS) enables simultaneous testing of multiple genes, either as a targeted gene list (also known as panel testing) or as an untargeted test interrogating the whole exome or even the whole genome. The ability to target up to an estimated 20 000 genes

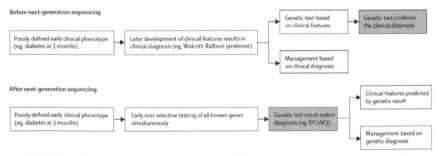

FIGURE 1.—The paradigm shift of genetic testing. Schematic representation of the steps involved in genetic testing before and after the introduction of next-generation sequencing. The red boxes indicate the role of genetic testing. (Reprinted from De Franco E, Flanagan SE, Houghton JA, et al. The effect of early, comprehensive genomic testing on clinical care in neonatal diabetes: an international cohort study. *Lancet.* 2015;386:957-963.)

contained within the exome in a single test or to select specific groups of genes for testing provides extraordinary flexibility. NGS tests can be tailored to almost any clinical scenario, with the only requirement being that the condition or phenotype exhibit genetic heterogeneity, meaning that the condition must be caused by deleterious sequence variants in more than 1 gene.

The adaptability and diagnostic power of NGS is revolutionizing genetic testing and clinical care. NGS simplifies genetic testing and increases the efficiency and cost-effectiveness of screening for common and rare causative genes, thus elevating diagnostic yield. As our knowledge of causative genes improves, relationships between genes and clinical presentations and between genes and treatment efficacy that impact clinical care are described. De Franco et al elegantly demonstrate the clinical utility of panel testing in a rare and imprecise clinical scenario, the development of neonatal diabetes. This condition can be caused by mutations in an impressive list of 21 genes and by methylation abnormalities at chromosome 6q24. Testing of the known pathogenic genes together with methylation status can provide a diagnosis in 82% of patients, a high yield that will undoubtedly increase in the future as the remaining causative genes are identified (Fig 1).

The phenotype of neonatal diabetes may resolve, persist, or evolve with the development of additional hepatic or skeletal findings that can lead to syndrome diagnoses such as Woolcott-Rallison syndrome. Thus, early testing can be clinically useful because it can predict the likelihood of neurological and other complications while patients are asymptomatic. An accurate genetic diagnosis is also particularly relevant to treatment for neonatal diabetes, in which the possibility of a therapeutic change, depending on the underlying genetic diagnosis, can occur in up to 40% of patients who are found to have a mutation in a potassium channel subunit gene, such as *ABCC8* or *KCNJ11*. Family structure may also be relevant to testing strategy because different causative genes are commoner in parents who are consanguineous compared with those who are unrelated.

The high diagnostic yield of NGS in neonatal diabetes and the development of gene-specific, therapeutic strategies have pushed the timing of genetic investigations for this disorder close to the initial presentation because performing the test will likely achieve a genetic diagnosis that has a real possibility of improving medical management. De Franco et al were able to use a targeted panel to dramatically shorten the time required to achieve a diagnosis and then preemptively treat patients with appropriate agents, rather than wait for additional clinical clues to guide therapies after the fact. The possibilities for combining Sanger sequencing for testing common genes with NGS for screening multiple, rarer genes are endless, and panel testing strategies or tiered genetic testing algorithms are being developed for a multitude of genetically heterogeneous conditions. Their usefulness is only likely to grow. As the authors conclude, "This model represents a new framework in which genetic testing defines, rather than just confirms, the clinical diagnosis."

A. Slavotinek, MBBS, PhD

Global Consensus Recommendations on Prevention and Management of Nutritional Rickets

Munns CF, Shaw N, Kiely M, et al (College of Medicine Univ of Lagos, Nigeria; Birmingham Children's Hosp, Birmingham, UK; Univ College Cork, Ireland; et al)

J Clin Endocrinol Metab 101:394-415, 2016

Background.—Vitamin D and calcium deficiencies are common worldwide, causing nutritional rickets and osteomalacia, which have a major impact on health, growth, and development of infants, children, and adolescents; the consequences can be lethal or can last into adulthood. The goals of this evidencebased consensus document are to provide health care professionals with guidance for prevention, diagnosis, and management of nutritional rickets and to provide policy makers with a framework to work toward its eradication.

Evidence.—A systematic literature search examining the definition, diagnosis, treatment, and prevention of nutritional rickets in children was conducted. Evidence-based recommendations were developed using the Grading of Recommendations, Assessment, Development and Evaluation (GRADE) system that describe the strength of the recommendation and the quality of supporting evidence.

Process.—Thirty-three nominated experts in pediatric endocrinology, pediatrics, nutrition, epidemiology, public health, and health economics evaluated the evidence on specific questions within five working groups. The consensus group, representing 11 international scientific organizations, participated in a multiday conference in May 2014 to reach a global evidence-based consensus.

Results.—This consensus document defines nutritional rickets and its diagnostic criteria and describes the clinical management of rickets and osteomalacia. Risk factors, particularly in mothers and infants, are ranked, and specific prevention recommendations including food fortification and supplementation are offered for both the clinical and public health contexts.

Conclusion.—Rickets, osteomalacia, and vitamin D and calcium deficiencies are preventable global public health problems in infants, children, and adolescents. Implementation of international rickets prevention programs, including supplementation and food fortification, is urgently required.

▶ Nutritional rickets is often associated with developing countries located in resource-poor areas of the world. However, recent epidemiologic data suggest that cases of nutritional rickets are increasing in both high- and low-income countries. In the United States, the incidence of nutritional rickets may be as high as 24 cases per 100 000, the majority of which affect the growing immigrant populations originating from Africa, Asia, and the Middle East. Contributors include regional diets that may be low in calcium, such as in West Africa (250–300 mg/day), compared with the average dietary calcium intake in the

United States, which can be as much as 2000 mg/day. However, special diets such dairy-free, vegan, and macrobiotic diets, and soy or rice milk products not specifically formulated for infants or children are additional risk factors for the development of nutritional rickets in infancy and childhood. Furthermore, children with fat malabsorption, liver disease, renal insufficiency, and dependence on total parental nutrition are particularly vulnerable to nutritional rickets. In this era of increased indoor recreation and appropriate sun avoidance and protection, vitamin D deficiency is more relevant than ever. This article presents an important consensus formulated among an impressive multidisciplinary global group of experts regarding prevention and treatment of nutritional rickets.

Nutritional rickets and osteomalacia are disorders of mineralization of the growth plate and osteoid, respectively, that manifest broadly with potentially severe clinical features (Table 1 in the original article). They develop when both calcium and vitamin D intakes are inadequate for a prolonged period of time, leading to parathyroid hormone elevation and impaired phosphate conservation. The interplay between calcium intake and vitamin D status is such that normalcy of either will compensate for insufficiency of the other and maintain integrity of skeletal mineralization (Fig 1 in the original article). Although vitamin D status can be easily determined via serum 25-OH vitamin D levels (Table A), evaluation of adequate calcium intake relies on detailed, regionally specific diet histories. Biochemical data often reveal low levels of serum 25-OH vitamin D, serum phosphorus, serum calcium, and urinary calcium; serum PTH, alkaline phosphatase, and urinary phosphorus levels are typically elevated. Radiographs confirm the diagnosis.

In the past decade, vitamin D supplementation and testing have rapidly emerged at the forefront of both adult and pediatric clinical practice. In 2008, the American Academy of Pediatrics revised its 2003 recommendations for prevention of rickets and vitamin D deficiency in the pediatric population, doubling vitamin D supplementation recommendations and shifting timeframe of initiation to soon after birth for all infants, whether breastfed or formula fed.[1] In 2011, the Institute of Medicine published a report updating its 1997 recommendations that increased its recommended dietary intake of vitamin D and calcium.[2] Also in 2011, the Endocrine Society published clinical practice guidelines regarding diagnosis, treatment, and prevention of vitamin D deficiency.[3] This important updated 2016 global consensus statement is another resource for pediatricians to reference when making recommendations vital to

TABLE A.—Vitamin D Status

	Global Consensus	Institute of Medicine	The Endocrine Society
Vitamin D sufficiency	>20 ng/mL	>20 ng/mL	>30 ng/mL
Vitamin D insufficiency	12-20 ng/mL	12-20 ng/mL	21-29 ng/mL
Vitamin D deficiency	<12 ng/mL	<12 ng/mL	<20 ng/mL
Vitamin D toxicity	>100 ng/mL	>50 ng/mL	>100 ng/mL

Reprinted from Munns CF, Shaw N, Kiely M, et al. Global Consensus Recommendations on Prevention and Management of Nutritional Rickets. *J Clin Endocrinol Metab* 2016;101:394-415, with permission from the Endocrine Society and S. Karger, AG, Basel.

TABLE B.—Recommended Dietary Calcium and Vitamin D Intake

	Vitamin D			Dietary Calcium	
	Global Consensus	Institute of Medicine	The Endocrine Society	Global Consensus	Institute of Medicine
0-6 months	400 IU/day	400 IU/day	400 IU/day	200 mg/day	200 mg/day
6-12 months	400 IU/day	400 IU/day	400 IU/day	260 mg/day	260 mg/day
1-3 years	600 IU/day	600 IU/day	600 IU/day	>500 mg/day	700 mg/day
4-8 years	600 IU/day	600 IU/day	600 IU/day	>500 mg/day	1000 mg/day
9-18 years	600 IU/day	600 IU/day	600 IU/day	>500 mg/day	1300 mg/day

Reprinted from Munns CF, Shaw N, Kiely M, et al. Global Consensus Recommendations on Prevention and Management of Nutritional Rickets. *J Clin Endocrinol Metab* 2016;101:394-415, with permission from the Endocrine Society and S. Karger, AG, Basel.

preventing nutritional rickets and osteomalacia (Table B). Although serum 25-OH vitamin D levels are important when considering a diagnosis of vitamin D deficiency or nutritional rickets, they should not be part of routine screening unless there are particular concerns about these diagnoses. If a diagnosis of nutritional rickets is confirmed, this report offers treatment regimens for nutritional rickets that stress sufficient calcium intake and vitamin D intake that is equivalent to 5 to 10 times the daily maintenance dose for a minimum of 12 weeks. Additional therapeutic option includes "stoss therapy," which is the use of a single high dose of vitamin D (up to 300 000 IU) in lieu of daily dosing. Although there were no significant differences in the rate of improvement of rickets between the 2 dosing strategies, hypercalcemia occurred more frequently in children receiving stoss therapy.

This report is another indispensible set of recommendations to add to your armament of tools to prevent and treat nutritional rickets. The authors make the hopeful case that we will someday be able to eradicate nutritional rickets, as it truly is a preventable disease. Vitamin D deficiency is a major global health issue, and the morbidity and mortality related to nutritional rickets seem unnecessary when we have evidence that simply providing adequate calcium and vitamin D intake is effective in preventing the development of nutritional rickets.

J. Y. Lee, MD, MPH

R. Long, MD

References

1. Wagner CL, Greer FR. American Academy of Pediatrics Section on Breastfeeding, American Academy of Pediatrics Committee on Nutrition. Prevention of rickets and vitamin D deficiency in infants, children, and adolescents. *Pediatrics*. 2008; 122:1142-1152.
2. Institute of Medicine. *Dietary Reference Intakes for Calcium and Vitamin D*. Washington, DC: The National Academies Press; 2011.
3. Holick MF, Binkley NC, Bischoff-Ferrari HA, et al. Evaluation, treatment, and prevention of vitamin D deficiency: an Endocrine Society clinical practice guideline. *J Clin Endocrinol Metab*. 2011;96:1911-1930.

Timing of Puberty in Overweight Versus Obese Boys

Lee JM, Wasserman R, Kaciroti N, et al (Univ of Michigan, Ann Arbor; American Academy of Pediatrics, Elk Grove Village, IL; et al)
Pediatrics 137:e20150164, 2016

Background and Objective.—Studies of the relationship of weight status with timing of puberty in boys have been mixed. This study examined whether overweight and obesity are associated with differences in the timing of puberty in US boys.

Methods.—We reanalyzed recent community-based pubertal data from the American Academy of Pediatrics' Pediatric Research in Office Settings study in which trained clinicians assessed boys 6 to 16 years for height, weight, Tanner stages, testicular volume (TV), and other pubertal variables. We classified children based on BMI as normal weight, overweight, or obese and compared median age at a given Tanner stage or greater by weight class using probit and ordinal probit models and a Bayesian approach.

Results.—Half of boys (49.9%, $n = 1931$) were white, 25.8% ($n = 1000$) were African American, and 24.3% ($n = 941$) were Hispanic. For genital development in white and African American boys across a variety of Tanner stages, we found earlier puberty in overweight compared with normal weight boys, and later puberty in obese compared with overweight, but no significant differences for Hispanics. For TV (≥ 3 mL or ≥ 4 mL), our findings support earlier puberty for overweight compared with normal weight white boys.

Conclusions.—In a large, racially diverse, community-based sample of US boys, we found evidence of earlier puberty for overweight compared with normal or obese, and later puberty for obese boys compared with normal and overweight boys. Additional studies are needed to understand the possible relationships among race/ethnicity, gender, BMI, and the timing of pubertal development.

▶ Lee et al reported that the relationship between timing of puberty in boys and body mass index (BMI), and by association, body fat, may not represent a linear relationship. They noted that overweight boys tended to mature earlier than normal weight and obese boys, but this relationship was not consistent across all stages of puberty, nor completely consistent within race or ethnicity. Are these findings, and the consequent conclusion, reasonable? What are the underlying reasons? How has this influenced relative timing of puberty in boys? Could this trend continue?

Over the past several decades the age of onset of puberty in girls has dropped. The earlier onset of puberty in girls has been linked to greater BMI overall and greater rates of obesity. A recent publication noted that the impact of BMI was greater than race and ethnicity, although race/ethnicity still significantly influenced timing of puberty.[1] Unlike 2 decades ago when a group of experts concluded that there was insufficient evidence that boys were maturing earlier, there is sufficient evidence that boys of the 21st century are maturing earlier than their fathers and grandfathers, and some of the underlying reasons for earlier maturation in girls may affect pubertal timing in boys differently.

Earlier onset of puberty in girls has been related to greater BMI, resulting in greater levels of leptin (the factor necessary but not sufficient for initiation of puberty). The association of BMI and onset of puberty in boys is less consistent. Many studies report earlier onset of pubertal markers with greater BMI; many report later onset with greater BMI, and some report an inconsistent relationship.[2] Both Lee and Boyne[3] have noted the earlier onset of puberty with increasing BMI, until obese status or high mass of adipose tissue[3] are attained.

Greater BMI and fat mass, and some of the underlying reasons for changes in BMI in the population, could influence onset of puberty differently in males, in contrast to females. Overweight boys have greater energy stores than underweight and normal-weight boys and would have greater levels of leptin and potentially earlier onset of puberty. However, mechanisms relating obesity and pubertal onset could be gender specific. Studies have suggested that one reasons obese girls have breast development may be independent of the hypothalamic-pituitary-ovarian axis, through peripheral aromatization of adrenal androgens in the adipose tissue,[4,5] similar to postmenopausal women and similar to the mechanism of estrogen synthesis in males, noted by several researchers in the 1970s.[6]

If these mechanisms occur in peripubertal girls, postmenopausal women, and adult men, why not in obese peripubertal boys who may have reached an adequate mass of adipose tissue? The estrogens so produced would suppress the hypothalamic-pituitary-testicular axis in boys, leading to the delay in onset of puberty.

There is another potential reason for the finding of a nonlinear relationship between BMI and onset of puberty in boys. It is possible that the same environmental exposures that result in greater obesity in boys and girls would have a gender-specific impact on pubertal timing, especially if the chemical exposures belong to one of the groups of endocrine-disrupting chemicals (EDCs). EDCs interfere with hormone biosynthesis or metabolism, or act on hormone receptors; the effect may depend on timing and gender. We, as others, have noted that the families of chemicals identified as estrogenic often act as antiandrogens rather than estrogens.[7] Additionally, some of the EDC groups are obesogens, which modulate peroxisome proliferator-activated receptor-gamma (PPR-gamma, associated with insulin resistance) and aromatase (the enzyme that catalyzes conversion of androgens into estrogens).[8]

Several families of chemicals have been classified as obesogens, such as the organic tins and the phthalates. Phthalates have been noted in epidemiologic studies to be associated with central adiposity and insulin resistance, and both phthalates and organic tins have been reported in laboratory research to upregulate PPR-gamma and to activate adipogenic genes on less differentiated mesenchymal cell lines.[8]

It appears that overall rates of obesity have begun to decline in the United States, in part through public health efforts that have addressed the imbalance between caloric intake and physical activity. However, if a portion of the obesity epidemic is through exposure to obesogens, we will need to identify those obesogens that are very prevalent (such as monobenzyl phthalate), as well as those that are especially potent (such as tributyl tin), and to avoid exposure to these chemicals.

F. M. Biro, MD

References

1. Biro FM, Greenspan LC, Galvez MP, et al. Onset of breast development in a longitudinal cohort. *Pediatrics.* 2013;132:1019-1027.
2. Biro FM, Kiess W. Contemporary trends in onset and completion of puberty, gain in height and adiposity. *Endocr Dev.* 2016;29:122-133.
3. Boyne MS, Thame M, Osmond C, et al. Growth, body composition, and the onset of puberty: longitudinal observations in Afro-Caribbean children. *J Clin Endocrinol Metab.* 2010;95:3194-3200.
4. Aksglaede L, Sorensen K, Petersen JH, Skakkebaek NE, Juul A. Recent decline in age at breast development: the Copenhagen Puberty Study. *Pediatrics.* 2009;123: e932-e939.
5. Biro FM, Pinney SM, Huang B, Baker ER, Chandler DW, Dorn LD. Hormone changes in peripubertal girls. *J Clin Endocrinol Metab.* 2014;99:3829-3835.
6. Santen RJ, Brodie H, Simpson ER, Siiteri PK, Brodie A. History of aromatase: saga of an important biological mediator and therapeutic target. *Endocr Rev.* 2009;30: 343-375.
7. Wolff MS, Teitelbaum SL, McGovern K, et al. Phthalate exposure and pubertal development in a longitudinal study of US girls. *Hum Reprod.* 2014;29:1558-1566.
8. Grun F, Blumberg B. Environmental obesogens: organotins and endocrine disruption via nuclear receptor signaling. *Endocrinology.* 2006;147:50-55.

Is Hypospadias Associated with Prenatal Exposure to Endocrine Disruptors? A French Collaborative Controlled Study of a Cohort of 300 Consecutive Children Without Genetic Defect

Kalfa N, Paris F, Philibert P, et al (CHU de Montpellier et Université Montpellier 1, France; et al)

Eur Urol 68:1023-1030, 2015

Background.—Numerous studies have focused on the association between endocrinedisrupting chemicals (EDCs) and hypospadias. Phenotype variability, the absence of representative comparison groups and concomitant genetic testing prevent any definitive conclusions.

Objective.—To identify the role of occupational and environmental exposures to EDCs in nongenetic isolated hypospadias.

Design, Setting, and Participants.—A total of 408 consecutive children with isolated hypospadias and 302 normal boys were prospectively included (2009—2014) in a multiinstitutional study in the south of France, the area of the country with the highest prevalence of hypospadias surgery.

Outcome Measurements and Statistical Analysis.—In patients without AR, SRD5A2, and MAMLD1 mutations, parental occupational and professional exposures to EDCs were evaluated based on European questionnaire QLK4-1999-01422 and a validated jobexposure matrix for EDCs. Environmental exposure was estimated using the zip code, the type of surrounding hazards, and distance from these hazards. Multivariate analysis was performed.

Results.—Fetal exposure to EDCs around the window of genital differentiation was more frequent in the case of hypospadias (40.00% vs 17.55%, odds ratio 3.13, 95% confidence interval 2.11—4.65). The substances were paints/solvents/adhesives (16.0%), detergents (11.0%), pesticides (9.0%), cosmetics (5.6%), and industrial chemicals (4.0%). Jobs with exposure were more frequent in mothers of hypospadiac boys (19.73% vs 10.26%, $p = 0.0019$), especially cleaners, hairdressers, beauticians, and laboratory workers. Paternal job exposure was more frequent in the cases of hypospadias (40.13% vs 27.48%, $p = 0.02$). Industrial areas, incinerators, and waste areas were more frequent within a 3-km radius for mothers of hypospadiac boys (13.29% vs. 6.64%, $p < 0.00005$). Association of occupational and environmental exposures increases this risk.

Conclusions.—This multicenter prospective controlled study with a homogeneous cohort of hypospadiac boys without genetic defects strongly suggests that EDCs are a risk factor for hypospadias through occupational and environmental exposure during fetal life. The association of various types of exposures may increase this risk.

Patient Summary.—Our multi-institutional study showed that parental professional, occupational, and environmental exposures to chemical products increase the risk of hypospadias in children (Tables 1 and 2).

▶ Hypospadias is the second most common genital anomaly after undescended testes and occurs in approximately 4 in 1000 live male births. Hypospadias ranges from quite mild, characterized by an asymmetric foreskin to severe where the urethral opening is in the perineum, the penis severely curved, and there is associated penoscrotal transposition. In severe hypospadias, there may be a consideration of a diagnosis of a disorder of sexual development.

At present, the etiology of hypospadias remains unknown. The leading hypothesis is that hypospadias is caused by genetic susceptibility and maternal exposure to endocrine disruptors. Present evidence supporting this hypothesis remained retrospective until this unique prospective study by Kalfa et al. This work is from the south of France, which has the highest incidence of hypospadias in that country. The study is unique in that it controls for known genetic causes of hypospadias, separating out patients with genetic mutations in the androgen receptor, 5 alpha reductase, and the *MAMLD1* gene. The remaining patients with isolated hypospadias (without evidence of any other anomalies) were compared with an age-matched control group. The study was appropriately powered. Both the hypospadias group and control group underwent a battery of validated endocrine disruptor, environmental exposure, and occupational exposure questionnaires.

This prospective study design and large cohort of patients with hypospadias and age-matched controls for the first time supply meaningful evidence supporting the hypothesis that adverse maternal exposure to environmental agents can cause hypospadias.

TABLE 1.—Fetal Exposure to Endocrine-Disrupting Chemicals (EDCs) During Pregnancy

Exposure	Group, n (%)		Odds Ratio (95% CI)
	Hypospadias ($n = 300$)	Control ($n = 302$)	
Any EDC			
Exposure	120 (40.00)	53 (17.55)	3.13 (2.11–4.65)
No exposure	180 (60.00)	249 (82.45)	
Paints/solvents			
Exposure	48 (16.00)	15 (4.97)	3.63 (1.94–7.17)
No exposure	252 (84.00)	287 (95.03)	
Detergents			
Exposure	33 (11.00)	17 (5.63)	2.05 (1.08–4.02)
No exposure	267 (89.00)	285 (94.37)	
Pesticides			
Exposure	27 (9.00)	13 (4.30)	2.20 (1.07–4.74)
No exposure	273 (91.00)	289 (95.70)	
Cosmetics			
Exposure	17 (5.67)	7 (2.32)	2.53 (0.98–7.32)
No exposure	283 (94.33)	295 (97.68)	
Other industrial chemicals			
Exposure	12 (4.00)	6 (1.99)	2.05 (0.70–6.76)
No exposure	288 (96.00)	296 (98.01)	
Herbicides			
Exposure	2 (0.67)	2 (0.66)	1.00 (0.07–13.97)
No exposure	298 (99.33)	300 (99.34)	

Reprinted from Kalfa N, Paris F, Philibert P, et al. Is hypospadias associated with prenatal exposure to endocrine disruptors? A French collaborative controlled study of a cohort of 300 consecutive children without genetic defect. Eur Urol. 2015;68:1023-1030, with permission from European Association of Urology.

The agents of concern came from a ubiquitous group of chemical compounds that includes paints, solvents, adhesives, detergents, pesticides, cosmetics, and industrial chemicals (Table 1). Occupation risks include working as a domestic cleaner, hairdresser, beautician, or laboratory workers (Table 2).

Genital development can be divided into 2 stages, hormonal independent or the indifferent stage, which in humans is up to ~8 weeks' gestation. At that time, gonadal differentiation under the influence of *SRY* gene and TDF factor stimulate testicular development and the subsequent production of testosterone and dihydrotestosterone. The penis develops during the hormone-dependent stage from the indifferent external genitalia with complete formation of the urethra, corporal bodies, and glans and circumferential foreskin by ~19 to 20 weeks' gestation. Presumably, endocrine disruptors act during the hormone-dependent stage by interfering with either the production of androgens and androgen precursors or by interfering with the binding of androgens to the androgen receptor. Because many known endocrine disruptors have a similar chemical compositions to androgens (ie, steroids with 4-hexagon carbon rings), the latter mechanism of interfering with the androgen receptor seems the most likely. That the androgen receptor and 5a-reductase type II enzyme are expressed differentially in the stroma and epithelium during penile development also suggest that competition from chemicals mimicking androgens my interfere with normal development. Also consistent with this hypothesis is that in animal models of urethral development, it is known that phthalates, diethylstilbestrol, and synthetic estrogen can all cause hypospadias.

TABLE 2.—Substances Corresponding to Jobs with Exposure for Mothers and Fathers[a]

	Professional exposure, n (%)			
	Maternal		Paternal	
	Hypospadias	Control	Hypospadias	Control
Polyaromatic hydrocarbons	—	1 (0.33)	23 (7.67)	21 (7.00)
Polychlorinated compounds	—	—	—	—
Pesticides	7 (2.33)	6 (1.99)	24 (8.00)	19 (6.33)
Phthalates	11 (3.67)	8 (2.65)	33 (11.00)	14 (4.67)
Organic solvents	47 (15.67)	25 (8.28)	65 (21.67)	39 (13.00)
Bisphenol A	—	—	1 (0.33)	—
Alkylphenolic compounds	38 (64.41)	24 (7.95)	26 (8.67)	17 (5.67)
Flame retardants	—	—	2 (0.67)	—
Metals	7 (12.67)	5 (1.66)	52 (17.33)	44 (14.67)
Miscellaneous	10 (3.33)	5 (1.66)	2 (0.67)	—

Editor's Note: Please refer to original journal article for full references.

[a]Sums may exceed 100% since a job may involve exposure to several chemicals. Correspondence between the type of job and the exposure was established using the data reported by Van Tongeren et al [33,34].

Reprinted from Kalfa N, Paris F, Philibert P, et al. Is hypospadias associated with prenatal exposure to endocrine disruptors? A French collaborative controlled study of a cohort of 300 consecutive children without genetic defect. Eur Urol. 2015;68:1023-1030, with permission from European Association of Urology.

This multi-institutional prospective study has shown that parental professional, occupational, and environmental exposure to chemical products increases the risk of hypospadias in children. What's the next step? Based on the high quality of the study design and the data from this prospective cohort of patients and families with and without hypospadias, it appears that a reasonable approach is to reduce exposure of these potential endocrine disruptors that are associated with hypospadias. These data are also a wake-up call to continue animal and basic science experimentation to identify means to directly test present suspicious endocrine disruptors and newer chemicals as become available. For hypospadias, the best strategy for cure is upfront prevention.

L. S. Baskin, MD

10 Gastroenterology

Manifestations of Cow's-Milk Protein Intolerance in Preterm Infants

Cordova J, Sriram S, Patton T, et al (Univ of Chicago, IL)
J Pediatr Gastroenterol Nutr 62:140-144, 2016

Objectives.—Cow's-milk protein intolerance (CMPI) is poorly recognized in preterm infants. This study examined the clinical events that preceded the diagnosis of CMPI in preterm infants.

Methods.—This was a retrospective study of infants in a level-III neonatal intensive care unit of those who received parenteral nutrition (PN) support during a 12-month period. Parameters assessed included birth weight (g), diagnosis, duration and frequency on PN, type of enteral feeds at initiation, and achievement of enteral autonomy. CMPI was diagnosed based on persistent feeding intolerance that resolved after change of feeds from intact protein to a protein hydrolysate or crystalline amino acid formula.

Results.—Three hundred forty-eight infants with birth weight (median/range) 1618 g (425–5110) received PN. Fifty-one (14%) infants required multiple courses of PN, and 19 of 348 (5%) were diagnosed with CMPI. The requirement for multiple courses on PN versus single course was associated with a high likelihood of CMPI: 14 of 51 versus 5 of 297, $P < 0.001$. Nine of the 14 infants identified with CMPI were initially diagnosed with necrotizing enterocolitis (NEC) after a median duration of 22 days (19–57) on intact protein feeds. After recovery from NEC, they had persistent feeding intolerance including recurrence of "NEC-like illness" (N = 3) that resolved after change of feeds to a protein hydrolysate or crystalline amino acid formula.

Conclusions.—The requirement for multiple courses of PN because of persistent feeding intolerance after recovery from NEC and recurrence of "NEC-like illness" may be a manifestation of CMPI in preterm infants.

▶ Necrotizing enterocolitis (NEC) is clearly not one single disease, as has been suggested in previous reviews.[1,2] The manifestations and final outcome of what has been termed "NEC" in babies with congenital heart disease, such as a hypoplastic left ventricle and/or left-sided cardiac obstructions, clearly undergoes a pathophysiologic cascade that differs from the extremely low birth weight infant who develops the disease at 6 weeks after birth. In the infants with the cardiac anomalies, this is likely to be primarily associated intestinal ischemia, whereas the intestinal necrosis in most preterm infants is related to inflammatory processes, microbial-host interactions, which result in the final pathways leading to intestinal necrosis. Another entity, spontaneous intestinal perforation

(SIP), usually occurs within the first week after birth, is not associated with significant intestinal necrosis, and can no longer be diagnosed as NEC.

Trying to define NEC is therefore a challenge, and use of staging criteria developed in the 1970s should no longer be relevant. What is called Bell Stage 1 "NEC" depends on criteria such as abdominal distension, feeding intolerance (whatever that means), and other clinical signs including apnea and bradycardia. These signs are manifested in almost all extremely low birth weight infants at one time or another during their hospitalization. However, Stage 1 shows no definitive signs of intestinal necrosis, and we have no biomarkers such as pneumatosis intestinalis and portal venous gas that clearly define this entity. Other preterm infants may show signs of abdominal distension or hematochezia, with or without pneumatosis, and respond to a few days of withholding feedings (but are also often treated with antibiotics) and then are able to resume enteral feedings.

Whether these infants actually have NEC has been questioned, and the possibility of a food protein intolerance (FPIES) has previously been raised.[3] These infants may exhibit many of the signs of NEC including pneumatosis intestinalis. Thus, many babies who manifest similar signs are diagnosed as having NEC.

The article by Cordova et al extends on the concept of what is diagnosed as "NEC" as being several different diseases. They retrospectively evaluated 348 preterm infants who received parenteral nutrition (PN) and were admitted to a level III neonatal intensive care unit over a 12-month period. Of these infants, 51 had to undergo multiple bouts of PN; of these 51, 14 received a protein hydrolysate or amino acid formula, and 11 of 51 developed "NEC" or SIP. In the group that only received a single course of PN, only 5 received protein hydrolysate or amino acid formula, a much lower percentage than those undergoing multiple bouts of PN. Unfortunately, the accounting of subjects in this study is challenging and somewhat confusing, and it is not completely clear what criteria were used to make the diagnosis of "NEC." For example, the flow diagram shows 11 cases of NEC/SIP, the text mentions 9 cases of NEC, the table shows 2 cases of SIP, and the flow diagram then again states there were 7 cases of single NEC and 4 of multiple NEC.

Some of the babies who developed "NEC" may have had cow's milk protein intolerance (CMPI) based on the fact that these infants appeared to respond to feeding the protein hydrolysate or amino acid formulas by improved tolerance. This, unfortunately, may be an incorrect inference in that causality was not substantiated. Had these infants been placed back on a cow's milk protein formulation and regressed after the hydrolysate/amino acid formula feeding initiation showed improvement, the point would have been much stronger. However, understandably, if there is an improvement, one does not want to "rock the boat" and cause regression. As stated by the authors in the discussion section the diagnosis of CMPI is also made by a process of exclusion rather than being based on diagnostic laboratory tools.

Nevertheless, despite the challenges faced in proving causality of CMPI in some cases of what we diagnose as NEC, this study aptly raises an important question and as suggested by the authors, requires further, more intensive investigation. The impact of more clearly defining which babies actually have CMPI rather than NEC could lead to considerably less time in the hospital, time on PN, and less use of antibiotics commonly given to infants suspected of having NEC.

J. Neu, MD

References

1. Neu J. Necrotizing enterocolitis: the mystery goes on. *Neonatology.* 2014;106: 289-295.
2. Gordon P, Christensen R, Weitkamp JH, Maheshwari A. Mapping the new world of necrotizing enterocolitis (NEC): review and opinion. *EJ Neonatol Res.* 2012;2: 145-172.
3. Nash M, Russell AB, Holder G, Singh A, Murch S. G120(P) Food protein induced enterocolitis syndrome (fpies) is an important differential diagnosis of necrotizing enterocolitis in preterm infants. *Arch Dis Childhood.* 2015;100:A52.

Validating bifidobacterial species and subspecies identity in commercial probiotic products
Lewis ZT, Shani G, Masarweh CF, et al (Univ of California, Davis et al)
Pediatr Res 79:445-452, 2016

Background.—The ingestion of probiotics to attempt to improve health is increasingly common; however, quality control of some commercial products can be limited. Clinical practice is shifting toward the routine use of probiotics to aid in prevention of necrotizing enterocolitis in premature infants, and probiotic administration to term infants is increasingly common to treat colic and/or prevent atopic disease. Since bifidobacteria dominate the feces of healthy breast-fed infants, they are often included in infant-targeted probiotics.

Methods.—We evaluated 16 probiotic products to determine how well their label claims describe the species of detectable bifidobacteria in the product. Recently developed DNA-based methods were used as a primary means of identification, and were confirmed using culture-based techniques.

Results.—We found that the contents of many bifidobacterial probiotic products differ from the ingredient list, sometimes at a subspecies level. Only 1 of the 16 probiotics perfectly matched its bifidobacterial label claims in all samples tested, and both pill-to-pill and lot-to-lot variation were observed.

Conclusion.—Given the known differences between various bifidobacterial species and subspecies in metabolic capacity and colonization abilities, the prevalence of misidentified bifidobacteria in these products is cause for concern for those involved in clinical trials and consumers of probiotic products (Table 1).

▶ Probiotics are being used clinically, in both reasonably healthy and vulnerable patients.[1] One active area of research is the use of probiotics to prevent necrotizing enterocolitis. Probiotics have been shown to be efficacious,[2] but further research targeted toward optimizing the strain and dose of probiotics continues.

TABLE 1.—Label Claims vs. Observed Polymerase Chain Reaction–Based Results

	B. Longum Subsp. Infantis					B. Longum Subsp. Longum					B. Breve					B. animalis					B. bifidum				
Sample	Label	First Lot First Pill	First Lot Second Pill	Second Lot First Pill	Second Lot Second Pill	Label	First Lot First Pill	First Lot Second Pill	Second Lot First Pill	Second Lot Second Pill	Label	First Lot First Pill	First Lot Second Pill	Second Lot First Pill	Second Lot Second Pill	Label	First Lot First Pill	First Lot Second Pill	Second Lot First Pill	Second Lot Second Pill	Label	First Lot First Pill	First Lot Second Pill	Second Lot First Pill	Second Lot Second Pill
1	X	~									X						X	X	X	X	X	X	X	X	X
2	X	X	X								X						X	X	X	X	X	X	X	X	X
3		~		~												X	X	X	X	X	X	X	X	X	X
4							X	X	X	X									~		X	X	X	X	X
5																X		X	X	X	X	X	X	X	X
6	X					X					X														~
7		~	X	~	~		X	X	~	X	X	~	X		X		X	X	X	X	X	X	X	X	X
8	X	X	X	X	X		X	~	X	X	X	X	X	X	X		X	X	X	X		X	X	X	X
9	X	~														X	X	X	X	X					
10	X	X	X													X	X	X	X	X					
11	X	X	X													X	X	X	X	X					
12	X	~	X	X	X	~						~	X			X	X	N/A	N/A	N/A				N/A	N/A
13	X	X	X	N/A	N/A	X	X	N/A	X	N/A	X			N/A	N/A							N/A	N/A	N/A	N/A
14a	X					X											X								
14b											X														
15	X	~	~	~	~	X	X	X	X	X						X	X	X	N/A	X		N/A	X	N/A	N/A
16	X	X	N/A	N/A	N/A	X	X	N/A	X	N/A				N/A	N/A						X	X	X	N/A	N/A

Species mentioned as present on each label are marked with an X in the label column, along with the species detected in each sample in its column. ~ = present only in trace amounts. N/A = not applicable, no sample tested.

Reprinted from Lewis ZT, Shani G, Masarweh CF, et al. Validating bifidobacterial species and subspecies identity in commercial probiotic products. *Pediatr Res.* 2016;79:445-452, with permission from International Pediatric Research Foundation, Inc.

One type of *Bifidobacterium*, *Bifidobacterium longum* subspecies *infantis*, is especially of interest in such research because it appears to be particularly well suited to growth in the breastfed infant's gut.

A principle in the probiotic field is that health effects of probiotics should be considered strain-specific. Although for the most part this is correct, research in this field has identified characteristics at the species level that may be important to certain clinical effects. With this in mind, it is reasonable to expect that probiotic products be labeled with the correct nomenclature (ie, genus, species, and subspecies) for all strains in the product.

Until now a convenient method to reliably distinguish the *infantis* subspecies from the other *B longum* subspecies has been lacking. Lewis et al report a method to correctly identify *Bifidobacterium* strains to the subspecies level. In particular, this method distinguishes among *B longum* subspecies based on unique genetic loci found therein. They report use of this method to identify the *Bifidobacteria* present in 16 commercial probiotic products. They found that the labels of only 1 of 16 products tested matched the species or subspecies identified by this new method (Table 1). Some products listed species that were not found in the product, the method found species or subspecies that were not listed on the label, and discrepancies were found between different lots of the same product and between different samples from the same lot of the same product. These results suggest that most commercial probiotics containing *Bifidobacteria* did not accurately identify the species and subspecies of *Bifidobacteria* contained in the product.

It is important to put the results of this study in context, especially with regard to limitations of the method and what we can reasonably expect of commercial probiotic suppliers. One limit of the method is that it can only detect *Bifidobacteria* that comprise approximately 5% or more of the total population. The authors demonstrate with their own mock blends that the method cannot detect *Bifidobacteria* that are known to be present but at low levels. Some of the lot-to-lot and pill-to-pill variation observed among many of the products may be due to levels of certain species that hover at the detection limit and not due to large inconsistencies within products. Further, commercial products may contain inhibitors of the polymerase chain reaction reaction on which this method depends, resulting in false-negative results. This drives home the importance of the need for widespread validation of the method.

What should health care providers reasonably expect from commercial probiotic companies? Companies should make a good-faith effort to use the best methods available to properly identify, to the level of genus, species, subspecies, and strain, which probiotics are in their produc.[3] They should make reasonable efforts to update their product labels to be consistent with current nomenclature changes adopted by the scientific community. They should indicate on the product label the strain designation for each strain contained within the probiotic product, and that strain should be consistent over time in the product. Any strain changes made in the product should be accompanied by a strain designation change on the label so that the change is apparent to consumers and health care providers. Companies should be able to identify to the strain level the different probiotics in their product. (Typically, DNA-based methods are available and reliable for strain identification.) Product users should recognize that nomenclature changes on a label that are not accompanied by a strain designation change do not necessarily indicate that the product is different from a previous version.

The authors did not release the names of the products, so it is not possible for clinicians or researchers to know which products were tested. This is an understandable decision by the researchers because this method is new and not yet confirmed by other laboratories. Companies rely on current methods, which this article challenges as inadequate for differentiating *Bifidobacteria* to the subspecies level.

Lewis et al provide an important new method for reliably distinguishing among the subspecies of probiotic *Bifidobacteria*. Once further validated, this method could provide probiotic companies a useful new tool for confirming correct nomenclature for the strains used in their products. Perhaps more important than correct nomenclature, however, is that companies identify probiotics in their product to the strain level and consistently formulate their products with the same strains and doses over time.

This article may lead some to be skeptical about *Bifidobacteria* probiotics. However, many commercialized probiotic strains are well characterized, even down to the full genomic sequence. So a casual reading of this article risks exaggeration of the problem that might exist with commercial products.

Physicians and clinical researchers should restrict probiotic use to products that can demonstrate their manufacture under Good Manufacturing Practices (GMP), required by law for foods and dietary supplements; that are labeled with correct nomenclature to the subspecies level (methods should be disclosed); and that provide strain designations for all strains contained in the product. One action that could facilitate confidence in products would be for industry to begin to utilize high-quality, third-party verification programs. For example, the US Pharmacopeia (USP) offers a USP Verified program for dietary supplements through which properly labeling and adherence to GMP standards is verified. Such verification could be useful to consumers and health care providers in choosing high-quality probiotic products.

M. E. Sanders, PhD

D. J. Merenstein, MD

References

1. Yi SH, Jernigan JA, McDonald LC. Prevalence of probiotic use among inpatients: a descriptive study of 145 U.S. hospitals. *Am J Infect Control.* 2016;44:548-553.
2. AlFaleh K, Anabrees J. Probiotics for prevention of necrotizing enterocolitis in preterm infants. *Cochrane Database Syst Rev.* 2014;(4):CD005496.
3. Hill C, Scott K, Klaenhammer TR, Quigley E, Sanders ME. Probiotic nomenclature matters. *Gut Microbes.* 2016;7:1-2.

Early versus Late Parenteral Nutrition in Critically Ill Children

Fivez T, Kerklaan D, Mesotten D, et al (KU Leuven Univ Hosp, Leuven, Belgium; Erasmus-MC Sophia Children's Hosp, Rotterdam, the Netherlands)
N Engl J Med 374:1111-1122, 2016

Background.—Recent trials have questioned the benefit of early parenteral nutrition in adults. The effect of early parenteral nutrition on clinical outcomes in critically ill children is unclear.

Methods.—We conducted a multicenter, randomized, controlled trial involving 1440 critically ill children to investigate whether withholding parenteral nutrition for 1 week (i.e., providing late parenteral nutrition) in the pediatric intensive care unit (ICU) is clinically superior to providing early parenteral nutrition. Fluid loading was similar in the two groups. The two primary end points were new infection acquired during the ICU stay and the adjusted duration of ICU dependency, as assessed by the number of days in the ICU and as time to discharge alive from ICU. For the 723 patients receiving early parenteral nutrition, parenteral nutrition was initiated within 24 hours after ICU admission, whereas for the 717 patients receiving late parenteral nutrition, parenteral nutrition was not provided until the morning of the 8th day in the ICU. In both groups, enteral nutrition was attempted early and intravenous micronutrients were provided.

Results.—Although mortality was similar in the two groups, the percentage of patients with a new infection was 10.7% in the group receiving late parenteral nutrition, as compared with 18.5% in the group receiving early parenteral nutrition (adjusted odds ratio, 0.48; 95% confidence interval [CI], 0.35 to 0.66). The mean ($\pm$SE) duration of ICU stay was 6.5 $\pm$ 0.4 days in the group receiving late parenteral nutrition, as compared with 9.2 $\pm$ 0.8 days in the group receiving early parenteral nutrition; there was also a higher likelihood of an earlier live discharge from the ICU at any time in the late-parenteral-nutrition group (adjusted hazard ratio, 1.23; 95% CI, 1.11 to 1.37). Late parenteral nutrition was associated with a shorter duration of mechanical ventilatory support than was early parenteral nutrition ($P = 0.001$), as well as a smaller proportion of patients receiving renal-replacement therapy ($P = 0.04$) and a shorter duration of hospital stay ($P = 0.001$). Late parenteral nutrition was also associated with lower plasma levels of γ-glutamyltransferase and alkaline phosphatase than was early parenteral nutrition ($P = 0.001$ and $P = 0.04$, respectively), as well as higher levels of bilirubin ($P = 0.004$) and C-reactive protein ($P = 0.006$).

Conclusions.—In critically ill children, withholding parenteral nutrition for 1 week in the ICU was clinically superior to providing early parenteral nutrition. (Funded by the Flemish Agency for Innovation through Science and Technology and others; ClinicalTrials.gov number, NCT01536275.)

▶ Two nutritional questions that crop up during a pediatric intensive care unit (PICU) admission frequently are: How much should I feed this child? And should I give this child parenteral nutrition (PN)?

A large, multinational, multicenter study attempts to answer the second question. In this study, children who ranged from term neonates to 17 years were randomized to PN on day 1 of admission (early PN) or day 8 of admission (late PN). They found that a series of important outcomes including new infections and length of PICU stay were significantly better in the late PN group. In addition, the late PN group was likely to have an earlier live discharge from the PICU than the early PN group, shorter duration of mechanical ventilation, and lower odds of renal replacement therapy.

Does this mean that all children who are admitted to the PICU can wait for 8 days before being started on PN? Hardly. The first problem with this study is that early PN was started within 24 hours of admission. This is not the norm in most PICUs in the United States. Most studies suggest that enteral nutrition be optimized in critically ill children.[1,2] Even in this study, children were receiving a mean of 30 kcal/kg per day (300 kcal per day) enterally by day 4. One could argue that most of these children could have been sustained enterally using a robust enteral nutrition protocol.[3] Second, as would be expected in most PICUs, children were discharged at healthy rates. Almost 50% of children were discharged from the PICU by day 4 and 74% by day 8. Since only 24% of the late PN cohort was exposed to PN, one could argue that this trial is actually one of early PN versus mostly no PN at all. This would lead one to the one firm conclusion that PN within the first 24 hours of admission is the problem and should not be recommended.

Should anyone at all be given PN between days 1 and 8 of the study? The authors try to make a case that they have included all nutritionally vulnerable populations in the study—term neonates and malnourished children—and that early PN was worse in both populations. It is unclear if there were many malnourished children in the study. The tool used in the study (STRONGkids) has not been validated in critically ill children.[4] Also, evaluation of the body mass index (BMI) z-scores provided in the study suggests that most children were well nourished. Data specifically pertaining to children who were malnourished based on standard anthropometric measures are not provided and extension of the results of this study to malnourished children study only be done with caution. Given that almost 20% of children in PICUs are malnourished, this is a vulnerable population that needs to be given some consideration.[5]

Again, neonates may also be another group that needs to be approached with caution even though premature infants were excluded in this study. In this study, children under 10 kg, were receiving 30 kcal/kg per day enterally by day 4. So this was not a group of neonates that was receiving no enteral nutrition. Since the study does not provide analyses specific to the neonates included in the study, most physicians will rightly continue to remain uncomfortable about delaying PN until day 8 in a neonate that is receiving very little enteral nutrition.

Briefly, this study also fails with regard to how much an individual child should be fed. The equations used by 2 of the 3 institutions in this study have been discredited in critically ill children. Hence, it is likely that children were either under- or overfed throughout this study.

This well-done study answers 1 important question and that is that most children should not receive PN on day 1 of PICU admission. The burning question that we need an answer for is when should PN be initiated if the child is tolerating no enteral nutrition. This study unfortunately provides no answer to that question. Many children can probably be started on parenteral nutrition on day 8 of PICU admission, at a time when three-quarters of PICU admissions would have been discharged. With regard to nutritionally vulnerable populations—term neonates and malnourished children—at this point, enteral nutrition should be first resort and should be aggressively pursued, as it should be in all children in the PICU.

P. S. Goday, MBBS

References

1. Mikhailov TA, Kuhn EM, Manzi J, et al. Early enteral nutrition is associated with lower mortality in critically ill children. *JPEN J Parenter Enteral Nutr.* 2014;38: 459-466.
2. Mehta NM, Bechard LJ, Cahill N, et al. Nutritional practices and their relationship to clinical outcomes in critically ill children—an international multicenter cohort study. *Crit Care Med.* 2012;40:2204-2211.
3. Hamilton S, McAleer DM, Ariagno K, et al. A stepwise enteral nutrition algorithm for critically ill children helps achieve nutrient delivery goals. *Pediatr Crit Care Med.* 2014;15:583-589.
4. Huysentruyt K, Alliet P, Muyshont L, et al. The STRONG(kids) nutritional screening tool in hospitalized children: a validation study. *Nutrition.* 2013;29: 1356-1361.
5. de Betue CT, van Steenselen WN, Hulst JM, et al. Achieving energy goals at day 4 after admission in critically ill children; predictive for outcome? *Clin Nutr.* 2015; 34:115-122.

Early Enteral Nutrition and Aggressive Fluid Resuscitation are Associated with Improved Clinical Outcomes in Acute Pancreatitis
Szabo FK, Fei L, Cruz LA, et al (Cincinnati Children's Hosp Med Ctr, OH)
J Pediatr 167:397-402, 2015

Objectives.—To determine whether recommendations for treatment of acute pancreatitis (AP) in adults impact the outcomes of pediatric AP.

Study Design.—Adult guidelines regarding early management of AP were implemented through an admission order set at Cincinnati Children's Hospital Medical Center at the beginning of the year 2014. Recommendations included administering high rates of intravenous fluid (IVF) within 24 hours of admission and enteral nutrition within 48 hours of admission. A retrospective chart review of AP admissions before and after the implementation of the recommendations was undertaken. Outcomes studied were: hospital length of stay, intensive care unit transfer rates, development of severe AP, pulmonary complications, and readmission rates post discharge from the hospital.

Results.—The study included 201 patients. Children who received feeds within the first 48 hours and received greater than maintenance IVF within 24 hours had a shorter length of stay, less intensive care unit admissions and severe AP rates compared with the patients who remained nil per os during the first 48 hours and received lower rates of IVF.

Conclusion.—Our data support that early enteral nutrition and early aggressive IVF improve outcomes of pediatric AP.

▶ The incidence of acute pancreatitis in children is increasing, occurring in approximately 1 in 10 000 children and creating almost 2-fold higher hospitalization costs than children without acute pancreatitis.[1,2] Traditional acute pancreatitis management has comprised aggressive fluid hydration and prolonged periods of "pancreatic rest" with nil per os (NPO). Reinitiation of feeds has been slow, with gradual transition from clear liquids to soft and then low fat diets over a prolonged period. However, in recent years, there has been growing evidence in adults that initiation of early enteral nutrition (within 48 hours) is safe and decreases mortality and morbidity, including length of hospitalization.[3,4] With these data in hand, pediatric gastroenterologists are questioning whether the same is true for children with acute pancreatitis.

In an effort to address this, Szabo et al undertook a retrospective study to evaluate the impact of early enteral nutrition and aggressive intravenous hydration on pediatric acute pancreatitis outcomes and complications. Building on the initiation of a new admission order set for acute pancreatitis which recommended high rates of intravenous fluids (1.5–2 times maintenance rate) during the first 24 hours and initiation of enteral nutrition within 48 hours of admission, they examined medical records from 201 children to determine whether these recommendations in intravenous fluids and enteral nutrition affected length of hospitalization, incidence of severe acute pancreatitis, and readmission rates. In their study, 75% of patients received enteral nutrition within 48 hours and 50% within 24 hours. Of particular interest is that patients were started on clear liquid diets on admission and advanced to regular diets as early as 6 hours, with no NPO and no use of low fat diets. Although it should be noted that the findings by Szabo et al can only be applied to a subset of those with mild acute pancreatitis because they excluded those with multisystem organ failure, systemic inflammatory response syndrome (SIRS), pancreatic or respiratory complications, trauma, and those with other comorbidities (oncologic disease, cardiac, diabetes, kidney, or surgical conditions), this study stimulates reflection on our current practices.

In this cohort of children with mild acute pancreatitis without complicating comorbidities, the most important contributing factor to improved outcomes was early enteral nutrition, with decreased length of stay, rate of severe acute pancreatitis, and intensive care transfers. Despite earlier discharges, there was no difference in readmission rates based on timing of enteral nutrition. This study corroborates adult data that oral feedings are safe in acute pancreatitis, with no difference between oral versus nasogastric versus nasojejunal feeds.[4,5]

It also adds to evidence in pediatric patients that the composition of the diet (clear liquids vs low fat vs regular) may not be important in outcomes as previously hypothesized.[6] Studies in adults suggest that the benefit from enteral nutrition may be derived from improving intestinal integrity, leading to decreased bacterial translocation and less systemic inflammation.[4] This hypothesis has yet to be examined in children with acute pancreatitis. However, the Szabo et al study does suggest that eating provides a positive therapeutic effect.

In contrast to enteral nutrition, low versus high rates of intravenous fluids made no significant difference in outcomes. Although not statistically significant, the data presented with high rates of intravenous fluids appeared to halve the rates of severe acute pancreatitis in both the NPO and enteral nutrition groups. One caveat of interpreting the low versus high intravenous fluids effects is that they were not the same type of crystalloid solution, with the low being Dextrose 5% ½ normal saline and the high being Dextrose 5% normal saline. Thus, further research examining the best type and rate of intravenous hydration is necessary.

It remains to be seen what the best management of acute pancreatitis is in children with comorbidities or pancreatitis complications. Is aggressive hydration more important in these individuals, who may be more similar to many adults with pancreatitis who have a profound systemic response? What about those with acute recurrent and chronic pancreatitis? We certainly need to better characterize different presentations of pediatric pancreatitis to understand how they differ from adults and help determine the best medical practice.

This study by Szabo et al represents a step forward in identifying treatment strategies for pediatric pancreatitis that will decrease morbidity and minimize the burden of care on families and the health care system. There are several limitations, including being retrospective, it not being a true pre–post intervention analysis, having a relatively narrow patient cohort, and using heterogenous types of intravenous fluids. Additionally, there was no adjustment for severity of illness, and there were some important differences between groups (eg, increased white blood counts in the NPO group), causing one to wonder whether those who received oral feeds were simply less sick. However, the data provide a premise for future prospective trials that can address these limitations. The findings in this article may represent a paradigm shift in pediatrics and will cause many pediatric gastroenterologists to begin questioning their current clinical approach to acute pancreatitis.

K. T. Park, MD

Z. M. Sellers, MD, PhD

References

1. Pohl JF, Uc A. Paediatric pancreatitis. *Curr Opin Gastroenterol.* 2015;31:380-386.
2. Pant C, Deshpande A, Olyaee M, et al. Epidemiology of acute pancreatitis in hospitalized children in the United States from 2000. *PLoS One.* 2014;9:e95552.
3. Eckerwall GE, Tingstedt BB, Bergenzaun PE, Andersson RG. Immediate oral feeding in patients with mild acute pancreatitis is safe and may accelerate recovery—a randomized clinical study. *Clin Nutr.* 2007;26:758-763.
4. Olah A, Romics L Jr. Evidence-based use of enteral nutrition in acute pancreatitis. *Langenbecks Arch Surg.* 2010;395:309-316.

5. Moraes JM, Felga GE, Chebli LA, et al. A full solid diet as the initial meal in mild acute pancreatitis is safe and result in a shorter length of hospitalization: results from a prospective, randomized, controlled, double-blind clinical trial. *J Clin Gastroenterol.* 2010;44:517-522.
6. Abu-El-Haija M, Wilhelm R, Heinzman C, et al. Early enteral nutrition in children with acute pancreatitis. *J Pediatr Gastroenterol Nutr.* 2016;62:453-456.

A Phase 3 Trial of Sebelipase Alfa in Lysosomal Acid Lipase Deficiency

Burton BK, Balwani M, Feillet F, et al (Northwestern Univ Feinberg School of Medicine, Chicago, IL; Icahn School of Medicine, Mount Sinai, NY; Centre Hospitalier Universitaire Brabois—Hopital d'Enfants, Vandoeuvre-les-Nancy, France; et al)

N Engl J Med 373:1010-1020, 2015

Background.—Lysosomal acid lipase is an essential lipid-metabolizing enzyme that breaks down endocytosed lipid particles and regulates lipid metabolism. We conducted a phase 3 trial of enzyme-replacement therapy in children and adults with lysosomal acid lipase deficiency, an underappreciated cause of cirrhosis and severe dyslipidemia.

Methods.—In this multicenter, randomized, double-blind, placebo-controlled study involving 66 patients, we evaluated the safety and effectiveness of enzyme-replacement therapy with sebelipase alfa (administered intravenously at a dose of 1 mg per kilogram of body weight every other week); the placebo-controlled phase of the study was 20 weeks long and was followed by open-label treatment for all patients. The primary end point was normalization of the alanine aminotransferase level. Secondary end points included additional disease-related efficacy assessments, safety, and side-effect profile.

Results.—Substantial disease burden at baseline included a very high level of low-density lipoprotein cholesterol (≥ 190 mg per deciliter) in 38 of 66 patients (58%) and cirrhosis in 10 of 32 patients (31%) who underwent biopsy. A total of 65 of the 66 patients who underwent randomization completed the double-blind portion of the trial and continued with open-label treatment. At 20 weeks, the alanine aminotransferase level was normal in 11 of 36 patients (31%) in the sebelipase alfa group and in 2 of 30 (7%) in the placebo group ($P = 0.03$), with mean changes from baseline of -58 U per liter versus -7 U per liter ($P < 0.001$). With respect to prespecified key secondary efficacy end points, we observed improvements in lipid levels and reduction in hepatic fat content ($P < 0.001$ for all comparisons, except $P = 0.04$ for triglycerides). The number of patients with adverse events was similar in the two groups; most events were mild and were considered by the investigator to be unrelated to treatment.

Conclusions.—Sebelipase alfa therapy resulted in a reduction in multiple disease-related hepatic and lipid abnormalities in children and adults with lysosomal acid lipase deficiency. (Funded by Synageva BioPharma and others; ARISE ClinicalTrials.gov number, NCT01757184.)

▶ Lysosomal acid lipase deficiency (LAL-D) is a rare metabolic disorder formerly known as Wolman disease in infants and cholesterol ester storage disease in children and adults. Wolman disease was named after Moshe Wolman, MD, an Israeli neuropathologist. Characteristic of this disorder are lipid deposits (microvesicular fat) in the liver resulting in early-age cirrhosis; accumulation of fat in the walls of the intestines, which leads to diarrhea; malabsorption and growth failure; and lipid abnormalities that can cause cardiovascular events. In Wolman disease, calcification of the adrenal glands is another pathognomonic finding

In the current article, the results of enzyme replacement therapy for LAL-D are presented. Of note, this enzyme-replacement therapy significantly improved liver and lipid abnormalities proving the efficacy of the drug. In fact, the US Food and Drug Administration (FDA) on December 8, 2015, approved this drug, sebelipase alfa (Kanuma, Alexion Pharmaceuticals, Cheshire, CT) for use in both Wolman disease and cholesterol ester storage disease.[1] The study did not investigate intestinal, cardiovascular, or adrenal manifestations of the disorder.

Although this drug is life-saving for infants with the severe form of this disorder, controversy surrounds the use of this drug in adults with a much milder form of the condition. Clearly, the disease is not rapidly progressive in those individuals who have survived into adulthood. The drug is not cheap; it is estimated to cost approximately $711 000 per year. In fact, Alexion has an assistance program to limit copayments for those in need.[2]

What is interesting about production of this orphan drug is that it is produced in chicken eggs. Recombinant DNA was introduced into hens and the hens produce recombinant LAL in their egg whites. This product is then collected and prepared for the intravenous infusions. The Center for Veterinary Medicine (CVM) approved an application for a recombinant DNA (rDNA) construct in chickens that are genetically engineered (GE) to produce a recombinant form of human lysosomal acid lipase (rhLAL) protein in their egg whites. The FDA regulates GE animals under the new animal drug provisions of the Federal Food, Drug, and Cosmetic Act, because an rDNA construct introduced into an animal to change its structure or function meets the definition of a drug. The Center for Drug Evaluation and Research (CDER) approved the human therapeutic biologic (Kanuma), which is purified from those egg whites, based on its safety and efficacy in humans with LAL deficiency.

As a pediatric hepatologist, it is gratifying to see interest and approvals of orphan drugs for children with rare metabolic diseases such as LAL-D. Not too long ago, there were no treatments available for these patients. Liver transplantation and hematopoietic stem cell transplantation have been used for some of these patients, but long-term results of these procedures in this disorder have not been published.[3] Orphan drug designation provides financial incentives for rare disease drug development such as clinical trial tax credits, user fee waivers, and eligibility for market exclusivity to promote rare disease drug development.

Kanuma was also granted breakthrough therapy designation because it is the first and only treatment available for Wolman disease. The breakthrough therapy designation program encourages the FDA to work collaboratively with sponsors by providing timely advice and interactive communications, to help expedite the development and review of important new drugs for serious or life-threatening conditions. The Kanuma application was also underwent a priority review, which is granted to drug applications that show a significant improvement in safety or effectiveness in the treatment of a serious condition. The manufacturer of Kanuma was granted a rare pediatric disease priority review voucher, a provision intended to encourage development of new drugs and biologics for the prevention and treatment of rare pediatric diseases. Let's hope this voucher is used for the development and approval of a drug for children with another rare and fatal metabolic disorder.

P. Rosenthal, MD

References

1. United States Food and Drug Administration. FDA approves first drug to treat a rare enzyme disorder in pediatric and adult patients. http://www.fda.gov/NewsEvents/Newsroom/PressAnnouncements/ucm476013.htm. Accessed April 3, 2016.
2. Kanuma. http://www.kanuma.com/ Accessed April 3, 2016.
3. Bernstein DL, Hulkova H, Bialer MG, Desnick RJ. Cholesteryl ester storage disease: review of the findings in 135 reported patients with an underdiagnosed disease. *J Hepatol.* 2013;58:1230-1243.

11 Genitourinary Tract

Ibuprofen-associated acute kidney injury in dehydrated children with acute gastroenteritis

Balestracci A, Ezquer M, Elmo ME, et al (Hospital General de Niños Pedro de Elizalde, Ciudad Autónoma de Buenos Aires, Argentina)
Pediatr Nephrol 30:1873-1878, 2015

Background.—Non-steroidal anti-inflammatory drugs (NSAIDs) induce acute kidney injury (AKI) in volume-depleted patients; however the prevalence of this complication is likely underestimated. We assessed the impact of ibuprofen exposure on renal function among dehydrated children with acute gastroenteritis (AGE) to further characterize NSAID-associated AKI.

Methods.—Over a 1-year period dehydrated children with AGE ($n - 105$) were prospectively enrolled and grouped as cases, presenting with AKI ($n = 46$) or controls, not presenting with AKI ($n = 59$). AKI was defined by pediatric RIFLE (pRIFLE) criteria.

Results. Among the children enrolled in the study, AKI prevalence was 44%, and 34 (54%) of the 63 patients who received ibuprofen developed renal impairment. Relative to the controls, children presenting with AKI were younger (median age 0.66 vs. 1.74 years; $p < 0.001$) and received ibuprofen more frequently (74 vs. 49%, $p = 0.01$). After adjusting for the degree of dehydration, ibuprofen exposure remained an independent risk factor for AKI ($p < 0.001$, odds ratio 2.47, 95% confidence interval 1.78–3.42). According to the pRIFLE criteria, 17 patients were at the 'risk' stage of AKI severity, 24 were at the 'injury' stage, and five were at the 'failure' stage; none required dialysis. Distribution of patients within categories was similar regardless of ibuprofen exposure. All cases fulled recovered from AKI.

Conclusions.—Ibuprofen-associated AKI was 54% in our cohort of dehydrated children with AGE. Drug exposure increased the risk for developing AKI by more than twofold, independent of the magnitude of the dehydration.

▶ Ibuprofen is available over the counter and is commonly used by caregivers to treat pain or fever in children. Although ibuprofen is safely used in many children with or without the direction of a medical provider, it is not without risk. A previous single-center study of 1015 children with acute kidney injury (AKI) found that 2.7% of AKI cases were associated with nonsteroidal anti-inflammatory drugs (NSAIDs), primarily ibuprofen. The majority of patients with NSAID-associated AKI (67%) were also volume depleted.[1]

The danger of using NSAIDs in hypovolemic states has been recognized previously, and in the United States, the Food and Drug Administration requires all over-the-counter NSAIDs marketed for children less than 12 years to carry a warning that caregivers should "[a]sk a doctor before use if [...] child has not been drinking fluids, child has lost a lot of fluid due to vomiting or diarrhea [... or] child is taking a diuretic."[2] However, the risk for children who receive NSAIDs while dehydrated was not previously well studied, and data were limited to case series.[3,4] With their recent study, Balestracci et al enhance our understanding of ibuprofen-associated AKI.

In this case-control study, the investigators evaluated children aged 1 month to 18 years hospitalized with acute gastroenteritis over a 1-year period in Buenos Aires for AKI (outcome) and ibuprofen use (exposure). The Pediatric Risk, Injury, Failure, Loss and End-stage kidney disease (pRIFLE) criteria, which are accepted internationally as a way to characterize AKI in children based on serum creatinine and estimated glomerular filtration rate, were used. Ibuprofen use before hospitalization was determined based on the report of the caregiver. The prevalence of AKI in the 105 children meeting inclusion criteria was 44%, with 98% having acute tubular necrosis (ATN) and 2% having biopsy-proven acute interstitial nephritis (AIN).

Exposure to ibuprofen was significantly higher in patients with AKI versus those without (74% vs 49%, $P = .01$). In a multivariate analysis that adjusted for percentage of dehydration, another risk factor for AKI, ibuprofen exposure was associated with 2.47 times increased odds of AKI (95% confidence interval 1.78−3.42). All but 1 patient exhibited rapid recovery of serum creatinine levels with rehydration and withdrawal of ibuprofen. The patient who did not respond was found to have AIN and had normal renal function after 8 days of steroid treatment. The study is limited by lack of patient-specific baseline kidney function data and caregiver report of ibuprofen use, both of which could lead to the misclassification of patients.

Ibuprofen and other NSAIDs exert their anti-inflammatory, antipyretic, and analgesic effects by decreasing prostaglandin (PG) synthesis via the reversible inhibition of cyclooxygenase-1 and -2. Prostaglandins do not have a large effect on renal hemodynamics in euvolemic patients. However, hypovolemia leads to an upregulation of the renin-angiotensin system (RAS), which causes vasoconstriction of the systemic and renal vasculature. To maintain glomerular filtration in the setting of hypovolemia, RAS-mediated vasoconstriction is locally opposed in the kidney by increased intra-renal PG production. This local PG production in the setting of hypovolemia is stimulated in part by sympathetic nervous system stimulation of the kidney and leads to decreased resistance of the afferent arteriole, which supplies the glomerulus. In this setting, PG plays an important role in maintaining adequate perfusion of the kidneys and glomerular filtration. Inhibition of PG synthesis, including in the kidneys, by NSAIDs removes this protective effect and leads to decreased kidney perfusion and glomerular filtration.[5] Ultimately, this can lead to ischemia of the kidney tubular cells, causing ATN, which compounds the decrease in glomerular filtration. Acute tubular necrosis is the mechanism through which most patients in the study by Balestracci sustained AKI.

Less frequently, NSAIDs cause AIN. This is an idiosyncratic reaction, and risk factors for development have not been identified. In medication-related AIN, a medication acts as an antigen that stimulates a cell-mediated response against the kidney. Interstitial infiltration of T-lymphocytes leads to additional inflammatory processes that further amplify the injury to the kidney. Medication-related AIN is most common 2 to 3 weeks after starting a medication, but can occur within hours of initial exposure or after long-term use. There is also no association between medication dose and AIN. Patients who develop AIN should not receive the offending medication again.[6]

In this study, all subjects were reported as returning to normal renal function. However, the lack of baseline kidney function data may have prevented the investigators from determining whether patients with AKI truly recovered to baseline function. Although there are not long-term follow-up data in children who had NSAID-associated kidney injury, AKI in children has been associated with a long-term risk of chronic kidney disease.[7,8] Additionally, evidence from children with cardiopulmonary-bypass-associated AKI found that although these patients did not have conventional evidence of chronic kidney disease, 7 years after cardiopulmonary bypass, they had persistent elevations in novel urinary biomarkers for AKI compared with age-matched cardiopulmonary-bypass patients who did not experience AKI. Although the clinical significance of these elevations is not known, investigators postulated that it may be evidence of subclinical kidney impairment that results from reduced kidney function reserve.[9] Additional study on the long-term effects of AKI, including nephrotoxic-medication-associated AKI, in children is needed.

In this study, Balestracci et al found that in children with acute gastroenteritis and dehydration severe enough to lead to hospitalization, ibuprofen is associated with an increased risk of AKI. For children who receive other nephrotoxic medications, are unable to maintain adequate hydration, and/or may be at increased risk for AKI due to existing chronic diseases, it may be prudent to consider an alternative to ibuprofen, such as acetaminophen, when possible. In patients presenting with AKI, it is important to avoid further exposure to ibuprofen and other nephrotoxic medications as much as possible. It is important for pediatricians and other health care providers to educate patients and caregivers on the risks associated with over-the-counter therapies. Over-the-counter medications can cause harm to children and should only be used when truly needed. Caregivers should always follow labeled warnings and dosing instructions. Although ibuprofen may be safely used in many children, it is not always innocuous.

E. S. Goswami, PharmD
J. J. Fadrowski, MD, MHS

References

1. Misurac JM, Knoderer CA, Leiser JD, Nailescu C, Wilson AC, Andreoli SP. Nonsteroidal anti-inflammatory drugs are an important cause of acute kidney injury in children. *J Pediatr.* 2013;162:1153-1159.

2. U.S. Department of Health and Human Services Food and Drug Administration Center for Drug Evaluation and Research. Guidance for industry: organ-specific warnings: internal analgesic, antipyretic, and antirheumatic drug products for over-the-counter human use – small entity compliance guide. 2010. http://www.fda.gov/downloads/drugs/guidancecomplianceregulatoryinformation/guidances/ucm222733.pdf.
3. Krause I, Cleper R, Eisenstein B, Davidovits M. Acute renal failure with nonsteroidal anti-inflammatory drugs in healthy children. *Pediatr Nephrol.* 2005;20: 1295-1298.
4. John CM, Shukla R, Jones CA. Using NSAID in volume depleted children can precipitate acute renal failure. *Arch Dis Children.* 2007;92:524-526.
5. Patzer L. Nephrotoxicity as a cause of acute kidney injury in children. *Pediatr Nephrol.* 2008;23:2519-2573.
6. Alon US. Tubulointerstitial nephritis. In: Avner ED, Harmon WE, Niaudet P, Yoshikawa N, eds. *Pediatric nephrology.* 6th edition. Berlin: Springer-Verlag; 2009.
7. Askenazi DJ, Feig EI, Graham NM, Hui-Stickle S, Goldstein SL. 3–5 year longitudinal follow-up of pediatric patients after acute renal failure. *Kidney Int.* 2006; 69:184-189.
8. Mammen C, Al Abbas A, Skippen P, et al. Long-term risk of CKD in children surviving episodes of acute kidney injury in the intensive care unit: a prospective cohort study. *Am J Kidney Dis.* 2012;56:523-530.
9. Cooper DS, Claes D, Goldstein SL, et al. Follow-up assessment of injury long-term after acute kidney injury (FRAIL-AKI). *Clin J Am Soc Nephrol.* 2016;11:21-29.

Early Volume Expansion and Outcomes of Hemolytic Uremic Syndrome

Ardissino G, Tel F, Possenti I, et al (Fondazione IRCCS Ca' Granda Ospedale Maggiore Policlinico, Milan, Italy; et al)
Pediatrics 137:e20152153, 2016

Background.—Hemolytic uremic syndrome associated with Shiga toxin–producing *Escherichia coli* (STEC-HUS) is a severe acute illness without specific treatment except supportive care; fluid management is concentrated on preventing fluid overload for patients, who are often oligoanuric. Hemoconcentration at onset is associated with more severe disease, but the benefits of volume expansion after hemolytic uremic syndrome (HUS) onset have not been explored.

Methods.—All the children with STEC-HUS referred to our center between 2012 and 2014 received intravenous infusion targeted at inducing an early volume expansion (+10% of working weight) to restore circulating volume and reduce ischemic or hypoxic tissue damage. The short- and long-term outcomes of these patients were compared with those of 38 historical patients referred to our center during the years immediately before, when fluid intake was routinely restricted.

Results.—Patients undergoing fluid infusion soon after diagnosis showed a mean increase in body weight of 12.5% (vs 0%), had significantly better short-term outcomes with a lower rate of central nervous system involvement (7.9% vs 23.7%, $P =.06$), had less need for renal replacement therapy (26.3% vs 57.9%, $P =.01$) or intensive care support (2.0 vs. 8.5 days, $P =.02$), and needed fewer days of hospitalization (9.0 vs

12.0 days, $P = .03$). Long-term outcomes were also significantly better in terms of renal and extrarenal sequelae (13.2% vs 39.5%, $P = .01$).

Conclusions.—Patients with STEC-HUS had great benefit from early volume expansion. It is speculated that early and generous fluid infusions can reduce thrombus formation and ischemic organ damage, thus having positive effects on both short- and long-term disease outcomes.

▶ Ardissino et al show that children with early hemolytic uremic syndrome (HUS) can, contrary to concerns, tolerate large volumes of isotonic crystalloid (10-15 mL/kg/hour of normal saline to reach an "infused target" weight 7%-10% greater than their estimated preillness weight). This infusion is administered at a point in illness when many are inclined to restrict fluids, but aggressive volume intervention was strongly associated with a decreased rate of dialysis.

The importance of this outcome should not be overlooked: many studies teach that long-term renal sequelae after HUS are related to the need for, and duration of, dialysis during acute HUS[1-12] (dialysis being a proxy for oligoanuria). These data also reinforce the concept that the evolution of renal injury following Shiga toxin-producing *Escherichia coli* (STEC) infections is secondary to renal hypoperfusion and ischemia.

Volume depletion is a major threat to children with HUS. In 1991, Coad et al[13] reported that greater hemoglobin concentrations at presentation with HUS were associated with worse outcomes. Oakes et al[14] demonstrated that fatality in diarrhea-associated HUS was predicted by relative (hematocrit > 23%) hemoconcentration at the time of HUS diagnosis. Ake et al[15] determined that among children with HUS at a regional referral center, those who had received the least amount of pre-HUS intravenous sodium had the highest rates of oligoanuria. Hickey et al corroborated these findings in an 11-site study in the United States and Scotland.[16] Her group also reported that if a child with HUS does not become anuric by day 10 of illness (day 1 is the first calendar day of diarrhea), then that child is highly likely to continue to urinate throughout the episode of HUS. This finding is very useful in volume expansion management, as discussed later in this commentary.

Additional data converge on the conclusion that children with HUS whose kidneys are well perfused before HUS do better than those with greater degrees of volume compromise. Balestracci et al[17] and Ojeda et al[18] have determined that dehydration on admission with HUS, as suggested by elevated hemoglobin concentrations, was a risk factor for severe acute renal injury and for chronic renal injury during and following diarrhea-associated HUS. Mody et al[19] demonstrated again that elevated hemoglobin in the early phases of HUS posed a risk for death. Ardissino et al[20] have previously shown that hemoconcentration is a risk factor for central nervous system complications in HUS.

Ardissino et al find volume expansion during early HUS is associated with few complications, corroborating data from North America.[15,16] Only 3 of the 79 children in these 2 series required ventilator support, and 1 required thoracentesis for a pleural effusion. It is important to note that these HUS complications are common and not necessarily caused by fluid overload. For example, in 37 children with HUS from an era in which pre-HUS volume expansion was not used, serious cardiopulmonary complications (adult respiratory distress syndrome, and/or pleural effusions) occurred in 9.[21]

Clearly, there is value to early recognition of children at risk for HUS, and of aggressive intravenous volume expansion to prevent acute tubular necrosis. However, operationalizing good care requires education and cooperation between many providers and institutions. Here are elements of practice that we believe produce good outcomes:

- *Know the epidemiology in your region so you can identify patients at first encounter.* E coli O157:H7 infections are mostly sporadic, rural, and rare: a primary care doctor in even a high-incidence area can practice many years without encountering an infected patient and for a whole career before 1 such patient develops HUS. Fortunately, most infected patients have acute, painful bloody diarrhea, and their illness is sufficiently severe to warrant presentation to emergency facilities, at least in North America. These venues are less numerous than doctors' offices, staffed by a relatively limited set of providers, and have diagnostic and therapeutic resources to facilitate and accelerate care.

- *Educate the first "evaluators."* The initial presentation of an STEC infection offers an opportunity to provide nephroprotection by intravenous volume expansion. We attempt to reach out to regional centers to help them identify infected children early. The key to successful outreach is education. The most important concept to convey to first-evaluating physicians is that acute bloody diarrhea is a medical emergency. Much like care of myocardial infarctions or strokes, where everyone knows that time injures hearts or brains, we teach that time lost in bloody diarrhea may result in an infarcted kidney. Once this realization is accepted, community management is much easier.

- *Provide directive advice.* We encourage a parsimonious diagnostic approach to children with acute bloody diarrhea, because of our conviction that extraneous testing is more likely to be misleading than helpful and can even delay appropriate treatment. We suggest a circumscribed set of tests: complete blood count (CBC), blood chemistries, and rapid bacterial stool testing. We strongly discourage computed tomography (CT) scans, coagulation studies, lactate dehydrogenase (LDH) determinations, and urinalyses and urine cultures.

- *Open a dialogue with your microbiologist before each E coli season.* Although E coli O157:H7 infections can be profiled clinically (acute, painful bloody diarrhea after 1−3 days of nonbloody but usually painful diarrhea, and rarely with documented fevers in medical settings), microbiologic diagnosis still provides considerable clarity to these illnesses. We urge sorbitol-MacConkey agar screening to detect E coli O157:H7. Indeed, Ake et al[15] found that early microbiologic diagnosis was strongly associated with a milder course of HUS. Laboratories that use toxin assays to screen for the presence of all STEC and only then employ sorbitol-MacConkey agar testing on toxin-positive specimens to determine whether an E coli O157:H7 is present, are offering inferior services to their communities. Rapid nonculture diagnostics that apply nucleic acid testing directly to stool hold promise to accelerate the diagnostic time line.

- *Admit patients with possible or definite STEC infections to hospital, start intravenous volume expansion, and do not use antibiotics.* A child with an

STEC infection, and in particular one caused by *E coli* O157:H7, is at considerable risk for an adverse short-term outcome. Volume expansion early in illness is highly justified and safe. Our protocols are detailed in several publications.[22-25] A comprehensive analysis of the risk of treating STEC infections with antibiotics has recently been published.[26]

- *Maintain lines of communication between referral centers and the institutions where infected children present.* As community institutions identify infected children sooner and more frequently, tertiary centers are obliged to help them provide care. This means being available as telephone consultants, readily accepting transfers, and harmonizing the same message from specialists in gastroenterology, hospital medicine, infectious diseases, and nephrology, who also might be called on for advice. There is a spectrum of capacity in the community to provide the assiduous monitoring that is required when administering pre-HUS volume expansion, so at the earliest suggestion of microangiopathic injury, we encourage transfer to a tertiary center.

- *Concentrate expertise within your own center.* At St. Louis Children's Hospital, the 10 to 20 *E coli* O157:H7—infected patients we treat each year at the diarrhea phase of illness are admitted to a single medical floor. Nurses are experienced in these illnesses, provide consistent and reassuring information to families, and are vigilant for complications. A single set of providers that operates from the same fluid administration playbook provides ideal management for such patients. We believe that pediatric hospitalists or gastroenterologists are best for the integrated care such illnesses require before they either resolve (which occurs in more than 80% of cases) or progress to renal shutdown.

This commonsense, low-tech, approach to STEC infections has, in our hands, been associated with dialysis rates ($\sim30\%$[27]) that are similar to that reported by Ardissino et al. Our outcomes contrast favorably to dialysis rates in recent multicenter series of diarrhea-associated HUS, which remain well over 50%.[16.19] Nonetheless, despite our ability to identify infected children very early in illness, some patients still come to our center with early HUS, having received little or no intravenous volume expansion in the prior week. Even though their serum creatinine concentration is rising, they are still urinating, but they have not reached the 10th day of their illness, a point after which anuria rarely occurs.[16]

The work of Ardissino et al suggests we might be too cautious in providing fluids at this relatively late stage of the "prerenal" phase of HUS. Their data recommend that considerable nephroprotection can be safely and simply provided to such still-urinating children, especially if they have not yet received volume expansion early in illness (as appears to have been the case in this series). As we all work to refine the timing and volume of isotonic crystalloid intravenous therapy for children at risk of impending renal failure, we commend the Milan group for their immense, and elegant, contribution to those of us who manage these patients worldwide.

M. P. Turmelle, MD
P. I. Tarr, MD

References

1. Gianantonio CA, Vitacco M, Mendilaharzu F, Gallo GE, Sojo ET. The hemolytic-uremic syndrome. *Nephron.* 1973;11:174-192.
2. Gianantonio CA, Vitacco M, Mendilaharzu F, Gallo G. The hemolytic-uremic syndrome. Renal status of 76 patients at long-term follow-up. *J Pediatr.* 1968; 72:757-765.
3. Tonshoff B, Sammet A, Sanden I, Mehls O, Waldherr R, Scharer K. Outcome and prognostic determinants in the hemolytic uremic syndrome of children. *Nephron.* 1994;68:63-70.
4. Siegler RL, Pavia AT, Christofferson RD, Milligan MK. A 20-year population-based study of postdiarrheal hemolytic uremic syndrome in Utah. *Pediatrics.* 1994;94:35-40.
5. Mizusawa Y, Pitcher LA, Burke JR, Falk MC, Mizushima W. Survey of haemolytic-uraemic syndrome in Queensland 1979-1995. *Med J Aust.* 1996; 165:188-191.
6. Spizzirri FD, Rahman RC, Bibiloni N, Ruscasso JD, Amoreo OR. Childhood hemolytic uremic syndrome in Argentina: long-term follow-up and prognostic features. *Pediatr Nephrol.* 1997;11:156-160.
7. Mencia Bartolome S, Martinez de Azagra A, de Vicente Aymat A, Monleon Luque M, Casado Flores J. Uremic hemolytic syndrome. Analysis of 43 cases. *An Esp Pediatr.* 1999;50:467-470.
8. Huseman D, Gellermann J, Vollmer I, et al. Long-term prognosis of hemolytic uremic syndrome and effective renal plasma flow. *Pediatr Nephrol.* 1999;13: 672-677.
9. Loirat C. Post-diarrhea hemolytic-uremic syndrome: clinical aspects. *Arch Pediatr.* 2001;8:776s-784s.
10. Garg AX, Suri RS, Barrowman N, et al. Long-term renal prognosis of diarrhea-associated hemolytic uremic syndrome: a systematic review, meta-analysis, and meta-regression. *JAMA.* 2003;290:1360-1370.
11. Oakes RS, Kirkham JK, Nelson RD, Siegler RL. Duration of oliguria and anuria as predictors of chronic renal-related sequelae in post-diarrheal hemolytic uremic syndrome. *Pediatr Nephrol.* 2008;23:1303-1308.
12. Dolislager D, Tune B. The hemolytic-uremic syndrome: spectrum of severity and significance of prodrome. *Am J Dis Child.* 1978;132:55-58.
13. Coad NA, Marshall T, Rowe B, Taylor CM. Changes in the postenteropathic form of the hemolytic uremic syndrome in children. *Clin Nephrol.* 1991;35: 10-16.
14. Oakes RS, Siegler RL, McReynolds MA, Pysher T, Pavia AT. Predictors of fatality in postdiarrheal hemolytic uremic syndrome. *Pediatrics.* 2006;117:1656-1662.
15. Ake JA, Jelacic S, Ciol MA, et al. Relative nephroprotection during *Escherichia coli* O157:H7 infections: association with intravenous volume expansion. *Pediatrics.* 2005;115:e673-e680.
16. Hickey CA, Beattie TJ, Cowieson J, et al. Early volume expansion during diarrhea and relative nephroprotection during subsequent hemolytic uremic syndrome. *Arch Pediatr Adolesc Med.* 2011;165(10):884-889.
17. Balestracci A, Martin SM, Toledo I, Alvarado C, Wainsztein RE. Dehydration at admission increased the need for dialysis in hemolytic uremic syndrome children. *Pediatr Nephrol.* 2012;27:1407-1410.
18. Ojeda JM, Kohout I, Cuestas E. Dehydration upon admission is a risk factor for incomplete recovery of renal function in children with haemolytic uremic syndrome. *Nefrologia.* 2013;33:372-376.
19. Mody RK, Gu W, Griffin PM, et al. Postdiarrheal hemolytic uremic syndrome in United States children: clinical spectrum and predictors of in-hospital death. *J Pediatr.* 2015;166:1022-1029.
20. Ardissino G, Dacco V, Testa S, et al. Hemoconcentration: a major risk factor for neurological involvement in hemolytic uremic syndrome. *Pediatr Nephrol.* 2015; 30:345-352.

21. Brandt JR, Fouser LS, Watkins SL, et al. *Escherichia coli* O 157:H7-associated hemolytic-uremic syndrome after ingestion of contaminated hamburgers. *J Pediatr.* 1994;125:519-526.
22. Ahn CK, Holt NJ, Tarr PI. Shiga-toxin producing *Escherichia coli* and the hemolytic uremic syndrome: what have we learned in the past 25 years? *Adv Exp Med Biol.* 2009;634:1-17.
23. Davis TK, McKee R, Schnadower D, Tarr PI. Treatment of Shiga toxin-producing *Escherichia coli* infections. *Infect Dis Clin North Am.* 2013;27:577-597.
24. Davis TK, Van De Kar NC, Tarr PI. Shiga toxin/verocytotoxin-producing *Escherichia coli* infections: practical clinical perspectives. *Microbiol Spectr.* 2014;2. EHEC-0025-2014.
25. Holtz LR, Neill MA, Tarr PI. Acute bloody diarrhea: a medical emergency for patients of all ages. *Gastroenterology.* 2009;136:1887-1898.
26. Freedman SB, Xie J, Neufeld MS, Hamilton WL, Hartling L, Tarr PI. Alberta Provincial Pediatric Enteric Infection Team (APPETITE). Shiga toxin-producing *Escherichia coli* infection, antibiotics, and risk of developing hemolytic uremic syndrome: a meta-analysis. *Clin Infect Dis.* 2016;62:1251-1258.
27. Wong CS, Mooney JC, Brandt JR, et al. Risk factors for the hemolytic uremic syndrome in children infected with *Escherichia coli* O157:H7: a multivariable analysis. *Clin Infect Dis.* 2012;55:33-41.

Diagnostic Accuracy of the Urinalysis for Urinary Tract Infection in Infants <3 Months of Age

Schroeder AR, Chang PW, Shen MW, et al (Santa Clara Valley Med Ctr, San Jose, CA; Kaiser Permanente Northern California, Oakland, CA; Dell Children's Med Ctr, Austin, TX; et al)
Pediatrics 135:965-971, 2015

Background.—The 2011 American Academy of Pediatrics urinary tract infection (UTI) guideline suggests incorporation of a positive urinalysis (UA) into the definition of UTI. However, concerns linger over UA sensitivity in young infants. Infants with the same pathogenic organism in the blood and urine (bacteremic UTI) have true infections and represent a desirable population for examination of UA sensitivity.

Methods.—We collected UA results on a cross-sectional sample of 276 infants <3 months of age with bacteremic UTI from 11 hospital systems. Sensitivity was calculated on infants who had at least a partial UA performed and had ≥50 000 colony-forming units per milliliter from the urine culture. Specificity was determined by using a random sample of infants from the central study site with negative urine cultures.

Results.—The final sample included 245 infants with bacteremic UTI and 115 infants with negative urine cultures. The sensitivity of leukocyte esterase was 97.6% (95% confidence interval [CI] 94.5%—99.2%) and of pyuria (>3 white blood cells/high-power field) was 96% (95% CI 92.5%—98.1%). Only 1 infant with bacteremic UTI (Group B *Streptococcus*) and a complete UA had an entirely negative UA. In infants with negative urine cultures, leukocyte esterase specificity was 93.9% (95% CI 87.9 − 97.5) and of pyuria was 91.3% (84.6%—95.6%).

Conclusions.—In young infants with bacteremic UTI, UA sensitivity is higher than previous reports in infants with UTI in general. This finding can be explained by spectrum bias or by inclusion of faulty gold standards (contaminants or asymptomatic bacteriuria) in previous studies (Fig 1).

▶ There has been a long-standing debate regarding the necessity of an abnormal urinalysis, and specifically, the requirement that pyuria be present, when diagnosing urinary tract infections (UTI).[1] Most bacterial infections, including UTIs, are characterized by an inflammatory response. However, previous studies have consistently found that approximately 10% to 30% of children with UTI lack pyuria.[2] Schroeder et al hypothesized that this paradoxical finding could be due to misclassification of children with asymptomatic bacteriuria or contamination as having "true UTIs." To this end, the authors examined a population of neonates with both bacteremia and a positive urine culture, and found that > 96% of such children exhibited pyuria. Because pyuria was present in virtually all cases with true UTI, this was interpreted as support for the idea that pyuria should always be required when diagnosing a UTI. A second important finding reported by Schroeder et al was that approximately 5% of children with true UTIs (ie, with *Escherichia coli* bacteriuria, pyuria, and bacteremia) had colony counts less that 50000 colony forming units (CFU) per milliliter, which is generally used as the standard for a positive culture from a specimen obtained by bladder catheterization.

	Ideal world: No asymptomatic bacteriuria or contamination present				Read world: asymptomatic bacteriuria and contamination present**		
		True UTI				Observed UTI	
		Yes	No			Yes	No
Prevalence of UTI 5%	Pyuria	48	48		Pyuria	48	46
	No pyuria	2£	902		No pyuria	27¥	879
	Row Total	50	950		Row Total	75	925
		True UTI				Observed UTI	
		Yes	No			Yes	No
Prevalence of UTI 20%¥	Pyuria	192	40		Pyuria	192	39
	No pyuria	8£	760		No pyuria	33¥	736
	Row Total	200	800		Row Total	225	775

FIGURE 1.—Two by two tables in low- and high-risk populations according to presence of asymptomatic bacteriuria* and contamination§ assuming that the sensitivity and specificity of pyuria are 96% and 95%, respectively.* Previous population studies have found that 1% of asymptomatic children have bacteriuria confirmed by a suprapubic aspiration sometime during the first year of life; the point prevalence of bacteriuria, however, is never more than 0.5% (and often closer to 0.25%).[11][§] One previous small study of children undergoing both catheterization and suprapubic aspiration found that, approximately 2% of the time, catheterization could yield growth of uropathogens >50,000 CFU/mL when the SPA culture was negative.[12] ** In the "real world", 25 more patients (2.5% of 1000) would appear to have a UTI because of asymptomatic bacteriuria and contamination (0.5% + 2%), when in fact only 2 have true UTI. £ The Number of children with true UTI who would have been missed if pyuria was required for the diagnosis of UTI. ¥ The number of children who would not receive antibiotics if pyuria was required for the diagnosis of UTI. *Editor's Note*: Please refer to original journal article for full references. (Reprinted from Schroeder AR, Chang PW, Shen MW, et al. Diagnostic Accuracy of the Urinalysis for Urinary Tract Infection in Infants <3 Months of Age. *Pediatrics* 135:965-971, 2015, with permission from the American Academy of Pediatrics.)

To understand the implications of these data, let us compare the number of children treated with antimicrobials if pyuria was and was not required for the diagnosis of UTIs. Imagine a population of 1000 consecutive febrile "low-risk" neonates, all of whom have a urinalysis and urine culture performed from a specimen obtained by catheterization and of whom 5% have a true UTI. Assuming a prevalence of asymptomatic bacteriuria and contaminated specimens of 0.5% and 2%, respectively (see footnotes to the Fig 1), and assuming that the sensitivity (96%) and specificity (95%) reported by Schroeder et al are accurate, one can calculate the impact of requiring pyuria for the diagnosis of UTI (Fig 1). One can then repeat this exercise for a "high risk" group of female infants with a temperature > 39°C for more than 24 hours without an apparent source, in whom the prevalence of UTI is approximately 20%.[3] In the low-risk group of neonates, requiring pyuria to define UTI would result in 27 fewer children receiving antibiotics (48 vs 75 would have been treated if pyuria was and was not required, respectively), but 2 febrile children with true UTI would be missed. In the high-risk group, 33 fewer children would receive unnecessary antibiotics, but 8 febrile children with a true UTI would be missed. A missed febrile UTI may result in renal scarring, whereas the implications of an extra antibiotic course may be less serious. Accordingly, using the estimates provided by Schroeder et al, it is not clear that requiring pyuria for the diagnosis of UTI is beneficial in all cases.

The sensitivity estimates reported by Schroeder et al are substantially higher than almost all previous reports.[2] Particularly important is the discrepancy between results from this study and results from studies in which all urine samples were collected using suprapubic aspiration, therefore eliminating the possibility of contamination. In 2 such studies, 86% and 88% of children with UTI had pyuria (ie, ≥10 white blood cells/mm^3).[4,5] Even if one were to account for asymptomatic bacteriuria, no more than 90% of the children with UTI in these studies would be expected to have pyuria. Several explanations are possible for the discrepancy between the results reported by Schroeder et al and previous reports. The study by Schroeder et al. was a case-control study, a design known to falsely inflate sensitivity and specificity estimates.[6-9] Furthermore, young infants with bacteremia, who represent a very small fraction of all children with UTI, may systematically be more likely to exhibit pyuria than neonates without bacteremia (spectrum bias). Previous studies have shown that children with bacteremia tend to be younger, have a longer duration of fever, and have higher acute-phase reactants than children with negative blood cultures.[10] In our practice, we have encountered several children who did not have pyuria on presentation but developed pyuria during the ensuing hours. Thus, the longer duration of illness in children with bacteremia may be an important source of bias.

Finally, the authors used unconventional, post hoc definitions for pyuria. If one were to repeat the preceding calculations using a sensitivity of 90%, requiring pyuria for the diagnosis of UTI would result in 5 missed febrile UTI in low-risk infants and 20 missed febrile UTI in high-risk infants (to save 30 and 45 antibiotic prescriptions, respectively). Generally, the number of missed UTIs increases as the sensitivity of pyuria decreases and the pretest probability of UTI increases. In the outpatient setting, where most UTIs are diagnosed, a dipstick test is often used to decide on the initial treatment. Because the sensitivity of the dipstick test is less than the sensitivity of WBC count established using a hemocytometer (the method used in both studies that used suprapubic aspiration), the number of missed UTIs will most likely be even higher.

Although some may use the data from Schroeder et al to argue that pyuria should always be required for the diagnosis of UTI, such a change may not always be beneficial. We agree that the accuracy of diagnosis may increase if urine culture could be combined with a urinary biomarker and that pyuria is the best candidate test currently available. Nevertheless, the accuracy of pyuria is not high enough for it to serve as an ideal biomarker. With recent advances in laboratory technology and high-throughput methods, a more appropriate biomarker is likely to be identified in the near future. Requiring pyuria for the diagnosis of UTI may stifle some of this research.

At present, a reasonable approach to enhance diagnostic accuracy would be to first and foremost reduce the levels of contamination using the best available collection method. Second, instead of relying on a single test (pyuria), diagnostic accuracy may be improved by using a Bayesian approach in which the contribution of all available data is used to determine the likelihood of UTI for a given patient.[3] A child with fever without a discernable source, suprapubic tenderness, marked pyuria, and positive nitrites most likely has a UTI even if the bacterial colony count is slightly less than 50 000 CFU/mL. Similarly, if all evidence points toward a UTI, the absence of pyuria, albeit highly unusual, could be a reflection of the less than perfect sensitivity of the test or early infection. Although a simple schema for categorization of children into those with and without disease is often desirable, such oversimplification may sometimes result in more harm than benefit.

In summary, pyuria is present in most children with UTIs. Accordingly, if pyuria is absent, the provider should carefully review all available clinical information. This case-by-case approach is preferable to incorporating pyuria into the definition of UTI and results in the flexibility needed to best take of children with UTI.

N. Shaikh, MD

References

1. Hoberman A, Wald ER. Urinary tract infections in young febrile children. *Pediatr Infect Dis J*. 1997;16:11-17.
2. Williams GJ, Macaskill P, Chan SF, Turner RM, Hodson E, Craig JC. Absolute and relative accuracy of rapid urine tests for urinary tract infection in children: a meta-analysis. *Lancet Infect Dis*. 2010;10:240-250.
3. Shaikh N, Morone NE, Lopez J, et al. Does this child have a urinary tract infection? *JAMA*. 2007;298:2895-2904.
4. Aronson AS, Gustafson B, Svenningsen NW. Combined suprapubic aspiration and clean-voided urine examination in infants and children. *Acta Paediatr Scand*. 1973;62:396-400.
5. Lin DS, Huang SH, Lin CC, et al. Urinary tract infection in febrile infants younger than eight weeks of Age. *Pediatrics*. 2000;105:E20.
6. Lijmer JG, Mol BW, Heisterkamp S, et al. Empirical evidence of design-related bias in studies of diagnostic tests. *JAMA*. 1999;282:1061-1066.

7. Whiting P, Rutjes AW, Reitsma JB, Glas AS, Bossuyt PM, Kleijnen J. Sources of variation and bias in studies of diagnostic accuracy: a systematic review. *Lancet Infect Dis.* 2004;140:189-202.

8. Whiting PF, Rutjes AW, Westwood ME, et al. QUADAS-2: a revised tool for the quality assessment of diagnostic accuracy studies. *Ann Intern Med.* 2011;155: 529-536.

9. Whiting PF, Rutjes AW, Westwood ME, Mallett S. QUADAS-2 Steering Group. A systematic review classifies sources of bias and variation in diagnostic test accuracy studies. *J Clin Epidemiol.* 2013;66:1093-1104.

10. Hoberman A, Wald ER, Hickey RW, et al. Oral versus initial intravenous therapy for urinary tract infections in young febrile children [see comment]. *Pediatrics.* 1999;104:79-86.

11. Wettergren B, Jodal U. Spontaneous clearance of asymptomatic bacteriuria in infants. *Acta Paediatr Scand.* 1990;79:300-304.

12. Pryles CV, Atkin MD, Morse TS, Welch KJ. Comparative bacteriologic study of urine obtained from children by percutaneous suprapubic aspiration of the bladder and by catheter. *Pediatrics.* 1959;24:983-991.

Renal tract abnormalities missed in a historical cohort of young children with UTI if the NICE and AAP imaging guidelines were applied

Narchi H, Marah M, Khan AA, et al (United Arab Emirates Univ, Al Ain)
J Pediatr Urol 11:252.e1-252.e7, 2015

Objective.—In a historical cohort of children with a urinary tract infection (UTI) who had already undergone all the imaging procedures, the aim was to determine renal tract abnormalities which would have been missed had we implemented the new guidelines from the National Institute for Health and Care Excellence in the United Kingdom (NICE) or the American Academy of Pediatrics (AAP).

Material and Methods.—After a UTI episode, forty-three children (28 females, 65%) aged between 2 months and 2 years presenting at two general hospitals with a febrile UTI before 2008 underwent all the recommended imaging studies predating the new guidelines. Hydronephrosis was defined and graded according to the Society for Fetal Urology (SFU) classification. Hydronephrosis grade II (mild pelvicalyceal dilatation), grade III (moderate dilatation), and grade IV (gross dilatation with thinning of the renal cortex), duplication, vesicoureteral reflux (VUR) grade II and above, renal scarring and reduced renal uptake (<45%) on technetium-99m-labeled dimercaptosuccinic acid (DMSA) scintigraphy were considered significant abnormalities. We calculated the proportion of abnormalities which would have been missed had the new guidelines been used instead.

Results.—The median of age was 7.6 months (mean 8.7, range 2–24 months), with the majority (*n* = 37, 86%) being under 1 year of age. Ultrasound (US) showed hydronephrosis in 14 (32%), all grade II. A voiding cystourethrogram (VCUG) was performed in all and showed VUR ≥ grade II in 16 (37%), including eight children (19%) where it was bilateral. DMSA scan showed scarring in 25 children (58%) of whom 11 (26%) had bilateral scars. Reduced differential renal uptake was present in 10 children (23%). Of the 29 children with normal US, 18 (62%) had renal scarring and nine (31%) had VUR ≥ grade II. The NICE guidelines would have missed 63% of the children with VUR ≥ grade II, including a high proportion of grades IV and V VUR, 44% of the children with renal scarring, and 20% of the children with decreased renal uptake, including some children with bilateral renal scarring and with decreased renal uptake. The AAP guidelines would have missed 56% of the children with VUR ≥ grade II, including a high proportion of grades IV and V VUR, and all children with renal scarring as well as those with decreased renal uptake.

Conclusion.—The prevalence of renal tract abnormalities missed by the new guidelines is high. They should be used with full awareness of their limitations.

▶ National urinary tract infection (UTI) guidelines in Britain[1] and the United States,[2] promulgated in 2007 and 2011, respectively, discouraged the routine performance of voiding cystourethrography (VCUG) after the first febrile UTI in an infant or young child. The guidelines recommend a renal-bladder ultrasonogram (RBUS) as the primary imaging study, with VCUG being reserved for infants and young children with an abnormal RBUS or atypical clinical course. In response, multiple articles have challenged the recommendation on the basis of what is missed by the stepwise approach compared with performing the full array of imaging tests. Most of these articles point out that RBUS is a poor screening test for identifying vesicoureteral reflux (VUR). This is certainly the case when all grades of VUR are considered, but most infants and young children with a UTI have either no VUR or low-grade, nondilating VUR, generally considered not harmful. It stands to reason that ultrasonography could only detect VUR if there is dilatation of the upper tract, so identifying the RBUS as insensitive for detecting all grades of VUR is neither surprising nor particularly disturbing. High-grade VUR, however, generates more concern because, compared with low-grade VUR, it is more likely to be associated with recurrent UTIs and renal scarring and less likely to resolve on its own. Fortunately, only a small percentage of infants and children with a febrile UTI have high-grade VUR, and most of them—though not all—have an abnormal RBUS.[3] Narchi et al review their experience prior to the guidelines (2000-2008) with 43 infants and young children to whom the guidelines would have applied: 2- to 24-month-old children with a febrile UTI. Each of the 43 had all of the following imaging tests performed: RBUS, VCUG, and dimercaptosuccinic acid (DMSA) nuclear scan. Had the imaging recommendations of the guidelines been followed during those years, 63% of the cases of VUR greater than grade II would have been missed with the National Institute for Health and Care Excellence in the United Kingdom (NICE) guideline and 56% with the American Academy of Pediatrics (AAP) guideline; 44% with renal scarring would have been missed with the NICE guideline, all with renal scarring with the AAP guideline. It is clear that when more tests are performed, more abnormalities are found. But are these findings of clinical concern?

Narchi et al acknowledge that the higher yield of abnormalities "should be carefully balanced against using the prior guidelines that advocate more use of US, VCUG, and DMSA scintigraphy, which are costly, time-consuming, sometimes unpleasant, and associated with radiation exposure as well as prolonged clinic follow-up visits." Just how much more additional cost and radiation exposure? La Scola and associates[4] answered that question in 2013, comparing the performance of all tests with those that would be performed according to NICE and AAP guidelines. The cost of imaging performed according to the guidelines would be decreased by 60% to 65%, the amount of radiation by 74% with the NICE guideline, and by 93% (from 608 mSv to 42 mSv) with the AAP guideline. But the question lingers: despite these benefits, do the guidelines put patients at unacceptable risk of having what Narchi et al call "significant abnormalities" missed?

Taking the approach that renal damage is the greatest concern, Shaikh and colleagues[3] determined that RBUS—the pivotal imaging test recommended in the guidelines—actually performs well to identify infants and young children whose febrile UTI is likely to result in renal scarring, partly because it identifies the majority with high-grade VUR. Perhaps the most important take-home message in the article by Narchi et al is not in the title or the recognition that multiple imaging studies increase the yield of abnormalities detected but in the closing sentence of the article. The authors note that the collective downside of using all of the multiple imaging procedures (cost, time, discomfort, and radiation exposure) "... is particularly important as there is no evidence that such heavy burden on the patients, their families, and health-care resources has any clinical benefit for affected children." This perspective is a valuable reminder when assessing tests to focus on clinical benefit rather than yield. And to weigh benefit against the downside of testing, as we were all taught: "primum non nocere."

K. B. Roberts, MD

References

1. National Institute for Health and Clinical Excellence. Urinary tract infection in children: diagnosis, treatment and long term management. www.nice.org.uk/nicemedia/pdf/CG54fullguideline.pdf.
2. Roberts KB. Subcommittee on Urinary Tract Infection, Steering Committee on Quality Improvement and Management. Urinary tract infection: clinical practice guideline for the diagnosis and management of the initial UTI in febrile infants and children 2 to 24 months. *Pediatrics.* 2011;128:595-610.
3. Shaikh N, Craig JC, Rovers MM, et al. Identification of children and adolescents at risk for renal scarring after a first urinary tract infection. A meta-analysis with individual patient data. *JAMA Pediatr.* 2014;168:893-900.
4. La Scola C, De Mutiis C, Hewitt IK, et al. Different guidelines for imaging after first UTI in febrile infants: Yield, cost, and radiation. *Pediatrics.* 2013;131:e665-e671.

Risk Factors for Recurrent Urinary Tract Infection and Renal Scarring

Keren R, Shaikh N, Pohl H, et al (Children's Hosp of Philadelphia, Pennsylvania; Univ of Pittsburgh School of Medicine, Pennsylvania; Children's Natl Health System, Washington, DC; et al)
Pediatrics 136:e13-e21, 2015

Objectives.—To identify risk factors for recurrent urinary tract infection (UTI) and renal scarring in children who have had 1 or 2 febrile or symptomatic UTIs and received no antimicrobial prophylaxis.

Methods.—This 2-year, multisite prospective cohort study included 305 children aged 2 to 71 months with vesicoureteral reflux (VUR) receiving placebo in the RIVUR (Randomized Intervention for Vesicoureteral Reflux) study and 195 children with no VUR observed in the CUTIE (Careful Urinary Tract Infection Evaluation) study. Primary exposure was presence of VUR; secondary exposures included bladder and bowel dysfunction (BBD), age, and race. Outcomes were recurrent febrile or symptomatic urinary tract infection ($_{F/S}$UTI) and renal scarring.

Results.—Children with VUR had higher 2-year rates of recurrent $_{F/S}$UTI (Kaplan-Meier estimate 25.4% compared with 17.3% for VUR and no VUR, respectively). Other factors associated with recurrent $_{F/S}$UTI included presence of BBD at baseline (adjusted hazard ratio: 2.07 [95% confidence interval (CI): 1.09−3.93]) and presence of renal scarring on the baseline ^{99m}Tc-labeled dimercaptosuccinic acid scan (adjusted hazard ratio: 2.88 [95% CI: 1.22−6.80]). Children with BBD and any degree of VUR had the highest risk of recurrent $_{F/S}$UTI (56%). At the end of the 2-year follow-up period, 8 (5.6%) children in the no VUR group and 24 (10.2%) in the VUR group had renal scars, but the difference was not statistically significant (adjusted odds ratio: 2.05 [95% CI: 0.86−4.87]).

Conclusions.—VUR and BBD are risk factors for recurrent UTI, especially when they appear in combination. Strategies for preventing recurrent UTI include antimicrobial prophylaxis and treatment of BBD.

▶ Pediatric urinary tract infection (UTI) is a common condition, and the incidence of emergency room visits for UTI, as well as the mean charge for these visits, is increasing.[1] Vesicoureteral reflux (VUR) is the most common structural abnormality found during radiologic investigation for children with UTI. UTIs in children can be divided into (1) clinical pyelonephritis (febrile UTI, symptoms of flank/abdominal pain), (2) cystitis (dysuria, frequency, urgency, suprapubic pain), and (3) asymptomatic bacteriuria (positive urine culture without irritative symptoms). Children with clinical pyelonephritis who have a dimercaptosuccinic acid (DMSA) renal scan or CT scan that shows a perfusion defect have acute pyelonephritis. However, most children with clinical pyelonephritis do not undergo a DMSA scan or CT scan. Overall, 50% of children with a febrile UTI have acute pyelonephritis and, of these, 50% will subsequently have a renal scar in the area of pyelonephritic involvement. In children with grade III, IV, or V VUR and a febrile UTI, 90% have acute pyelonephritis. Children with febrile UTIs are at risk for renal scarring, whereas those with cystitis typically are not.

In 2010, the American Urological Association (AUA) published evidence-based treatment guidelines for VUR.[2] The authors of those guidelines coined a new term for dysfunctional elimination syndrome, *bladder and bowel dysfunction*, or *BBD*. BBD refers to (1) abnormalities in bladder filling or emptying, including urinary frequency, urgency, incontinence, holding maneuvers, prolonged voiding intervals or (2) abnormal bowel patterns, including constipation and encopresis. Pediatric urologists use the Bristol Stool scale to assess bowel habits. Often families report that the child's stool habits are normal, but with close questioning, we often find that children with UTIs or incontinence have clinical constipation. In the AUA analysis, BBD increased the risk of persistent VUR and reduced the success rate of endoscopic injection therapy for VUR. The guidelines recommended that children with VUR and BBD receive antibiotic prophylaxis. A subsequent analysis found that BBD also increases the risk of breakthrough UTI and postoperative UTI following successful antireflux surgery.[3]

The RIVUR trial is the largest recent pediatric urology/pediatric nephrology prospective randomized trial. The results showed that trimethoprim-sulfamethoxazole prophylaxis was effective in reducing the risk of UTI (febrile and afebrile) in children with VUR, although the rate of renal scarring was similar between the groups that received trimethoprim-sulfamethoxazole or placebo. In RIVUR, 71 of 126 (56%) of toilet-trained children with VUR had BBD. Children with BBD who received prophylaxis had an 80% reduction in UTI.

This article offers a unique insight into the impact of VUR and BBD on the risk of recurrent UTI in children age 2 months to 6 years following their first or second UTI. The study combined the placebo arm of the RIVUR study and a sideline group, termed the *CUTIE group* (children who were evaluated for RIVUR but who did not qualify because they did not have VUR). The CUTIE children were monitored for 2 years without antibiotic prophylaxis and underwent similar follow-up evaluations, including renal scans, to determine the long term risk of recurrent UTI and renal scarring. At baseline, 46% of the CUTIE group (UTI and no VUR) had BBD, and only 2% had renal scarring.

This report shows that VUR and BBD are separate risk factors for recurrent UTI. At 2 years, children with BBD and any degree of VUR (not receiving prophylaxis) had a 56% risk of having another UTI, and children with BBD and no VUR had a 35% risk of recurrent UTI. Furthermore, children with grade 0 to II VUR and no BBD had a 29% incidence of recurrent UTI, indicating the importance of close monitoring of these children. Unfortunately, whether the recurrent UTIs were febrile or afebrile was not reported. This factor is important, because cystitis does not result in new renal scarring. Nevertheless, in this report, the rate of new renal scarring was twice as high in the VUR group as in the non-VUR group, although the difference was not statistically significant, probably because of low patient numbers.

A factor that was not assessed in RIVUR and CUTIE was the effect of BBD treatment, which is individualized. Therapy may include (1) timed voiding, (2) anticholinergic medication for overactive bladder, (3) α-adrenergic medication for detrusor-sphincter discoordination, and (4) polyethylene glycol powder for constipation. It is possible that treatment for BBD might obviate the need for prophylaxis.

An interesting sidebar to this study is that the second author published a study in 2003 on the long-term incidence of dysfunctional elimination syndrome (ie, BBD) in children who had a UTI or were found to have VUR before 2 years of age.[4] They found that when these children were toilet trained, there was not a higher incidence of BBD than in a control group of children. This is an interesting finding that deserves further study. More recently, the same author published another analysis of BBD in children in the RIVUR and CUTIE studies showing that children with VUR and BBD were at greater risk of having recurrent UTIs than those with VUR or BBD alone.[5]

It seems clear from this report that VUR is a risk factor for recurrent UTI. In my opinion, the most recent American Academy of Pediatrics Guidelines on UTI in children 2 months to 2 years should be revised to recommend that children undergo a renal ultrasound scan and voiding cystourethrogram following their first febrile UTI. In addition, in children with VUR and UTI, prophylaxis should be considered. Children with VUR and BBD should receive antimicrobial prophylaxis and undergo individualized treatment for BBD.

J. S. Elder, MD, FACS

References

1. Sood A, Penna FJ, Elder JS. Incidence, admission rates, and economic burden of pediatric emergency department visits for urinary tract infection: data from the nationwide emergency department sample. *J Pediatr Urol.* 2015;11: 246.e1-246.e8.
2. Peters CA, Skoog SJ, Arant BS Jr, et al. Summary of the AUA guidelines on management of primary vesicoureteral reflux in children. *J Urol.* 2010;184:1133-1144.
3. Elder JS, Diaz M. Vesicoureteral reflux—the role of bladder and bowel dysfunction. *Nat Rev Urol.* 2013;10:640-648.
4. Shaikh N, Hoberman A, Wise B, et al. Dysfunctional elimination syndrome: is it related to urinary tract infection or vesicoureteral reflux diagnosed early in life? *Pediatrics.* 2003;112:1134-1137.
5. Shaikh N, Hoberman A, Keren R, et al. Recurrent urinary tract infections in children with bladder and bowel dysfunction. *Pediatrics.* 2015;137.

Kidney Disease Progression in Autosomal Recessive Polycystic Kidney Disease

Dell KM, on behalf of the Chronic Kidney Disease in Children (CKiD) Study (Case Western Reserve Univ, Cleveland, OH; et al)
J Pediatr 171:196-201, 2016

Objective.—To define glomerular filtration rate (GFR) decline, hypertension (HTN), and proteinuria in subjects with autosomal recessive polycystic kidney disease (ARPKD) and compare with 2 congenital kidney disease control groups in the Chronic Kidney Disease in Children cohort.

Study Design.—GFR decline (iohexol clearance), rates of HTN (ambulatory/casual blood pressures), antihypertensive medication usage, left ventricular hypertrophy, and proteinuria were analyzed in subjects with ARPKD (n = 22) and 2 control groups: aplastic/hypoplastic/dysplastic disorders (n = 44) and obstructive uropathies (n = 44). Differences between study groups were examined with the Wilcoxon rank sum test.

Results.—Annualized GFR change in subjects with ARPKD was −1.4 mL/min/1.73 m^2 (−6%), with greater decline in subjects age ≥10 years (−11.5%). However, overall rates of GFR decline did not differ significantly in subjects with ARPKD vs controls. There were no significant differences in rates of HTN or left ventricular hypertrophy, but subjects with ARPKD had a greater percent on ≥3 blood pressure medications (32% vs 0%, $P < .0001$), more angiotensin-converting enzyme inhibitor use (82% vs 27% vs 36%, $P < .0005$), and less proteinuria (urine protein: creatinine = 0.1 vs 0.6, $P < .005$).

Conclusions.—This study reports rates of GFR decline, HTN, and proteinuria in a small but well-phenotyped ARPKD cohort. The relatively slow rate of GFR decline in subjects with ARPKD and absence of significant proteinuria suggest that these standard clinical measures may have limited utility in assessing therapeutic interventions and highlight the need for other ARPKD kidney disease progression biomarkers.

▶ Autosomal recessive polycystic kidney disease (ARPKD), formerly described by the renal phenotype and recessive mode of inheritance, is now being ascribed to more than 300 underlying gene mutations in the *PKHD1* gene. The gene product fibrocystin has been localized to primary ciliary bodies. This has improved the description of the spectrum of organ-specific and clinical manifestations; however, no clear genotype-phenotype correlations can be defined. Prenatal manifestations endanger survival through lung hypoplasia, early renal failure, and early liver disease with cholangitis and portal hypertension. At age 10 years, 60% of patients require renal replacement or kidney transplantation, whereas about 10% of patients may need liver transplantation, mainly sequential liver-kidney transplantation, with favorable results.

For those not yet requiring renal replacement therapy, it would be of major importance to define new therapies slowing the progression to end-stage renal failure. Molecular targeted therapies (eg, mTor-inhibitors, vasopressin receptor antagonist, or somatostatin analogs in adult ADPKD) need clearly defined end points to demonstrate clinical relevance. In ARPKD, decline of GFR would be a key end point; however, no longitudinal data are available to plan for a study.

Dell and colleagues at the Chronic Kidney Disease in Children (CKiD) Study Group have tried to answer the important question on the annual decline of GFR in children with ARPKD compared with children with chronic kidney diseases due to hypoplastic/dysplastic renal disease and obstructive uropathy. The study is strengthened by the prospective design as well as the standardized measurement and calculation of the GFR. The control group with mainly hereditary diseases is well chosen, because immune-mediated kidney diseases and glomerulopathies with proteinuria with a more rapid progression to end-stage renal failure were excluded. In the ARPKD group, decline of GFR was astonishingly low and did not differ from the other groups; however, children with ARPKD older than 10 years of age seem to suffer from a more rapid decline.

The study confirms what clinicians already know. Nearly all children with ARPKD had severe arterial hypertension, which was well controlled with 3 or more drugs. In addition, in 82% of cases, an angiotensin-converting enzyme (ACE) inhibitor was used. On the other hand, proteinuria in this group was low.

What can be extracted from the study and what remains unanswered? The GFR decline in this selected ARPKD patients was low with 1.4 mL/min/ 1.73 m^2 per year only, but the decline intensified as children grew older. Arterial hypertension seems to be well controlled; however, the effect of ACE inhibitors on nephron-protection, GFR, fluids, electrolytes, and proteinuria remains an open question.

There are some points that need more clarification in this study:

- There is no information of the renal phenotype with relative kidney size and the distribution pattern of cysts.
- A comparison of decline of GFR in percentage between groups with GFR <45 and >45 mL/min/1.73 m^2 may be skewed and can lead to an artifact due to data misclassification.
- No genetic information is provided to confirm the diagnosis of ARPKD. Other mutations, such as *HNF1β*, *PKD1*, and *PKD2*, might have a phenotype in young children indistinguishable from each other.
- Information about the hepatic phenotype is completely missing but should be of relevance in many ways. Portal hypertension with splenomegaly is of concern because it may lead to poor nutritional status and more pronounced muscle wasting. A nephrology-centered view may miss important clinical aspects.
- The number of patients with ARPKD included seems to be small compared with the number of participating CKiD sites, which can increase the likelihood of a selection bias.

What is the outlook? Because of the great phenotypic heterogeneity of the disease, it may be unrealistic to search for simplified therapeutic approaches. A more individualized approach is needed. With respect to this point, the study is unable to answer this question; however, the study does highlight the need for further research to define biomarkers for disease progression. Given the frequency to the disease and the fact that there are 52 participating CKiD Study Group centers, one should be optimistic that in the near future, this group will provide more robust numbers and new approaches to care.

P. F. Hoyer

Differences between the pediatric and adult presentation of fibromuscular dysplasia: results from the US Registry

Green R, Gu X, Kline-Rogers E, et al (Univ of Pennsylvania, Philadelphia; Univ of Michigan, Ann Arbor; et al)
Pediatr Nephrol 31:641-650, 2016

Background.—Fibromuscular dysplasia (FMD) is a noninflammatory arteriopathy that causes significant morbidity in children.

Methods.—The clinical features, presenting symptoms, and vascular beds involved are reviewed in the first 33 patients aged <18 years who are enrolled in the United States Registry for FMD from five registry sites and compared with 999 adult patients from 12 registry sites.

Results.—Mean age at diagnosis was 8.4 + 4.8 years (16 days to 17 years). Compared with adults, pediatric FMD occurs in more males (42.4 vs 6 %, p < 0.001) Children with FMD have a stronger previous history of hypertension (93.9 vs 69.9 %, p = 0.002). Hypertension (100 %), headache (55 %), and abdominal bruits (10.7 %) were the most common presenting signs and symptoms. FMD affects renal vasculature in almost all children (97 vs 69.7 %, p = 0.003). The extra-cranial carotid vessels are less commonly involved in children (23.1 vs 73.3 %, p < 0.001). The mesenteric arteries (38.9 vs 16.2 %, p = 0.02) and aorta (26.3 vs 2.4 %, p < 0.001) are more commonly involved in children.

Conclusions.—In the United States Registry for FMD, pediatric FMD affects children from infancy throughout childhood. All children presented with hypertension and many presented with headache and abdominal bruits. In children, FMD most commonly affects the renal vasculature, but also frequently involves the mesenteric arteries and abdominal aorta; the carotid vessels are less frequently involved (Table 2).

▶ Fibromuscular dysplasia (FMD) is a very uncommon condition in children mainly presenting with very severe renovascular hypertension (RVH). Together with Takayasu arteritis (TA), it is the most common cause for childhood renovascular disease worldwide. In the Western world, it is the dominating cause.

The knowledge on the presentation and treatment of FMD, in particular in childhood, is limited and comes from a number of case series. The authors are therefore to be congratulated on their effort to also include children in the United States registry for their analysis of patients with FMD.

Nine pediatric centers included data. The number of included children (n = 33), despite the rarity of FMD, is surprisingly low, as the register already has been in place for eight years. Thus, there is a chance for a selection bias, which the use of the registry was meant to overcome.

One potential cause for the low inclusion rate might be the lack of knowledge about FMD in the general pediatric community. There is also a lot of confusion regarding the differential diagnosis between FMD and TA. The criteria that have been published for TA are so wide that all children with FMD would also qualify for the TA diagnosis. It is always important to have solid findings of inflammation to make the diagnosis of a vasculitis; these might be typical symptoms of an

TABLE 2.—Presenting Signs and Symptoms

Presenting Signs/Symptoms at Time of Diagnosis	Age <18	Age ≥18	p Value
None of the symptoms/signs below	0/33 (0)	19/973 (2.0)	1.0
Symptoms			
Headache	17/31 (54.8)	551/918 (60.0)	0.56
Claudication	1/29 (3.4)	61/876 (7.0)	0.71
Weight loss	1/31 (3.2)	49/870 (5.6)	1.0
Post-prandial abdominal pain	1/29 (3.4)	61/866 (7.0)	0.71
Chest pain/SOB	2/29 (6.9)	165/868 (19.0)	0.14
Flank/abdominal pain	2/28 (7.1)	126/848 (14.9)	0.41
Neck pain	1/27 (3.7)	246/846 (29.1)	0.002
Dizziness	2/27 (7.4)	283/837 (33.8)	0.003
Tinnitus	1/29 (3.4)	175/838 (20.9)	0.002
Pulsatile tinnitus	0/28 (0)	319/864 (36.9)	<0.001
Signs			
Stroke	1/32 (3.1)	75/902 (8.3)	0.51
Amaurosis fugax	0/29 (0)	46/879 (5.2)	0.39
Hemispheric TIA	0/29 (0)	75/885 (8.5)	0.16
Horner's	0/30 (0)	48/848 (5.7)	0.40
Cervical bruit	2/27 (5.3)	218/850 (25.6)	0.039
Carotid artery dissection	0/30 (0)	149/896 (16.6)	0.01
Vertebral artery dissection	0/13 (0)	12/185 (6.5)	1.0
Renal artery dissection	0/32 (0)	21/892 (2.4)	1.0
Aortic dissection	0/25 (0)	6/568 (1.1)	1.0
Hypertension	33/33 (100)	601/942 (63.8)	<0.001
Renal infarction	2/24 (8.3)	13/527 (2.5)	0.14
Renal failure	0/25 (0)	1/528 (0.2)	1.0
Azotemia	0/32 (0)	25/875 (2.9)	1.0
Abdominal bruit	3/28 (10.7)	74/832 (8.9)	0.73
Mesenteric ischemia	0/30 (0)	8/879 (0.9)	1.0
Myocardial infarction	0/32 (0)	24/900 (2.7)	1.0
Coronary revascularization	0/25 (0)	16/534 (3.0)	1.0
Aneurysms	2/32 (6.3)	148/905 (16.4)	0.21
Venous thrombosis	0/24 (0)	14/533 (2.6)	1.0

SOB shortness of breath, TIA transient ischemic attack

Reprinted from Green R, Gu X, Kline-Rogers E, et al. Differences between the pediatric and adult presentation of fibromuscular dysplasia: results from the US Registry. *Pediatr Nephrol.* 2016;31:641-650, with permission from IPNA.

inflammatory disease or raised inflammatory markers. A positron emission tomography (PET) scan can also be used to define inflammation in the vascular wall. We see several cases of misdiagnosis where the child unnecessarily has been given corticosteroids and immunosuppressive treatment for TA when the true diagnosis is likely to have been FMD.

The children in this article display some quite unusual features compared to the literature. The most striking is that the children were treated with a median of only 1 drug. Our experience is that they need 5 to 7 drugs, despite not achieving acceptable blood pressure control. I suspect that the children in this study were left with quite high blood pressures.

All children in this report displayed symptoms. This is markedly different from the previous literature in which a significant proportion, 30% to 40%, of the children showed no symptoms at all. Their very significantly raised blood pressures were discovered at routine screening, often during treatment of a concomitant unrelated condition.

The authors compare the presentation of the children to that of the adult patients (Table 2). The most striking difference was the much higher rate of cerebral involvement in the adult patients. This is reflected as a large proportion in the adult group presenting with transient ischemic attack (TIA) or stroke but with normal blood pressure. All the children were hypertensive. Consequently, 73% of the adult patients showed extracranial carotid involvement while this was found only in 23% of the children.

Renal, aortic, and mesenteric involvement was found much more often among the children, in 97%, 26%, and 39%, respectively, compared with 70%, 2%, and 16% of the adults. There were thus clear signs of a much more widespread vascular disease in the children despite their younger age. The disease in children is often progressive, so one has to suspect that those children, when they reach adulthood, will differ even more significantly from the adult patients presented in this study.

Most other differences that were found between the pediatric and adult patients were merely related to age; clearly, the children were significantly younger than the adults. They also smoked and used contraceptive pills less often. No big surprise here.

Potentially interesting information on the outcome of the different treatment procedures, angioplasty with or without stenting or surgery, is not given in the article. We do know that these interventions are generally effective but that a significant proportion of the children are not at all or only partly helped by the procedures. Many require several repeated interventions. Such information would be very valuable to have.

FMD is a disease in which very little research has been undertaken during several decades. We do not have any knowledge of its causes even if most of us suspect it to be a developmental disorder of the blood vessel wall. It has for decades been suggested that there are 3 forms of FMD depending on which layer in the blood vessel wall that is involved. In this article, the authors narrow this down to 2 forms: medial and intimal hyperplasia. They suggest that intimal hyperplasia mostly causes a focal disease and that medial hyperplasia usually is multifocal.

In my experience, there seems to be a small group with isolated focal RVD. These children respond well to angioplasty, and if they experience recurrent hypertension, they do so after many years. Unfortunately, very few of the children in this publication were defined according to extent of their disease and this would have been very interesting to see.

In summary, I strongly endorse the authors' effort to describe a potentially unbiased group of children with FMD. This should give us more solid knowledge about this severe condition. I hope that the authors will be able to include significantly more children in the future and also that they will be able to collect more data on the extent of the disease, how the children were treated, and what their long term outcomes were.

K. Tullus, MD, PhD, FRCPCH

Female genital mutilation in children presenting to a London safeguarding clinic: a case series

Hodes D, Armitage A, Robinson K, et al (Univ College London Hosp, UK, The Whittington Hosp, London, UK)
Arch Dis Child 101:212-216, 2016

Objective.—To describe the presentation and management of children referred with suspected female genital mutilation (FGM) to a UK safeguarding clinic.

Design and Setting.—Case series of all children under 18 years of age referred with suspected FGM between June 2006 and May 2014.

Main Outcome Measures.—These include indication for referral, demographic data, circumstances of FGM, medical symptoms, type of FGM, investigations and short-term outcome.

Results.—Of the 47 girls referred, 27 (57%) had confirmed FGM. According to the WHO classification of genital findings, FGM type 1 was found in 2 girls, type 2 in 8 girls and type 4 in 11 girls. No type 3 FGM was seen. The circumstances of FGM were known in 17 cases, of which 12 (71%) were performed by a health professional or in a medical setting (medicalisation). Ten cases were potentially illegal, yet despite police involvement there have been no prosecutions.

Conclusions.—This study is an important snapshot of FGM within the UK paediatric population. The most frequent genital finding was type 4 FGM with no tissue damage or minimal scarring. FGM was performed at a young age, with 15% reported under the age of 1 year. The study also demonstrated significant medicalisation of FGM, which matches recent trends in international data. Type 4 FGM performed in infancy is easily missed on examination and so vigilance in assessing children with suspected FGM is essential (Box 1, Fig 1).

▶ In February 2016, the United Nations International Children's Emergency Fund (UNICEF) estimated that more than 200 million girls and women worldwide (including 44 million at or under the age of 14 years) are currently living with female genital mutilation (FGM), also called cutting or female circumcision.[1] FGM is defined by the World Health Organization (WHO) as injury to, or partial or complete removal of, the female genitalia without medical indication (Box 1 and Fig 1).[2] This tradition has long been practiced in girls throughout Africa, the Middle East, and Asia but has only recently come to the attention of clinicians who practice in places that receive immigrants from these countries.

In an important article, Hodes and colleagues have published one of the first case series of FGM from a developed country. Although it reports only a small number of cases (27 in 8 years), may be subject to selection bias, and thus may not be generalizable, this retrospective audit of a tertiary pediatric "safeguarding" clinic in London highlights the urgent need for education and up-skilling of pediatricians about FGM.

Box 1: WHO classification of female genital mutilation

Type 1: Clitoridectomy: partial or total removal of the clitoris (a small sensitive and erectile part of the female genitals) and, in rare cases, removal of the prepuce only (the fold of skin surrounding the clitoris).

Type 2: Excision: partial or total removal of the clitoris and labia minora with or without removal of the labia majora (the labia are 'the lips' that surround the vagina).

Type 3: Infibulation: narrowing of the vaginal opening through the creation of a covering seal. The seal is formed by cutting and repositioning the labia minora or majora with or without removal of the clitoris.

Type 4: Other: all other harmful procedures to the genitals for non-medical reasons, for example, pricking, piercing, incision, scraping and cauterising the genital area.

Reprinted from Hodes D, Armitage A, Robinson K, et al. Female genital mutilation in children presenting to a London safeguarding clinic: a case series. *Arch Dis Child.* 2016;101:212-216, with permission.

Type 1 FGM

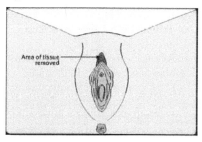

Type 2 FGM

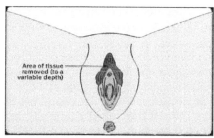

Type 3 FGM

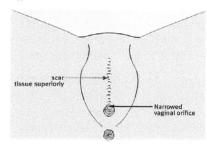

Type 4 FGM

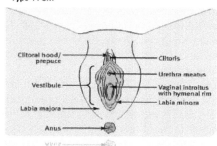

FIGURE. 1.—WHO classification of female genital mutilation. (Reprinted from Hodes D, Armitage A, Robinson K, et al. Female genital mutilation in children presenting to a London safeguarding clinic: a case series. *Arch Dis Child.* 2016;101:212-216, with permission.)

The article reminds us that as pediatricians we need to know about FGM for several important reasons. First, immigration continues to occur to developed countries, including the United States, Canada, United Kingdom, and Australia, from countries in which FGM is widely accepted. All but 1 case in this series came from Africa, although the practice is widespread in Asia. For example, UNICEF estimates that 50% of girls at or under age 11 years and living in

Indonesia have been subject to FGM.[1] Although FGM was not performed in the United Kingdom in any case reported by Hodes, there is evidence from the United Kingdom and other developed countries that FGM continues to be requested and practiced within some communities in the adopted country and that some children are taken "home" to their country of origin or to countries nearby for the procedure.

Second, FGM is usually performed in young girls; hence, is likely to be seen by pediatricians. In this study, most girls were under age 10 years at the time of the procedure and 15% of children had been subjected to FGM before 1 year of age. This finding is in line with an international trend documented by the WHO and UNICEF and suggests that we need a high index of suspicion for the child at risk, particularly if that child's mother or sibling has undergone FGM.

Third, FGM is associated with serious physical and psychological complications, some of which may present in childhood. One-third of girls reported by Hodes et al had problems, including recurrent urinary tract infection, difficulty with menstruation and micturition, pain, and bleeding. Importantly, Hodes recognized that some children were suffering from posttraumatic stress disorder. Adolescent and adult survivors of FGM frequently report mental health concerns including depression and anxiety, difficulty establishing intimate relationships, sexual problems, and difficulties with fertility and childbirth. Early recognition of FGM and its complications by pediatricians and their appropriate management may help minimize these many adverse secondary outcomes.

Fourth, pediatricians may be asked to perform FGM or arrange for referral for the procedure and must be aware that the conduct or procurement of FGM is illegal in most developed countries.[3] In some developed countries, reporting to child protection authorities is mandated for doctors who identify a child in whom the procedure has been performed or whom they consider at risk. The latter enables provision of sensitive education and support to families and may protect some children from FGM. No prosecutions have occurred in the United Kingdom where FGM has been illegal since 2003: the process is complex, and children are often too young or unwilling to testify, often against a family member or friend.

Hodes et al also raised the issue of "medicalization" of FGM—that is, when FGM is performed by a medical practitioner in a clinic or hospital or with use of analgesia or antibiotics. This approach has been used in some settings as justification for continuation of FGM but is condemned by UNICEF, which clearly states that regardless of the type and how it is performed, FGM is a violation of human rights.

As pediatricians we have an important role in the identification, management and prevention of FGM, but 2 recent studies suggest we have first to overcome considerable barriers. A systematic review by Zurynski et al revealed sparse good quality information about pediatricians' knowledge, attitudes, and practice regarding FGM and identified variable knowledge of FGM types and child protection laws.[3]

Sureshkumar et al surveyed Australian pediatricians and found that 10% had seen a child with FGM in their career in Australia and 3.3% had seen a case in the previous 5 years.[4] Despite this, there were knowledge gaps. Although more than half the pediatricians believed that FGM was performed in Australia, many were unaware of the groups at most risk, and some wrongly thought FGM was a practice required by religion. Few ever asked about or examined for FGM. In addition, only 22% knew the WHO classification for FGM, and only half were aware of local policy regarding FGM. Fewer than 15% had received any training in FGM, and more than half requested educational materials for themselves and their patients.

In summary, FGM is a human rights issue. It represents gender-based violence and is a form of child abuse that has become mandatory business for pediatricians. It is likely underrecognized in the developed world, through a lack of knowledge and the secrecy that surrounds a traditional practice hidden in minority communities. For girls living with FGM and for their families and communities, FGM is a particularly sensitive issue, and we must work together and support them to discuss and abandon the procedure. Men also have a crucial role. In September 2015, the United Nations agreed on the Sustainable Development Goal 5: to eliminate all FGM/C by 2030. Many affected countries are rising to the challenge. Pediatricians must also do their part.

E. J. Elliott, AM, MD, MPhil, MBBS, FRACP, FRCPCH, FRCP

References

1. UNICEF. At least 200 million girls and women alive today living in 30 countries have undergone FGM/C. 2016. http://data.unicef.org/child-protection/fgmc.html. Accessed May 16, 2016.
2. World Health Organisation. Female Genital Mutilation. http://www.who.int/mediacentre/factsheets/fs241/en/. Accessed May 16, 2016.
3. Zurynski Y, Sureshkumar P, Phu A, Elliott E. Female genital mutilation and cutting: a systematic literature review of health professionals' knowledge, attitudes and clinical practice. *BMC Int Health Hum Rights*. 2015;15:32.
4. Sureshkumar P, Zurynski Y, Moloney S, Raman S, Varol N, Elliott EJ. Female genital mutilation: Survey of paediatricians' knowledge, attitudes and practice. *Child Abuse Negl*. 2016;55:1-9.

12 Health Policy and Economics

Effect of Attribution Length on the Use and Cost of Health Care for a Pediatric Medicaid Accountable Care Organization
Christensen FW, Payne NR (Children's Hosps and Clinics of Minnesota, Minneapolis)
JAMA Pediatr 170:148-154, 2016

Importance.—Little is known about the effect of pediatric accountable care organizations (ACOs) on the use and costs of health care resources, especially in a Medicaid population.

Objective.—To assess the association between the length of consistent primary care (length of attribution) as part of an ACO and the use and cost of health care resources in a pediatric Medicaid population.

Design, Setting, and Participants.—A retrospective study of Medicaid claims data for 28 794 unique pediatric patients covering 346 277 patient-attributed months within a single children's hospital. Data were collected for patients attributed from September 1, 2013, to May 31, 2015. The effect of the length of attribution within a single hospital system's ACO on the use and costs of health care resources were estimated using zero-inflated Poisson distribution regression models adjusted for patient characteristics, including chronic conditions and a measure of predicted patient use of resources.

Exposures.—Receiving a plurality of primary care at an ACO clinic during the preceding 12 months (attribution to the ACO).

Main Outcomes and Measures.—The primary outcome measure was the length of attribution at an ACO clinic compared with subsequent inpatient hospitalization and subsequent use and cost of outpatient and ancillary health care resources.

Results.—Among the 28 794 pediatric patients receiving treatment covering 346 277 patient-attributed months during the study period, continuous attribution to the ACO for more than 2 years was associated with a decrease (95% CI) of 40.6% (19.4%-61.8%) in inpatient days but an increase (95% CI) of 23.3% (2.04%-26.3%) in office visits, 5.8% (1.4%-10.2%) in emergency department visits, and 15.3% (12.5%-18.0%) in the use of pharmaceuticals. These changes in the use of health care resources combined resulted in a cost reduction of 15.7% (95% CI, 6.6%-24.8%). At the population level, the impact of consistent primary

183

care was muted by the many patients in the ACO having shorter durations of participation.

Conclusions and Relevance.—These findings suggest significant and durable reductions of inpatient use and cost of health care resources associated with longer attribution to the ACO, with attribution as a proxy for exposure to the ACO's consistent primary care. Consistent primary care among the pediatric Medicaid population is challenging, but these findings suggest substantial benefits if consistency can be improved.

▶ "She could no longer borrow from the future to ease her present grief."
—Nathaniel Hawthorne, *The Scarlet Letter*

Although Hester Prynne and her accusing neighbors in Hawthorne's classic certainly knew what her scarlet "A" stood for, those in the business of Accountable Care Organization (ACO) operations know that the future financial success or failure of an ACO largely begins with the "A" of attribution method chosen by the payer rather than the "A" of accountability for health outcomes. Because the assignment of patients and families to an ACO is critical to costs, attribution of patients during contracting may take precedence over all because of adverse selection with some high cost patients. Unfortunately, current methods encourage contracts that focus on patients linked to primary care providers rather than total populations of children in Medicaid.

In traditional managed care systems like health maintenance organizations (HMOs), patients are assigned to a plan, and care inside the network with any provider is managed, but care outside the network is often not the responsibility of the plan or providers. In contrast, an ACO and its network of providers assumes both clinical and some degree of financial risk for an attributed group of patients wherever they receive care; how those patients are identified, though, makes all the difference for financial outcomes. Two primary forms of attribution[1] have been employed in assigning patients to ACOs in Medicare ACOs: retrospective attribution and prospective attribution. The first employs prior year's claims data to identify primary care clinicians providing the bulk of outpatient care and assigns patients to the ACOs of those clinicians for managing care going forward. The second method uses panels of patients currently seen in primary care groups to attribute patients to primary care physicians and include them within an ACO network. The ACO is then held "accountable" for costs and use incurred by the population during a fixed time period and measured against some standard cost growth or savings target. Retrospective attribution is thought to be less accurate because many patients change primary care clinicians.[2] In both systems, primary care clinicians are the entry point into ACOs and therein lies the motivation for the large number of massive health care systems that have consolidated primary care networks.

The article by Christiansen and Payne in *JAMA Pediatrics* and a very similar article in *Journal of Pediatrics*[3] by the same authors using the same data set both focused on attribution and cost savings in a Medicaid pediatric ACO in Minnesota, 1 of 14 ACOs operated in partnership with children's hospitals nationally.[4] As noted in their articles and 2 accompanying editorials,[5,6] the authors demonstrate modest cost savings over time in those patients who persistently received care in the network as contrasted with those who were not persistently "attributed" to the network. Unfortunately, this was a vanishingly small number of patients as more than 70% of patients were no longer attributable at two years and the agreement stipulated only 15 000 children enrolled in Medicaid to start.

The take-home message from this study depends on your vantage point. For providers and hospital systems engaged in ACOs, a modest risk proposal with shared savings/losses for a prospectively attributed population of children enrolled in Medicaid can generate savings as has been previously noted in Cleveland.[7] The ACO clearly benefited from the prospective attribution method employed by Medicaid and is a reassuring message to pediatric networks not accustomed to taking risk.

In contrast, Medicaid and child advocates should be concerned that accountability for long term costs and linkages of the highest risk children who are not tightly linked to a network and medical home is unclear in such models. Attribution methods inherently dependent on existing primary care medical homes will often leave out the most vulnerable and even when initially included, families at risk of housing instability and impermanence among others, will be likely to be the first to leave a practice. The highest costs were among patients not longitudinally connected to the primary care network in the Minnesota studies to no one's surprise. To the extent that primary care clinicians and their ACOs are only accountable for patients well known and connected to them, they will have limited incentives to engage in community health with high-risk families or neighborhoods.

So how can we make delivery systems focus on population health and the care of all children, regardless of whether those children are strongly connected to a primary care practice? The most logical method is to attribute all children in Medicaid in a given geography to the healthcare system with some form of accountability for overall health. There are a limited number of such examples out there now. Oregon's Coordinated Care Organization's Medicaid waiver encourages shared population health activities among diverse payers and providers and represents one of the most innovative because it focuses on all children in a given geography enrolled in Medicaid. Similarly, the intermediary model of Partners For Kids[8] in Ohio covers all children enrolled in Medicaid managed care across 34 counties, making them accountable regardless of plan churn or provider switching. Although much remains to be done in setting population health measures and determining how much responsibility for improvement collaborating healthcare systems have in their communities, it is only when we move beyond the Medicare-derived attribution methods focused on practices to broader Medicaid geographic inclusion that the "A" on pediatric ACOs will focus less on attribution for financial success and more on accountability for child health.

K. J. Kelleher, MD, MPH

References

1. Luft H. Assignment, attribution, and accountability: new responsibilities and relationships in accountable care organizations. *Virtual Mentor.* 2012;14:407-410.
2. Lewis VA, McClurg AB, Smith J, Fisher ES, Bynum J. Attributing patients to accountable care organizations: performance year approach aligns stakeholders' interests. *Health Aff.* 2013;32:587-595.
3. Christensen EW, Payne NR. Pediatric inpatient readmissions in an accountable care organization. *J Pediatr.* 2016;170:113-119.
4. Makni N, Rothenburger A, Kelleher K. Survey of twelve children's hospital-based accountable care organizations. *J Hosp Admin.* 2015;4:64-73.
5. Gleeson S, Kelleher KJ, Gardner WP. Evaluating a pay-for-performance program for medicaid children in an accountable care organization. *JAMA Pediatr.* 2016; 170:259-266.
6. Eisen M, Rubin D. Breaking new ground in health services research effect of attribution length in a pediatric Medicaid accountable care organization. *JAMA Pediatr.* 2016;170:114-115.
7. Bieber EJ, Hertz A. Pushing the Boundaries of Population Health Management: How University Hospitals Launched Three ACOs. University Hospital Summit Presentation. July 26, 2013.
8. Kelleher KJ, Cooper J, Deans K, et al. Cost saving and quality of care in a pediatric accountable care organization. *Pediatrics.* 2015;135:e582-e589.

Urgent Care and Emergency Department Visits in the Pediatric Medicaid Population

Montalbano A, Rodean J, Kangas J, et al (Children's Mercy Hosps and Clinics, Kansas City, MO; Children's Hosp Association, Overland Park, KS)
Pediatrics 137:e20153100, 2016

Background.—Urgent care (UC) is one of the fastest growing venues of health care delivery. We compared clinical and cost attributes of pediatric UC and emergency department (ED) visits that did not result in admission.

Methods.—Our study examined 5 925 568 ED and UC visits of children under 19 years old in the 2010 through 2012 Marketscan Medicaid Multi-State Database. Basic demographics, diagnoses, severity, and payments were compared. Between ED and UC visits, χ^2 tests were used for proportions and Wilcoxon rank-sum tests were used for continuous variables.

Results.—The UC and ED had the same most common diagnoses. Over half the UC visits were low severity. The ED had a higher rate of return within 7 days (8.4% vs 6.9%, $P < .001$) and follow-up with their primary care physician (22% vs 17.2%, $P < .001$). Few (<1%) were admitted on return visits from the ED or UC. Payments for UC were significantly less (median $76.90 vs $186.20, $P < .001$). This continued to hold true when comparing payments for selected diagnoses and each severity level. By extrapolating the cost savings, a national Medicaid per-year savings, if all lowest severity level visits were seen in UC, was more than $50 million.

Conclusions.—UC and ED Medicaid visits have similar most common diagnoses, rate of return, and admission. Severity level and payments were lower in UC. There is potential significant cost savings if lower acuity cases can be transitioned from the ED to UC.

▶ "Invent a better mousetrap and the world will beat a path to your door." Oh, if only it were as true in health care as it is in consumer goods!

This article shows, to no one's surprise, that urgent care clinics (UCs) provide less-expensive care to patients with mild and nonurgent illnesses than emergency departments (ED's), with no apparent loss of quality. One wonders, then, if it should be surprising is that EDs are still handling the bulk of urgent care in the United States. Is this what economists call a *market failure*? If so, why has this market failed?

One answer is that it is not in the economic interest of those who would set up and run UCs to do so. Who would the agents of change be? Not hospitals; they would be cutting their own throats. It is easy to set up a UC side by side with an ED, staff it with midlevel providers supervised by physicians, and divert urgent but nonsevere cases from ED to UC at ED triage. The result is less-expensive care, true, but who experiences the savings? Not the hospital; the hospital experiences primarily decreased revenues and less profit per patient to subsidize the expensive ED equipment and staffing. Instead, the savings are experienced by insurance companies and patients. Why, then, would a hospital do it?

Although the article does not explore alternative arrangements, private practices and clinics could establish UCs on their own, either by simply extending their hours to evenings and weekends or cooperating among themselves to set up and staff a UC for out-of-hours care. This method comes at a cost to themselves of convenience, because it means working less-attractive hours or hiring others to do so. There are common procedural terminology codes that would be applicable for extra compensation for out-of-hours care, but the payment is modest, and moreover, many payers choose not to honor those codes. As a result, once again, out-of-hours care savings redound to the benefit of government, insurance companies, and patients but not sufficiently to practices for them to answer the bell for potential profits.

Perhaps more tellingly, the article calculates that roughly $50 million a year could be saved by Medicaid if UCs replaced EDs for these pediatric cases. Although $50 million sounds like a lot of money, how significant would that really be? Total Medicaid spending for the United States in 2014 was about $476 billion. The projected savings to government would thus be 0.01%. The savings, then (like pediatric care overall in the nation's health care budget) would be "budget dust." By contrast, Medicaid is said to lose $29 billion to fraud, which would be 6%. It is no wonder government appears not to care much about the apparent ED waste.[1]

Moreover, one unit's waste is another unit's profit. By reducing the acute care income from an ED, the hospital ED would become less profitable. In effect, this extra remuneration for the ER subsidizes the cost of having ready a unit to service the true emergencies that appear there, which in themselves would not be financially worthwhile to serve. It might be true that if UCs proliferate, hospitals would be impelled to centralize their true emergency services to one hospital per city. But would that be optimal care? It is not clear that it would be.

Thus, the case for UCs replacing EDs for common acute care seems to be shaky. On the other hand, extending out-of-hours care at pediatric patient—centered medical homes seems to be a better choice. True, the savings for Medicaid would still appear to be small. The savings for private insurance might be larger, as private payments are usually higher than Medicaid payments. But even if the economic advantage were small, the improved quality of care and simplified communications conferred by better continuity might impel change. Convenience for the patient could also be enhanced, as waiting times are so much higher in EDs than in an office or many clinics. In addition, because accountable care organizations are ever in search of even small financial advantages, they might encourage pediatric practices to become PPCMHs and to provide the out-of-hours care that are part of the PPCMH charter. An accountable care organization would also be in a position to make out-of-hours care financially attractive for a PPCMH, rather than a sacrifice.

If there was more research on the economics of replacing routine acute care now performed in the ED, considering the PPCMH might be a better alternative to consider than a UC. The PPCMH is, after all, the American Academy of Pediatrics' preferred solution for transforming the organization of pediatric health care. Despite the small economic advantage of diverting patients from the ED, there is still reason for hope.

B. N. Shenkin, MD, MAPA

Reference

1. Medicaid Program Integrity: Improved Guidance Needed to Better Support Efforts to Screen Managed Care Providers. GAO-16%13402. 2016. http://www.gao.gov/products/GAO-16–402. Accessed May 9, 2016.

Measuring patient-perceived quality of care in US hospitals using Twitter

Hawkins JB, Brownstein JS, Tuli G, et al (Harvard Med School, Boston, MA; Virginia Tech, Blacksburg; et al)

BMJ Qual Saf 25:404-413, 2016

Background.—Patients routinely use Twitter to share feedback about their experience receiving healthcare. Identifying and analysing the content of posts sent to hospitals may provide a novel real-time measure of quality, supplementing traditional, survey-based approaches.

Objective.—To assess the use of Twitter as a supplemental data stream for measuring patientperceived quality of care in US hospitals and compare patient sentiments about hospitals with established quality measures.

Design.—404 065 tweets directed to 2349 US hospitals over a 1-year period were classified as having to do with patient experience using a machine learning approach. Sentiment was calculated for these tweets using natural language processing. 11 602 tweets were manually categorised into patient experience topics. Finally, hospitals with ≥50 patient experience tweets were surveyed to understand how they use Twitter to interact with patients.

Key Results.—Roughly half of the hospitals in the US have a presence on Twitter. Of the tweets directed toward these hospitals, 34 725 (9.4%) were related to patient experience and covered diverse topics. Analyses limited to hospitals with ≥50 patient experience tweets revealed that they were more active on Twitter, more likely to be below the national median of Medicare patients ($p < 0.001$) and above the national median for nurse/patient ratio ($p = 0.006$), and to be a nonprofit hospital ($p < 0.001$). After adjusting for hospital characteristics, we found that Twitter sentiment was not associated with Hospital Consumer Assessment of Healthcare Providers and Systems (HCAHPS) ratings (but having a Twitter account was), although there was a weak association with 30-day hospital readmission rates ($p = 0.003$).

Conclusions.—Tweets describing patient experiences in hospitals cover a wide range of patient care aspects and can be identified using automated approaches. These tweets represent a potentially untapped indicator of quality and may be valuable to patients, researchers, policy makers and hospital administrators.

► The array of social media sites and mobile applications is dizzying—Twitter, Facebook, Yelp, Instagram, Snapchat, to name a few. Social media mostly seems to be put on earth (or in the "cloud") to entice us with frothy swaths of cotton-candy-like bits (and bytes) of distraction.

However, over the past few years, an accumulating body of research has delved into whether we can harness the power of social media to learn something useful about the world, in particular about health and health care.[1-6] That was the goal of the study by Hawkins et al, who looked at Twitter as a potential data stream on hospital care. Twitter, an online community that allows user to send messages (a.k.a. tweets) to followers using a max of 140 characters, has an international presence, and 1 in 5 adults were actively using Twitter in 2014.

There are a few memorable aspects to the study: the use of natural language processing techniques to analyze a massive dataset of 404 065 tweets; the finding that some hospitals actively monitor and react to tweets; and the finding that positive tweets were correlated with hospital 30-day readmissions but not with patient satisfaction measures.

Natural language processing techniques are being touted as solutions to mining the electronic medical record for any sort of data. This study is an interesting case and entertaining in its innovation but also points out that these techniques are still limited in providing useful information—they can be used to identify sentiment (positive or negative) as a binary metric, but identifying topics of the tweets is difficult using machine learning. For instance, only 9.4% of comments could be identified as patient experience comments, the topic categories were broad (eg, "money concerns," "treatment side effects," "medication instructions"), and some categories had poor interrater reliability even for human readers (kappa of 0.18 for "communication" "discharge" and "medication instructions," with a kappa of 0.70 considered to be a scientifically acceptable minimum). The limitations of natural language processing to identify real meaning is not totally surprising and is likely a combined effect of the fact that machines have not yet achieved the human ability for nuanced contextual interpretation of language, coupled with the fact that tweets are limited to 140 characters, which can make comments difficult to interpret for humans and machines alike.

When the authors surveyed hospitals with at least 50 tweets (n = 297 hospitals, ~10% of all the hospitals with a twitter account and ~5% of all hospitals in the United States), they found that the hospitals all monitored Twitter closely, actively interacted with patients, and were aware that patients post about their experiences. One survey respondent commented: "We've had patients tweet us from waiting rooms, we've even had patients tweet us from their hospital beds!"

Monitoring Twitter accounts allows hospitals to do more timely service recovery for patients (while being mindful of the Health Insurance Portability and Accountability Act [HIPAA]). One hospital commented: "[O]ur goal is to respond to patient comments within an hour of their post. If the comment can be addressed via Twitter, we direct them to appropriate resources online. We are extremely careful to abide by HIPAA guidelines and the protection of patient privacy." Interestingly, the hospitals that were actively using the platform were not more experienced with Twitter; their accounts were the same age as other hospitals. The implication to these findings is that hospitals can make an active decision to leverage social media and that they may view Twitter as an innovative new method to cultivate connections with their patients and the larger community.

The relationship between positive sentiment and lower 30-day hospital readmissions echoes similar findings on other social media sites (eg, Yelp, Facebook).[2,7,8] However, it is unexpected that they did not find a relationship between positive sentiment on Twitter and patient experience scores, which one would think would be the stronger a priori hypothesis. On a cynical day, this raises the question for me as to whether the natural language processing techniques have produced random noise that we interpret as meaningful. On a cheerful day, I agree with the authors that further work is warranted, that Twitter is a potentially useful source of information and communication between hospitals and consumers and that natural language processing techniques are well suited to help analyze this "big data" set, allowing us to glean meaning from social media activity that would otherwise just be a live-chirping soundtrack.

N. S. Bardach, MD, MAS

References

1. Greaves F, Laverty AA, Cano DR, et al. Tweets about hospital quality: a mixed methods study. *BMJ Qual Saf.* 2014;23:838-846.
2. Greaves F, Pape UJ, King D, et al. Associations between Web-based patient ratings and objective measures of hospital quality. *Arch Intern Med.* 2012;172:435-436.
3. Lagu T, Goff SL, Hannon NS, Shatz A, Lindenauer PK. A mixed-methods analysis of patient reviews of hospital care in England: implications for public reporting of

health care quality data in the United States. *Jt Comm J Qual Patient Saf.* 2013;39: 7-15.

4. Lagu T, Hannon NS, Rothberg MB, Lindenauer PK. Patients' evaluations of health care providers in the era of social networking: an analysis of physician-rating websites. *J Gen Intern Med.* 2010;25:942-946.

5. Brownstein JS, Freifeld CC, Madoff LC. Digital disease detection—harnessing the Web for public health surveillance. *N Engl J Med.* 2009;360:2153-2155. 2157.

6. Verhoef LM, Van de Belt TH, Engelen LJ, Schoonhoven L, Kool RB. Social media and rating sites as tools to understanding quality of care: a scoping review. *J Med Internet Res.* 2014;16:e56.

7. Bardach NS, Asteria-Peñaloza R, Boscardin WJ, Adams Dudley R. The relationship between commercial website ratings and traditional hospital performance measures in the USA. *BMJ Qual Saf.* 2012;22:194-202.

8. Timian A, Rupcic S, Kachnowski S, Luisi P. Do patients "like" good care? Measuring hospital quality via Facebook. *Am J Med Qual.* 2013;28:374-382.

The Influence of Sugar-Sweetened Beverage Health Warning Labels on Parents' Choices

Roberto CA, Wong D, Musicus A, et al (Univ of Pennsylvania, Philadelphia; Harvard T.H. Chan School of Public Health, Boston, MA; et al)
Pediatrics 137:e20153185, 2016

Background and Objectives.—US states have introduced bills requiring sugar-sweetened beverages (SSBs) to display health warning labels. This study examined how such labels may influence parents and which labels are most impactful.

Methods.—In this study, 2381 demographically and educationally diverse parents participated in an online survey. Parents were randomly assigned to 1 of 6 conditions: (1) no warning label (control); (2) calorie label; or (3–6) 1 of 4 text versions of a warning label (eg, Safety Warning: Drinking beverages with added sugar[s] contributes to obesity, diabetes, and tooth decay). Parents chose a beverage for their child in a vending machine choice task, rated perceptions of different beverages, and indicated interest in receiving beverage coupons.

Results.—Regression analyses controlling for frequency of beverage purchases were used to compare the no warning label group, calorie label group, and all warning label groups combined. Significantly fewer parents chose an SSB for their child in the warning label condition (40%) versus the no label (60%) and calorie label conditions (53%). Parents in the warning label condition also chose significantly fewer SSB coupons, believed that SSBs were less healthy for their child, and were less likely to intend to purchase SSBs. All *P* values <.05 after correcting for multiple comparisons. There were no consistent differences among different versions of the warning labels.

Conclusions.—Health warning labels on SSBs improved parents' understanding of health harms associated with overconsumption of such beverages and may reduce parents' purchase of SSBs for their children.

▶ One of the key recommendations of the US Department of Agriculture (USDA) Dietary Guidelines for America 2015 was to limit calories from added sugars to less than 10% per day.[1] Sources of added sugar in Western diet are sugar sweetened beverages (SSBs), snacks, and varied sweets. SSBs account for 47% of all added sugars consumed by the United States population, especially in children, adolescents, and young adults.[2] Therefore, they constitute a plurality, if not majority, of added sugar consumption in the pediatric age group.

Sugar has been shown to be causative for type 2 diabetes, heart disease, fatty liver disease, and tooth decay, unrelated to its calories or its effects on weight gain.[3] Thus, sugar is a specific and independent risk factor for chronic disease, especially in children. Similar to cigarettes and alcohol, public health advocates have proposed adding a warning label to SSBs to attempt to reduce consumption.

This study is the first to examine the potential impact of SSB warning labels on consumption. The authors used highly visible and salient labels (either calorie or warning labels; Fig 1 in the original article) to investigate the influence of the presence or absence of labels on parents who are shopping for their children. Previously, the California legislature proposed (but did not adopt) warning label criteria, which identified any sweetened nonalcoholic beverages with added sweeteners that contain 75 or more calories per 12 fluid ounces.[4] The California warning label was used as a template to generate the other test warning labels to make them more salient. Despite their high glycemic load (ie, high sugar, low fiber content), natural fruit or vegetable juices, milk, and electrolyte solutions and other liquid products used for oral nutrition therapy without added sugar were not delineated as SSBs for this study because they did not meet the California proposed criteria. This trial was conducted with a large sample size, including a large proportion of racial and ethnic minority with different education levels. However, these results cannot be generalized to other populations due to the lack of a nationally representative sample.

The authors did not see any difference in outcomes between different warning labels. This result prompted a combined analysis of data for the warning labels. They reported a reduction in parental perception of SSBs as healthy, and an increase in perception of consuming SSBs as a risk for weight gain, heart disease, and diabetes. All participants supported the warning label policy regardless of their political view. The authors found a "barely" significant and nonsignificant interaction between education versus warning or calorie labels, respectively.

Others have previously reported that people with higher education and income were more likely to use calorie information provided in restaurant menus as compared to those with lower education and income.[5,6] When participants were asked to make an at-the-moment hypothetical purchasing decision for their child, caregivers who saw warning labels were significantly less likely to choose an SSB relative to those who saw calorie or no labels on beverages. But that does not mean that they will be purchasing fewer SSBs in the future because education and retention are 2 different entities. We know we can educate the public about the risks of consuming SSBs; but the retention of this information and the availability of these products will be the determinant of future behavior.

The experience with warning labels for SSBs is not likely to be different from that of experiences with warning labels for tobacco and alcohol. The evidence suggests that warning labels about the health effects of alcohol have had little effect on total consumption (although there is a limited effect on risky drinking patterns such as driving while intoxicated).[7,8] Rather, there is robust evidence supporting the effectiveness of environmentally focused, regulatory controls that impact the pricing, marketing, and distribution of alcohol,[9-11] and now for sugar-laden products as well, such as the Mexican soda tax.[12] These data suggest that if societies wish to mitigate the adverse sequelae caused by commodities, the best way to do this is by reducing their overall availability and ease of accessing such products.[13]

A. Erkin-Cakmak, MD, MPH

R. Lustig, MD

References

1. Dietary Guidelines for Americans. US Department of Agriculture. 2015. http://health.gov/dietaryguidelines/2015/default.asp.
2. What we eat in America, NHANES 2007–2010 for average intakes by age and sex group.
3. Lustig RH. Debate: Sickeningly sweet: does sugar cause diabetes? YES. *Can J Diab.* In press.
4. Senate Bill-1000. Public Health: sugar sweetened beverages: safety warnings. http://leginfo.legislature.ca.gov/faces/billNavClient.xhtml?bill_id=201320140SB 1000. Accessed March 21, 2016.
5. Breck A, Cantor J, Martinez O, Elbel B. Who reports noticing and using calorie information posted on fast food restaurant menus? *Appetite.* 2014;81:30-36.
6. Chen R, Smyser M, Chan N, Ta M, Saelens BE, Krieger J. Changes in awareness and use of calorie information after mandatory menu labeling in restaurants in King County, Washington. *Am J Public Health.* 2015;105(3):546-553.
7. Greenfield TK, Graves KL, Kaskutas LA. Alcohol warning labels for prevention: National survey results. *Alcohol Health Res World.* 1993;17:67-75.
8. Greenfield TK, Johnson SP, Giesbrecht NA. *The Alcohol Policy Development Process: Policy Makers Speak.* Washington, DC: American Public Health Association; 1998.
9. Edwards G, Anderson P, Babor TF, et al. *Retail Price Influences on Alcohol Consumption, and Taxation on Alcohol as a Prevention Strategy. Alcohol Policy and the Public Good.* New York, NY: Oxford University Press; 1994:109-213.
10. Moore M, Gerstein D, eds. Alcohol and Public Policy: In the Shadow of Prohibition. Washington, DC: National Academy Press; 1981.
11. Osterberg E. Do alcohol prices affect consumption and related problems?. In: Holder HD, Edwards G, eds. *Alcohol and Public Policy: Evidence and Issues.* Oxford, UK: Oxford University Press; 1995:145-163.
12. Colchero MA, Salgado JC, Unar-Munguía M, Molina M, Ng S, Rivera-Dommarco JA. Changes in prices after an excise tax to sweetened and sugar beverages was implemented in Mexico: evidence from urban areas. *PLoS One.* 2015; 10:e0144408.
13. Schmidt LA, Patel A, Brindis CD, Lustig RH. Towards evidence-based policies for reduction of dietary sugars: lessons from the alcohol experience. In: Goran MI, Tappy L, Le KA, eds. *Dietary Sugars and Health.* Taylor and Francis; 2014. Chapter 26:371-390.

Effect of the Healthy Hunger-Free Kids Act on the Nutritional Quality of Meals Selected by Students and School Lunch Participation Rates
Johnson DB, Podrabsky M, Rocha A, et al (Univ of Washington, Seattle)
JAMA Pediatr 170:e153918, 2016

Importance.—Effective policies have potential to improve diet and reduce obesity. School food policies reach most children in the United States.

Objective.—To assess the nutritional quality of foods chosen by students and meal participation rates before and after the implementation of new school meal standards authorized through the Healthy Hunger-Free Kids Act.

Design, Setting, and Participants.—This descriptive, longitudinal study examined changes in the nutritional quality of 1 741 630 school meals at 3 middle schools and 3 high schools in an urban school district in Washington state. Seventy two hundred students are enrolled in the district; 54% are eligible for free and reduced-price meals. Student food selection data were collected daily from January 2011 through January 2014 during the 16 months prior to and the 15 months after implementation of the Healthy Hunger-Free Kids Act.

Exposure.—The Healthy Hunger-Free Kids Act.

Main Outcomes and Measures.—Nutritional quality was assessed by calculating monthly mean adequacy ratio and energy density of the foods selected by students each day. Six nutrients were included in the mean adequacy ratio calculations: calcium, vitamin C, vitamin A, iron, fiber, and protein. Monthly school meal participation was calculated as the mean number of daily meals served divided by student enrollment. Mean monthly values of mean adequacy ratio, energy density, and participation were compared before and after policy implementation.

Results.—After implementation of the Healthy Hunger-Free Kids Act, change was associated with significant improvement in the nutritional quality of foods chosen by students, as measured by increased mean adequacy ratio from a mean of 58.7 (range, 49.6-63.1) prior to policy implementation to 75.6 (range, 68.7-81.8) after policy implementation and decreased energy density from a mean of 1.65 (range, 1.53-1.82) to 1.44 (range, 1.29-1.61), respectively. There was negligible difference in student meal participation following implementation of the new meal standards with 47% meal participation (range, 40.4%-49.5%) meal participation prior to the implemented policy and 46% participation (range, 39.1%-48.2%) afterward.

Conclusions and Relevance.—Food policy in the form of improved nutrition standards was associated with the selection of foods that are higher in nutrients that are of importance in adolescence and lower in energy density. Implementation of the new meal standards was not associated with a negative effect on student meal participation. In this district, meal standards effectively changed the quality of foods selected by children.

▶ The Healthy Hunger-Free Kids Act of 2010 required the US Department of Agriculture (USDA) to update regulations for the school food environment, including the National School Lunch Program (NSLP). The changes to the NSLP were extensive, including requirements for more whole grains, a greater variety of vegetables, calorie maximums (not just minimums) for meals, and a new policy that all reimbursable meals must include a fruit or vegetable.

One might think that improving the nutrition quality of school meals would be a noncontroversial issue. After all, who would argue against improving school nutrition when our country is facing an epidemic of childhood obesity? As it turns out, certain players with a financial stake in the program (ie, segments of the food industry that sell to schools) and some of those responsible for implementing these much stronger standards without losing money (ie, food service directors) were quite unhappy with the new, stronger nutrition standards. To be clear, many food service professionals and segments of the food industry were completely supportive of the changes, but enough were complaining about them to bring significant negative press to the process and risk damaging the reputation of the NSLP.

A particularly low point was when Representative Collin C. Peterson (Seventh Congressional District of Minnesota) and Senator Amy Klobuchar from Minnesota (home to the Schwan Food Company, which sells 70% of all pizza sold in schools) argued that the tomato paste in pizza sauce should continue to count as a full vegetable serving, which was a loophole that the USDA had attempted to close with these new regulations.[1] This led to the memorable headline: "Congress Says Pizza Is a Vegetable." This did not help reassure the American public that school meals are healthy.

It was within this context that the Johnson paper was published. This is 1 of a handful of studies that have been able to take advantage of the real-time experiment by comparing data from before the changes were implemented in the fall of 2012 to data from subsequent years. One considerable strength of the Johnson study is its size: they were able to get all of the production records from 6 schools in an urban district for 16 months before and 15 months after the regulations were implemented, resulting in a sample size of more than 1.7 million meals. They were also able to assess student participation using daily data from the district during this time frame.

The findings about improved nutrition quality and lower energy density were very encouraging. This suggests that the food service professionals, at least in Washington State, are following the new rules, and the lunches are indeed better than they used to be. As the authors note, they did not assess consumption and plate waste, so one might still wonder if the students are eating these healthier lunches. But work by our group and another group at Harvard found that while plate waste in school meals is a problem, it is not more of a problem now than it has ever been in the past.[2,3] So, taken together, the picture looks promising.

The meal participation data were not quite as encouraging. Participation varies considerably from month to month, and although there was not a statistically significant change from before to after, the *P* value was .10, which some researchers might call a trend. Improving participation is an important area for future research on school meals. There are factors that may help, such as removing the competitive foods, which are the a la carte or snack foods sold in the cafeteria or vending machines. Another strategy that increases participation is instituting universal free meals, which can be done through a process called Community Eligibility in low-income districts. Because the business model of the NSLP depends on maximum participation, future work is needed to identify strategies to increase the number of students who eat the school lunch.

One implication of this study is that health professionals who work directly with families, such as pediatricians, can comfortably encourage patients to eat the school lunch. In the past, some physicians may have discouraged patients from eating the school lunch out of concerns about its nutritional quality. This study, as well as knowledge about the considerable changes to the NSLP and the rest of the school food environment in recent years, should provide reassurance that the meals provided by schools are an asset to student health.

M. B. Schwartz, PhD

References

1. Confessore N. How school lunch became the latest political battleground. *New York Times Magazine*. 2014.
2. Cohen JF, Richardson S, Parker E, Catalano PJ, Rimm EB. Impact of the new US Department of Agriculture school meal standards on food selection, consumption, and waste. *Am J Prev Med*. 2014;46:388-394.
3. Schwartz MB, Henderson KE, Read M, Danna N, Ickovics JR. New school meal regulations increase fruit consumption and do not increase total plate waste. *Child Obes*. 2015;11:242-247.

Promoting Physical Activity With the Out of School Nutrition and Physical Activity (OSNAP) Initiative: A Cluster-Randomized Controlled Trial
Cradock AL, Barrett JL, Giles CM, et al (Harvard T. H. Chan School of Public Health, Boston, MA) *JAMA Pediatrics* 170:155-162, 2016

Importance.—Millions of children attend after-school programs in the United States. Increasing physical activity levels of program participants could have a broad effect on children's health.

Objective.—To test the effectiveness of the Out of School Nutrition and Physical Activity (OSNAP) Initiative in increasing children's physical activity levels in existing after-school programs.

Design, Setting, and Participants.—Cluster-randomized controlled trial with matched program pairs. Baseline data were collected September 27 through November 12, 2010, with follow-up data collected April 25 through May 27, 2011. The dates of our analysis were March 11, 2014, through August 18, 2015. The setting was 20 after-school programs in Boston, Massachusetts. All children 5 to 12 years old in participating programs were eligible for study inclusion.

Interventions.—Ten programs participated in a series of three 3-hour learning collaborative workshops, with additional optional opportunities for training and technical assistance.

Main Outcomes and Measures.—Change in number of minutes and bouts of moderate to vigorous physical activity, vigorous physical activity, and sedentary activity and change in total accelerometer counts between baseline and follow-up.

Results.—Participants with complete data were 402 racially/ethnically diverse children, with a mean age of 7.7 years. Change in the duration of physical activity opportunities offered to children during program time did not differ between conditions (-1.2 minutes; 95% CI, -14.2 to 12.4 minutes; $P = .87$). Change in moderate to vigorous physical activity minutes accumulated by children during program time did not differ significantly by intervention status (1.0; 95% CI, 3.3 to 1.3, $P = .40$). Total minutes per day of vigorous physical activity (3.2; 95% CI, 1.8-4.7; $P < .001$), vigorous physical activity minutes in bouts (4.1; 95% CI, 2.7-5.6; $P < .001$), and total accelerometer counts per day (16 894; 95% CI, 5101-28 686; $P = .01$) increased significantly during program time among intervention participants compared with control participants.

Conclusions and Relevance.—Although programs participating in the OSNAP Initiative did not allot significantly more time for physical activity, they successfully made existing time more vigorously active for children receiving the intervention.

Trial Registration.—clinicaltrials.gov Identifier: NCT01396473.

▶ Increasing the amount of moderate-to-vigorous physical activity (MVPA) children accumulate daily is a public health priority. In this study, the authors sought to increase children's MVPA in a setting that has emerged over the past decade as one of the most important locations, outside of the regular school day, to promote physical activity: afterschool programs. What the authors found has important implications for practitioners seeking to increase the amount of MVPA children accumulate while attending their program and for the intervention scientific community.

For practitioners, this study provides convincing evidence for a strategy they could adopt to get children more active. The authors' data clearly demonstrated that doing simple modifications to a program—namely, increasing the amount of time scheduled for children to be active, leads to an impressive increase in the amount of MVPA children accumulate. Specifically, the authors reported that both intervention and control programs increased the amount of time scheduled for physical activity from baseline to posttest by +23 and +24 minutes per day. Correspondingly, children in both conditions increased their MVPA by approximately +9 minutes per day or an increase of 37% and 30% from baseline.

This finding has major implications for practitioners who are seeking to increase physical activity in their programs but who are unable to purchase expensive curricula and equipment or pay for quality professional development training. Thus, making small changes, like increasing the amount of time allotted for children to be active, can have a major impact on children's MVPA. Moreover, this does not require a formal intervention. This finding alone should push the field forward in terms of substantiating the impact of a simple, practical strategy can have on the amount of activity children accumulate.

For the intervention scientific community, this study clearly suggests areas where we need improvements. The improvements largely surround the interpretation of intervention effects, statistical analyses, the reliance on P values to make judgements, and examining one's data. In the conclusion, the authors' state they "made existing time more vigorously active for children receiving the intervention." However, a quick review of their study findings show that what actually happened is they made the 2 groups equal in vigorous physical activity (VPA) by posttest, with the intervention and control groups accumulating 12.1 versus 13.5 minutes of VPA per day at posttest, respectively.

The authors also claim "the programs participating in the OSNAP Initiative did not make significant changes in time allotted for physical activity compared with controls." This statement implies that neither control nor intervention programs increased the amount of time allotted for activity opportunities, when they in fact both increased by approximately 20 minutes at posttest. Specifically, scheduled time for activity increased by 67% and 49% in the intervention and control programs, respectively.

To uncover changes from baseline to posttest or a lack of differences between groups at posttest, however, does not require statistical analyses and P values. A review of the raw means presented in the tables should have signaled that activity opportunities increased from baseline to posttest and that change in VPA over time occurred but did not result in differences between the groups at posttest. This indicates that those involved in the review process, as well as the authors, have interpreted the group × time interaction incorrectly: no changes at all occurred (for scheduled physical activity opportunities) nor were the groups different at posttest (for VPA). An interaction effect, however, only provides information on differential change over time between groups, not whether the groups are different at posttest. These misinterpretations are highly problematic, not only for this field, but for many others in which inaccurate conclusions are made about the effectiveness of an intervention.

I suggest to readers that there is a lot of value in this study, just not for the reasons the authors indicate. Increasing children's MVPA is not overly complicated, as demonstrated in this study, and can be accomplished by elongating the time allotted for children to be active. Moreover, our field needs to do a better job of training intervention scientists in understanding how interventions work (or do not work) and also ensure that we interpret the results from statistical tests correctly.

M. W. Beets, MEd, MPH, PhD

Progression to Traditional Cigarette Smoking After Electronic Cigarette Use Among US Adolescents and Young Adults

Primack BA, Soneji S, Stoolmiller M, et al (Univ of Pittsburgh School of Medicine, PA; Dartmouth Univ, Hanover, NH; Univ of Oregon, Eugene; et al)
JAMA Pediatr 169:1018-1023, 2015

Importance.—Electronic cigarettes (e-cigarettes) may help smokers reduce the use of traditional combustible cigarettes. However, adolescents and young adults who have never smoked traditional cigarettes are now using e cigarettes, and these individuals may be at risk for subsequent progression to traditional cigarette smoking.

Objective.—To determine whether baseline use of e-cigarettes among nonsmoking and nonsusceptible adolescents and young adults is associated with subsequent progression along an established trajectory to traditional cigarette smoking.

Design, Setting, and Participants.—In this longitudinal cohort study, a national US sample of 694 participants aged 16 to 26 years who were never cigarette smokers and were attitudinally nonsusceptible to smoking cigarettes completed baseline surveys from October 1, 2012, to May 1, 2014, regarding smoking in 2012-2013. They were reassessed 1 year later. Analysis was conducted from July 1, 2014, to March 1, 2015. Multinomial logistic regression was used to assess the independent association between baseline e-cigarette use and cigarette smoking, controlling for sex, age, race/ethnicity, maternal educational level, sensation-seeking tendency, parental cigarette smoking, and cigarette smoking among friends. Sensitivity analyses were performed, with varying approaches to missing data and recanting.

Exposures.—Use of e-cigarettes at baseline.

Main Outcomes and Measures.—Progression to cigarette smoking, defined using 3 specific states along a trajectory: nonsusceptible nonsmokers, susceptible nonsmokers, and smokers. Individuals who could not rule out smoking in the future were defined as susceptible.

Results.—Among the 694 respondents, 374 (53.9%) were female and 531 (76.5%) were non-Hispanic white. At baseline, 16 participants (2.3%) used e-cigarettes. Over the 1-year follow-up, 11 of 16 e-cigarette users and 128 of 678 of those who had not used e-cigarettes (18.9%) progressed toward cigarette smoking. In the primary fully adjusted models, baseline e-cigarette use was independently associated with progression to smoking (adjusted odds ratio [AOR], 8.3; 95%CI, 1.2-58.6) and to susceptibility among nonsmokers (AOR, 8.5; 95% CI, 1.3-57.2). Sensitivity analyses showed consistent results in the level of significance and slightly larger magnitude of AORs.

Conclusions and Relevance.—In this national sample of US adolescents and young adults, use of e-cigarettes at baseline was associated with progression to traditional cigarette smoking. These findings support regulations to limit sales and decrease the appeal of e-cigarettes to adolescents and young adults.

▶ Electronic cigarettes (e-cigarettes) are increasingly used by adolescents in the United States. These devices vaporize and deliver to the lungs a chemical mixture typically composed of nicotine, propylene glycol, and flavorings, although some products claim to contain no nicotine. In 2014, for the first time, the prevalence of e-cigarette use among US adolescents surpassed that of traditional cigarettes. Of great importance, a growing number of adolescents have used e-cigarettes but have never tried traditional cigarettes.

Using aerosolized nicotine rather than combustion, e-cigarettes likely produce fewer toxins than traditional cigarettes and are even marketed as a safer alternative to traditional cigarettes. As such, research in adult established smokers is largely focused on whether these products may be a form of harm reduction or even tools for cessation. At the other end of the spectrum, among adolescent nonsmokers, there is concern that these products may serve as a gateway to traditional cigarettes smoking.

With almost no research in the area, it is unclear whether e-cigarettes pose differential harms to teens than to adults. However, 2 points have been made relatively clear in the extant literature: (1) nicotine (contained in many e-cigarette solutions) has adverse effects on the developing brain and (2) the younger that children begin smoking traditional cigarettes, the more likely they are to become nicotine-dependent, lifelong smokers, and have trouble quitting smoking. Thus, a key question related to e-cigarette use among teens is whether their use is associated with increased likelihood of cigarette smoking initiation.

Primack and colleagues directly addressed this question with a longitudinal study design. The study's main finding is that, among adolescents and young adults, use of e-cigarettes is associated with an 8-fold greater risk of progression to traditional cigarette use compared with not using e-cigarettes first. A novel aspect of this article was the examination of "susceptibility" to smoking (ie, not ruling out smoking in the next year). E-cigarette use was also associated with an 8-fold greater risk of susceptibility to smoking, highlighting a further vulnerability of their use among never-smokers.

These findings have important implications as the US Food and Drug Administration (FDA) considers how to regulate e-cigarettes. Currently, there are no restrictions on "child-friendly" marketing, flavoring or labeling of e-cigarettes or related products. For example, it is currently legal to market bubblegum-flavored e-cigarettes and even call them vape pens instead of electronic cigarettes, which may be more appealing to children who feel that cigarettes are "bad." In fact, as nicotine-delivery devices, e-cigarettes likely pose the same risk for dependence as traditional cigarettes, but with fewer regulatory controls, their use could be undermining some of the important gains in the tobacco control movement made over the past decade where we actually saw a decrease in adolescent tobacco use. Findings by Primack and colleagues support regulations that limit access to e-cigarettes by youth.

This study is an important start to understanding what effect e-cigarette use may have on subsequent smoking among young people. Nevertheless, there are a few important limitations that should be considered. First, of the 694 young people aged 16 to 26 enrolled in the study, just 16 (2%) used only e-cigarettes at baseline. With such a small sample size, the confidence that the findings would be replicated in a future study is quite low. Further, the exact wording of the terms used to assess e-cigarette use are not reported in the study. There are many different terms for e-cigarettes. If "e-cigarette" was the only term used, there was likely underreporting of use. Young people have increasingly adopted other terms to describe products used to vaporize nicotine solution such as vape pens, e-hookahs, and others and, as such, may not have identified as having used an "e-cigarette." Finally, the US-based Dartmouth Media, Advertising, and Health Study recruited via random digit dialing with two-thirds landline and one-third cellular phone numbers. Given that 98% of young adults age 18 to 29 own a cellular phone[1] and more than half of households with young adults do not have landlines,[2] the study design likely missed a huge proportion of teens and young adults. Any study seeking a representative sample of young people should be recruiting primarily through cellular phones.

Despite these concerns, the study is an important contribution to the literature on how e-cigarettes are affecting nicotine use among young people and informing the regulatory landscape of these products. There is still quite a bit of controversy over whether e-cigarettes are harmful or helpful among those who currently smoke. For example, many are championing their use to support quitting among long-term, nicotine-dependent smokers. However, the evidence is growing that, in the absence of regulations limiting access to minors, their use is a public health threat to children. As the FDA considers regulations of e-cigarettes, effects of their use on subsequent uptake of smoking are of utmost importance to the public's health.

D. E. Ramo, PhD

M. L. Rubinstein, MD

References

1. Pew Internet and American Life Project. http://www.pewinternet.org/2015/10/29/technology-device-ownership-2015/. Accessed March 20, 2016.
2. Pew/CDC. http://www.pewresearch.org/fact-tank/2014/07/08/two-of-every-five-u-s-households-have-only-wireless-phones/. Accessed March 20, 2016.

Symptomatic Dengue in Children in 10 Asian and Latin American Countries
L'Azou M, for the CYD14 and CYD15 Primary Study Groups (Sanofi Pasteur, Lyon, France; et al) *N Engl J Med* 374:1155-1166, 2016

Background.—The control groups in two phase 3 trials of dengue vaccine efficacy included two large regional cohorts that were followed up for dengue infection. These cohorts provided a sample for epidemiologic analyses of symptomatic dengue in children across 10 countries in Southeast Asia and Latin America in which dengue is endemic.

Methods.—We monitored acute febrile illness and virologically confirmed dengue (VCD) in 3424 healthy children, 2 to 16 years of age, in Asia (Indonesia, Malaysia, the Philippines, Thailand, and Vietnam) from June 2011 through December 2013 and in 6939 children, 9 to 18 years of age, in Latin America (Brazil, Colombia, Honduras, Mexico, and Puerto Rico) from June 2011 through April 2014. Acute febrile episodes were determined to be VCD by means of a nonstructural protein 1 antigen immunoassay and reverse-transcriptase–polymerase-chain-reaction assays. Dengue hemorrhagic fever was defined according to 1997 World Health Organization criteria.

Results.—Approximately 10% of the febrile episodes in each cohort were confirmed to be VCD, with 319 VCD episodes (4.6 episodes per 100 person-years) occurring in the Asian cohort and 389 VCD episodes (2.9 episodes per 100 person-years) occurring in the Latin American cohort; no trend according to age group was observed. The incidence of dengue hemorrhagic fever was less than 0.3 episodes per 100 person-years in each cohort. The percentage of VCD episodes requiring hospitalization was 19.1% in the Asian cohort and 11.1% in the Latin American cohort. In comparable age groups (9 to 12 years and 13 to 16 years), the burden of dengue was higher in Asia than in Latin America.

Conclusions.—The burdens of dengue were substantial in the two regions and in all age groups. Burdens varied widely according to country, but the rates were generally higher and the disease more frequently severe in Asian countries than in Latin American countries. (Funded by Sanofi Pasteur; CYD14 and CYD15 ClinicalTrials.gov numbers, NCT01373281 and NCT01374516.)

▶ Dengue is the most important mosquito-borne viral disease, with approximately half of the world population at risk of transmission and outbreaks increasing in magnitude and geographic range.[1-3] The disease and economic burden of dengue are substantial, with 50 to 100 million symptomatic cases per year, and economic losses of about $8.9 billion.[1,2,4]

With the first dengue vaccine licensed in Mexico, the Philippines, and Brazil late in 2015 and new vector control approaches under development, accurate estimates of dengue burden are critical to inform evidence-based health policy. However, estimates of dengue burden have vast uncertainty, mostly because of variation in the availability, quality, and use of reported data.[5] One of the main challenges to estimate disease burden comes from underreporting of dengue episodes,[6] including fatal cases.[7,8] Prospective cohort studies with active surveillance across diverse settings are a key input to estimating the disease and economic burden of dengue.[2,4,5] Unfortunately, high-quality prospective cohort studies are scarce because they are expensive, time-consuming, and present several challenges in their implementation. The report by L'Azou and others based on 10 063 children in the control group of trials across 10 countries in Asia and Latin America with about 2 years of follow-up each, is one of the largest cohort studies of dengue to date.

Designers of clinical trials generally prefer settings and age groups with high expected incidence rates because these features tend to minimize the number of participants required. L'Azou et al. estimated the incidence (and 95% confidence interval) of virologically confirmed dengue (VCD) per 100 person years of 4.6 (4.1-5.1) in Asia (ages 2-16 years) and 2.9 (2.6-3.2) in Latin America (ages 9-18). Stanaway et al[2] estimated the incidence by comparable super-regions across all ages. Their estimated rates (and uncertainty intervals) were 3.4 (1.7-8.0) for Southeast Asia and 1.0 (0.4-2.0) for Tropical Latin America.[2] The fact that the rates observed by L'Azou et al are about twice those from the model suggest that the study designers succeeded in situating their trials in age groups and settings with above average risk.

L'Azou et al's study is extremely valuable for examining age-specific incidence of clinical disease across 2 regions. To clarify these patterns, Fig 1 plots incidence rates by age and region and associated trend lines. It shows higher dengue risk in Southeast Asia than Latin America as previously known[9] and declining risk with age in both regions.

Another key contribution of this study is the estimated percentage of virologically confirmed dengue episodes that were hospitalized. They averaged 19.1% (15.0%-23.9%) in Asia and 11.1% (8.1%-14.6%) in Latin America. These rates are valuable because surveillance of hospitalized dengue tends to be more complete than that for dengue overall.[6] The inverses of these hospitalization rates 5.2 (4.2-6.7) for Southeast Asia and 9.0 (6.8-12.3) for Latin America provide approximate regional factors. Multiplying the regional factor times the number of hospitalized confirmed dengue cases provides a rough estimate of overall confirmed dengue cases in a region or subregion.

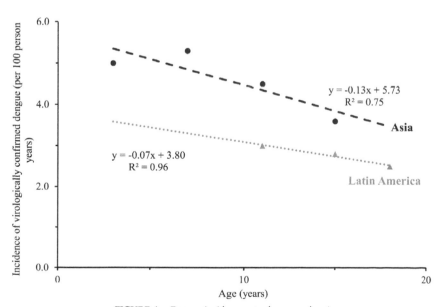

FIGURE 1.—Dengue incidence rates by age and region.

Finally, data from L'Azou et al show that most (77%) of the confirmed dengue hospitalizations did not meet the criteria for dengue hemorrhagic fever. This pattern, likely reflecting the risk that the condition of a dengue patient could deteriorate quickly, contributes to dengue's substantial economic burden.

L'Azou et al confirm the validity of Shepard et al's recent estimates of global dengue burden, which were developed from earlier data.[4] Shepard et al.'s estimated share of dengue cases hospitalized were 19.0% (8.9%-56.6%) for Asia and 3.8% (1.6%-8.3%) for Latin America, so the uncertainty intervals and confidence intervals of the 2 studies overlap.

Despite the great quality of the study design and implementation, there is always room for additional work. Longer follow-up periods of illness episodes would improve understanding of persistent symptoms of dengue, which may affect people's quality of life and ability to work way beyond the acute phase of the infection.[10] Detailed comparisons between VCD incidence and reported cases, building on a publication for Latin America,[11] would strengthen policy-makers' ability to infer the total burden of dengue. Overall, the study provides valuable data to reinforce previous estimates of the global burden of dengue, inform age-specific incidence, and we hope will help inform evidence-based health policy.

D. S. Shepard, PhD

E. A. Undurraga, PhD

References

1. Bhatt S, Gething PW, Brady OJ, et al. The global distribution and burden of dengue. *Nature*. 2013;496:504-507.
2. Stanaway JD, Shepard DS, Undurraga EA, et al. The global burden of dengue: a systematic analysis from the Global Burden of Disease Study 2013. *Lancet Infect Dis*. 2016;16:712-723.
3. Simmons CP, Farrar JJ, Nguyen VVC, Wills B. Current concepts: dengue. *N Engl J Med*. 2012;366:1423-1432.
4. Shepard DS, Undurraga EA, Halasa YA, Stanaway JD. The global economic burden of dengue: a systematic analysis. *Lancet Infect Dis*. 2016;16:935-941.
5. Shepard DS, Undurraga EA, Betancourt-Cravioto M, et al. Approaches to refining estimates of global burden and economics of dengue. *PLoS Negl Trop Dis*. 2014;8:e3306.
6. Undurraga EA, Halasa YA, Shepard DS. Use of expansion factors to estimate the burden of dengue in Southeast Asia: a systematic analysis. *PLoS Negl Trop Dis*. 2013;7:e2056.
7. Pamplona LG, de Melo Braga DN, da Silva LMA, et al. Postmortem diagnosis of dengue as an epidemiological surveillance tool. *Am J Trop Med Hyg*. 2016;94:187-192.
8. Tomashek KM, Gregory CJ, Rivera Sánchez A, et al. Dengue deaths in Puerto Rico: lessons learned from the 2007 epidemic. *PLoS Negl Trop Dis*. 2012;6:e1614.
9. Halstead SB. Dengue in the Americas and Southeast Asia: do they differ? *Rev Panam Salud Publica*. 2006;20:407-415.
10. Tiga DC, Undurraga EA, Ramos-Castañeda J, Martínez-Vega R, Tschampl CA, Shepard D. Persistent symptoms of dengue: estimates of the incremental disease and economic burden in Mexico. *Am J Trop Med Hyg*. 2016;94:1085-1089.
11. Sarti E, L'Azou M, Mercado M, et al. A comparative study on active and passive epidemiological surveillance for dengue in five countries of Latin America. *Int J Infect Dis*. 2016;44:44-49.

13 Heart and Blood Vessels

Radiofrequency Catheter Ablation of Accessory Atrioventricular Pathways in Infants and Toddlers ≤ 15 kg

Backhoff D, Klehs S, Müller M.J, et al (Georg August Univ, Göttingen, Germany)
Pediatr Cardiol 37:892-898, 2016

Accessory atrioventricular pathways (AP) are the most common substrate for paroxysmal supraventricular tachycardia in infants and small children. Up-to-date data on AP ablation in infants and small children are limited. The aim of the present study was to gain additional insight into radiofrequency (RF) catheter ablation of AP in infants and toddlers focusing on efficacy and safety in patients with a body weight of ≤ 15 kg. Since 10/2002, RF ablation of AP was performed in 281 children in our institution. Indications, procedural data as well as success and complication rates in children with a body weight ≤ 15 kg (n = 22) were compared with children > 15 kg (n = 259). Prevalence of structural heart anomalies was significantly higher among children ≤ 15 kg (27 vs. 5.7 %; $p = 0.001$). Procedure duration (median 262 vs. 177 min; $p = 0.001$) and fluoroscopy time (median 20.6 vs. 14.0 min; $p = 0.007$) were significantly longer among patients ≤ 15 kg. Procedural success rate did not differ significantly between the two groups (82 vs. 90 %).More RF lesions were required for AP ablation in the smaller patients (median 12 vs. 7; $p = 0.019$). Major complication rate was significantly higher in children ≤ 15 kg (9 vs. 1.1 %; $p = 0.05$) with femoral vessel occlusion being the only major adverse event in patients ≤ 15 kg. Catheter ablation of AP in children was effective irrespective of body weight. In children ≤ 15 kg, however, procedures were more challenging and time-consuming. Complication rate and number of RF lesions in smaller children were higher when compared to older children.

► Since the introduction of radiofrequency catheter ablation (RFCA) for the treatment of pediatric tachyarrhythmias in 1989, the procedure has evolved into the standard approach for many rhythm disorders. With user experience, success rates have been improving, and complication rates have been steadily declining. According to data from the pediatric RFCA registry assessing outcomes of initial cases of supraventricular tachycardia (SVT), a success rate of

95% and complication rate of 3% were achieved, with the most common complications being atrioventricular block, cardiac perforation with or without pericardial effusion, and thromboembolic events.[1,2]

SVT is the most common arrhythmia in the pediatric population, and RFCA has evolved into a safe and effective treatment option in older children and adolescents. However, controversy remains with respect to the safety of RFCA in smaller children. The consensus statement from the European Heart Rhythm Association/ Association for European Pediatric and Congenital Cardiology considered RFCA of SVT in children younger than 5 years as a class IIa recommendation if antiarrhythmic medications were ineffective or intolerable and a class I recommendation in cases of life-threatening arrhythmias regardless of age.[3]

Multiple studies across the literature assessed RFCA outcome in small children with SVT with varying results. The general consensus is that RFCA is a viable treatment option in selected cases with acceptable success and complication rates. These studies were not uniform in their definition of small children. This study by Backhoff et al, utilizing a weight of less than 15 kg to describe small patients, contributes to the body of evidence with certain unique features. Their study is one of the few that compares outcomes in smaller patients with institutional data on older children as a control. Additionally, they assess patients with SVT caused by accessory pathways only, excluding SVT caused by other substrates in an attempt to form a homogenous group of patients for comparison.

Although a significantly higher major complication rate was evident in patients who were ≤ 15 kg in this study, other comparative studies have not found a significant difference in smaller children.[4,5] Also, the complications encountered were related to catheter access rather than the ablation process per se. The prolonged procedure and fluoroscopy times are reflective of the challenges involved in performing RFCA on patients with smaller anatomy. In using nonfluoroscopic catheter navigation systems, accuracy is impaired when the patch electrodes are placed in closer proximity, as is the case in smaller patients, with resultant increased use of fluoroscopy for guiding catheter advancement. In addition, the need for increased numbers of lesions for successful ablation shows the technical challenges of the procedure in children ≤ 15 kg.

Given the prolonged procedure and fluoroscopy times, intermittent reports of increased complications, and the technical challenges in performing RFCA in smaller children, we recommend a judicious approach with a transparent conversation with the family reflective of the concerns seen in this study and others. However, in the setting of life-threatening arrhythmias, impending hemodynamic compromise, and medically refractive cases, RFCA has an adequate safety profile and success rate to justify its use in small children. With continued operator experience, institutions devoted to procedural and postprocedural care of small children and access to imaging systems and equipment tailored for pediatric patients, the safety and efficacy of RFCA will continue to improve.

D. Menon, MD

P. F. Aziz, MD

References

1. Van Hare GF, Javitz H, Carmelli D, et al. Prospective assessment after pediatric cardiac ablation: demographics, medical profiles, and initial outcomes. *J Cardiovasc Electrophysiol.* 2004;15:759-770.
2. Kugler JD, Danford DA, Houston K, Felix G. Radiofrequency catheter ablation for paroxysmal supraventricular tachycardia in children and adolescents without structural heart disease. Pediatric EP Society, Radiofrequency Catheter Ablation Registry. *Am J Cardiol.* 1997;80:1438-1443.
3. Brugada J, Blom N, Sarquella-Brugada G, et al. Pharmacological and non-pharmacological therapy for arrhythmias in the pediatric population: EHRA and AEPC-Arrhythmia Working Group joint consensus statement. *Europace.* 2013;15:1337-1382.
4. Blaufox AD, Felix GL, Saul JP. Radiofrequency catheter ablation in infants </−18 months old: when is it done and how do they fare? Short-term data from the pediatric ablation registry. *Circulation.* 2001;104:2803-2808
5. Aiyagari R, Saarel EV, Etheridge SP, et al. Radiofrequency ablation for supraventricular tachycardia in children < or =15 kg is safe and effective. *Pediatr Cardiol.* 2005;26:622-626.

Availability of Automated External Defibrillators in Public High Schools
White MJ, Loccoh EC, Goble MM, et al (Univ of Michigan, Ann Arbor; et al)
J Pediatr 172:142-146.e1, 2016

Objectives.—To assess automated external defibrillator (AED) distribution and cardiac emergency preparedness in Michigan secondary schools and investigate for association with school sociodemographic characteristics.

Study Design.—Surveys were sent via electronic mail to representatives from all public high schools in 30 randomly selected Michigan counties, stratified by population. Association of AED-related factors with school sociodemographic characteristics were evaluated using Wilcoxon rank sum test and χ^2 test, as appropriate.

Results.—Of 188 schools, 133 (71%) responded to the survey and all had AEDs. Larger student population was associated with fewer AEDs per 100 students ($P < .0001$) and fewer staff with AED training per AED ($P = .02$), compared with smaller schools. Schools with >20% students from racial minority groups had significantly fewer AEDs available per 100 students than schools with less racial diversity ($P = .03$). Schools with more students eligible for free and reduced lunch were less likely to have a cardiac emergency response plan ($P = .02$) and demonstrated less frequent AED maintenance ($P = .03$).

Conclusions.—Although AEDs are available at public high schools across Michigan, the number of AEDs per student varies inversely with minority student population and school size. Unequal distribution of AEDs and lack of cardiac emergency preparedness may contribute to outcomes of sudden cardiac arrest among youth (Tables 3 and 5).

▶ I am heartened by the fact that studies such as this are bringing increased awareness to medical professionals, school personnel, and laypeople on the

TABLE 3.—AED Distribution and Training by School Characteristics

School Characteristics	Number of AEDs per 100 Students		Number of School Staff Trained per AED	
	Median (IQR)	P Value*	Median (IQR)	P Value*
School population				
Small (<600 students)	0.65 (0.41-1.05)		5.5 (2.8-10.0)	
Medium (600-1500 students)	0.34 (0.25-0.57)	<.0001†	3.2 (1.3-7.5)	.02†
Large (>1500 students)	0.20 (0.14-0.78)		1.5 (1.0-4.5)	
Proportion of students of minority race/ethnicity, %				
>20	0.34 (0.23-0.62)	.03	5 (1.5-16)	.57
≤20	0.57 (0.35-0.90)		5 (1.7-8.6)	
Proportion of students eligible for free or reduced lunch, %				
>50	0.52 (0.34-0.90)	.72	6 (3.0-10)	.24
≤50	0.45 (0.32-0.90)		4 (1.6-8.0)	

*P value from χ^2 test for categorical variables and Wilcoxon rank sum test for continuous variables.
†Comparison of small vs medium or large.
Reprinted from White MJ, Loccoh EC, Goble MM, et al. Availability of automated external defibrillators in public high schools. *J Pediatr.* 2016;172:142-146.e1, with permission Elsevier.

TABLE 5.—Cardiac Emergency Response Plan by School Characteristics (N = 132)

School Characteristics	Cardiac Emergency Response Plan*			
	Yes (N = 63)	No (N = 34)	Unknown (N = 35)	P Value†
School population				
Small (<600 students)	35 (41.7)	24 (28.6)	25 (29.8)	
Medium (600-1500 students)	25 (56.8)	9 (20.5)	10 (22.7)	.07‡
Large (>1500 students)	3 (75.0)	1 (25.0)	0 (0.0)	
Proportion of students of minority race/ethnicity, %	7.6 (5.0-12.8)	6.6 (4.4-18.2)	6.6 (4.8-9.8)	.45
Proportion of students eligible for free or reduced lunch, %	44.6 (28.3-52.4)	45.0 (36.5-53.9)	49.2 (37.4-62.0)	.02

*Data are presented as N (%) for categorical variable and median (IQR) for continuous variables.
†P value from χ^2 test or Wilcoxon rank sum test, as appropriate, for the comparison of yes vs no or unknown for cardiac emergency response plan.
‡Comparison of small vs medium or large; P value from χ^2 test.
Reprinted from White MJ, Loccoh EC, Goble MM, et al. Availability of automated external defibrillators in public high schools. *J Pediatr.* 2016;172:142-146.e1, with permission Elsevier.

importance of dissemination of automated external defibrillators (AED) and the need for cardiopulmonary resuscitation (CPR) training and cardiac emergency response plans (CERP).

I write this commentary as a general pediatrician but also as a sudden cardiac arrest (SCA) rescuer. In 2013, my incredibly physically fit husband suffered an SCA at the height of an intense workout. Luckily I was present and able to respond quickly and identify what was likely happening. Unfortunately, there was no AED nearby, and I performed CPR with another trained and wickedly strong individual, who also happened to be working out that morning. When the paramedics arrived about 10 minutes after the event, my husband was shocked back to life on the gym floor with a defibrillator.

After 4 days in intensive care with substantial support, we are incredibly fortunate that he woke up, neurologically intact. He has since made a full recovery. Without getting into the specifics of our situation, our family now feels incredibly blessed, and we work within our community to increase awareness on the prevalence and signs and symptoms of heart attack and SCA, increase CPR and AED training and hopefully work to save lives.

By now everyone has probably seen the updated American Heart Association CPR Guidelines from 2015.[1] This guideline makes the recommendation, for adult basic life support and CPR in a witnessed arrest, to defibrillate as soon as possible. The guideline reaffirmed the recommended C-A-B sequence, circulation-airway-breathing, for pediatric CPR and continued to recommend AED use in pediatric patients if a patient is unresponsive and not breathing normally.

Whereas the 2010 Guidelines recommended the establishment of AED programs in public locations where there is a relatively high likelihood of witnessed cardiac arrest, the updated 2015 guidelines recommended that these Public Access Defibrillator (PAD) programs be implemented. The guidelines emphasize that deployment of an AED should not be limited to trained individuals (although training is still recommended). If instructor-led AED training is not available, a combination of self-directed training may be considered for lay providers learning AED skills.

In this article, the focus on health disparities associated with AED availability and maintenance as well as the presence of a CERP unfortunately mirrors other health disparities well documented in our society (Tables 3 and 5). Although important to discuss, I would like to use this commentary as an opportunity to advocate for a higher level focus both from the legislative side and medical side of the house on AED distribution, CPR training, and CERP implementation.

The authors appropriately report on the prevalence of sudden cardiac death (SCD) of 5% to 10% in children aged 5 to 10 years of age and 75% of sudden deaths among young athletes. Some data purport that more than 400 000 people die each year of SCD with 10 000 of those being children. These numbers are staggering and yet lifesaving, safe, and easy to use AEDS are not yet deployed ubiquitously in our country.

Similarly to the public health initiatives of the 1960s and 70s with fire extinguishers and smoke detectors mandated under widespread legislative efforts with insurance oversight, so too should we focus on public access and availability of AEDs and hands-only CPR training within our schools and communities.

I was struck by the highly successful survival rates of up to 71% for out-of-hospital cardiac arrest (OHCA) in schools. Similarly I am scared that 1 in 73 schools will have a sudden cardiac arrest on campus each year, and yet we have not yet mandated that each of those schools have an appropriate number of AEDs, well maintained and highly accessible, with students and staff trained and prepared to use them when needed with an active CERP.

I am in total agreement with the authors that we need more specific recommendations, legislative mandates, funding, and oversight of public access defibrillators as well as CPR training in our schools, and in our communities. With these more specific recommendations and mandates, we will hopefully see improvement in the health disparities specifically for SCD in children and young athletes.

C. L. Johnson, MD

Reference

1. 2015 American Heart Association Guidelines Update for cardiopulmonary resuscitation and emergency cardiovascular care. *Circulation.* 2015;132.

Comprehensive Versus Targeted Genetic Testing in Children with Hypertrophic Cardiomyopathy
Bales ND, Johnson NM, Judge DP, et al (Johns Hopkins Univ School of Medicine, Baltimore, MD; Invitae Corporation, San Francisco, CA)
Pediatr Cardiol 37:845-851, 2016

Hypertrophic cardiomyopathy (HCM) is a genetic disease of the sarcomere that can be found in both children and adults and is associated with many causative mutations. In children who are not the index case of HCM in their families, current recommendations call only for targeted genetic testing for familial mutations. However, clinical experience suggests that de novo mutations are possible, as are mutations inherited from apparently an unaffected parent. A chart review was conducted of all patients who received HCM genetic testing at Johns Hopkins from 2004 to 2013. In total, 239 patient charts were analyzed for personal and familial genetic findings. Eighty-one patients with sarcomere gene mutations were identified, of which 66 had a clinical diagnosis of HCM. Importantly, eight patients had >1 pathogenic or likely pathogenic mutation, including six patients who were diagnosed with HCM as children (18 or younger). In this analysis, when a sarcomere mutation is identified in a family, the likelihood of a child with HCM having >1 mutation is 25% (6/24), compared to 4.8% (2/42) for adults. The large number of children with multiple mutations suggests that broad panel rather than targeted genetic testing should be considered in HCM presenting during childhood even if the child is not the index case.

▶ Comprehensive genetic testing for hypertrophic cardiomyopathy (HCM), which commonly includes the 9 myofilament, HCM-associated genes (*ACTC, MYBPC3, MYH7, MYL2, MYL3, TNNC1, TNNI3, TNNT2,* and *TPM1*), has been available clinically since about 2005. The addition of genetic information to the evaluation of this disease has had a significant impact across the diagnostic, prognostic, and therapeutic triad of medicine.[1] Besides the exceptional circumstance in which the genetic test result directly alters the treatment of the index case with manifest disease, it significantly aids in the diagnosis and clinical management of family members. Specifically, a relative who is mutation positive but phenotype negative (no signs of disease) will be followed with careful scrutiny, while a mutation-negative relative who also has a normal echocardiogram could potentially be dismissed. Additionally, several studies have shown a prognostic value to genetic testing as long-term outcome studies have shown genotype-positive patients have worse outcome than their genotype-negative counterparts with regard to progression to heart failure, stroke or cardiac-related death.[2]

Clinically, the genetic screening strategy usually involves comprehensive testing of most to all known HCM-associated genes for the index case followed by mutation-specific testing for first-degree family members (and concentric circles of relatedness if positive) if a putative pathogenic mutation has been identified—so-called cascade testing. In this article, Bales et al pose an interesting and important implication and possible flaw in the cascade screening strategy: what if an additional mutation(s) is missed because a relative, especially offspring, was only tested for the sentinel variant implicated in the index case? In light of the low penetrance and extreme variability in expression of HCM, it is not unthinkable that the other parent might host a possible HCM-causing mutation, while not demonstrating the clinical phenotype of HCM, or that, although this would be rare, an additional de novo mutation has occurred in the tested relative.

In their retrospective study, Bales et al report a positive genetic test result of 35% among their HCM patients tested. More important, they found that among the 66 genotype- and phenotype-positive patents, patients diagnosed as children were significantly more likely to have a second mutation (6/24; 25%) compared with adults (2/42; 4.2%). And although the adult multiple-mutation frequency is very similar to previous studies, their contemplation that additional variants might have been or would be missed because of cascade screening is a fair consideration. Then again, should this always lead to full comprehensive testing in children or all family members rather than a targeted strategy? Or is there a way to select which patients might need to have additional testing performed?

To answer this question, one first has to determine whether mutations were in fact missed. Although their study was not set-up to effectively address this question, their results do illustrate 2 situations where a family members indeed had different genetic profiles: a sister and brother with 2 and 4 HCM mutations respectively, and a father and son with 2 and 3 respectively. And while the authors don't indicate whether how these variants were identified (comprehensive vs cascade screening) and whether parent(s) were tested as a result, it does point toward potential misses.

There is, however, a lot we can do in our clinical evaluation that might help us to decide a priori whether additional comprehensive genetic testing is indicated. First and foremost, we can look at the clinical phenotype of the affected individual(s). For instance, previous research has established clinical indicators that can guide this decision process, while several studies have also shown that there seems to be dosing with sarcomeric mutations. Therefore, when evaluating a family of patients with genotype positive HCM, comprehensive screening of the child could indeed be considered if the phenotype especially regarding age of diagnosis, degree of hypertrophy, and septal morphology[3] is significantly discordant with the phenotype of the affected parent. In fact, genotype prediction tools could herein aid in establishing whether the phenotype is vastly different than the parent, thereby prompting the consideration of additional genetic testing rather than simply confirming the presence or absence of the variant of interest that was established in the affected parent.

If in fact a second (or third) mutation is identified, this would change the genetic screening strategy for the family as (1) the unaffected parent should be tested and possibly enter periodic screening and (2) additional children (or children's children) should be tested for both variants. Lastly, especially in children diagnosed before age 1 year, a concomitant diagnosis of syndromic HCM should be considered.[4] Full clinical evaluation with particular attention to extracardiac features fitting 1 of these diagnoses can help in establishing this possible (rare) co-occurrence. However, aside from the need for supporting data on the exact miss rate, there are reasons to "stick with the old," such as cost for the additional genetic test and potential screening, absence of a genetic therapeutic options, and the fact that it would not result in a change in treatment, and, not in the least, the possible discovery of a variant of uncertain significance, also called "genetic purgatory." As has been shown, there is an approximate 5% background noise rate in HCM, as well as a continuing challenge to fully classify identified mutations.[5] Herein, the expanded screen could very well reveal an uninterpretable variant that only complicates the genetic evaluation of this family, without significant changes in diagnostic management.

With their article, Bales et al have raised an interesting question regarding a potential pitfall of cascade genetic testing strategy for families, and future research will show the true scope of this problem and whether we should alter our approach in certain cases. Despite some anecdotal exceptions and excepting those scenarios where the manifest phenotype in "a to be tested relative" ought to compel an independent comprehensive genetic test, the current strategy of variant-specific cascade testing of the appropriate relatives of solely the variant implicated as the probable root cause in the index case is likely to be validated as the best in practice approach.

J. M. Bos, MD, PhD

M. J. Ackerman, MD, PhD

References

1. Ackerman MJ, Priori SG, Willems S, et al. HRS/EHRA expert consensus statement on the state of genetic testing for the channelopathies and cardiomyopathies this document was developed as a partnership between the Heart Rhythm Society (HRS) and the European Heart Rhythm Association (EHRA). *Heart Rhythm.* 2011;8:1308-1339.
2. Olivotto I, Girolami F, Ackerman MJ, et al. Myofilament protein gene mutation screening and outcome of patients with hypertrophic cardiomyopathy. *Mayo Clin Proc..* 2008;83:630-638.
3. Bos JM, Will ML, Gersh BJ, Kruisselbrink TM, Ommen SR, Ackerman MJ. Characterization of a phenotype-based genetic test prediction score for unrelated patients with hypertrophic cardiomyopathy. *Mayo Clin Proc.* 2014;89:727-737.
4. Lipshultz SE, Orav EJ, Wilkinson JD, et al. Risk stratification at diagnosis for children with hypertrophic cardiomyopathy: an analysis of data from the Pediatric Cardiomyopathy Registry. *Lancet.* 2013;382:1889-1897.
5. Kapplinger JD, Landstrom AP, Bos JM, Salisbury BA, Callis TE, Ackerman MJ. Distinguishing hypertrophic cardiomyopathy-associated mutations from background genetic noise. *J Cardiovasc Transl Res.* 2014;7:347-361.

Physical Activity, Obesity Status, and Blood Pressure in Preschool Children
Vale S, Trost SG, Rêgo C, et al (Univ of Porto, Portugal; Queensland Univ of Technology, Brisbane, Australia)
J Pediatr 167:98-102, 2015

Objective.—To examine the combined effects of physical activity and weight status on blood pressure (BP) in preschool-aged children.

Study Design.—The sample included 733 preschool-aged children (49% female). Physical activity was objectively assessed on 7 consecutive days by accelerometry. Children were categorized as sufficiently active if they met the recommendation of at least 60 minutes daily of moderate-to-vigorous physical activity (MVPA). Body mass index was used to categorize children as nonoverweight or overweight/obese, according to the International Obesity Task Force benchmarks. BP was measured using an automated BP monitor and categorized as elevated or normal using BP percentile-based cut-points for age, sex, and height.

Results.—The prevalence of elevated systolic BP (SBP) and diastolic BP was 7.7% and 3.0%, respectively. The prevalence of overweight/obese was 32%, and about 15% of children did not accomplish the recommended 60 minutes of daily MVPA. After controlling for age and sex, overweight/obese children who did not meet the daily MVPA recommendation were 3 times more likely (OR 3.8; CI 1.6-8.6) to have elevated SBP than nonoverweight children who met the daily MVPA recommendation.

Conclusions.—Overweight or obese preschool-aged children with insufficient levels of MVPA are at significantly greater risk for elevated SBP than their nonoverweight and sufficiently active counterparts (Fig 2).

▶ The pediatric obesity epidemic has increased significantly over the past 3 decades. This increase represents a problem for the health care system because being overweight is directly associated with an increased probability of developing metabolic syndrome and high blood pressure (BP). In a systematic review, which evaluated more than 55 studies of the 5 continents and included 122 053 adolescents, our research group noted a higher prevalence (1 in 10 of adolescents) of hypertension.[1]

The study by Vale et al is based on data from preschool children, who are scarcely represented in the literature. The authors analyze the combined effects of physical activity (PA) and weight status on blood pressure (BP) in 1566 Portuguese children.

Body mass index and body fat are important risk indices for the development of hypertension (independent of the age and gender). In addition, obese children have a lower PA level than normal weight children. As a result, there is probably a double effect on blood pressure levels, due to weight status plus lower PA levels (Fig 2). An important contribution of this study was to demonstrate the high prevalence of obesity and high BP in children in a higher income country.

The current PA guidelines from the World Health Organization recommend that children have at least 60 minutes per day of moderate-to-vigorous of PA

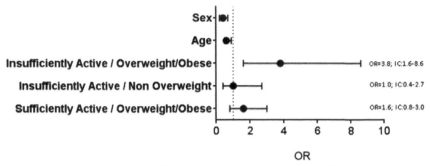

FIGURE 2.—ORs and 95% CIs from multivariate logistic regression analysis of the association between combined physical activity. Weight status grouping and elevated BP (≥90th percentile). (Reprinted from Vale S, Trost SG, Rêgo C, et al. Physical activity, obesity status, and blood pressure in preschool children. *J Pediatr.* 2015;167:98-102, with permission from Elsevier.)

(MVPA) to promote cardiovascular health. The main benefit of PA on the cardiovascular system is that the sheer stress caused by regular PA has a powerful effect on the release of vasodilator factors produced by the vascular endothelium, such as nitric oxide and endothelium-derived hyperpolarizing factor (EDHF).[2] Children who perform less than < 60 minutes per day of PA have lower vasodilation capacity of the endothelium, and this could be a biological mechanism through which they develop HBP.[3]

This article delivers the message that the obese children who are insufficiently active (< 60 minutes/day of MVPA) are 4 times more likely to have elevated systolic BP compared with those who were nonoverweight and meeting the daily 60 minutes of MVPA recommendation. These findings are relevant because higher blood pressure (HBP) is considered the risk factor with the highest attributable fraction for cardiovascular diseases (CVD) mortality (40.6%).

Recently, our research group also found that a low level of PA is not the only important risk factor to increase BP in children, but the frequency of sedentary behavior (time spent on computers, TV, and video games) is also important. In children from 8 European countries children who maintained sedentary behavior > 2 hours/day during a 2-year follow-up showed a high incidence of HBP. They also had a 30% increased risk to develop HBP.[4] In this article, the authors did not assess the sedentary behavior, which is strongly associated with the risk of development of obesity in children and adolescents.

It is important to focus on the combined effect of obesity and lifestyle variables (eg, PA and sedentary behavior). These findings suggest that interventions in children to prevent hypertension should begin early in life and include not only weight control but also interventions to increase the PA levels and reduce the sedentary behavior, even among those with a normal body mass index. In addition, these interventions should preferably address multiple behaviors, not just single factors. Integrated approaches targeting PA, sedentary behavior, and healthy dietary patterns which consider the family and home environment are currently considered to be the most promising approaches to tackle overweight and obesity, as well as BP control.

A. C. F. de Moraes, BSc, MSc, PhD

References

1. de Moraes AC, Lacerda MB, Moreno LA, Horta BL, Carvalho HB. Prevalence of high blood pressure in 122,053 adolescents: a systematic review and meta-regression. *Medicine (Baltimore)*. 2014;93:e232.
2. Bond B, Hind S, Williams CA, Barker AR. The acute effect of exercise intensity on vascular function in adolescents. *Med Sci Sports Exerc*. 2015;47:2628-2635.
3. de Moraes AC, Fernández-Alvira JM, Carvalho HB, et al. Physical activity modifies the associations between genetic variants and blood pressure in European adolescents. *J Pediatr*. 2014;165:1046-1049.e1-2.
4. de Moraes AC, Carvalho HB, Siani A, et al. Incidence of high blood pressure in children - effects of physical activity and sedentary behaviors: the IDEFICS study: high blood pressure, lifestyle and children. *Int J Cardiol*. 2015;180:165-170.

Hypertension Prevalence, Cardiac Complications, and Antihypertensive Medication Use in Children

Dobson CP, Eide M, Nylund CM (Tripler Army Med Ctr, Honolulu, HI; Uniformed Services Univ of the Health Sciences, Bethesda, MD)
J Pediatr 167:92-97, 2015

Objective.—To determine the prevalence of hypertension diagnosis in children of US military members and quantify echocardiography evaluations, cardiac complications, and antihypertensive prescriptions in the post-2004 guideline era.

Study Design.—Using billing data from military health insurance (TRICARE) enrollees, hypertension cases were defined as 2 or more visits with a primary or unspecified hypertension diagnosis during any calendar year or 1 such visit if with a cardiologist or nephrologist.

Results.—During 2006-2011, the database contained an average 1.3 million subjects aged 2-18 years per year. A total of 16 322 met the definition of hypertension (2.6/1000). The incidence of hypertension increased by 17% between 2006 and 2011 (from 2.3/1000 to 2.7/1000; $P < .001$). Hypertension was more common in adolescents aged 12-18 years than in younger children (5.4/1000 vs 0.9/1000). Among patients with hypertension, 5585 (34%) underwent echocardiography. The frequency of annual echocardiograms increased from 22.7% to 27.7% ($P < .001$). In patients with echocardiography, 8.0% had left ventricular hypertrophy or dysfunction. Among the patients with hypertension, 6353 (38.9%) received an antihypertensive medication.

Conclusion.—The prevalence of hypertension in children has increased. Compliance with national guidelines is poor. Of pediatric patients with hypertension who receive an echocardiogram, 1 in 12 had identified cardiac complications, supporting the current recommendations for echocardiography in children with hypertension. Less than one-half of children with hypertension are treated with medication (Fig 1).

▶ The prevalence of elevated blood pressure (BP) in children and adolescents has increased over recent decades, with the main contributing factors being the

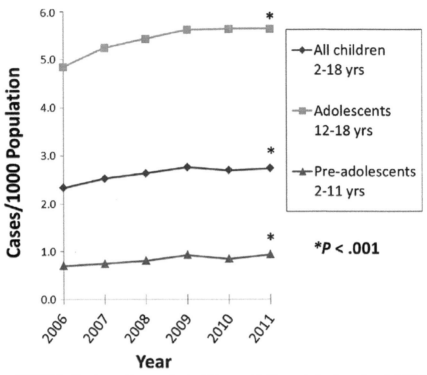

FIGURE 1.—Prevalence of hypertension in children aged 2-18 years during the study period 2006-2011. Hypertension was defined as requiring 2 visits with any primary or unspecified hypertension ICD-9-CM code or a single visit with a nephrologist or cardiologist who assigned the diagnosis. (Reprinted from Dobson CP, Eide M, Nylund CM. Hypertension prevalence, cardiac complications, and antihypertensive medication use in children. *J Pediatr.* 2015;167:92-97, with permission from Elsevier.)

childhood obesity epidemic, excessive dietary sodium intake, and the decreased physical activity. Although there can be immediate complications of high BP in childhood, such as left ventricular hypertrophy (LVH), abnormal vascular function, and impaired cognitive function, the major concern is that these hypertensive children will become hypertensive adults and will be at increased risk of premature cardiovascular disease (CVD). Although there has been some recent controversy as to the utility of detection of high BP in the young as a strategy for prevention of adult CVD, current consensus recommendations endorse routine BP measurement in children and adolescents and outline strategies for evaluation and management of high BP when it is found.

Few studies have actually examined the extent to which such consensus recommendations are followed in routine clinical practice. Dobson and colleagues examined the billing database of TRICARE, the main insurer for military families, to identify whether publication of the National High Blood Pressure Education Program (NHBPEP) Fourth Report, issued in 2004, has resulted in an increased diagnosis of hypertension (HTN) among children and adolescents enrolled in TRICARE, and whether specific recommendations contained in the Fourth

Report pertaining to diagnostic tests and prescribing of antihypertensive medications are being followed.

The authors did find an increase in the number of children diagnosed with HTN over the study period (2006–2011), with the greatest prevalence being 0.54% in adolescents in 2011 (Fig 1). Of note, this figure is only about one-eighth of the expected prevalence of HTN based on data collected in school screening studies. Why is this? There are 2 potential reasons: First, insurance billing data obviously do not contain detailed clinical information; therefore, we do not know how many children may have had an elevated BP reading that was going to be followed up at a future visit or how many had an elevated BP reading identified but did not return for the recommended repeat BP determinations. Second, several studies published since the Fourth Report was issued have highlighted the failure of many clinicians to correctly identify children and adolescents with high BP, so there may be many children enrolled in TRICARE who did not have the recommended follow-up visits for confirmation of the diagnosis of HTN.

Unfortunately, although the authors did show an increase in the number of children diagnosed with HTN over the study, period, there is no way to know whether this increase was actually attributable to clinicians following the new Fourth Report recommendations. The increase in pediatric enrollees in TRICARE diagnosed with HTN is more likely a reflection of the secular trends in BP among American children and adolescents, which as noted earlier has been primarily fueled by the childhood obesity epidemic. Thus, this finding of Dobson et al is interesting, but it actually does not answer the question they posed as one of the rationales for their study.

What about diagnostic testing and antihypertensive medication use? Here the study's findings are more informative. About one-third of children and adolescents with HTN had echocardiography performed, about 40% were prescribed antihypertensive medications, and nearly 80% of those children with LVH were prescribed an antihypertensive. While other investigators have previously shown that performance of echocardiography in children and adolescents is less frequent than what the Fourth Report would recommend, the present study shows an increase in the percentage of hypertensive youth who did actually undergo echocardiography, which is reassuring—but again, there is no way to know whether this increase occurred as a consequence of publication of the Fourth Report. Other investigators have also shown that medication use is less frequent than perhaps expected, but here Dobson et al are correct when they say that the guidelines also recommend lifestyle changes as the first step in treatment, so the relatively low rate of medication use may actually be consistent with the Fourth Report.

Clinical practice guidelines are well intentioned but can be difficult to implement successfully in the primary care setting. Specific to pediatric HTN, much has been made of the complexity of making an accurate diagnosis given the need to consult the detailed tables of normative BP values found in the Fourth Report. Dobson et al have provided a snapshot view of how the current pediatric BP guidelines appear to be performing in a large population of pediatric outpatients. Whether the flaws of this study could ever be overcome to get better information is uncertain. In the meantime, the information contained in this report should serve to stimulate self-examination among clinicians and should help to identify further research questions related to pediatric and adult CVD.

J. T. Flynn, MD, MS

Turner Syndrome in Girls Presenting with Coarctation of the Aorta
Eckhauser A, South ST, Meyers L, et al (Univ of Utah, Salt Lake City)
J Pediatr 167:1062-1066, 2015

Objective.—To evaluate the frequency of Turner syndrome in a population-based, statewide cohort of girls with coarctation of the aorta.

Study Design.—The Utah Birth Defects Network was used to ascertain a cohort of girls between 1997 and 2011 with coarctation of the aorta. Livebirths with isolated coarctation of the aorta or transverse arch hypoplasia were included and patients with complex congenital heart disease not usually seen in Turner syndrome were excluded.

Results.—Of 244 girls with coarctation of the aorta, 77 patients were excluded, leaving a cohort of 167 girls; 86 patients (51%) had chromosomal studies and 21 (12.6%) were diagnosed with Turner syndrome. All patients were diagnosed within the first 4 months of life and 5 (24%) were diagnosed prenatally. Fifteen patients (71%) had Turner syndrome-related findings in addition to coarctation of the aorta. Girls with mosaicism were less likely to have Turner syndrome-associated findings (3/6 mosaic girls compared with 12/17 girls with non-mosaic 45,X). Twelve girls (57%) diagnosed with Turner syndrome also had a bicommissural aortic valve.

Conclusion.—At least 12.6% of girls born with coarctation of the aorta have karyotype-confirmed Turner syndrome. Such a high frequency, combined with the clinical benefits of an early diagnosis, supports genetic screening for Turner syndrome in girls presenting with coarctation of the aorta (Table 2).

▶ Turner syndrome (TS), a condition caused by loss of or abnormality in the second X chromosome in an individual who is phenotypically female, is commonly associated with short stature, primary ovarian failure, and other health problems including autoimmune thyroid dysfunction, celiac disease, hearing deficits, cardiovascular (including aortic dilatation leading to dissection), and metabolic morbidity. Clearly, these health complications may not be identified early if TS itself remains undiagnosed. In addition, it is known that families in which adolescents receive a late diagnosis often struggle to deal with issues relating to difficulties with fertility, a particularly emotionally charged issue.[1] Unfortunately, late diagnosis of TS is still not uncommon, with recent audits suggesting that about a quarter are still diagnosed later in adolescence and adulthood.[2,3] Current expert consensus recommends that karyotype analysis should be performed in girls with short stature, delayed puberty, webbed neck, lymphedema, and coarctation of the aorta (CoA).[4]

TABLE 2.—Associated Turner Syndrome Related Findings

Phenotypic Anomaly	n
WN	11/21
Low or posteriorly set ears	4/21
Renal anomalies	4/21
WSN	3/21
Cystic hygroma	3/21
Deep-set/hypoplastic nails	2/21
Single umbilical artery	2/21

Reprinted from Eckhauser A, South ST, Meyers L, et al. Turner syndrome in girls presenting with coarctation of the aorta. *J Pediatr.* 2015;167:1062-1066, with permission from Elsevier.

However, what is the likelihood that a girl presenting with CoA has TS; therefore, what is the evidence base for CoA as the impetus for karyotype analysis in all girls presenting with CoA? The study by Eckhauser et al uses data from the Utah Birth Defect Network, looking at live born girls (1997 to 2011) with a diagnosis of CoA to address this issue. This question has recently been considered in a cohort of 140 girls with CoA presenting to one tertiary pediatric institution in Australia (1975-2010).[5] The true strength of the study by Eckhauser et al is the stringent and careful review by geneticists and cardiologists of this clinical database. In addition, the cases were re-reviewed by a geneticist and cardiothoracic surgeon, ensuring that the diagnoses of both CoA and Turner syndrome are appropriate.

Of 167 girls with CoA, only 86 had a karyotype analysis in this study (51%), in contrast to 41.7% reported by Wong et al.[5] Wong et al[5] found that karyotype analysis was more frequently requested for girls presenting with CoA in recent years (53% from 2000-2010). Both studies, therefore, confirm nonadherence to expert consensus. There could be multiple reasons for this finding, including more urgent life-threatening cardiac issues at diagnosis of CoA, lack of awareness of the consensus guidelines, or a lack of evidence-based/perceived benefit for screening karyotypes in all girls with CoA.

Eckhauser et al identified 21 of 167 (12.6%) girls with TS in their cohort with CoA. However, given that only 86 girls with CoA had karyotype analysis, we believe that the prevalence of TS should be 24.4%, although a minimum prevalence of 12.6% as suggested by the authors is not inaccurate. This figure is in contrast to the prevalence of 5.3% in the Australian study,[5] one of whom was diagnosed at the age of 2.5 years after presenting with CoA in the neonatal period. Wong et al[5] also went on to conduct a research study to perform karyotype analysis in those girls with CoA who did not have the test performed clinically (51.4% response rate). None of those who were recalled for a research study karyotype with a 50-cell count had TS diagnosed.

What are the possible reasons for the discrepancy between these 2 studies? The method used to diagnose TS may theoretically be a possible reason. Eckhauser et al did not report the number of cells counted for the karyotype analysis, but it is likely to be 15 to 30 cells, as is the case in routine clinical practice. This count is also likely to be the same in those who had clinical karyotyping performed in the Australian study.[5] Low-level mosaicism may be missed by counting 15 to 30 cells, hence, the current recommendation to increase cell counts if this is suspected.[6] If anything, one should expect more low-level mosaic girls with TS to be diagnosed in the Australian cohort, given that those who did not have a clinical karyotype had a research karyotype analysis with 50-cell count.[5]

However, the number of girls with TS in any cohort depends on the number of girls who survived to live birth. A total of 99% of 45,X embryos are thought to terminate in the first 2 trimesters.[7] A recent study reviewing the characteristics of pregnancies with a prenatal diagnosis of TS via amniocentesis or chorionic villous sampling in Scotland over a 10-year period found that only 21 of 60 (35%) resulted in a live birth.[8] The other interesting observation in this study by Lucas-Herald et al[8] is that 28 of 30 (94%) TS fetuses with abnormalities on ultrasound scanning were associated with termination of pregnancy, although it is not known how many had CoA specifically. The rate of TS in CoA could be associated with local differences in termination of pregnancy rates.

How should a clinician encountering a girl with CoA interpret the results of these 2 studies to answer the question of whether a screening karyotype should be performed in all girls with CoA? In this study by Eckhauser et al and in the study by Wong et al,[5] 14 of 21 (67%) and 4 of 6 (67%) of the girls with CoA and TS had lymphedema or neck abnormalities, respectively. Therefore, the likelihood of TS maybe greater if those clinical features are present in an infant with CoA, although absence of those signs does not rule TS out (Table 2).

Does it matter what the prevalence of TS in CoA is? To put things in context, studies have found that performing a karyotype analysis in girls with short stature, a well-accepted practice in pediatrics, will only identify 2% to 4% of TS.[9,10] If we do not challenge the practice of performing karyotype analysis in all short girls, like Dr Eckhauser and colleagues, then we believe that all girls with CoA should have a screening karyotype. If the idea is to diagnose TS early, screening in girls with CoA allows the perfect opportunity. We feel that it is not an issue of how many cases we will diagnose but the fact that early and timely treatment is found to lead to optimal growth and pubertal outcome. Early diagnosis as mentioned also offers the opportunity for earlier identification of the other comorbidities associated with TS, including prophylactic gonadectomy in TS with a karyotype with Y material. The emotional devastation of late diagnosis in adolescence and even in adulthood should be avoided.

Unfortunately, late diagnosis of TS still happens in current clinical practice. Studies such as this by Eckhauser et al are important in ensuring that health professionals from a wider group than purely pediatric endocrinology have a lower threshold to think about TS in their clinical practice. Undiagnosed girls with TS present to general practitioners, general/community pediatricians, pediatric otorhinolaryngologists, cardiologists, gastroenterologists, and neonatologists. There should be a push to increase awareness and to ensure adherence for screening in situations recommended in the consensus guidelines. The question of whether a screening karyotype should be performed in girls with bicuspid aortic valves (the most common cardiac abnormality in TS, seen in about 30%) or those with recurrent/complicated ear infections (extremely common and troublesome in girls with TS) warrants future research or incorporation into clinical practice.

A. K. Lucas-Herald, MRCPCH

S. C. Wong, DMedSci, MRCPCH

References

1. Starke M, Wikland KA, Moller A. Parents' experiences of receiving the diagnosis of Turner syndrome: an explorative and retrospective study. *Patient Education and Counselling*. 2002;47:347-354.
2. Massa G, Verlinde F, De Schepper J, et al. Belgian Study Group for Pediatric Endocrinology. Trends in age at diagnosis of Turner syndrome. *Arch Dis Child*. 2005;90:267-268.
3. Savendahl L, Davenport ML. Delayed diagnoses of Turner's syndrome: proposed guidelines for change. *J Pediatr*. 2000;137:455-459.
4. Bondy CA, Turner Syndrome Study Group. Care of girls and women with Turner syndrome: a guideline of the Turner Syndrome Study Group. *J Clin Endocrinol Metab*. 2007;92:10-25.
5. Wong SC, Burgess T, Cheung M, Zacharin M. The prevalence of turner syndrome in girls presenting with coarctation of the aorta. *J Pediatr*. 2014;164:259-263.
6. Wolff DJ, Van Dyke DL, Powell CM, Working Group of the ACMG Laboratory Quality Assurance Committee. Laboratory guideline for Turner syndrome. *Genet Med*. 2010;12:52-55.
7. Urbach A, Benvenisty N. Studying early lethality of 45,XO (Turner's syndrome) embryos using human embryonic stem cells. *PLoS One*. 2009;4:e4175.
8. Lucas-Herald AK, Cann F, Crawford L, et al. The outcome of prenatal identification of sex chromosome abnormalities. *Arch Dis Child*. 2016 [Epub ahead of print].
9. Gicquel C, Gaston V, Cabrol S, Le Bouc Y. Assessment of Turner's syndrome by molecular analysis of the X chromosome in growth-retarded girls. *J Clin Endocrinol Metab*. 1998;83:1472-1476.
10. Grote FK, Oostdijk W, De Muinck Keizer-Schrama SM, et al. The diagnostic work up of growth failure in secondary health care; an evaluation of consensus guidelines. *BMC Pediatr*. 2008;13:8-21.

Management Options and Outcomes for Neonatal Hypoplastic Left Heart Syndrome in the Early Twenty-First Century
Kane JM, Canar J, Kalinowski V, et al (Univ of Chicago Medicine and Comer Children's Hosp, IL; Rush Univ Med Ctr, Chicago, IL; et al)
Pediatr Cardiol 37:419-425, 2016

Without surgical treatment, neonatal hypoplastic left heart syndrome (HLHS) mortality in the first year of life exceeds 90 % and, in spite of improved surgical outcomes, many families still opt for non-surgical management. The purpose of this study was to investigate trends in neonatal HLHS management and to identify characteristics of patients who did not undergo surgical palliation. Neonates with HLHS were identified from a serial cross-sectional analysis using the Healthcare Cost and Utilization Project's Kids' Inpatient Database from 2000 to 2012. The primary analysis compared children undergoing surgical palliation to those discharged alive without surgery using a binary logistic regression model. Multivariate logistic regression was conducted to determine factors associated with treatment choice. A total of 1750 patients underwent analysis. Overall hospital mortality decreased from 35.3 % in 2000 to 22.9 % in 2012. The percentage of patients undergoing comfort care discharge without surgery also decreased from 21.2 to 14.8 %. After controlling for demographics and comorbidities, older patients at presentation were less likely to undergo surgery (OR 0.93, 0.91–0.96), and patients in 2012 were more likely to undergo surgery compared to those in prior years (OR 1.5, 1.1–2.1). Discharge without surgical intervention is decreasing with a 30 % reduction between 2000 and 2012. Given the improvement in surgical outcomes, further dialogue about ethical justification of nonoperative comfort or palliative care is warranted. In the meantime, clinicians should present families with surgical outcome data and recommend intervention, while supporting their option to refuse (Table 1).

▶ Hypoplastic left heart syndrome (HLHS) is uniformly fatal without staged surgical palliation or heart transplantation. In 1983, Dr William Norwood developed a way to utilize the single right ventricle to provide both unobstructed systemic blood flow and a controlled amount of pulmonary blood flow, thus reporting the first patient with HLHS to survive staged palliation.[1] In 1985, Dr Leonard Bailey performed the first successful infant heart transplantation on Baby Moses with HLHS who survived 24 years. Over the past 35 years, 2 important developments have dramatically changed outcomes for HLHS: (1) results of surgical palliation have greatly improved, although the associated morbidity and mortality remain significant, and (2) early diagnosis by fetal echocardiography has facilitated both pregnancy termination and a more stable preoperative course for those pursuing surgery.

Outcomes for patients with HLHS are widely published due in part to the complexity of the newborn palliative surgery, commonly referred to as the Norwood procedure. Management and survival of infants with HLHS are often used to benchmark institutional success with complex neonatal heart disease. Published data include single-center outcomes, administrative databases (eg, Pediatric Health Information Systems, PHIS; Kids Inpatient Database, KID; Nationwide Inpatient Sample, NIS), clinical registries (Society of Thoracic Surgeons, STS; Extracorporeal Life Support Organization, ELSO; National Pediatric Cardiology Quality Improvement Collaborative, NPCQIC), multi-institutional prospective cohorts (Congenital Heart Surgeons' Society, CHSS, borderline LV) and multi-institutional prospective randomized clinical trials (Single Ventricle Reconstruction, SVR, trial) (Table 1).

The highest mortality risk is during the initial hospitalization for the Norwood procedure. More granular analyses have demonstrated that higher institutional Norwood volume is associated with lower mortality and shorter hospital length of stay,[2] early survival seems to favor the right ventricular to pulmonary artery shunt over the modified Blalock Taussig shunt,[3,4] later survival does not differ between shunt types,[5] and higher risk patients tend to undergo the hybrid procedure (ductal stent with bilateral pulmonary artery bands).[6,7] Historically, the period between discharge and the second surgical procedure (interstage period)

TABLE 1.—Reported Outcomes for Hypoplastic Left Heart Syndrome

Dataset	Type of Dataset	N	Year	Palliative Care	Norwood Mortality, (%)	Interstage Mortality, (%)	Long-term Transplant free Survival, Years, (%)
CHOP Tabbutt,[16] 2005 Ballweg,[17] 2010	SC	149	2002-2004	n/r	15%	13.5%	5 years, 61%
CHW Tweddell[18] 2002	SC	115	1996-2001	n/r	7%	19%	n/r
STS Jacobs,[19] 2016	CR	2828	2011-2014	n/r	15.6%	n/r	n/r
CHSS Ashburn[20] 2003	CR	710	1994-2000	n/r	1 month, 72%	n/r	5 years, 54%
NPCQIC Oster,[9] 2015	CR	494	2008-2012	n/r	n/r	8.1%	n/r
ELSO Jolley 2014	CR	307	1998-2013	n/r	Norwoods requiring ECMO, 64%	n/r	n/r
SVR Ohye[3] 2010 Tabbutt[22] 2012 Newburger,[5] 2014	RCT	549	2005-2008	n/r	12%	6.3%	3 years, 36%
NIS Karamlou,[10] 2010	AD	3286	1998-2005	57%	30%	n/r	n/r
KIDS Kane, 2015	AD	1750	2000-2012	32%	21%	n/r	n/r

SC, single center; CR, clinical registry; RCT, randomized clinical trial; AD, administrative database CHOP, Children's Hospital of Philadelphia; CHW, Children's Hospital of Wisconsin; STS, Society of Thoracic Surgeons; CHSS, Congenital Heart Surgeons Society; NPCQIC, National ; ELSO, Extracorporeal Life Support Organization; SVR, Single Ventricle Reconstruction; NIS, Nationwide Inpatient Sample; KIDS, Kids Inpatient Database; n/r, not recorded.

has been another period of high risk. More recently, the development of interstage home monitoring programs has been demonstrated to effectively decrease the rate of interstage mortality in single-center reports.[8] An attempt by the NPCQIC registry to replicate the success at single centers was not successful.[9] Despite numerous publications, most report outcomes following surgical palliation, therefore excluding newborns with HLHS for whom only comfort care is provided.

Two recent studies used administrative databases to describe outcomes for newborns with HLHS inclusive of comfort care. Karamlou et al analyzed data from the NIS database (1988–2005), and Kane et al analyzed the KID database (2000–2012).[10] Karamlou et al reported on 3286 neonates with HLHS, of which 16% underwent the Norwood procedure, 2% received heart transplantation, and 57% received comfort care (discharged alive or died in hospital without surgery). In-hospital mortality for patients undergoing the Norwood procedure decreased from 86% in 1988 to 1990 to 24% in 2003 to 2005. The frequency of the Norwood procedure increased over time, from 2% in 1988 to 1990 to 24% in 2003 to 2005. Included in the analysis were the patients transferred without surgery (25%); the authors attempted to account for those transferred to institutions in the KID database, but potentially some were double-counted. Patients undergoing the hybrid procedure were excluded.

Kane et al analyzed data from 1750 neonates with HLHS; patients receiving heart transplantation or transferred to another hospital were excluded and patients undergoing hybrid procedure were included. Of this cohort, 62% underwent Norwood procedure, 5.8% underwent a hybrid procedure, 13.7% died in the hospital without intervention, and 18.6% were discharged alive without surgery. They found a significant decrease over time in all-cause in-hospital mortality among children with HLHS, from 35.3% in 2000 to 22.9% in 2012. Some of this improvement reflects a decrease in the percentage of children receiving comfort care (discharged or died in hospital without surgery) from 37.7% in 2000 to 26.6% in 2012. Presumably this also reflects a decrease in operative mortality. Extrapolating from the data provided, operative mortality (Norwood and hybrid combined) was 28.3% in 2000 and 15.1% in 2012. The frequency of the Norwood procedure did not change notably, remaining between 60% and 63%, while the frequency of hybrid palliation increased from 1.1% in 2000 to 10.4% in 2012.

There is a notable difference in the observed frequency of the Norwood procedure (16% and 62%) and comfort care (57% and 32%) between the Karamlou and Kane studies, respectively. This may be due to the different time periods analyzed and thus may represent a change in practice patterns in the direction of more surgical intervention. It may also reflect differences in the sampling population or coding accuracy between the 2 administrative databases. Both the KID and NIS databases are part of the Healthcare Cost and Utilization Project. The KID is an 80% sample of all pediatric discharges from hospitals within the registry; the NIS (before 2012) sampled 20% of the hospitals within the registry but included all discharges from the sampled hospitals.

Both studies used multivariate analysis to identify factors associated with nonoperative management, finding that higher risk and older patients and those presenting to rural hospitals[10] were more likely to receive comfort care.

Although not directly addressed, one might assume that patients who were older at presentation were not diagnosed in utero and more likely to have hemodynamic compromise and probable associated end-organ dysfunction.

Missing from all outcome papers for patients with HLHS are the prenatally diagnosed fetuses with HLHS for whom the pregnancy is terminated. The prevalence of termination would likely influence the incidence of newborns receiving comfort care. Similarly, the absence of a prenatal diagnosis may suggest the mother/child did not have access to tertiary or quaternary care, which would potentially increase the likelihood of a recommendation of comfort care. This missing information underscores the importance of complete data sets or merging of databases to accurately describe the outcomes of HLHS and make accurate recommendations. Merging of registries and databases has been reported,[11,12] and computational analysis of big data has contributed significantly to advancing care in other areas of medicine.[13]

Finally, what are the comparative strengths and weaknesses of administrative databases, clinical registries, and randomized clinical trials? A limitation of administrative databases is inaccuracy due to inherent coding errors, for example, the lack of an *International Classification of Diseases* (Ninth Revision) code for the Norwood procedure or hybrid procedure. In addition, the inability to track patients transferred to another institution is a significant limitation as the administrative databases will double count the patient transferred to another facility within the registry and lose the patient transferred to a nonregistry facility. This simple insufficiency in the data (inclusive vs not inclusive of transfers) could easily explain the some of the differences in the frequency of the Norwood procedure and comfort care. Routine institutional audits have demonstrated excellent accuracy in data entry for clinical registries.[14] Comparative analyses demonstrated a significant difference in mortality rates for congenital heart surgery between administrative databases and clinical registries.[15] Thus, caution is warranted when interpreting data from administrative databases; appropriately audited clinical registries and randomized clinical trials are likely to present more accurate data.

M. J. Cisco, MD

S. Tabbutt, MD, PhD

References

1. Norwood WI, Lang P, Hansen DD. Physiologic repair of aortic atresia-hypoplastic left heart syndrome. *N Engl J Med.* 1983;308:23-26.
2. Anderson BR, Ciarleglio AJ, Cohen DJ, et al. The Norwood operation: relative effects of surgeon and institutional volumes on outcomes and resource utilization. *Cardiol Young.* 2016;26:683-692.
3. Ohye RG, Sleeper LA, Mahony L, et al. for the Pediatric Heart Network Investigators. Comparison of shunt types in the Norwood procedure for single-ventricle lesions. *N Engl J Med.* 2010;362:1980-1992.
4. Wilder TJ, McCrindle BW, Phillips AB, et al. Survival and right ventricular performance for match children after stage-1 Norwood: modified Blalock-Taussig shunt versus right-ventricle-to-pulmonary-artery conduit. *J Thorac Cardiovasc Surg.* 2015;150:1440-1452.
5. Newburger JW, Sleeper LA, Frommelt PC, et al. for the Pediatric Heart Network Investigators: Transplantation-free survival and interventions at 3 years in the single ventricle reconstruction trial. *Circulation.* 2014;129:2013-2020.

6. Karamlou T, Overman D, Hill KD, et al. Stage 1 hybrid palliation for hypoplastic left heart syndrome—assessment of contemporary patterns of use: an analysis of the Society of Thoracic Surgeons Congenital Heart Surgery Database. *J Thorac Cardiovasc Surg.* 2015;149:195-202.

7. Malik S, Bird TM, Jaquiss RDB, Morrow WR, Robins JM. Comparison of in-hospital and longer-term outcomes of hybrid and Norwood stage 1 palliation of hypoplastic left heart syndrome. *J Thorac Cardiovasc Surg.* 2015;150:474-480.

8. Ghanayem NS, Hoffman GM, Mussatto KA, et al. Home surveillance program prevents interstage mortality after the Norwood procedure. *J Thorac Cardiovasc Surg.* 2003;126:1367-1377.

9. Oster M, Ehrlich A, King E, et al. Association of interstage home monitoring with mortality, readmissions, and weight gain. A multicenter study from the National Pediatric Cardiology Quality Improvement Collaborative. *Circulation.* 2015; 132:502-508.

10. Karamlou T, Diggs BS, Ungerleider RM, Welke KF. Evolution of treatment options and outcomes for hypoplastic left heart syndrome over an 18-year period. *J Thorac Cardiovasc Surg.* 2010;139:119-127.

11. Jacobs JP, Pasquali SK, Austin E, et al. Linking the Congenital Heart Surgery Databases of the Society of Thoracic Surgeons and the Congenital Heart Surgeons' Society: Part 1—rationale and methodology. *World J Pediatr Congenit Heart Surg.* 2014;5:256-271.

12. Jacobs JP, Pasquali SK, Austin E, et al. Linking the congenital heart surgery databases of the Society of Thoracic Surgeons and the Congenital Heart Surgeons' Society: Part 2—lessons learned and implications. *World J Pediatr Congenit Heart Surg.* 2014;5:272-282.

13. Li L, Ruau DJ, Patel CJ, et al. Disease risk factors identified through shared genetic architecture and electronic medical records. *Sci Translational Med.* 2014;6:234ra57.

14. Gaies M, Donohue JE, Willis GM, et al. Data integrity of the Pediatric Cardiac Critical Care Consortium (PC4) clinical registry. *Cardiol Young..* 2015;26:1-7.

15. Pasquali SK, Peterson ED, Jacobs JP, et al. Differential case ascertainment in clinical registry versus administrative data and impact on outcomes assessment for pediatric cardiac operations. *Ann Thorac Surg.* 2013;95:197-203.

16. Tabbutt S, Dominguez TE, Ravishankar C, et al. Outcomes after the stage i reconstruction comparing the right ventricular to pulmonary artery conduit with the modified Blalock Taussig shunt. *Ann Thorac Surg.* 2005;80:1582-1591.

17. Ballweg JA, Dominguez TE, Ravishankar C, et al. A contemporary comparison of the effect of shunt type in hypoplastic left heart syndrome on the hemodynamics and outcome at Fontan completion. *J Thorac Cardiovasc Surg.* 2010;140:537-544.

18. Tweddell JS, Hoffman GM, Mussatto KA, et al. Improved survival of patients undergoing palliation of hypoplastic left heart syndrome: lessons learned from 115 consecutive patients. *Circulation.* 2002;106:182-189.

19. Jacobs JP, Mayer JE Jr, Mavroudis C, et al. The Society of Thoracic Surgeons Congenital Heart Surgery Database: 2016 update on outcomes and quality. *Ann Thorac Surg.* 2016;101:850-862.

20. Ashburn DA, McCrindle BW, Tchervenkov CI, et al. Outcomes after the Norwood operation in neonates with critical aortic stenosis or aortic valve atresia. *J Thorac Cardiovasc Surg.* 2003;125:1070-1082.

21. Jolley M, Yarlagadda VV, Rajagopal SK, Almodovar MC, Rycus PT, Thiagarajan RR. Extracorporeal membrane oxygenation-supported cardiopulmonary resuscitation following stage 1 palliation for hypoplastic left heart syndrome. *Pediatr Crit Care Med.* 2014;15:538-545.

22. Tabbutt S, Ghanayem N, Ravishankar C, et al. for the Pediatric Heart Network Investigators. Risk factors for hospital morbidity and mortality after the Norwood procedure a report from the Pediatric Heart Network Single Ventricle Reconstruction trial. *J Thorac Cardiovasc Surg.* 2012;144:882-895.

14 Hospital Critical Care

A Cost-Effectiveness Analysis of Obtaining Blood Cultures in Children Hospitalized for Community-Acquired Pneumonia

Andrews AL, Simpson AN, Heine D, et al (Med Univ of South Carolina, Charleston, East Cobb Pediatrics, Marietta, GA)
J Pediatr 167:1280-1286, 2015

Objective.—To determine the clinical utility and cost-effectiveness of universal vs targeted approach to obtaining blood cultures in children hospitalized with community-acquired pneumonia (CAP).

Study Design.—We conducted a cost-effectiveness analysis using a decision tree to compare 2 approaches to ordering blood cultures in children hospitalized with CAP: obtaining blood cultures in all children admitted with CAP (universal approach) and obtaining blood cultures in patients identified as high risk for bacteremia (targeted approach). We searched the literature to determine expected proportions of high-risk patients, positive culture rates, and predicted bacteria and susceptibility patterns. Our primary clinical outcome was projected rate of missed bacteremia with associated treatment failure in the targeted approach. Costs per 100 patients and annualized costs on the national level were calculated for each approach.

Results.—The model predicts that in the targeted approach, there will be 0.07 cases of missed bacteremia with treatment failure per 100 patients, or 133 annually. In the universal approach, 118 blood cultures would need to be drawn to identify 1 patient with bacteremia, in which the result would lead to a meaningful antibiotic change compared with 42 cultures in the targeted approach. The universal approach would cost $5178 per 100 patients or $9 214 238 annually. The targeted approach would cost $1992 per 100 patients or $3 545 460 annually. The laboratory-related cost savings attributed to the targeted approach would be projected to be $5 668 778 annually.

Conclusions.—This decision analysis model suggests that a targeted approach to obtaining blood cultures in children hospitalized with CAP may be clinically effective, cost-saving, and reduce unnecessary testing.

▶ Despite efforts to universally vaccinate children for the most frequent causative bacterial agents, community acquired pneumonia (CAP) remains one of the most common reasons for hospitalization in children in the United States.[1] In 2011, the Pediatric Infectious Disease Society (PIDS) and the Infectious Disease Society of America (IDSA) published guidelines titled "The Management of Community-Acquired Pneumonia in Infants and Children Older Than 3 Months of Age," becoming the first national guideline in the United States for children with CAP.[2] Among the many recommendations is the endorsement to obtain blood cultures in all children hospitalized for community-acquired pneumonia with moderate or severe disease, a recommendation that has been interpreted by some to include any child hospitalized with CAP.[3] The IDSA and PIDS use the GRADE criteria for guideline development and the recommendation for inpatient blood cultures was described as a "strong" recommendation with "low" quality of evidence.[2]

Several years before the new pediatric guidelines were published, IDSA published similar guidelines for adults with CAP. These included the analogous recommendation to obtain blood cultures for hospitalized patients.[4] Similar to the pediatric recommendation, the quality of evidence was reported by IDSA as "low." Several publications, made available after the adult IDSA CAP guidelines were issued, questioned the validity of this recommendation in adults.[5] Despite the controversy over this topic, the blood culture recommendation became adopted as a reportable quality indicator for adults hospitalized with CAP. However, given the consistency of evidence contradicting this recommendation, clinicians questioned the validity of this recommendation as a quality indicator, leading to eventual retirement by government agencies.[6]

Following the example of researchers in adult medicine, several pediatric investigators have examined the role of universal blood cultures for children hospitalized with CAP. In a recent comprehensive review that included most of these studies, investigators from Minnesota analyzed the results of 21 publications regarding blood cultures obtained in children evaluated in the hospital setting for CAP.[7] Their analysis revealed that the rate of positive pathogenic blood cultures is low at an adjusted rate of 4.71% and the rate of contaminants is similar at 4.1%. If only patients with severe pneumonia are included, the yield of positive blood cultures jumps to a rate of 9.8%. Although only 3 studies overtly examined this question, the utility of blood cultures in aiding antibiotic adjustment (narrowing or widening coverage) was not consistent among the studies.

In December 2015, investigators from the Medical University of South Carolina published the first cost-effective analysis of blood cultures specifically tailored to inpatient pediatric CAP. Andrews et al performed a decision analysis model that examined the cost-effectiveness of 2 approaches to obtaining blood cultures in children with CAP. The first was a universal approach in which all children admitted to the hospital with the diagnosis of CAP would have a blood culture obtained. The second strategy used a targeted approach in which only patients with CAP at high risk of having bacteremia would have a blood culture obtained. "High risk" was defined by 6 patient characteristics: (1) age less than 6 months, (2) having a central catheter in place, (3) immunocompromised status, (4) ill or "toxic" appearing at presentation or admitted to an ICU setting, (5) chronic medical conditions, and (6) effusion or empyema on chest radiograph.9.

The 2 main clinical outcomes measured by the model depended on the arm. For the universal approach the investigators assessed the number of true bacteremia cases that led to meaningful antibiotic change per 100 hypothetical patients. In the targeted approach, the number of patients with missed bacteremia associated with treatment failure was calculated per 100 hypothetical patients. The primary cost outcome was the difference in cost per 100 patients between both arms.

The result of this model favored the targeted approach, which resulted in an estimated cost savings of $3186 per 100 patients. The number needed to test (NNT) in the universal approach to identify 1 case of bacteremia that leads to a clinically meaningful change in antibiotic was 122, whereas the targeted approach would have an NNT of 42. Using the Health Cost and Utilization Project database1 as their reference, Andrews et al performed a secondary cost analysis on a population wide level. If only laboratory costs are included, the targeted approach would save approximately $5 668 778 annually. If hospital charges are included, the cost savings of the targeted approach jump to $187 669 983 annually, although this estimate is based on the 0.8 difference in LOS between patients who have blood cultures obtained versus those who do not, which infers a causal association between obtaining a blood culture and a longer LOS.

Because of the hypothetical model approach (despite its basis on evidence-based assumptions), this study has several limitations. The assumptions depend on generalizations that may not reflect real-world practices. The quality of the literature directly reflects the quality of the assumptions of a decision analysis, and although there has been much evidence published since the PIDS-IDSA CAP guidelines, the quality of this evidence is limited. For example, the guidelines used to identify high-risk patients are based on a single-center study.[8] Costs may also be underestimated as the cost-analysis for the primary outcome was limited to direct costs, which ignore such costs as nursing or other ancillary medical professionals' time. Nevertheless, this study, along with other work published since the dissemination of PIDS-IDSA CAP guidelines, adds to the growing body of evidence that the recommendation of obtaining a blood cultures in children hospitalized for CAP should be reevaluated.

R. A. Quinonez, MD, FAAP, FHM

References

1. HCUP Kids' Inpatient Database (KID). *Healthcare Cost and Utilization Project (HCUP)*. Rockville, MD: Agency for Healthcare Research and Quality; 2006 and 2009, www.hcup-us.ahrq.gov/kidoverview.jsp.
2. Bradley JS, Byington CL, Shah SS, et al. Pediatric Infectious Diseases Society and the Infectious Diseases Society of America. The management of community-acquired pneumonia in infants and children older than 3 months of age: clinical practice guidelines by the Pediatric Infectious Diseases Society and the Infectious Diseases Society of America. *Clin Infect Dis*. 2011;53:e25-e76.
3. Murtagh Kurowski E, Shah SS, Thomson J, et al. Improvement methodology increases guideline recommended blood cultures in children with pneumonia. *Pediatrics*. 2015;135:e1052-e1059.

4. Bartlett JG, Breiman RF, Mandell LA, File TM Jr. Community-acquired pneumonia in adults: guidelines for management. The Infectious Diseases Society of America. *Clin Infect Dis.* 1998;26:811-838.

5. Afshar N, Tabas J, Afshar K, Silbergleit R. Blood cultures for community-acquired pneumonia: are they worthy of two quality measures? A systematic review. *J Hosp Med.* 2009;4:112-123. Review.

6. Wilson KC, Schünemann HJ. An appraisal of the evidence underlying performance measures for community-acquired pneumonia. *Am J Respir Crit Care Med.* 2011; 183:1454-1462.

7. Iroh Tam PY, Bernstein E, Ma X, Ferrieri P. Blood culture in evaluation of pediatric community-acquired pneumonia: a systematic review and meta-analysis. *Hosp Pediatr.* 2015;5:324-336.

8. Heine D, Cochran C, Moore M, Titus MO, Andrews AL. The prevalence of bacteremia in pediatric patients with community acquired pneumonia: guidelines to reduce the frequency of obtaining blood cultures. *Hosp Pediatr.* 2013;3:92-96.

Use of Procalcitonin Assays to Predict Serious Bacterial Infection in Young Febrile Infants

Milcent K, Faesch S, Gras-Le Guen C, et al (Antoine Béclère Univ Hosp, Clamart, France; Paris Descartes Univ, France; Nantes Univ Hosp, France; et al)
JAMA Pediatr 170:62-69, 2016

Importance.—The procalcitonin (PCT) assay is an accurate screening test for identifying invasive bacterial infection (IBI); however, data on the PCT assay in very young infants are insufficient.

Objective.—To assess the diagnostic characteristics of the PCT assay for detecting serious bacterial infection (SBI) and IBI in febrile infants aged 7 to 91 days.

Design, Setting, and Participants.—A prospective cohort study that included infants aged 7 to 91 days admitted for fever to 15 French pediatric emergency departments was conducted for a period of 30 months (October 1, 2008, through March 31, 2011). The data management and analysis were performed from October 1, 2011, through October 31, 2014.

Main Outcomes and Measures.—The diagnostic characteristics of the PCT assay, C-reactive protein (CRP) concentration, white blood cell (WBC) count, and absolute neutrophil cell (ANC) count for detecting SBI and IBI were described and compared for the overall population and subgroups of infants according to the age and the duration of fever. Laboratory test cutoff values were calculated based on receiver operating characteristic (ROC) curve analysis. The SBIs were defined as a pathogenic bacteria in positive culture of blood, cerebrospinal fluid, urine, or stool samples, including bacteremia and bacterial meningitis classified as IBIs.

Results.—Among the 2047 infants included, 139 (6.8%) were diagnosed as having an SBI and 21 (1.0%) as having an IBI (11.0%and 1.7%of those with blood culture (n = 1258), respectively). The PCT assay offered an area under the curve (AUC) of ROC curve similar to that for CRP concentration for the detection of SBI (AUC, 0.81; 95%

CI, 0.75-0.86; vs AUC, 0.80; 95% CI, 0.75-0.85; $P = .70$). The AUC ROC curve for the detection of IBI for the PCT assay was significantly higher than that for the CRP concentration (AUC, 0.91; 95% CI, 0.83-0.99; vs AUC, 0.77; 95% CI, 0.65-0.89; $P = .002$). Using a cutoff value of 0.3 ng/mL for PCT and 20 mg/L for CRP, negative likelihood ratios were 0.3 (95% CI, 0.2-0.5) for identifying SBI and 0.1 (95% CI, 0.03-0.4) and 0.3 (95% CI, 0.2-0.7) for identifying IBI, respectively. Similar results were obtained for the subgroup of infants younger than 1 month and for those with fever lasting less than 6 hours.

Conclusions and Relevance.—The PCT assay has better diagnostic accuracy than CRP measurement for detecting IBI; the 2 tests perform similarly for identifying SBI in febrile infants aged 7 to 91 days.

▶ The febrile young infant less than 90 days of age is commonly encountered in both the emergency department and primary care office. These febrile infants are at high risk for serious bacterial infection (SBI), most commonly urinary tract infection (UTI), although bacteremia and bacterial meningitis, coined *invasive bacterial infection* (IBI), are the most feared. As opposed to older infants and children, clinical appearance alone is not adequate to distinguish which febrile infants will have bacterial infection versus benign viral infection. Therefore, these young infants often undergo extensive laboratory evaluation, including lumbar puncture.

For this high-risk and commonly encountered population, it would be sensible to have a standardized laboratory approach to diagnosis and management. More than 20 years ago, 3 sets of criteria (Rochester, Philadelphia, and Boston) were developed to identify febrile infants at low risk of infection, the so-called *low-risk criteria*. Using a combination of clinical and laboratory factors, these criteria have a sensitivity of 92% to 100% for SBI with a specificity around 50%. Therefore, a similarly sensitive diagnostic test with higher specificity would have clinical utility to accurately identify infants with bacterial infection while reducing the number of infants who are hospitalized and empirically treated as false-positive non—low-risk patients. Additionally, because of differing age ranges and requirement for cerebrospinal fluid testing among the criteria, and no currently published guidelines that offer explicit management recommendations, wide variation exists in the evaluation and management of febrile infants.[1] A unified diagnostic testing strategy with improved specificity is necessary.

Procalcitonin has been studied previously alone and in combination with other clinical and laboratory markers as a diagnostic tool in febrile infants. In the only prior prospective study, Maniaci et al[2] reported that a procalcitonin level of 0.12 ng/mL had a sensitivity of 95.2%, but the specificity was unacceptably low at 25.5%. Subsequent studies reported lower sensitivity but higher specificity for SBI with procalcitonin of 0.5 ng/mL, with better performance characteristics for IBI; Gomez et al[3] reported a positive likelihood ratio of 11.14 for IBI with a procalcitonin level of 2 ng/mL. Procalcitonin has also been incorporated into algorithms with C-reactive protein and urine dipstick (the Lab score) and sequentially with both clinical factors, urine dipstick, C-reactive protein, and absolute neutrophil cell (the sequential approach) with favorable test characteristics compared with the low-risk criteria.[4] Interestingly, most of these studies were conducted in Europe where procalcitonin is used more widely; adoption in the United States has been sparse for febrile infants. The question is why—inertia, lack of timely availability, need for larger prospective study?

The 2015 *Journal of the American Medical Association Pediatrics* study by Milcent et al may move the needle forward on procalcitonin use in febrile infants. The authors conducted the largest prospective study of procalcitonin in febrile infants to date. Similar to prior investigations, procalcitonin showed favorable test characteristics for detection of bacterial infection, IBI in particular, with a high area under the curve (AUC) for both: 0.81 (95% confidence interval [CI]: 0.75-0.86) for definite SBI and 0.91 (95% CI: 0.83-0.99) for IBI. The AUCs were similarly high in the subset of infants age 7 to 30 days. A nice feature of the study is the determination of the sensitivity, specificity, and likelihood ratios for procalcitonin at different values. At a level of ≥0.3 ng/mL, procalcitonin showed a sensitivity of 90% (although with a wide 95% CI: 68-99) and specificity of 78% (95% CI: 75-80) for IBI; the negative likelihood ratio of 0.1 (95% CI: 0.03-0.4) is clinically useful for identification of infants at low risk of IBI.

The specificity of procalcitonin for detection of SBI was similar, as high as 94% (95% CI: 92-95) for procalcitonin ≥2 ng/mL. However, the sensitivity for SBI was notably lower, only 74% (95% CI: 62-84) for a procalcitonin level of ≥0.3 ng/mL. This low sensitivity likely represents missed UTI, which accounted for most SBIs in the study. Conceivably, the systemic inflammatory response may be less to UTI, producing a lower procalcitonin level than with IBI. However, both urine dipstick and urinalysis are sensitive with high negative predictive value for UTI among febrile infants,[5] and a combination of urine testing with procalcitonin may identify most SBIs.

A few lingering questions remain from this study. Clinicians may view a sensitivity of 90% for IBI as unacceptably low, as one missed case of bacteremia or bacterial meningitis is viewed by many as one too many. The devil is in the details, however. The one missed IBI in the Milcent study was an 83-day-old infant who was described as becoming "spontaneously afebrile" after emergency department discharge and had a blood culture positive for *Streptococcus pneumoniae*, which may have represented transient pneumococcal bacteremia. More telling, the studies of the low-risk criteria included relatively few cases of IBI, and the sensitivity for IBI has varied from as low as 80% up to 100%. Furthermore, the prevalence of the most feared IBI, bacterial meningitis, is very low among febrile infants, particularly those who are well appearing and older than 28 days. Given that the largest outpatient investigation on management and outcomes of febrile infants reported even missed infants (1 with bacteremia, 1 with meningitis) did well with close follow-up,[6] procalcitonin at a level of ≥0.3 ng/mL has an acceptable sensitivity with the added benefit of higher specificity for IBI.

A notable limitation of the Milcent study is that the test characteristics of procalcitonin were calculated for the 1258 infants in whom a blood culture was obtained, not the entire cohort. There is a risk of spectrum bias with this potentially sicker subgroup the cohort. Additionally, the study included both ill-appearing and well-appearing febrile infants, and there is a need for assessment of procalcitonin at 0.3 ng/mL limited to well-appearing infants. Future prospective investigation should also directly compare the existing low-risk criteria with an algorithm of urine dipstick/urinalysis and procalcitonin by month of life and stratified by clinical appearance. In particular, robust evidence that well-appearing infants 7 to 30 days of age with procalcitonin less than 0.3 ng/mL and normal urinalysis are at low risk for SBI could potentially reduce iatrogenic risks associated with hospitalization or empiric antibiotic therapy in this age group.

P. L. Aronson, MD

References

1. Aronson PL, Thurm C, Alpern ER, et al. Variation in care of the febrile young infant <90 days in US pediatric emergency departments. *Pediatrics.* 2014;134: 667-677.
2. Maniaci V, Dauber A, Weiss S, Nylen E, Becker KL, Bachur R. Procalcitonin in young febrile infants for the detection of serious bacterial infections. *Pediatrics.* 2008;122:701-710.
3. Gomez B, Bressan S, Mintegi S, et al. Diagnostic value of procalcitonin in well-appearing young febrile infants. *Pediatrics.* 2012;130:815-822.
4. Mintegi S, Bressan S, Gomez B, et al. Accuracy of a sequential approach to identify young febrile infants at low risk for invasive bacterial infection. *Emerg Med J.* 2014;31.e19-e24.
5. Glissmeyer EW, Korgenski EK, Wilkes J, et al. Dipstick screening for urinary tract infection in febrile infants. *Pediatrics.* 2014;133:e1121-e1127.
6. Pantell RH, Newman TB, Bernzweig J, et al. Management and outcomes of care of fever in early infancy. *JAMA.* 2004;291:1203-1212.

Double-Blind Prospective Randomized Controlled Trial of Dopamine Versus Epinephrine as First-Line Vasoactive Drugs in Pediatric Septic Shock

Ventura AMC, Shieh HH, Bousso A, et al (Hospital Universitário da Universidade de São Paulo, Brazil)

Crit Care Med 43:2292-2302, 2015

Objectives.—The primary outcome was to compare the effects of dopamine or epinephrine in severe sepsis on 28-day mortality; secondary outcomes were the rate of healthcare—associated infection, the need for other vasoactive drugs, and the multiple organ dysfunction score.

Design.—Double-blind, prospective, randomized controlled trial from February 1, 2009, to July 31, 2013.

Setting.—PICU, Hospital Universitário da Universidade de São Paulo, Brazil.

Patients.—Consecutive children who are 1 month to 15 years old and met the clinical criteria for fluid-refractory septic shock. Exclusions were receiving vasoactive drug(s) prior to hospital admission, having known cardiac disease, having already participated in the trial during the same hospital stay, refusing to participate, or having do-not-resuscitate orders.

Interventions.—Patients were randomly assigned to receive either dopamine (5—10 μg/kg/min) or epinephrine (0.1—0.3 μg/kg/min) through a peripheral or intraosseous line. Patients not reaching predefined stabilization criteria after the maximum dose were classified as treatment failure, at which point the attending physician gradually stopped the study drug and started another catecholamine.

Measurements and Main Results.—Physiologic and laboratory data were recorded. Baseline characteristics were described as proportions and mean (± SD) and compared using appropriate statistical tests. Multiple regression analysis was performed, and statistical significance was defined as a *p* value of less than 0.05. Baseline characteristics and therapeutic interventions for the 120 children enrolled (63, dopamine; 57, epinephrine) were similar. There were 17 deaths (14.2%): 13 (20.6%) in the dopamine group and four (7%) in the epinephrine group ($p = 0.033$). Dopamine was associated with death (odds ratio, 6.5; 95% CI, 1.1—37.8; $p = 0.037$) and healthcare—associated infection (odds ratio, 67.7; 95% CI, 5.0—910.8; $p = 0.001$). The use of epinephrine was associated with a survival odds ratio of 6.49.

Conclusions.—Dopamine was associated with an increased risk of death and healthcare—associated infection. Early administration of peripheral or intraosseous epinephrine was associated with increased survival in this population. Limitations should be observed while interpreting these results.

▶ Three questions seem to consistently arise in the minds of clinicians during the resuscitation of pediatric septic shock. Should I give fluid, and if so how much and what should I give? What vasoactive agent, and how much should I give? Should I give steroids, and if so how much hydrocortisone? The Brazilians have approached these questions in a systematic fashion. Back in 2001, I was privileged to visit our Brazilian colleagues to give a 3-day course on pediatric advanced life support (PALS)/American College of Critical Care Medicine (ACCM) guidelines for hemodynamic support of pediatric septic shock.[1] Six months after a thoroughly enjoyable time with my new Brazilian friends, I received an e-mail telling me that they had tried the guidelines, and they did not work. If I had been in their shoes, I probably would have left it at that, but thankfully the brilliant and dedicated Dr Claudio de Olivera came to spend time in Pittsburgh. At the end of his 6 months, he concluded that the same things were being done in Brazil as in Pittsburgh, but at a different pace. He performed a cohort study showing that time to fluid boluses and amount of fluid boluses were related to outcome. Having overcome barriers to fluid bolus implementation, he then performed a randomized controlled trial showing that targeting fluid and vasoactive therapies to normal perfusion pressure and ScVO$_2$ (after central line access was attained on average 2 hours after pediatric intensive care unit admission) reduced mortality from fluid refractory septic shock from 40% to 11%.[2] This goal-directed therapy resulted in use of more fluid boluses, more blood transfusions, and more inotrope and vasodilator infusions in the intensive care unit.

Although well and good, Dr Nelly Ninis at the same time noted that UK deaths from meningococcemia in children were related to lack of experienced physician care, giving too little fluid, but also giving too much fluid (hmmm . . .), and, most important, delay in giving inotropes.[3] In response to these findings, the next set of guidelines[4] continued to emphasize fluid status monitoring but also newly recommended beginning inotropes peripherally, rather than waiting for central access (2 hours in the de Oliveira study),[2] with transitioning to central administration of vasoactive agents once attained. Dr Ventura performed the present study to determine whether to start with peripheral dopamine or epinephrine.[5] Dopamine is the darling of the neonatal intensive care unit (NICU), and indeed randomized trials in the NICU have demonstrated no differences in outcome when comparing dopamine to other vasoactive agents in the treatment of hypotension.[6] Conversely, adult studies have shown that dopamine is associated with more arrhythmias than norepinephrine.[7] Dr Ventura shows that epinephrine is superior to dopamine as the first-line peripheral agent in fluid refractory pediatric septic shock reducing mortality from 20% to 7% ($P = .033$).[5] Biological plausibility for the finding lies in the observations that epinephrine increased systolic blood pressure and perfusion pressure as well as reduced health care infection rates compared with dopamine. Epinephrine is a more potent inotrope than dopamine, which could explain more effective shock resuscitation. Dopamine prevents prolactin secretion, which can lead to stress (cortisol)-induced immune depression and might explain more health care infections. As always, more trials are needed, but for now it is reasonable to start with peripheral epinephrine infusion until central access is attained when resuscitating fluid refractory pediatric septic shock.

J. Carcillo, MD

References

1. Carcillo JA, Fields AI. American College of Critical Care Medicine Task Force Committee Members Clinical practice parameters for hemodynamic support of pediatric and neonatal patients in septic shock. *Crit Care Med.* 2002;30: 1365-1378.
2. de Oliveira CF, de Oliveira DS, Gottschald AF, et al. ACCM/PALS haemodynamic support guidelines for paediatric septic shock: an outcomes comparison with and without monitoring central venous oxygen saturation. *Intensive Care Med.* 2008; 34:1065-1075.
3. Ninis N, Phillips C, Bailey L, et al. The role of healthcare delivery in the outcome of meningococcal disease in children: case-control study of fatal and non-fatal cases. *BMJ.* 2005;330:1475. Erratum in: BMJ 2005;331(7512):323.
4. Brierley J, Carcillo JA, Choong K, et al. Clinical practice parameters for hemodynamic support of pediatric and neonatal septic shock: 2007 update from the American College of Critical Care Medicine. *Crit Care Med.* 2009;37:666-688. Erratum in: Crit Care Med 2009;37(4):1536.
5. Noori S, Seri I. Neonatal blood pressure support: the use of inotropes, lusitropes, and other vasopressor agents. *Clin Perinatol.* 2012;39:221-238.
6. Dellinger RP, Levy MM, Rhodes A, et al. Surviving Sepsis Campaign Guidelines Committee including the Pediatric Subgroup. Surviving sepsis campaign: international guidelines for management of severe sepsis and septic shock: 2012. *Crit Care Med.* 2013;41:580-637.

Oxygen saturation targets in infants with bronchiolitis (BIDS): a double-blind, randomised, equivalence trial

Cunningham S, for the Bronchiolitis of Infancy Discharge Study (BIDS) group
(Univ of Edinburgh, UK; et al)
Lancet 386:1041-1048, 2015

Background.—The American Academy of Pediatrics recommends a permissive hypoxaemic target for an oxygen saturation of 90% for children with bronchiolitis, which is consistent with the WHO recommendations for targets in children with lower respiratory tract infections. No evidence exists to support this threshold. We aimed to assess whether the 90% or higher target for management of oxygen supplementation was equivalent to a normoxic 94% or higher target for infants admitted to hospital with viral bronchiolitis.

Methods.—We did a parallel-group, randomised, controlled, equivalence trial of infants aged 6 weeks to 12 months of age with physician-diagnosed bronchiolitis newly admitted into eight paediatric hospital units in the UK (the Bronchiolitis of Infancy Discharge Study [BIDS]). A central computer randomly allocated (1:1) infants, in varying length blocks of four and six and without stratification, to be clipped to standard oximeters (patients treated with oxygen if pulse oxygen saturation [SpO_2] <94%) or modified oximeters (displayed a measured value of 90% as 94%, therefore oxygen not given until SpO_2 <90%). All parents, clinical staff, and outcome assessors were masked to allocation. The primary outcome was time to resolution of cough (prespecified equivalence limits of plus or minus 2 days) in the intention-to-treat population. This trial is registered with ISRCTN, number ISRCTN28405428.

Findings.—Between Oct 3, and March 30, 2012, and Oct 1, and March 29, 2013, we randomly assigned 308 infants to standard oximeters and 307 infants to modified oximeters. Cough resolved by 15·0 days (median) in both groups (95% CI for difference −1 to 2) and so oxygen thresholds were equivalent. We recorded 35 serious adverse events in 32 infants in the standard care group and 25 serious adverse events in 24 infants in the modified care group. In the standard care group, eight infants transferred to a high-dependency unit, 23 were readmitted, and one had a prolonged hospital stay. In the modified care group, 12 infants were transferred to a high-dependency unit and 12 were readmitted to hospital. Recorded adverse events did not differ significantly.

Interpretation.—Management of infants with bronchiolitis to an oxygen saturation target of 90% or higher is as safe and clinically effective as one of 94% or higher. Future research should assess the benefits and risks of different oxygen saturation targets in acute respiratory infection in older children, particularly in developing nations where resources are scarce (Table 1).

▶ Efforts to improve value in health care often target high-resource practices that are generally accepted but not backed by solid evidence. Bronchiolitis

TABLE 1.—: Baseline Clinical Data

	Standard Group (n = 308)	Modified Group (n = 307)
Age (weeks)	21·3 (12·6—31·1)	21·1 (11·1—32·0)
Boys	186 (60%)	166 (54%)
Preterm (<37 weeks')	28/278 (10%)	45/279 (16%)
Eczema	51/305 (17%)	44/303 (15%)
Food allergy	8/305 (3%)	11/302 (4%)
Household smoking	133/303 (44%)	130/304 (43%)
1 or more siblings	221/304 (73%)	211/304 (69%)
Primary care visits in previous 4 weeks	1 (1—2)	1 (0—2)
Heart rate on arrival (bpm)	159 (146—173)	158 (148—172)
Respiratory rate on arrival (breaths per min)	50 (44—58)	49 (42—58)
Antibiotics on arrival	24/305 (8%)	23/304 (8%)
Bronchodilator on arrival	17/305 (6%)	16/304 (5%)
Length of Illness (days) on arrival	4 (3—5)	4 (3—5)
Apnoea on arrival	3/303 (1%)	3/304 (1%)
SpO$_2$ on arrival (%)	95% (93 97)	95% (93 97)
SpO$_2$ on arrival ≤94%	121/304 (40%)	119/303 (39%)

Data are n (%), n/N (%), or median (IQR). On arrival relates to arrival at the emergency department. Data were missing for the following numbers of patients (standard group, modified): primary care attendances (7, 4), heart rate (3, 4), respiratory rate (9, 5), length of illness (3, 5), and SpO$_2$ (4, 4). SpO$_2$ = pulse oxygen saturation.

Reprinted from Cunningham S, for the Bronchiolitis of Infancy Discharge Study (BIDS) group. Oxygen saturation targets in infants with bronchiolitis (BIDS): a double-blind, randomised, equivalence trial. *Lancet.* 2015;386:1041-1048, with permission from Cunningham et al.

has always been an easy target: it's common; it's morbid; it costs the health care system a lot of money; and few, if any, of our commonly used interventions actually benefit patients in meaningful ways. One of the hottest and more controversial issues surrounding bronchiolitis management is the use of the pulse oximeter (pulse ox) and the establishment of appropriate oxygen saturation thresholds.

The pulse ox came into widespread use in the late 1980s at which time bronchiolitis hospitalizations in infants tripled in the United States, with no impact on mortality.[1] Infants who previously would not have been recognized as hypoxemic were now being hospitalized simply because of a pulse ox reading that indicates a "low" oxygen saturation, although the benefit of detection of hypoxemia in these infants, to this day, remains uncertain. Once hospitalized, infants are often kept on a continuous pulse ox, and discharge may be delayed because of intermittent hypoxemia. This overreliance on the pulse ox has triggered recommendations from groups such as the American Academy of Pediatrics (AAP) and the Choosing Wisely Campaign to limit continuous pulse oximetry use. Arguably, these recommendations can be viewed as an indictment of health care practitioners' clinical judgment, conveying a message that because we impulsively overreact to information, we should be shielded from it. Nonetheless, the movement away from continuous pulse oximetry in convalescing bronchiolitis patients appears to be underway.[2,3]

Whether the pulse ox is used continuously or intermittently, most institutions require an oxygen saturation threshold for initiation and discontinuation of supplemental oxygen. Recommended thresholds differ: 90% in the United States (AAP) versus 94% in the United Kingdom (National Institute for Health and

Care Excellence [NICE]), a potentially meaningful difference given the frequency of desaturation to the low 90s among infants with bronchiolitis. Until the recent randomized trial by Cunningham et al there was no solid evidence to support any particular saturation threshold.

The Cunningham trial is now the second large trial in bronchiolitis that utilized an altered pulse ox machine to compare, in blinded fashion, the impact of 2 saturation thresholds. The earlier trial by Schuh et al[4] (reviewed in last year's YEAR BOOK OF PEDIATRICS) randomized bronchiolitis patients in the emergency department to a true pulse ox versus a pulse ox altered to read 3% higher. Subjects in the altered pulse ox group were approximately 40% less likely to be hospitalized (absolute risk difference of 16%), with no difference in revisit rates, indicating that hypoxemia is indeed overdiagnosed in bronchiolitis.

In the Cunningham trial, investigators from the United Kingdom compared the AAP saturation threshold of 90% to the NICE threshold of 94% in 615 infants 6 weeks to 12 months of age hospitalized with bronchiolitis. Infants were randomized to true pulse oximeters versus oximeters that were altered to reflect saturations that were 4% higher, and 94% was used as a threshold for discontinuation of oxygen (such that the threshold for the infants in the altered group was actually 90%). The authors demonstrated that the altered and true pulse ox groups met criteria for equivalence in terms of the primary outcome—time to resolution of cough. The choice of this primary outcome is somewhat peculiar because it is hard to understand how different oxygen saturations would affect cough duration. In terms of secondary outcomes, not surprisingly, infants in the 90% group received oxygen for approximately 1 less day ($P = .002$) and were discharged approximately 10 hours sooner ($P = .003$) but did not have a significantly increased risk of pediatric intensive care unit transfers, deaths, readmissions, or other adverse outcomes, although the study lacked power to detect differences in most of these rare outcomes.

Somewhat unexpectedly, infants in the 90% saturation group were deemed by their parents to be back to normal and resume normal feeding more quickly than the 94% group, differences that were statistically significant using a Cox regression model. These differences could still be explained by chance; alternatively, there may be some negative effects of hospitalization and/or oxygen therapy that are poorly characterized.

One other noteworthy finding from the study, unrelated to pulse oximetry: per Table 1, the use of bronchodilators (5%—6%) and antibiotics (8%) was strikingly low in contrast to comparable US studies where the use of these agents has traditionally been much more common. The relatively infrequent use of these therapies, coupled with a reasonable length of stay (approximately 2 days), serves as a reminder that we can do less, safely, in bronchiolitis.

With demonstration of no clear harm from a 90% threshold compared with a 94% threshold, and some potential clinical benefit in terms of a reduced duration of oxygen therapy and length of hospitalization, as well as other clinical findings such as feeding and general convalescence, the AAP's 90% threshold seems reasonable. But additional questions linger: Is 90% still too high? How rigid should this threshold be? Why do we need a threshold for oxygen saturation when we don't have firm thresholds for other vital signs such as heart rate, respiratory rate, and temperature? Hopefully the next decade of bronchiolitis research will attack these critical questions.

A. R. Schroeder, MD

References

1. Shay DK, Holman RC, Newman RD, et al. Bronchiolitis-associated hospitalizations among US children, 1980–1996. *JAMA*. 1999;282:1440-1446.
2. McCulloh R, Koster M, Ralston S, et al. Use of intermittent vs continuous pulse oximetry for nonhypoxemic infants and young children hospitalized for bronchiolitis: a randomized clinical trial. *JAMA Pediatr*. 2015;169:898-904.
3. Schondelmeyer AC, Simmons JM, Statile AM, et al. Using quality improvement to reduce continuous pulse oximetry use in children with wheezing. *Pediatrics*. 2015; 135:e1044-e1051.
4. Schuh S, Freedman S, Coates A, et al. Effect of oximetry on hospitalization in bronchiolitis: a randomized clinical trial. *JAMA*. 2014;312:712-718.

Risk factors for mechanical ventilation and reintubation after pediatric heart surgery

Gupta P, Rettiganti M, Gossett JM, et al (Univ of Arkansas for Med Sciences, Little Rock; et al)
J Thorac Cardiovasc Surg 151:451-458.e3, 2016

Objective.—To determine the prevalence of and risk factors associated with the need for mechanical ventilation in children following cardiac surgery and the need for subsequent reintubation after the initial extubation attempt.

Methods.—Patients younger than 18 years who underwent cardiac operations for congenital heart disease at one of the participating pediatric intensive care units (ICUs) in the Virtual PICU Systems (VPS), LLC, database were included (2009-2014). Multivariable logistic regression models were fitted to identify factors likely associated with mechanical ventilation and reintubation.

Results.—A total of 27,398 patients from 62 centers were included. Of these, 6810 patients (25%) were extubated in the operating room (OR), whereas 20,588 patients (75%) arrived intubated in the ICU. Of the patients who were extubated in the OR, 395 patients (6%) required reintubation. In contrast, 2054 patients (10%) required reintubation among the patients arriving intubated postoperatively in the ICU. In adjusted models, patient characteristics, patients undergoing high-complexity operations, and patients undergoing operations in lower-volume centers were associated with higher likelihood for the need for postoperative mechanical ventilation and need for reintubation. Furthermore, the prevalence of mechanical ventilation and reintubation was lower among the centers with a dedicated cardiac ICU in propensity-matched analysis among centers with and without a dedicated cardiac ICU.

Conclusions.—This multicenter study suggests that proportion of patients extubated in the OR after heart operation is low. These data further suggest that extubation in the OR can be done successfully with a low complication rate.

▶ The care of children recovering from cardiac surgery continues to see exceptional advances. However, despite this evolution of postoperative care, the optimal time to separate patients from mechanical ventilation remains a subject of significant debate. Clearly, surgical repair of congenital cardiac defects cannot be accomplished without an endotracheal tube and a ventilator. But, once such a repair is completed, how soon can these devices be removed from the child in question? Can children undergo safe extubation in the operating theater, or does this simply ensure that they will require replacement of the endotracheal tube (and all of the associated risks of that procedure) in the intensive care unit? Several individual centers have reported useful results,[1-4] but their broad applicability is questionable. Variations in surgical and anesthetic approach, the expertise of operating room (OR) and intensive care unit (ICU) providers, and the complexity of case load are among a multitude of factors that may influence an institution's extubation practice. In this article, Gupta et al use the Virtual PICU Systems, LLC database, a Web-based repository of information from diverse hospitals caring for critically ill children, to analyze a large, multi-institutional approach to mechanical ventilation following pediatric cardiac surgery.

The authors' analysis of 27 398 patients from 62 centers in the United States is observational but certainly robust. The results show what many in the field would expect: most pediatric patients (75%) undergoing surgery for congenital heart disease arrive in the ICU following surgery with an endotracheal tube still in place and a mechanical ventilator supplying positive-pressure ventilation. After arrival in the ICU, these patients continued to receive mechanical ventilation for an average of 2 days with the associated increased risk for barotrauma, pneumonia, and infection, among others. Once extubated, 10% of patients in this group required reintubation. Of the approximately 7000 patients undergoing extubation in the OR, only 6% required reintubation during their hospital course. This is similar to the findings of other single-center studies, suggesting that extubation in the operating room can be safe and successful in select patients following pediatric heart surgery.[5,6] This practice results not only in shorter durations of mechanical ventilation but in shorter ICU and hospital lengths of stay as well.[5,7] In an era of medicine in which a premium is placed on cost-effective practice and minimization of days spent in the hospital, such results are clearly beneficial.

The question, therefore, becomes how best to select patients for early extubation with an eye toward minimizing both their duration of mechanical ventilation and their risk for reintubation. While we do not know why individual patients in this study required reintubation, several factors appear useful for future prospective screening. In high-complexity cases such as the Norwood procedure or the arterial switch procedure (Society of Thoracic Surgeons and the European Association for Cardiothoracic Surgery [STS-EACTS] category 4 and 5), reintubation rates were higher for OR extubations (26%) than for those patients extubated in the ICU (17%). Although these statistics show that 74% of patients undergoing complex repairs were successfully extubated in the OR, the difference in success implies that caution is warranted when considering early extubation for this population. Conversely, for low-complexity cases such as aortic stenosis repair, ventricular septal defect repair, or Fontan procedure (STS-EACTS category 1-3), the incidence of reintubation after OR extubation (4%) was actually lower than the incidence of reintubation after arriving in the ICU with an endotracheal tube in place (7%). Although causality cannot be readily assigned based on this analysis, this finding suggests that early extubation may prevent repeat manipulation of the airway in addition to limiting exposure to mechanical ventilation. The STS-EACTS category of the planned procedure is known in advance and could, theoretically, be used to help inform decisions or protocols regarding extubation timing. Similarly, age less than 1 year, weight-for-age Z score of -1 or less, higher Pediatric Index of Mortality—2 scores, and the presence of pulmonary hypertension or underlying genetic disorders are all factors that can be screened for preoperatively and, in this review, were independent risk factors correlated with the need for reintubation. Finally, it should be noted that the likelihood of successful OR extubation improved if the extubation was performed in a center with a dedicated cardiovascular ICU. What role the cardiovascular ICU played in avoiding reintubation, however, remains unclear. While other factors (ie, postoperative sepsis, development of chylothorax, and the postoperative recognition of diaphragmatic paralysis) may also contribute to the likelihood of success or failure, these cannot be reliably predicted and, therefore, become of questionable use in the patient selection process.

Should children undergoing surgical repair of congenital heart disease be extubated in the OR? The data from single-center and multicenter retrospective reviews argue that, for at least a subset of these patients, doing so would decrease their length of stay without significantly increasing their likelihood of reintubation. While other, unknown factors may mitigate the benefits of this undertaking, prospective studies with appropriate patient selection criteria are clearly needed for further evaluation. This practice can (and should) be considered for a subset of patients, especially those receiving care in high-volume centers and whose recovery will take place in a dedicated pediatric cardiovascular ICU.

L. D. Sacks, MD

References

1. Harrison AM, Cox AC, Davis S, Piedmonte M, Drummond-Webb JJ, Mee RB. Failed extubation after cardiac surgery in young children: Prevalence, pathogenesis, and risk factors. *Pediatr Crit Care Med.* 2002;3:148-152.
2. Davis S, Worley S, Mee RB, Harrison AM. Factors associated with early extubation after cardiac surgery in young children. *Pediatr Crit Care Med.* 2004;5:63-68.
3. Mittnacht AJ, Thanjan M, Srivastava S, et al. Extubation in the operating room after congenital heart surgery in children. *J Thorac Cardiovasc Surg.* 2008;136:88-93.
4. Howard F, Brown KL, Garside V, Walker I, Elliott MJ. Fast-track paediatric cardiac surgery: the feasibility and benefits of a protocol for uncomplicated cases. *Eur J Cardiothorac Surg.* 2010;37:193-196.
5. Harris KC, Holowachuk S, Pitfield S, et al. Should early extubation be the goal for children after congenital cardiac surgery? *J Thorac Cardiovasc Surg.* 2014;148:2642-2647.

6. Laudato N, Gupta P, Walters HL 3rd, Delius RE, Mastropietro CW. Risk factors for extubation failure following neonatal cardiac surgery. *Pediatr Crit Care Med.* 2015;16:859-867.
7. Garg R, Rao S, John C, et al. Extubation in the operating room after cardiac surgery in children: a prospective observational study with multidisciplinary coordinated approach. *J Cardiothorac Vasc Anesth.* 2014;28:479-487.

Parental Sources of Support and Guidance When Making Difficult Decisions in the Pediatric Intensive Care Unit

Madrigal VN, Carroll KW, Faerber JA, et al (George Washington Univ School of Medicine, DC; Univ of Pennsylvania School of Medicine, Philadelphia)
J Pediatr 169:221-226, 2016

Objective.—To assess sources of support and guidance on which parents rely when making difficult decisions in the pediatric intensive care unit and to evaluate associations of sources of support and guidance to anxiety, depression, and positive and negative affect.

Study Design.—This was a prospective cohort study of 86 English-speaking parents of 75 children in the pediatric intensive care unit at The Children's Hospital of Philadelphia who were hospitalized greater than 72 hours. Parents completed standardized instruments and a novel sources of support and guidance assessment.

Results.—Most parents chose physicians, nurses, friends, and extended family as their main sources of support and guidance when making a difficult decision. Descriptive analysis revealed a broad distribution for the sources of support and guidance items related to spirituality. Parents tended to fall into 1 of 2 groups when we used latent class analysis: the more-spiritual group (n = 47; 55%) highly ranked "what my child wants" ($P = .023$), spouses ($P = .002$), support groups ($P = .003$), church community ($P < .001$), spiritual leader ($P < .001$), higher power ($P < .001$), and prayer ($P < .001$) compared with the less-spiritual group (n = 39; 45%). The more-spiritual parents had greater positive affect scores ($P = .005$). Less-spiritual parents had greater depression scores ($P = .043$).

Conclusions.—Parents rely most on physicians, nurses, and friends and extended family when making difficult decisions for their critically ill child. Respondents tended to fall into 1 of 2 groups where the more-spiritual respondents were associated with greater positive affect and may be more resistant to depression.

▶ More than 50 000 children die annually in the Unites States, and the majority of these deaths occur in the intensive care unit.[1,2] How we support children and families experiencing such challenges, suffering, and loss is of great importance to all pediatric health care providers. The article by Mardrigal builds on the limited understanding we have of this subject.

The aim of this study was to understand the sources of support and guidance families seek in making difficult decisions for their seriously ill child in the intensive care setting. What the authors found is that all parents look to physicians, nurses, and extended family/friends to help with decision making. What varied was the relative importance parents gave to the "spiritual" aspects of these decisions. Although acknowledgment of the general use of spiritual, religious, and faith communities to guide decisions was around 50%, the impact this had on the psychological well-being of parents was significant. Parents who felt they had spiritual guidance self-reported lower rates of depression and higher rates of positive mood/affect despite these immensely difficult circumstances. Interestingly, measures of parent's hopefulness did not change regardless of the importance of spiritual guidance.

Assisting families with end-of-life decision making is clearly a heartbreaking and challenging area for pediatric providers. We know that every child's life is precious and that nothing can truly make the difficulties of decision making for a seriously ill child vanish for families.[3] We also know that maintaining hope is critical to a family's well-being, even in times of a child's death.[1] As providers, we claim that families are "not ready to hear bad news" or we worry that they "will lose hope when given poor prognostic information."[5] We have since learned that these assumptions are misleading and that families want honest and clear information from health care providers.[6,7] Studies of parents of children with cancer have shown that parents want to continue being a "good parent" to their child throughout their life and even at the end of life.[3] What being a "good parent" means and how health care providers support this is the challenging part. The authors of this study point us toward "spirituality" as a way of supporting families in these unimaginable circumstances.

Most health care providers are not trained to handle spiritual issues and are often hesitant to ask about the spiritual needs of the families they care for. Providers also are not expert in how to think about the broad definition of "spiritual practice" and how truly vast experiences of "spiritual practice" can be. For example, spiritual practice can include observing cultural activities, honoring parental instinct, or connecting with nature. It is possible that "spirituality" was too narrowly defined in this study and with a broader understanding the authors would have seen that more parents invoked "spiritual practice" in their decision making. This may be true especially given the increase in people who identify as "spiritual but not religious" in the United States today.[8]

Opportunities to learn from those more expert in this area exist. Professionally trained, interfaith hospital-based chaplains often can carefully and respectfully elicit information about a family's "spirituality." Understanding how a particular family uses "spiritual" guidance in a broad sense can be helpful in aligning families and providers before discussing difficult decisions. For example, when families indicate prayer is important to them, inviting a chaplain to offer a prayer of hope and peace at the beginning of an advance care planning discussion can put families and providers on a shared foundation of hopes. This technique is often used by palliative care teams to incorporate family values, priorities, and meaningfulness into everyday care when cure is not possible. Unfortunately, only 4 of the 86 parents in this study received palliative care services.

The issues of meaningfulness and being a "good parent" are closely tied together. Using the skills and expertise of chaplains and palliative care teams can help to draw out these aspects of parenting even in the most difficult of circumstances. Connecting parents and families to their "spirituality" whatever it may be, may help them to access their own strengths, priorities, and meaning even when their child is critically ill and even when a child dies.

J. F. Bogetz, MD

References

1. National Vital Statistics System Centers for Disease Control and Prevention. www.cdc.gov. http://www.cdc.gov/nchs/nvss/mortality_tables.htm. Accessed March 17, 2016.
2. Feudtner C, Kang TI, Hexem KR, et al. Pediatric palliative care patients: a prospective multicenter cohort study. *Pediatrics.* 2011;127:1094-1101.
3. Feudtner C, Walter JK, Faerber JA, et al. Good-parent beliefs of parents of seriously Ill children. *JAMA Pediatr.* 2015;169:39.
4. Feudtner C. The breadth of hopes. *N Engl J Med.* 2009;361:2306-2307.
5. Davies B, Sehring SA, Partridge JC, et al. Barriers to palliative care for children: perceptions of pediatric health care providers. *Pediatrics.* 2008;121:282-288.
6. Contro N, Larson J, Scofield S, Sourkes B, Cohen H. Family perspectives on the quality of pediatric palliative care. *Arch Pediatr Adolesc Med.* 2002;156:14.
7. Hinds PS, Kelly KP. Helping parents make and survive end of life decisions for their seriously ill child. *Nursing Clinics of North America.* 2010;45:465-474.
8. Pew Research Center: Religion & Public Life. pewforum.org. http://www.pewforum.org. Accessed March 17, 2016.

Intern and Resident Workflow Patterns on Pediatric Inpatient Units: A Multicenter Time-Motion Study

Starmer AJ, Destino L, Yoon CS, et al (Harvard Med School, Boston, MA; Stanford Univ School of Medicine, CA; Brigham and Women's Hosp, Boston, MA)

JAMA Pediatrics 169:1175-1177, 2015

▶ Medical training has had a long-standing tradition of learning from patients. Every patient is unique, every patient tells a story. We "practice" medicine, and the purpose of medicine is to serve the patient. Or has this changed?

We have seen medical education evolve to adapt to growing societal demands, increasing complexity of patients as new innovations emerge, volumes of data whether historical or predictive, growing collaborations across the world, and the reexamination of duty hours and the medical trainee's well-being. With this, we have seen increased electronic health record (EHR) systems, decreased resident duty hours, and increased e-learning and simulation training.

The time-motion study by Starmer et al paints the current state of events in pediatrics residency training. Research assistants monitored resident activities through a sampling of 3452 hours across 9 pediatric institutions, which is the first multicenter study of its kind. Not surprisingly, the findings demonstrated a marked skew of the percentage of time spent in front of a computer (20.5%) and in interprofessional communication (34.7%) versus in patient or family contact (12.0%) and educational activities (4.7%); the rest of the time is spent on paper (~5%), telephone (~5%), personal time (including walking, talking, restroom use, ~18%), and looking for items (~2%). Although the article shows that pediatric residents spend less time in front of the computer than in previous similar internal medicine studies, the results still show almost double the amount of time in front of the computer than with patients. Although the EHR has allowed for more efficient order entry, enhanced provider communication, and rapid transmission of pertinent information to the entire health care team for expedited execution of care, this study suggests that it may be shunting providers away from the patient's bedside.

We can easily blame the computer, but institutional priorities and safety audits from national organizations likely have an equally heavy hand in impacting trainees' educational activities that involve direct patient contact. Institutional priorities add to the responsibilities of a trainee through endeavors such as medication reconciliation, "chart biopsies," exhaustive sign-out lists for the increasing number of handoffs, or added notes in the chart for procedures and events with a new emphasis on documentation integrity to assure the safety of not only the patient, but also the safety of hospital systems against litigation, liability, and risk.

This time-motion analysis has its limitations with categorization because it does not take into account category overlaps or establish causation. Interdisciplinary communication has the highest percentage (38.3%) of time winning over the time in front of the computer, but arguably, can this also be a consequence of the computer-shunted resident workflow? Specifically, what percentage of this interdisciplinary communication is for order clarifications, order corrections, requests for updates for nursing/families, requests for interteam communication and coordination that results from directing patient care with the ease of a remote click in the resident workroom?

As pediatricians, we spend a considerable amount of time counseling families about avoidance of excessive "screen time." Should this counseling also be directed to our trainees? Although the solution certainly doesn't lie in a global return to paper charts or restrictions on Internet searches for valuable medical information, many challenges loom for our academic community. How might graduate medical education evolve so that it can continue to incorporate direct patient/family interactions into its educational activities? How can the computer become part of medical education without completely detracting from patient interaction? We are already seeing the growth of mobile workstations, telemedicine, EHR systems that incorporate evidence-based guidelines and suggestions to add to patient's care plans, and the advent of patient experience departments fully centered at engaging patients and families in their care. As evidenced by this important article by Starmer et al, the digital age has had the unintended consequence of a shift away from important patient/family interactions for trainees. We must evolve as a community to creatively utilize these untapped educational opportunities that continue to refocus resident training on patients and families.

Part of the solution may need to come from above. Attendings and even resident supervisors have the power to relieve younger trainees from their less patient-centered tasks to enable them, for example, to return to the patients' rooms in the afternoon even if just to learn to connect. Perhaps the senior resident or attending could hold the pager or complete the sign-out list to allow trainees to have follow-up conversations with their patients.

New curricula and electives have emerged to provide trainees other opportunities to interface with patients even beyond the bedside. Towle et al highlight programs aimed at empowering patients as health mentors serving as teachers for residents as experts of their own diseases.[1,2] Similarly, Bogetz et al discuss educational opportunities and programs with pediatric complex care patients and their parents, allowing trainees to have a glimpse into their everyday lives.[3] Palliative care panels and patient family advisory council guest speakers are also becoming more ingrained into teaching conferences.

Role modeling, an "oldie but goodie" tool in medical education, plays a central role as a solution to this highlighted problem. Supervisors have the capability of engaging patients in bedside teaching—whether it's talking about physical exam findings, asking the patient about their illness, or demonstrating professional skills and bedside etiquette. Perhaps more important, this growing shift away from patients should remind more senior physicians to take a pause because if they lead the team in a task-driven, workhorse-centric manner where the main goal is checking all the boxes and getting all the orders in, then trainees will follow in that example. However, if leaders put words into practice, pause to teach at the bedside, and actively engage the patients as an example for trainees, the importance of the physician-patient-family relationship is emphasized, and trainees are reminded where priorities should be: the patient.

I. S. Chua, MD

References

1. Towle A, Brown H, Hofley C, Kerston RP, Lyons H, Walsh C. The expert patient as teacher: an interprofessional health mentors programme. *Clin Teach*. 2014;11:6.
2. Towle A, Godolphin W. Patients as educators: interprofessional learning for patient-centred care. *Med Teach*. 2013;35:219-225.
3. Bogetz JF, Bogetz AL, Rassback CE, Gabhart JM, Blankeburg RL. Caring for children with medical complexity: challenges and educational opportunities identified by pediatric residents. *Acad Pediatr*. 2015;15:621-625.

Physicians and Physician Trainees Rarely Identify or Address Overweight/Obesity in Hospitalized Children

King MA, Nkoy FL, Maloney CG, et al (Saint Louis Univ, MO; Univ of Utah, Salt lake City)
J Pediatr 167:816-820, 2015

Objectives.—To determine how frequently physicians identify and address overweight/obesity in hospitalized children and to compare physician documentation across training level (medical student, intern, resident, attending).

Study Design.—We conducted a retrospective chart review. Using an administrative database, Centers for Disease Control and Prevention body mass index calculator, and random sampling technique, we identified a study population of 300 children aged 2-18 years with overweight/obesity hospitalized on the general medical service of a tertiary care pediatric hospital. We reviewed admission, progress, and discharge notes to determine how frequently physicians and physician trainees identified (documented in history, physical exam, or assessment) and addressed (documented in hospital or discharge plan) overweight/obesity.

Results.—Physicians and physician trainees identified overweight/ obesity in 8.3% (n = 25) and addressed it in 4% (n = 12) of 300 hospitalized children with overweight/obesity. Interns were most likely to document overweight/ obesity in history (8.3% of the 266 patients they followed). Attendings were most likely to document overweight/ obesity in physical examination (8.3%), assessment (4%), and plan (4%) of the 300 patients they followed. Medical students were least likely to document overweight/obesity including it in the assessment (0.4%) and plan (0.4%) of the 244 hospitalized children with overweight/obesity they followed.

Conclusions.—Physicians and physician trainees rarely identify or address overweight/obesity in hospitalized children. This represents a missed opportunity for both patient care and physician trainee education (Fig 2, Table 2).

▶ Pediatric obesity is a chronic disease that affects nearly 13 million children and adolescents.[1] American Academy of Pediatrics policy statements affirm that outpatient pediatricians should address pediatric obesity,[2] but similar recommendations do not exist for inpatient providers who have the opportunity to address overall health during admissions. This article builds on existing literature that

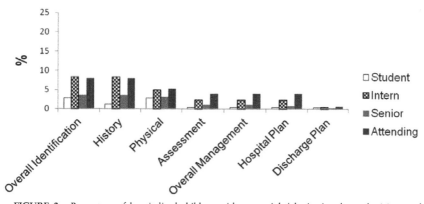

FIGURE 2.—Percentage of hospitalized children with overweight/obesity in whom physicians and physician trainees documented overweight/obesity. Items documented by specific physician and physician trainee providers (medical student, intern, resident, attending) involved in the care of the patient at any point during his/her hospitalization (admission, progress note, or discharge). Total overweight/obesity identification, history, and physical exam were documented more frequently by attendings and interns ($P < .05$). Assessment was documented more frequently by attendings ($P < .05$). Overweight/obesity management, hospital plan, and discharge plan documentation did not differ by physician training level. (Reprinted from King MA, Nkoy FL, Maloney CG, et al. Physicians and physician trainees rarely identify or address overweight/obesity in hospitalized children. *J Pediatr*. 2015;167:816-820, with permission from Elsevier Inc.)

TABLE 2.—Frequency of Physicians and Physician Trainee Overweight/Obesity Documentation in Hospitalized Children with Overweight/Obesity*

	Overweight and Obese Patients (n = 300)	
	%	n
Overall identification	8.3	25
History	8	24
Diet	8	24
Physical activity	1.7	5
Screen time	0.7	2
Family history	0.7	2
Physical examination	8.3	25
BMI	5.3	16
BMI percentile for age/sex	2.7	8
Physical examination findings	8.3	25
Assessment	4.3	13
Overall management	4	12
Hospital plan	4	12
Inpatient nutrition consultation	2.7	8
Diet counseling by physician team	2	6
Laboratory evaluation (discussed or ordered)	1.7	5
Activity counseling by physician team	0.7	2
Discharge plan	0.7	2
Referral to weight management program	0.7	2
Referral to primary care physician	0.7	2

*Items documented by any physician or physician trainee (medical student, intern, senior, or attending) involved in the care of the patient at any point during his/her hospitalization (admission, progress note, or discharge).

Reprinted from King MA, Nkoy FL, Maloney CG, et al. Physicians and physician trainees rarely identify or address overweight/obesity in hospitalized children. *J Pediatr.* 2015;167:816-820, with permission from Elsevier Inc.

identifies obesity recognition and management during acute hospitalization as a potential area for improvement.

Although other researchers[3-6] have recognized a lack of physician identification of overweight/obesity status during acute hospitalization, the study by King et al is unique in that it includes a broader range of pediatric ages and assesses both provider identification of and intention to treat overweight/obesity using an electronic medical records (EMR) that automatically calculates body mass index (BMI) and BMI percentile. The observation that providers across the medical training level rarely identify and address pediatric overweight/obesity is a new finding that adds another layer of poor teaching and role-modeling to the issue (Fig 2, Table 2).

There are a variety of arguments to support physician identification and initiation of treatment of childhood obesity during acute hospitalization. Any admission represents an opportunity to address patient health needs. This may be particularly so for patients who do not frequently follow-up with a primary care provider. Acute hospitalization may be a period when patients and families are focused on health and more amenable to new diagnoses and treatment recommendations. Contrary to the opinion of the majority of pediatric hospitalists, surveys demonstrate that parents of hospitalized children are interested in knowing if their child is overweight/obese and feel providers should address the issue.[3,7,8] Finally, providers should identify overweight children during admission because overweight/obese children are at risk of worse outcomes,[9–13] because increased complexity can improve reimbursements and because these patients may require unique resources to create a safe hospitalization, such as healthy diets, medical equipment, or adjusted medication dosing.[14]

Although the article by King et al certainly supports the notion that inpatient provider identification and treatment of overweight/obesity leaves room for improvement, we highlight some additional issues to consider. For providers to identify overweight/obesity during hospitalization, accurate measurement of height and weight at the time of hospitalization is imperative. In this study, patients with physiologically impossible weight and/or height data were excluded and previous studies have also observed inaccurate measurement of height and weight in the medical record.[6] Although there are many possible benefits of obesity treatment initiation during acute hospitalization, it is also useful to consider unintended costs, which might include increased provider time spent eliciting daily habits to effectively counsel patients and their families, increased utilization of potentially scarce resources such as dieticians, and increased training for inpatient providers (such as in motivational interviewing skills).

Some adult literature cautions against addressing chronic diseases during an inpatient hospitalization because changes in medication regimens may lead to adverse drug reactions and/or medication non-compliance (especially in patients without a stable medical home)[15]; however, we feel this may be less relevant in a pediatric population on few medications. Principal interventions such as healthy eating recommendations, increased physical activity and dietary referrals are unlikely to pose harm to patients. Ultimately, it remains to be seen is whether identification and treatment of childhood obesity during an acute hospitalization leads to improved patient outcomes.

Despite these considerations, we agree that the inpatient setting presents an important opportunity to address a significant threat to child health and the study by King et al highlights the limited impact in our current state. There is a need to develop the systems and supports to identify and treat obesity in the inpatient setting; one study suggests that only 37% of pediatric hospitals currently have a system in place to do so.[13] Identification is the first step in management and an EMR trigger/alarm systems can assist providers in identifying overweight/obese children, but more needs to be done. We need to develop efficient and effective methods to engage patients and families in behavior change that can be delivered in the inpatient setting. In situations where recommended lab work is obtained to screen for obesity comorbidities and sequelae,[16] challenges will include preventing redundant testing, comprehensively following results, and address abnormal values when there is suboptimal transfer of information between inpatient and outpatient providers.[17] More than 30% of children are overweight or obese,[1] and the development of strategies to improve recognition and management of this epidemic in the inpatient setting could be impactful. We look forward to future studies that evaluate the effect of these strategies on trainee education and patient outcomes.

E. Aragona, MD

E. Schainker, MD, MSc

References

1. Ogden CL, Carroll MD, Kit BK, Flegal KM. Prevalence of childhood and adult obesity in the United States, 2011–2012. *JAMA.* 2014;311:806.
2. Krebs NF, Jacobson MS, American Academy of Pediatrics Committee on Nutrition. Prevention of pediatric overweight and obesity. *Pediatrics.* 2003;112:424-430.
3. McLean K, Wake M, McCallum Z. Overweight in medical paediatric inpatients: detection and parent expectations. *J Paediatr Child Health.* 2007;43:256-261.
4. Azhdam DB, Reyhan I, Grant-Guimaraes J, Feinstein R. Prevalence and documentation of overweight and obesity in hospitalized children and adolescents. *Hosp Pediatr.* 2014;4:377-381.
5. Sleeper EJ, Ariza AJ, Binns HJ. Do hospitalized pediatric patients have weight and blood pressure concerns identified? *J Pediatr.* 2009;154:213-217.
6. O'Connor J, Youde LS, Allen JR, Hanson RM, Baur LA. Outcomes of a nutrition audit in a tertiary paediatric hospital: implications for service improvement. *J Paediatr Child Health.* 2004;40:295-298.
7. Bradford K, Kihlstrom M, Pointer I, et al. Parental attitudes toward obesity and overweight screening and communication for hospitalized children. *Hosp Pediatr.* 2012;2:126-132.
8. Lee DS, Gross E, Rinke ML. Physician perspectives on obesity screening in hospitalized children. *Clin Pediatr (Phila).* 2015; http://dx.doi.org/10.1177/0009922815617976.
9. Shanley LA, Lin H, Flores G. Factors associated with length of stay for pediatric asthma hospitalizations. *J Asthma.* 2015;52:471-477.
10. Ross E, Burris A, Murphy JT. Obesity and outcomes following burns in the pediatric population. *J Pediatr Surg.* 2014;49:469-473.
11. Woolford SJ, Gebremariam A, Clark SJ, Davis MM. Incremental hospital charges associated with obesity as a secondary diagnosis in children. *Obesity.* 2007;15:1895-1901.
12. Fleming-Dutra KE, Mao J, Leonard JC. Acute care costs in overweight children: a pediatric urban cohort study. *Child Obes Print.* 2013;9:338-345.
13. Young KL, Demeule M, Stuhlsatz K, et al. Identification and treatment of obesity as a standard of care for all patients in children's hospitals. *Pediatrics.* 2011;128:S47-S50.
14. Ross EL, Heizer J, Mixon MA, et al. Development of recommendations for dosing of commonly prescribed medications in critically ill obese children. *Am J Health Syst Pharm.* 2015;72:542-556.
15. Steinman MA, Auerbach AD. Managing chronic disease in hospitalized patients. *JAMA Intern Med.* 2013;173:1857.
16. Barlow SEthe Expert Committee. Expert committee recommendations regarding the prevention, assessment, and treatment of child and adolescent overweight and obesity: summary report. *Pediatrics.* 2007;120:S164-S192.
17. Harlan G, Srivastava R, Harrison L, McBride G, Maloney C. Pediatric hospitalists and primary care providers: a communication needs assessment. *J Hosp Med.* 2009;4:187-193.

Who's My Doctor? Using an Electronic Tool to Improve Team Member Identification on an Inpatient Pediatrics Team

Singh A, Rhee KE, Brennan JJ, et al (Stanford Univ School of Medicine, Palo Alto, CA; Univ of California San Diego School of Medicine)

Hosp Pediatr 6:157-165, 2016

Objectives.—Increase parent/caregiver ability to correctly identify the attending in charge and define terminology of treatment team members

(TTMs). We hypothesized that correct TTM identification would increase with use of an electronic communication tool. Secondary aims included assessing subjects' satisfaction with and trust of TTM and interest in computer activities during hospitalization.

Methods.—Two similar groups of parents/legal guardians/primary caregivers of children admitted to the Pediatric Hospital Medicine teaching service with an unplanned first admission were surveyed before (Phase 1) and after (Phase 2) implementation of a novel electronic medical record (EMR)-based tool with names, photos, and definitions of TTMs. Physicians were also surveyed only during Phase 1. Surveys assessed TTM identification, satisfaction, trust, and computer use.

Results.—More subjects in Phase 2 correctly identified attending physicians by name (71% vs. 28%, $P < .001$) and correctly defined terms intern, resident, and attending ($P \leq .03$) compared with Phase 1. Almost all subjects (>79%) and TTMs (>87%) reported that subjects' ability to identify TTMs moderately or strongly impacted satisfaction and trust. The majority of subjects expressed interest in using computers to understand TTMs in each phase.

Conclusions.—Subjects' ability to correctly identify attending physicians and define TTMs was significantly greater for those who used our tool. In our study, subjects reported that TTM identification impacted aspects of the TTM relationship, yet few could correctly identify TTMs before tool use. This pilot study showed early success in engaging subjects with the EMR in the hospital and suggests that families would engage in computer-based activities in this setting.

▶ In academic medical centers, the number of caregivers on a single patient's treatment team is often expressed in double digits. On weekday mornings, gaggles of white coats and scrubs are seen roaming the hallways with computers on wheels in tow. The herd of clinicians moves slowly down the hallway, periodically stopping for a patient presentation or teaching. And then, from the hallway viewer's perspective, they vanish—one by one ritualistically rubbing their hands together with antiseptic gel and disappearing into an open doorway. Now imagine the patient's perspective, alone in his or her own room just a moment before and now surrounded by a wall of uninvited, stern-looking inpatient team members who all are purportedly all connected in some way to why the patient is in the hospital.

In a crucially important effort to humanize this orchestrated interaction, repeated thousands of times a day throughout academic hospitals, Rady Children's Hospital in San Diego started by putting names and roles to faces. And as we would predict, from the patient and family perspective, knowing who is walking into your room and what he or she does on the treatment team can make a significant difference in terms of trust and empowerment.

Rady Children's Hospital made the decision to leverage its investment in electronic health record software to engage patients by providing online access to a photo representation of each member of their treatment team and definitions of each member's role. This intervention resulted in a dramatic rise in the ability of patients and family to name their attending physician—the doctor in charge of their care—as well as increased knowledge about the identity and role of other treatment team members. Because the providers entering inpatient rooms—the patients' spaces for healing—were more recognizable, patients felt more empowered and satisfied and trusted their caregivers to a greater degree.

This patient engagement innovation study is important to share and has important limitations. The acknowledged limitation that postintervention patient surveys may have been biased by the help of bedside nurses and others necessitates that we take the reported numbers with a grain of salt. And although the postintervention data presented certainly show a trend of improved patient and family subjective assessments of care, no statistical significance is reported. Therefore, it is impossible for us know whether these trends toward greater postintervention scores are statistically significant for satisfaction (84%/95%), communication (87%/93%), and trust (79%/93%). Still, these data are useful to share, even though the study was not necessarily powered to measure these secondary outcomes definitively.

As is the key for most digital health interventions, incorporating innovation into the clinician's and family's day-to-day activity with minimal inconvenience is important. This exercise is often termed "workflow analysis." The authors tell us that the manual process for keeping the treatment team up-to-date was mandatory but do not discuss how this practice is monitored and enforced. It is also important to consider how patients and families can best access patient-engagement technology.

At a high level, there are 3 models of providing inpatients with access to electronic data and digital engagement tools. First, medical centers are increasingly providing patients with their own in-room connected device to use while in the hospital (eg, a tablet that is tethered to the bedside of the patient, secure and wipe-able in between patients). A second strategy is for the nurse or some other member of the care team to bring patient-facing devices into the room upon request. The third method is to rely on patients to bring their own devices to interact online with the hospital systems (ie, "bring your own device" strategy). Each of the strategies has its own advantages and disadvantages, which are important for providers to consider as they learn from this publication and implement digital inpatient engagement tools.

We are now in the midst of a patient empowerment revolution. Providers are increasingly looking to digital health tools to meet consumer expectations from other industries, health policy regulations, and changing reimbursement incentives. Patient engagement tools can serve to bridge gaps in knowledge, communication, and language as this publication indicates. We are only in the early days of using technology to enable and delight patients.

S. Bokser, MD, MPH

15 Infectious Diseases

Zika Virus Infection in Pregnant Women in Rio de Janeiro — Preliminary Report

Brasil P, Pereira JP Jr, Raja Gabaglia C, et al (Fundação Oswaldo Cruz, Rio de Janeiro; Biomedical Res Institute of Southern California, Oceanside, CA)

N Engl J Med 2016 [Epub ahead of print]

Background.—Zika virus (ZIKV) has been linked to neonatal microcephaly. To characterize the spectrum of ZIKV disease in pregnancy, we followed patients in Rio de Janeiro to describe clinical manifestations in mothers and repercussions of acute ZIKV infection in fetuses.

Methods.—We enrolled pregnant women in whom a rash had developed within the previous 5 days and tested blood and urine specimens for ZIKV by reverse-transcriptase—polymerasechain-reaction-assays. We followed the women prospectively and collected clinical and ultrasonographic data.

Results.—A total of 88 women were enrolled from September 2015 through February 2016; of these 88 women, 72 (82%) tested positive for ZIKV in blood, urine, or both. The timing of acute ZIKV infection ranged from 5 to 38 weeks of gestation. Predominant clinical features included pruritic descending macular or maculopapular rash, arthralgias, conjunctival injection, and headache; 28% had fever (short-term and low-grade). Women who were positive for ZIKV were more likely than those who were negative for the virus to have maculopapular rash (44% vs. 12%, $P = 0.02$), conjunctival involvement (58% vs. 13%, $P = 0.002$), and lymphadenopathy (40% vs. 7%, $P = 0.02$). Fetal ultrasonography was performed in 42 ZIKV-positive women (58%) and in all ZIKV-negative women. Fetal abnormalities were detected by Doppler ultrasonography in 12 of the 42 ZIKV-positive women (29%) and in none of the 16 ZIKV-negative women. Adverse findings included fetal deaths at 36 and 38 weeks of gestation (2 fetuses), in utero growth restriction with or without microcephaly (5 fetuses), ventricular calcifications or other central nervous system (CNS) lesions (7 fetuses), and abnormal amniotic fluid volume or cerebral or umbilical artery flow (7 fetuses). To date, 8 of the 42 women in whom fetal ultrasonography was performed have delivered their babies, and the ultrasonographic findings have been confirmed.

Conclusions.—Despite mild clinical symptoms, ZIKV infection during pregnancy appears to be associated with grave outcomes, including fetal death, placental insufficiency, fetal growth restriction, and CNS injury.

▶ Zika virus is an arbovirus of the Flaviviridae family transmitted by mosquitos of the *Aedes* genus that was originally described as an infection of primates in Uganda in 1947[1] and subsequently of humans in tropical Africa and southern Asia.[2] Since 2007 an Asian lineage of Zika virus has spread through the Western Pacific to Polynesia,[3,4] appearing in the Americas first in Easter Island, Chile, in 2014[5] and later that year in Brazil.[6,7] The disease itself is relatively benign, causing a febrile rash illness in approximately 20% of acutely infected individuals.[4,8] However, as it has spread through Latin America and the Caribbean in 2014 and 2015, it has been temporally and geographically associated with an outbreak of fetal microcephaly, presumably from in utero encephalitis and arrested brain growth.[9-13] As of April 2016, more than 40 countries without prior documented transmission are experiencing an ongoing Zika virus outbreak, which the World Health Organization has categorized as a Public Health Emergency of International Concern.

Brasil and colleagues from the Fundação Oswaldo Cruz (FIOCRUZ) in Rio de Janeiro, provided some of the most compelling early evidence of a causal association between maternal infection and fetal anomalies. From the acute febrile illness clinic at FIOCRUZ, the Brazilian equivalent of the National Institutes of Health's Clinical Center, the authors enrolled self-referred pregnant women who had had a rash illness within the preceding 5 days. They recruited 88 women between 5 and 38 weeks' gestation and tested them for Zika virus infection using serum and urine polymerase chain reaction (PCR). Of the 88 women, 72 (82%) had confirmed Zika virus infection. Compared with the 16 women who had other causes for their rash illnesses, women with Zika virus infection were more likely to have a maculopapular rash, conjunctival injection, and lymphadenopathy.

Forty-two (58%) of the 72 women with confirmed infection, and all 16 without infection, consented to fetal ultrasonography. Fetal anomalies were found in 12 (29%) of the 42 women with infection, and in none of the 16 who had other causes for their rash illnesses. Fetal abnormalities included 2 intrauterine fetal deaths, 5 cases with intrauterine growth restriction (IUGR; 4 with associated microcephaly), 6 fetuses with cerebral calcifications or other structural central nervous system (CNS) lesions, and 5 with abnormal amniotic fluid volume or cerebral or umbilical artery flow. At the time of publication, 8 of the 42 fetuses had been delivered, and the ultrasonographic findings were confirmed in all but 1 newborn.

This is a sobering report. The attack rate seems high, with 82% of pregnant women with acute rash illness having confirmed Zika virus infection. This underlies the virus's rapid spread through tropical and subtropical Brazil. It also reflects the expanding distribution of the daytime-biting Aedes vectors, considered eradicated from South America by 1965 only to reinfest the continent beginning 1 decade later.[14] Also alarming is the high incidence of clinical disease in fetuses of infected mothers; nearly one-third had sonographically detectable abnormalities, corroborated at birth. In many ways, the most startling finding was that pathology occurred across gestation. Two mothers with Zika virus infection suffered miscarriage in the first trimester, 2 additional intrauterine fetal deaths occurred after infection at 25 and 32 weeks' gestation, while IUGR and CNS structural abnormalities were noted across all trimesters. This is quite different from other systemic congenital viral infections such as rubella and cytomegalovirus, where infection appears to be most severe when early in gestation.[15,16] What remains unknown from this study is what factors led to fetal transmission and infection, whether exposed neonates without overt signs of disease are harboring undetected deficits, and whether pregnant women with asymptomatic infection (excluded from this study) can transmit virus to their fetuses as well.

Parallel work suggests that Zika virus has tropism for neural crest cells, which may explain its devastating effect on brain growth and development.[17,18] But why have we not seen this before it spread to the Americas? A retrospective survey in French Polynesia, where Zika arrived in 2013, has found an excess of cases of microcephaly, suggesting that it has happened before.[19] Phylogenetic studies comparing strains isolated during the current epidemic with banked genomes from African, Asian, and Americas-Pacific lineages have detected several nucleotide differences.[20,21] These mutations' effects on neurotropism or virulence remain to be clarified.

It has been more than 50 years since the devastating pandemic of rubella virus infection in 1964 that led to as many as 20 000 cases of congenital rubella syndrome in the United States alone.[22]

The lessons learned may be useful here. First, the spectrum of clinical disease was broad and ranged from intrauterine fetal deaths and the classical clinical presentation of cataracts, heart defects, and deafness with or without mental retardation to much more subtle findings, such as late-onset hearing loss.[23] We will likely have to wait several years to understand the full range of symptoms in children congenitally infected with Zika virus. Second, our emphasis needs to be on prevention. We were not able to deploy rubella vaccine in time to stop the spread of disease in 1964, but it was available by 1968 and has prevented countless exposures. With all candidate Zika vaccines still in the predevelopment phase, control will hinge on advanced methods of vector control specifically targeting *Aedes aegypti* to limit spread and density of infection.[24,25] Prevention campaigns will also need to educate the public effectively regarding transmission risks stemming from travel and local exposures as well as from sexual transmission.[26,27] Meanwhile, recent reports of transfusion-mediated transmission in Brazil and viral detection in donated blood underscore the need for expanded bank screening.[28]

Finally, this is yet another example of the Columbian exchange. The transfer of organisms, beneficial and harmful, between Old World and New World ecosystems has occurred since the late 15th century. The latest Zika virus epidemic in the Americas represents another instance of the introduction of a pathogenic virus into a receptive environment inhabited by a previously unexposed population, just as we have seen in the 16th century with yellow fever virus and more recently with Chikungunya virus, Dengue virus, and West Nile virus (where the unexposed population was *Corvidae* birds). Intensive biosurveillance for new and emerging pathogens, with transnational sharing of data from relevant clinical sites and registries, remains our best hope for recognizing importations as they occur and controlling them at the source.[29]

G. W. Rutherford, MD, AM

O. Medzihradsky, MD, MPH, MSc

References

1. Dick GW, Kitchen SF, Haddow AJ. Zika virus. I. Isolation and serological specificity. *Trans R Soc Trop Med Hyg.* 1952;46:509-520.
2. Haddow AD, Schuh AJ, Yasuda CY, et al. Genetic characterization of Zika virus strains; geographic expansion of the Asian lineage. *PLoS Negl Trop Dis.* 2012;6: e1477.
3. Musso D, Nilles EJ, Cao-Lormeau VM. Rapid spread of emerging Zika virus in the Pacific area. *Clin Microbiol Infect.* 2014;20:O595-O596.
4. Duffy MR, Chen TH, Hancock WT, et al. Zika virus outbreak on Yap Island, Federated States of Micronesia. *N Engl J Med.* 2009;360:2536-2543.
5. Tognarelli J, Ulloa S, Villagra E, et al. A report of the outbreak of Zika virus on Easter Island, South Pacific, 2014. *Arch Virol.* 2016;161:665-668.
6. Musso D. Zika virus transmission from French Polynesia to Brazil. *Emerg Infect Dis.* 2015;21:1887.
7. Zanhuca C, de Melo VC, Mosimann AL, dos Santos GI, dos Santos CN, Luz K. First report of autochthonous transmission of Zika virus in Brazil. *Mem Inst Oswaldo Cruz.* 2015;100:569-572.
8. Hayes EB. Zika virus outside Africa. *Emerg Infect Dis.* 2009;15:1347-1350.
9. Driggers RW, Ho C-Y, Korhonen EM, et al. Zika virus infection with prolonged maternal viremia and fetal brain abnormalities. *N Engl J Med.* 2016;374: 2142-2151.
10. Oliveira Melo AS, Malinger G, Ximenes R, et al. Zika virus intrauterine infection causes fetal brain abnormality and microcephaly: tip of the iceberg? *Ultrasound Obstet Gynecol.* 2016;47:6-7.
11. Mlakar J, Korva M, Tul N, et al. Zika virus associated with microcephaly. *N Engl J Med.* 2016;374:951-958.
12. Rasmussen SA, Jamieson DJ, Honein MA, Peterson LR. Zika virus and birth defects—reviewing the evidence for causality. *N Engl J Med.* 2016;374: 1981-1987.
13. Teixeira MG, da Conceição N, Costa M, de Oliveira WK, Nunes ML, Rodrigues LC. The epidemic of Zika virus—related microcephaly in Brazil: detection, control, etiology, and future scenarios. *Am J Public Health.* 2016;106: 601-605.
14. Vezzani D, Carbago AE. Aedes aegypti, Aedes albopictus, and dengue in Argentina: current knowledge and future directions. *Mem Inst Oswaldo Cruz.* 2008; 103:66-74.
15. Zgórniak-Nowosielska I, Zawilińska B, Szostek S. Rubella infection during pregnancy in the 1985—86 epidemic: follow-up after seven years. *Eur J Epidemiol.* 2006;12:303-308.
16. Ahlfors K, Ivarsson SA, Harris S. Report on a long-term study of maternal and congenital cytomegalovirus infection in Sweden. Review of prospective studies available in the literature. *Scand J Infect Dis.* 1999;31:443-457.
17. Garcez PP, Loiol WX, Madeiro da Costa R, et al. Zika virus impairs growth in human neurospheres and brain organoids. *Science.* 2016;352:816-818.
18. Tang H, Hammack C, Ogden SC, et al. Zika virus infects human cortical neural progenitors and attenuates their growth. *Cell Stem Cell.* 2016;18:1-4.
19. Cauchemez S, Besnard M, Bompard P, et al. Association between Zika virus and microcephaly in French Polynesia, 2013—15: a retrospective study. *Lancet.* 2016; 387:2125-2132.

20. Faria NR, Azevedo Rdo S, Kraemer MU, et al. Zika virus in the Americas: early epidemiological and genetic findings. *Science.* 2016;352:345-349.
21. Wang L, Valderamos SG, Wu A, et al. From mosquitos to humans: genetic Evolution of Zika virus. *Cell Host Microbe.* 2016;19:561-565.
22. Lambert N, Strebel P, Orenstein W, Icenogle J, Poland GA. Rubella. *Lancet.* 2015;385:2297-2307.
23. Dudgeon JA. Congenital rubella. *J Pediatr.* 1975;87:1078-1086.
24. Caragata EP, Dultra HL, Moreira LA. Exploiting intimate relationships: controlling mosquito-transmitted disease with Wolbachia. *Trends Parasitol.* 2016;32:207-218.
25. Adelman ZN, Tu Z. Control of mosquito-borne infectious diseases: sex and gene drive. *Trends Parasitol.* 2016;32:219-229.
26. Centers for Disease Control and Prevention. Update: interim guidance for health care providers caring for women of reproductive age with possible Zika virus exposure – United States, 2016. *MMWR Morb Mortal Wkly Rep.* 2016;365:315-322.
27. Centers for Disease Control and Prevention. Update: interim guidance for prevention of sexual transmission of Zika virus—United States, 2016. *MMWR Morb Mortal Wkly Rep.* 2016;365:323-325.
28. Musso D, Nhan T, Robin E, et al. Potential for Zika virus transmission through blood transfusion demonstrated during an outbreak in French Polynesia, November 2013 to February 2014. *Euro Surveill.* 2014;19. pii:20761.
29. Heymann DL, Chen L, Takemi K, et al. Global health security: the wider lessons from the west African Ebola virus disease epidemic. *Lancet.* 2015;385:1884-1901.

Clinical Management of Ebola Virus Disease in the United States and Europe

Uyeki TM, for the Working Group of the U.S.–European Clinical Network on Clinical Management of Ebola Virus Disease Patients in the U.S. and Europe (Ctrs for Disease Control and Prevention, Atlanta, GA; et al)

N Engl J Med 374:636-646, 2016

Background.—Available data on the characteristics of patients with Ebola virus disease (EVD) and clinical management of EVD in settings outside West Africa, as well as the complications observed in those patients, are limited.

Methods.—We reviewed available clinical, laboratory, and virologic data from all patients with laboratory-confirmed Ebola virus infection who received care in U.S. and European hospitals from August 2014 through December 2015.

Results.—A total of 27 patients (median age, 36 years [range, 25 to 75]) with EVD received care; 19 patients (70%) were male, 9 of 26 patients (35%) had coexisting conditions, and 22 (81%) were health care personnel. Of the 27 patients, 24 (89%) were medically evacuated from West Africa or were exposed to and infected with Ebola virus in West Africa and had onset of illness and laboratory confirmation of Ebola virus infection in Europe or the United States, and 3 (11%) acquired EVD in the United States or Europe. At the onset of illness, the most common signs and symptoms were fatigue (20 patients [80%]) and fever or feverishness (17 patients [68%]). During the clinical course, the predominant findings included diarrhea, hypoalbuminemia, hyponatremia, hypokalemia, hypocalcemia, and hypomagnesemia; 14 patients (52%) had hypoxemia, and 9

(33%) had oliguria, of whom 5 had anuria. Aminotransferase levels peaked at a median of 9 days after the onset of illness. Nearly all the patients received intravenous fluids and electrolyte supplementation; 9 (33%) received noninvasive or invasive mechanical ventilation; 5 (19%) received continuous renal-replacement therapy; 22 (81%) received empirical antibiotics; and 23 (85%) received investigational therapies (19 [70%] received at least two experimental interventions). Ebola viral RNA levels in blood peaked at a median of 7 days after the onset of illness, and the median time from the onset of symptoms to clearance of viremia was 17.5 days. A total of 5 patients died, including 3 who had respiratory and renal failure, for a mortality of 18.5%.

Conclusions.—Among the patients with EVD who were cared for in the United States or Europe, close monitoring and aggressive supportive care that included intravenous fluid hydration, correction of electrolyte abnormalities, nutritional support, and critical care management for respiratory and renal failure were needed; 81.5% of these patients who received this care survived.

▶ The emergence of the largest Ebola virus disease (EVD) outbreak in global history in West Africa in 2014 and subsequent secondary cases in the United States and other developed countries was unprecedented. Before this summary, the World Health Organization (WHO) reported an average case fatality rate (CFR) of 50%, and the range of reported mortality rates for EVD varied from 25% to 90% in prior outbreaks. However, all previously published data were largely in resource-limited settings.

Uyeki et al summarize the experience of 27 patients cared for in 15 hospitals across the United States and 8 European countries during the recent West African outbreak. The report is the first to summarize and highlight the substantially lower mortality rate of 18.5% in these settings. The authors' summary of the clinical data for these patients notes that aggressive intravenous fluid hydration and electrolyte management may improve outcomes and be the major contributor to these lower fatality rates.

Of note, all 27 patients were adults with an age range of 25 to 75, and consistent with other Ebola literature, all deaths were in patients older than 42 years. In contrast, a March 2015 *New England Journal of Medicine* correspondence summarized pediatric Ebola cases from the West Africa outbreak and reported a high CFR of 80-90% in children less than 5 years old, and the lowest age group mortality rate across all ages of 52% in 10- to 15-year-olds.[1]

Other key clinical findings noted in this article include associations of clinical signs with mortality. Longer duration from onset of illness to hospitalization, increased creatinine and bilirubin, and higher EVD RNA viral levels were all seen among those who died compared with survivors. The median duration of viremia was 17.5 days. Authors also noted that while historically EVD has not typically been reported to have a significant respiratory component, almost one-third of patients had respiratory symptoms such as cough or dyspnea on presentation. The article also summarizes the various experimental drugs and combinations used to treat Ebola patients in the United States and

Europe but also notes that determining which of the treatments are effective or most effective is extremely difficult to assess with small numbers and no established protocols.

As a public health official who has been working with US hospitals and providers to prepare for the unusual but potential case of EVD or other viral hemorrhagic fever diseases presenting here, this commentary also brings the opportunity to increase awareness of clinicians preparing to care for EVD patients with a few additional key points. In addition to the paramount importance of appropriate infection control equipment and practices, planning for EVD care should include the logistics and equipment to provide continuous renal-replacement therapy for an EVD patient and consider what other imaging, diagnostic, and large equipment can be provided within an Ebola treatment room and how it would be cleaned and decontaminated later.

Another challenging issue is providing point-of-care testing in the patient's room for priority laboratory data needed to care for the patient. This includes complete blood counts (CBCs), coagulation tests, and other important assessment tests that are not typical point-of-care tests in the hospital setting. This facet of EVD response requires extensive preparation and coordination with clinical and public health laboratories. Hospitals planning for EVD care should also involve ethicists early on in a patient's course to discuss decisions and criteria for resuscitation in advance to balance provider safety and the likelihood of improving patient outcome.

While understanding clinical presentation and likely progression, including potential mortality, predictors are important for EVD care, this article does not address the crucial importance of prevention measures while caring for isolated EVD patients. This includes availability of appropriate personal protective equipment and staff training for donning and doffing the equipment safely, as well as any of the social factors and measures to contain and prevent additional cases, such as contact monitoring (including health care providers) and contact tracing. Although for adult EVD care, it is clear that no visitors or family members should be in the patient's room, pediatric care planning should work with hospital administration, pediatric health care providers, and public health to coordinate and establish protocols regarding potential benefits versus risks of certain children having an informed parent or guardian in the room with the child with appropriate personal protective equipment and training.

This summary of EVD patients in well-developed countries is encouraging with a lower mortality rate than noted in West Africa and prior studies, but it cannot be generalized to pediatric patients. It is unknown if and how much pediatric mortality rate may be decreased with aggressive care in the United States or other countries with well-resourced health care settings. The article provides an excellent summary of clinical findings and potential mortality associations, but the small total number of cases and deaths was underpowered to detect statistically significant differences between survivors and those that died. In addition, most of these cases were health care workers or others healthy enough to travel to West Africa. It would be interesting to assess whether these individuals had any comorbidities and any contribution of comorbidities to mortality rates among the several thousand cases and deaths among the larger population affected by this Ebola outbreak in West Africa.

Ebola is an extremely difficult infectious disease to manage both at the individual care level as well as from a public health perspective of measures to prevent of secondary cases. Although aggressive fluid and electrolyte management likely do improve outcomes, additional studies and data need to be collected to understand the best treatment regimens, and, as with other infectious diseases, vaccine development is really what we need to respond to this significant infectious disease with high morbidity and mortality.

E. Pan, MD, MPH, FAAP

Reference

1. WHO Ebola Response Team, Agua-Agum J, Ariyarajah A, Blake IM, et al. Ebola virus disease among children in West Africa. *N Engl J Med.* 2015;372:1274-1277.

Dexamethasone Therapy for Septic Arthritis in Children
Fogel I, Amir J, Bar-On E, et al (Tel Aviv Univ, Israel)
Pediatrics 136:e776-e782, 2015

Background and Objective.—Prospective studies of children with septic arthritis report that adding dexamethasone to antibiotic therapy contributes significantly to clinical and laboratory improvement. This study sought to evaluate the effect of this regimen outside of a randomized controlled trial.

Methods.—The sample consisted of children with septic arthritis hospitalized at a tertiary pediatric medical center in 2008 to 2013. Disease course and outcome were compared between children treated with antibiotics alone or with adjuvant dexamethasone, according to the admitting department policy.

Results.—The cohort included 116 patients, 90 treated with antibiotics alone and 26 treated with antibiotics+dexamethasone. The groups were similar for age, symptom duration before hospitalization, body temperature, acute-phase reactant levels, and rate of positive fluid cultures (21.6% total). Compared with monotherapy, antibiotics+dexamethasone treatment was associated with a shorter duration of fever (mean 2.3 vs 3.9 days, $P = .002$), more rapid clinical improvement (mean 6.3 vs 10.0 days to no pain/limitation, $P < .001$), more rapid decrease in C-reactive protein level to <1 mg/dL (mean 5.3 vs 8.4 days, $P = .002$), shorter duration of parenteral antibiotic treatment (mean 7.1 vs 11.4 days, $P < .001$), and shorter hospital stay (mean 8.0 vs 10.7 days, $P = .004$). Recurrent symptoms of fever and joint pain occurred in 4 patients in the antibiotics+dexamethasone group after completion of the steroid course.

Conclusions.—Children with septic arthritis treated early with a short course of adjuvant dexamethasone show earlier improvement in clinical and laboratory parameters than children treated with antibiotics alone.

▶ Septic arthritis, also referred to as acute bacterial arthritis (ABA), is a relatively common occurrence in children, with an annual incidence between 4 and 10 per

100 000 children. Although there is some overlap in presentation and pathogens, acute bacterial osteomyelitis (ABO) occurs somewhat more frequently. Between 15% and 50% of osteoarticular infections involve both the joint and adjacent bone. Initially, ABA or ABO was treated with 4- to 6-week intravenous (IV) courses of antibiotics. Very good data from North America and Europe now support early transition from IV to oral therapy for children who have good clinical recovery, are afebrile and have a significant drop in C-reactive protein (CRP). Ultra-short treatment courses, some as short as 10 days for ABA, have been studied with success in very low-risk patients in Europe. The use of corticosteroids for ABA has now become a point of discussion as well.

There is precedence for the use of corticosteroids for acute bacterial infections. Early initiation of dexamethasone for children with *Haemophilus* influenza meningitis reduces hearing loss, and survival of pneumococcal meningitis is improved with corticosteroids. These outcomes are predicated on giving the dexamethasone before or within hours of the first antibiotic dose. Somewhat less well-founded uses of corticosteroids for acute bacterial infections include pharyngitis and deep neck infections.

The classic premise of the use of corticosteroids for meningitis is that the immune system damages the brain and blunting the immune response early in treatment limits the damage and leads to fewer sequelae. A commonly noted clinical consequence is ablation of fever and decreasing inflammatory markers, which could mask the clinical signs of a worsening disease process. Even for short-term use of corticosteroids, there is also the concern for the side-effect profile, which includes increasing the risk for gastric ulcers in critically ill patients, decreasing antibiotic penetration into the affected site, and delaying the diagnosis of an uncommon presentation of leukemia.

At the intersection of the risks and benefits of steroids for acute bacterial infections are 2 previously published prospective, randomized studies and a recent article in *Pediatrics* that retrospectively reported the clinical outcomes of 116 patients who presented to the hospital with ABA, 26 of whom were treated with antibiotics and steroids. The recent *Pediatrics* article by Fogel and colleagues describes faster resolution of fever, fewer IV days, and fewer hospital days in the antibiotic plus steroid group. Patients were followed for no less than 9 months (average of 53 months) and no side effects from steroids or sequelae of the infections were noted. The conclusion was that steroids are a safe adjunct to antibiotic therapy for uncomplicated ABA. The authors note the significant methodologic gaps, which include the retrospective design, potential selection bias, and the low rate of positive cultures.

Is it time to start adding a 4-day course of dexamethasone to our ABA order sets? If so, why were only 26 of the 116 patients treated with steroids? A more detailed look at surgical practices and pathogen distribution and a discussion of risks and benefits is needed.

First, there is clearly a trend toward less invasive treatment of ABA, especially outside North America. The study group led by Peltola and colleagues published a series of articles on a randomized trial of different durations of antibiotics for ABO or ABA, and the ABA arms often included a simple needle aspiration. In this *Pediatrics* article, Fogel et al present a series of 116 patients in whom only a needle aspiration was done in most cases. Furthermore, magnetic resonance imaging was not part of the routine evaluation, so the true rate of coinfected bone is not known. One of the main concerns with the use of steroids is that it could mask the symptoms and signs associated with a clinical treatment failure, and both nonsurgical therapy and the potential to miss a concomitant osteomyelitis may increase that risk. Although the 26 patients in this report did not suffer any adverse consequence or treatment failure from the use of steroids, this is a small number on which to draw such a conclusion. Many clinicians are uncomfortable with nonsurgical treatment of ABA, and the concept of both treating nonsurgically and obscuring the objective data from which clinical failure can be presumed may make physicians more reticent.

Another potential issue is the generalizability of the results. In the very well-designed Peltola series, the now rare *H influenza* was the pathogen in 17% of the patients, and there were no cases of methicillin-resistant *Staphylococcus aureus* (MRSA). In the *Pediatrics* article, there was a predominance of *Kingella kingae*, followed by methicillin-sensitive *Staphylococcus aureus* (MSSA), with no MRSA. Because of its fastidious nature, *K kingae* is probably underdiagnosed North America although there is no doubt that MRSA is a major cause of ABA and ABO, accounting for 25% or more of invasive *S aureus* infections in some areas of the United States. Multiple studies suggest that MRSA infections have more complications and longer treatment durations.

Finally, we are back to the benefits derived from dexamethasone adjunctive therapy for ABA. The data available unanimously support fewer days of symptoms and fewer IV antibiotic days. However, all patients with ABO plus ABA were in the nondexamethasone group, as were a higher percentage of the patients who had irrigation and debridement of the hip. Combined ABA plus ABO are known to have more severe presentations and a higher percent of open hip surgery could also suggest a more severe population. The average IV antibiotic duration of 11.4 days in the antibiotics only group seems somewhat long for an uncomplicated ABA, which raises the question of the benefit attributable to dexamethasone. Additionally, the vast majority of the ABA treated with dexamethasone occurred in the knee with only 20% being hip infections.

There is strong evidence that combined dexamethasone and antibiotics improves symptoms faster and is associated with shorter IV antibiotic courses for ABA. This article raises practical considerations of adding dexamethasone to our treatment of ABA. In young children (average age of 2 years) with knee ABA without ABO, most likely to be caused by *K kingae*, the treatment was effective with no sequelae. Whether this can be applied more broadly to other anatomic locations, combined ABO plus ABA, and for those at risk for MRSA, remains a question, as does the unasked question of whether there might actually be lower rates of rare complications, such as permanent joint damage, with the use of steroids as we have seen with meningitis.

J. C. Arnold, MD

Outbreaks of Invasive *Kingella kingae* Infections in Closed Communities

Yagupsky P, Ben-Ami Y, Trefler R, et al (Soroka Univ Med Ctr, Beer-Sheva, Israel; Israel Defense Forces Med Corps)

J Pediatr 169:135-139, 2016

Objectives.—To describe the results of the epidemiologic investigation of outbreaks of invasive *Kingella kingae* infections among attendees at daycare facilities located in 4 closed communities in Israel.

Study Design.—The preschool-aged population of communities with clusters of *Kingella* cases had oropharyngeal cultures performed. *K kingae* isolates from infected patients and healthy contacts were genotyped by pulsed field gel electrophoresis to determine the spread of outbreak strains.

Results.—The affected closed communities (3 military bases and 1 "kibbutz" commune) were characterized by tight social and family networks and intensive mingling. The outbreaks affected 9 of 51 attendees (attack rate: 17.6%) age 8-19 months (median: 12 months), within a 21-day period. Cases included skeletal system infections (n = 8) and bacteremia (n = 1); *K kingae* isolates were confirmed by the use of blood culture vials and selective media. Clinical presentation was mild and acute-phase reactants were usually normal or only moderately elevated. Thirty out of 55 (54.5%) asymptomatic children carried the outbreak strains. Analysis of the 3 clusters in which the entire preschool-aged population was cultured revealed that 31 of 71 (43.7%) children younger than 24 months of age were colonized with *K kingae* organisms compared with 8 of 105 (7.6%) older children (*P* < .001).

Conclusions.—Clusters of invasive *K kingae* infections characterized by sudden onset, high attack rate, and wide dissemination of the outbreak strain can occur in daycare facilities and closed communities. Because the mild clinical presentation of invasive *K kingae* infections and the fastidious nature of the organism, a high index of suspicion and use of sensitive detection methods are recommended (Table 2).

▶ *Kingella kingae* is a gram-negative coccobacillus that belongs to the Neisseriaceae family and is recognized increasingly as an important etiology of septic arthritis, osteomyelitis, intervertebral diskitis, and occult bacteremia in young children, generally between 6 months and 3 years of age. The increased incidence of *K kingae* disease is a consequence of enhanced culture techniques and application of polymerase chain reaction (PCR) assays for analysis of joint fluid and bone aspirates, reflecting the fact that *K kingae* is a fastidious organism and is often refractory to standard culture techniques, similar to other members of the Neisseriaceae family. Like other invasive bacterial pathogens in children (such as *Neisseria meningitidis* and *Haemophilus influenzae* type b), *K kingae* appears to be transmitted efficiently from person to person among young children, resulting in occasional clusters of *K kingae* invasive disease among children in daycare centers.

The report by Yagupsky and colleagues draws additional attention to the risk of outbreaks of *K kingae* disease in daycare facilities and highlights the increased risk

TABLE 2.—Case Categories and clinical presentation of children involved in clusters of invasive *K kingae* infections in closed communities

Day-Care Center Location	Proven (n)	Highly Presumptive (n)	Presumptive (n)	Age Range (mo)	Cases features			
					Osteomyelitis (n)	Arthritis (n)	Spondylodiscitis (n)	Bacteremia (n)
2005 Military base A	1	0	2	8-12	3	0	0	0
2014 Military base B	0	0	2	11-14	0	1	0	0
2014 Military base C	0	2	0	17-19	0	1	1	0
2014 Kibbutz	1	1	0	8-16	0	1	0	1
Total	2	3	4	8-19	3	4	1	1

Reprinted from Yagupsky P, Ben-Ami Y, Trefler R, et al. Outbreaks of invasive *Kingella kingae* infections in closed communities. *J Pediatr.* 2016;169:135-139, with permission from Elsevier.

in closed communities. The affected communities included 3 military bases and 1 kibbutz commune in Israel and were characterized by tight social and family networks and intensive mingling of members of the communities. As a consequence of the close and intensive contact, oropharyngeal colonization with *K kingae* was approximately 40% and the attack rate of *K kingae* invasive disease was nearly 20% among attendees at the involved daycare facilities. This publication also highlights the fact that the clinical presentation with *K kingae* disease is often mild, with no fever and with normal or only modestly elevated acute phase reactants. Consistent with other reports, one outbreak was preceded by an outbreak in the facility of a nonspecific viral upper respiratory infection, and another was preceded by an outbreak in the daycare center of hand-foot-and-mouth disease.

Although this report describes critical observations regarding *K kingae* invasive disease associated with daycare facilities, it is important to appreciate several caveats. In particular, the authors did not compare the 4 outbreaks in closed communities with outbreaks in open communities, precluding conclusions about the relative risk of outbreaks in closed versus open communities. In addition, among the 9 cases in the 4 daycare centers, only 5 cases were proven (based on positive cultures of normally sterile body fluids) or highly presumptive (based on a compatible clinical picture such as a joint, bone, or intervertebral disk infection and a positive oropharyngeal culture or PCR result). The remaining 4 cases were only presumptive (based on a compatible clinical picture such as a joint, bone, or intervertebral disk infection plus occurrence of another case in the same center within a 1-month period), raising the possibility that the attack rate was lower than calculated (Table 2).

This publication underscores that clinicians should have a high index of suspicion for *K kingae* invasive disease in children attending a daycare facility with an index case, regardless of whether the daycare center exists in a closed community. Suspicion should be high even if fever is lacking and laboratory evaluation is normal or only moderately abnormal, especially if presentation is preceded by a viral respiratory infection or oral infection. It is likely that *K kingae* invasive disease will be diagnosed more often if PCR assays for *K kingae* are used routinely for analysis of joint fluid and bone aspirates in clinical microbiology laboratories.

J. W. St. Geme III, MD

Lack of Accuracy of Body Temperature for Detecting Serious Bacterial Infection in Febrile Episodes
De S, Williams GJ, Teixeira-Pinto A, et al (The Univ of Sydney, Australia; et al)
Pediatr Infect Dis J 34:940-944, 2015

Background.—Body temperature is a time-honored marker of serious bacterial infection, but there are few studies of its test performance. The aim of our study was to determine the accuracy of temperature measured on presentation to medical care for detecting serious bacterial infection.

Methods.—Febrile children 0–5 years of age presenting to the emergency department of a tertiary care pediatric hospital were sampled consecutively. The accuracy of the axillary temperature measured at presentation was evaluated using logistic regression models to generate receiver operating characteristic curves. Reference standard tests for serious bacterial infection were standard microbiologic/radiologic tests and clinical follow-up. Age, clinicians' impression of appearance of the child (well versus unwell) and duration of illness were assessed as possible effect modifiers.

Results.—Of 15,781 illness episodes 1120 (7.1%) had serious bacterial infection. The area under the receiver operating characteristic curve for temperature was 0.60 [95% confidence intervals (CI): 0.58–0.62]. A threshold of $\geq$38°C had a sensitivity of 0.67 (95% CI: 0.64–0.70), specificity of 0.45 (95% CI: 0.44–0.46), positive likelihood ratio of 1.2 (95% CI: 1.2–1.3) and negative likelihood ratio of 0.7 (95% CI: 0.7–0.8). Age and illness duration had a small but significant effect on the accuracy of temperature increasing its "rule-in" potential.

Conclusion.—Measured temperature at presentation to hospital is not an accurate marker of serious bacterial infection in febrile children. Younger age and longer duration of illness increase the rule-in potential of temperature but without substantial overall change in its test accuracy.

▶ The evaluation and management of fever in infants and young children has been a source of consternation for pediatricians and parents alike for many decades. Clinical investigators have invested a great deal of time and energy pursuing methods of identifying clinical or laboratory markers that might identify those with fever who either are at higher risk or at lower risk of having treatable causes of illness.

Along the way, much has been learned about the relationship of fever to etiology of illness. Certain groups of children, such as those in the first months of life or those otherwise immunocompromised, have been proven to be at higher risk of having bacterial illnesses associated with fever than their older otherwise normal counterparts. Well appearance in younger infants has been shown to not eliminate the possibility of serious bacterial infection as the cause of fever. Two-thirds of young febrile infants with associated bacterial infection appear well to clinicians. Likewise, presence of documented viral illness in young infants and toddlers has not been shown to eliminate the possibility of concurrent infection with bacteria. Approximately 6% to 7% of febrile infants and a smaller percentage toddlers with test-positive viral illnesses have concurrent test-positive bacterial infection.

During the past several decades, there has also been an international trend toward less invasive means of evaluation and management of illnesses. Novel devices that measure different surface temperatures as a surrogate for core temperature have been developed and marketed. These newer methods of measurement of fever have been investigated many times and compared with more traditional methods of measurement of body temperature, such as rectal thermometry.

These investigations have yielded a range of results and conclusions. Yet none have conclusively demonstrated that any surface temperature measurements are as reliable or accurate as rectal temperature measurement with regard to estimating core body temperature. Among the less reliable means of measurement of body temperature is axillary thermometry. Even less reliable is empirical (qualitative, nonmeasured) assessment reported by family members. These 2 parameters form the basis of the methodology of this study.

In this article, the authors ask a reasonable primary question: is elevated body temperature at presentation to the hospital an accurate clinical marker of serious bacterial infection? They also consider secondary factors, including the influence of duration of fever and age of subject. The study sample size is encouragingly large (n = 15 702), representing nearly 80% of those eligible for enrollment. The age range of those enrolled is also large (0—5 years), which serves as somewhat of a confounder. Prior studies have shown that youngest febrile infants are at substantially higher risk of having associated serious bacterial infection than older infants, toddlers and preschool-age children. Extent of laboratory or radiological investigation of cause of fever was not prescribed by the investigators. Only 22% to 23% of study subjects had assessment of blood or urine for presence of bacteria. Approximately 7% of study subjects were lost to follow-up, thereby eliminating any follow-up means of verification of outcome of febrile illness. Nearly two-thirds of enrolled subjects had received antipyretic medication before enrollment, possibly altering the results of measurement of body temperature. One of every 6 patents enrolled had received antibiotics before presentation, thereby contaminating any body fluid culture results. Family members proved to be unreliable (inconsistent) when answering a simple question regarding magnitude of body temperature measured at home.

Despite these methodological issues, the data reinforce some findings published by others. Most importantly, different types of associated infections were not distinguished by lower range body temperatures, higher range body temperatures, or maximum magnitude of reported body temperatures. Although children with higher range temperatures of longer duration (> 39 degrees, > 96 hours) were more likely to have (discovered) associated bacterial infections than children with similar temperatures of lesser duration (< 25 hours), the type of and extent of testing was not uniform for all subjects.

The authors' conclusions are just. Body temperature is an inaccurate marker of serious bacterial infection in children who present to the hospital with fever. Low or high magnitude of body temperature does not rule in or rule out presence of bacterial disease. Other clinical parameters, such as age and duration of fever, should be considered when evaluating fever in young children. It is important also to consider that not all means of assessment or measurement of body temperature are equally reliable, and that empirical impressions of elevated body temperature are no more than guesses.

M. Douglas Baker, MD

Efavirenz-Based Antiretroviral Therapy Among Nevirapine-Exposed HIV-Infected Children in South Africa: A Randomized Clinical Trial
Coovadia A, Abrams EJ, Strehlau R, et al (Univ of the Witwatersrand, Johannesburg, South Africa; Columbia Univ. NY; et al)
JAMA 314:1808-1817, 2015

Importance.—Advantages of using efavirenz as part of treatment for children infected with human immunodeficiency virus (HIV) include once-daily dosing, simplification of co-treatment for tuberculosis, preservation of ritonavir-boosted lopinavir for second-line treatment, and harmonization of adult and pediatric treatment regimens. However, there have been concerns about possible reduced viral efficacy of efavirenz in children exposed to nevirapine for prevention of mother-to-child transmission.

Objective.—To evaluate whether nevirapine-exposed children achieving initial viral suppression with ritonavir-boosted lopinavir—based therapy can transition to efavirenz-based therapy without risk of viral failure.

Design, Setting, and Participants.—Randomized, open-label noninferiority trial conducted at Rahima Moosa Mother and Child Hospital, Johannesburg, South Africa, from June 2010 to December 2013, enrolling 300 HIV-infected children exposed to nevirapine for prevention of mother-to-child transmission who were aged 3 years or older and had plasma HIV RNA of less than 50 copies/mL during ritonavir-boosted lopinavir—based therapy; 298 were randomized and 292 (98%) were followed up to 48 weeks after randomization.

Interventions.—Participants were randomly assigned to switch to efavirenz-based therapy (n = 150) or continue ritonavir-boosted lopinavir—based therapy (n = 148).

Main Outcomes and Measures.—Risk difference between groups in (1) viral rebound (ie, $\geq$1 HIV RNA measurement of >50 copies/mL) and (2) viral failure (ie, confirmed HIV RNA >1000 copies/mL) with a noninferiority bound of −0.10. Immunologic and clinical responses were secondary end points.

Results.—The Kaplan-Meier probability of viral rebound by 48 weeks was 0.176 (n = 26) in the efavirenz group and 0.284 (n = 42) in the ritonavir-boosted lopinavir group. Probabilities of viral failure were 0.027 (n = 4) in the efavirenz group and 0.020 (n = 3) in the ritonavir-boosted lopinavir group. The risk difference for viral rebound was 0.107 (1-sided 95% CI, 0.028 to ∞) and for viral failure was −0.007 (1-sided 95% CI, −0.036 to ∞). We rejected the null hypothesis that efavirenz is inferior to ritonavir-boosted lopinavir ($P < .001$) for both end points. By 48 weeks, CD4 cell percentage was 2.88% (95% CI, 1.26%-4.49%) higher in the efavirenz group than in the ritonavir-boosted lopinavir group.

Conclusions and Relevance.—Among HIV-infected children exposed to nevirapine for prevention of mother-to-child transmission and with initial viral suppression with ritonavir-boosted lopinavir—based therapy, switching to efavirenz-based therapy compared with continuing ritonavir-boosted lopinavir—based therapy did not result in significantly higher rates of viral rebound or viral failure. This therapeutic approach may offer advantages in children such as these.

Trial Registration.—clinicaltrials.gov Identifier: NCT01146873.

▶ On a global scale, treating infants and young children diagnosed with human immunodeficiency virus (HIV) has been logistically more problematic than treating adults. Infants require special drug formulations, which may require refrigeration and have poor palatability. They are a relative minority compared with the worldwide population of people living with HIV, and stock outs of medications are a greater issue. As a result, of the estimated 2.6 million children under age 15 years living with HIV in 2014, only 32% had access to antiretroviral therapy. Although this situation is better than it was in 2010, when only 14% had access, it means that more than two-thirds of children in need of antiretroviral therapy cannot obtain it.[1]

Adults and adolescents newly diagnosed with HIV now have single tablet, highly effective, once daily options for treatment. The World Health Organization (WHO) has harmonized first-line treatment for all infected patients aged 3 years and older with tenofovir/emtricitabine or lamivudine, and efavirenz.[2] Formulations have been created that allow for dispersability in liquid, so that scored adult tablets can be given to younger patients, thus decreasing stock-out issues by allowing a single set of drugs in several tablet strengths to be purchased. However, a once-daily regimen for our youngest patients remains elusive.

Efavirenz concentrations in those younger than 3 years of age remain highly variable and will probably require therapeutic drug monitoring to be effective. This monitoring is unlikely to be widely available even in the United States and Europe. Currently, the most readily available potential combination in the youngest patients for once-daily use would be abacavir/emtricitabine or lamivudine, and extended release nevirapine.

There are several major issues with this approach. First, trial data indicate that for children diagnosed under age 3 years, a lopinavir/ritonavir-based regimen is preferred at least initially. Second, nevirapine is still used in many areas to prevent perinatal and breastfeeding transmission, potentially making it a less attractive treatment option. Third, HIV plasma RNA monitoring should be available if a non—nucleoside-exposed infant is switched to a non—nucleoside-based treatment after suppression with lopinavir/ritonavir because the potential for virologic failure may be greater. Finally, extended release nevirapine has not been adequately studied in this population.

Enter the paper by Coovadia et al.[3] This group previously studied the use of nevirapine in children who were exposed to single-dose nevirapine for prophylaxis after they were fully suppressed on a lopinavir/ritonavir regimen.[3] The NEVEREST study led to the WHO recommendation of nevirapine as a consideration after viral suppression with lopinavir/ritonavir as long as plasma RNA monitoring could be performed, thus potentially resolving points 1 and 2 above. However, points 3 and 4 remain. Now the same group has performed a similar study with efavirenz. Efavirenz remains an attractive treatment option because it would allow once-daily dosing, it can be used in children receiving therapy for active tuberculosis, it would preserve lopinavir/ritonavir for later use, and it would harmonize with the WHO guidelines as they currently stand. Again, children—all older than 3 years, all exposed to nevirapine to try to prevent perinatal transmission, and all virologically suppressed—were randomized either to continue lopinavir/ritonavir or switch to efavirenz-based therapy. The investigators found efavirenz to be noninferior to lopinavir/ritonavir through 48 weeks of study, indicating that children exposed to nevirapine in infancy could be placed on a standard WHO regimen at 3 years of age.

This option would have great advantages to national HIV treatment programs. In addition, it creates an opportunity for younger children already exposed to antiretroviral therapy to receive a simplified, once-daily treatment regimen. Nevirapine resistance did not appear to affect the efficacy of efavirenz. Most infants receiving single-dose nevirapine develop the Y181C mutation by population sequencing that confers high-level resistance to nevirapine.[4] However, this mutation only confers a 2-fold resistance to efavirenz. In this study, efavirenz mutations that developed during virologic failure were all K103N mutations, which led to high-level resistance to efavirenz.[5] Archived nevirapine resistance did not appear to play an active role in virologic failure.

Unfortunately, this study could not address once-daily treatment in children younger than 3 years for the pharmacokinetic reasons described earlier. This issue may have to wait for alternative medications with appropriate pharmacokinetic parameters in younger children or possibly for studies of extended release nevirapine in these age groups. However, this study remains a major advance in our ability to treat children globally that have already been exposed to and failed nonnucleoside prophylaxis.

M. D. Foca, MD

References

1. http://www.unaids.org/sites/default/files/media_asset/FactSheet_Children_en.pdf.
2. http://www.who.int/hiv/pub/guidelines/arv2013/art/whatregimentostart/en/.
3. Coovadia A, Abrams EJ, Strehlau R, et al. Reuse of nevirapine in exposed HIV-infected children after protease inhibitor-based viral suppression: a randomized controlled trial. *JAMA*. 2010;304:1082-1090.
4. Eshleman SH, Mracna M, Guay LA, Deseyve M, Cunningham S, Mirochnick M, et al. Selection and fading of resistance mutations in women and infants receiving nevirapine to prevent HIV-1 vertical transmission (HIVNET 012). *AIDS*. 2001;15: 1951-1957.
5. http://hivdb.stanford.edu/DR/NNRTIResiNote.html.

16 Musculoskeletal

Primary Care Physician Follow-up of Distal Radius Buckle Fractures

Koelink E, Schuh S, Howard A, et al (McMaster Univ Med Centre and McMaster Univ, Hamilton, Ontario, Canada; The Hosp for Sick Children and Univ of Toronto, Ontario, Canada)
Pediatrics 137:e20152262, 2016

Objectives.—Our main objective was to determine the proportion of children referred abstract to a primary care provider (PCP) for follow-up of a distal radius buckle fracture who subsequently did not deviate from this reassessment strategy.

Methods.—This prospective cohort study was conducted at a tertiary care pediatric emergency department (ED). Eligible children were aged 2 to 17 years with a distal radius buckle fracture treated with a removable splint and referred to the PCP for reassessment. We telephoned families 28 days after their ED visit. The primary outcome was the proportion who received PCP follow-up exclusively. We also measured the proportion who received PCP anticipatory guidance and those children who reported returning to usual activities "always" by 4 weeks.

Results.—We enrolled 200 children, and 180 (90.0%) received telephone follow-up. Of these, 157 (87.2% [95% confidence interval: 82.3 to 92.1]) received PCP follow-up exclusively. Specifically, 11 (6.1%) families opted out of physician follow-up, 5 (2.8%) self-referred to an ED, and the PCP requested specialty consultation in 7 (3.9%) cases. Of the 164 with a PCP visit, 77 (47.0%) parents received anticipatory guidance on return to activities for their child, and 162 (98.8%) reported return to usual activities within 4 weeks.

Conclusions.—The vast majority of children with distal radius buckle fractures presented to the PCP for follow-up and did not receive additional orthopedic surgeon or ED consultations. Despite a suboptimal rate of PCP advice on return to activities, almost all parents reported full return to usual activities within 4 weeks.

▶ Buckle fractures of the distal radius in children are minor, stable, nonangulated, compression injuries of the metaphyseal area of the bone. Buckle fractures do not displace and do not involve the growth plate. In a sense, buckle fractures of the distal radius are "boo-boo" injuries. Treatment of a buckle fracture is a brief, 3-week period of immobilization for comfort.

The outcome of treating a buckle fracture of the distal radius is the excellent and equivalent whether treated in a traditional manner with a cast by an orthopedic surgeon including a follow-up visit for cast removal and a follow-up radiograph, treated by a pediatrician with a removable splint and follow-up with a pediatrician for anticipatory guidance on splint use and return to activities instructions, or treated in the emergency department with a removable splint and splint removal at about 3 weeks with no physician follow-up.[1,2]

Noted Harvard health economist Michael Porter[3] has written that
Value = Outcomes/Cost.

In the case of a buckle fracture of the distal radius, outcomes are equivalent with pediatric care without additional orthopedic consultation, therefore, cost is reduced and value is increased. Follow-up radiographs do not alter treatment for buckle fractures. Minimalistic, but appropriate, treatment of buckle fractures of the distal radius in children by pediatricians will potentially save millions of health care dollars annually. Additional potential advantage of splint treatment and follow-up by the pediatrician include less anxiety and skin burn risk associated with use of the cast saw. A removable splint offers a safe and cost-effective alternative to traditional casting for buckle fractures of the distal radius in children.

This elegant study by Boutis and colleagues simplifies treatment and lowers cost of a common musculoskeletal injury in children.

W. Hennrikus, MD

References

1. Plint A, Perry J, Correll R, Gaboury I, Lawton L. A randomized, controlled trial of removable splitting versus casting for wrist buckle fractures in children. *Pediatrics*. 2006;117:691-697.
2. West S, Andrews J, Bebbington A, Ennis O, Alderman P. Buckle fractures of the distal radius are safely treated in a soft bandage: a randomized prospective trial of bandage versus plaster cast. *J Pediatr Orthop*. 2005;25:322-325.
3. Porter M. What is value in health care? *N Engl J Med*. 2010;363:2477-2481.

Celiac Disease Does Not Influence Fracture Risk in Young Patients with Type 1 Diabetes
Reilly NR, Lebwohl B, Mollazadegan K, et al (Columbia Univ Med Ctr, NY; Karolinska Institutet, Stockholm, Sweden; et al)
J Pediatr 169:49-54, 2016

Objectives.—To examine the risk of any fractures in patients with both type 1 diabetes (T1D) and celiac disease (CD) vs patients with T1D only.

Study Design.—We performed a population-based cohort study. We defined T1D as individuals aged ≤30 years who had a diagnosis of diabetes recorded in the Swedish National Patient Register between 1964 and 2009. Individuals with CD were identified through biopsy report data between 1969 and 2008 from any of Sweden's 28 pathology departments. Some 958 individuals had both T1D and CD and were matched for sex, age, and calendar period with 4598 reference individuals with T1D only. We then used a stratified Cox regression analysis, where CD was modeled as a time-dependent covariate, to estimate the risk of any fractures and osteoporotic fractures (hip, distal forearm, thoracic and lumbar spine, and proximal humerus) in patients with both T1D and CD compared with that in patients with T1D only.

Results.—During follow-up, 12 patients with T1D and CD had a fracture (1 osteoporotic fracture). CD did not influence the risk of any fracture (adjusted hazard ratio = 0.77; 95% CI = 0.42-1.41) or osteoporotic fractures (adjusted hazard ratio = 0.46; 95% CI = 0.06-3.51) in patients with T1D. Stratification for time since CD diagnosis did not affect risk estimates.

Conclusion.—Having a diagnosis of CD does not seem to influence fracture risk in young patients with T1D. Follow-up in this study was, however, too short to ascertain osteoporotic fractures which traditionally occur in old age.

▶ It is well known that persons with type 1 diabetes (T1D) have an increased risk for developing other autoimmune diseases, such as thyroid disease and celiac disease (CD). However, it is less commonly appreciated that persons with T1D are also at higher risk for low bone mineral density (BMD) and fracture. For persons with T1D diagnosed as children, reducing this risk begins in childhood with optimizing nutrition and physical activity.

The reasons for the osteopenia and osteoporosis observed in adults with T1D are incompletely understood and are likely multifactorial. Literature suggests an imbalance between bone formation and resorption.[1] While markers of calcium metabolism and bone turnover are generally normal, studies have shown lower serum phosphorus levels and insulin-like growth factor-1 (IGF-1) levels in persons with T1D compared with controls.[1] Advanced glycation end products may also accumulate in bone and make it brittle. Although it does not appear that T1D-related bone disease is directly related to glycemic control, some studies have demonstrated an association with other diabetic complications such as retinopathy, neuropathy, and nephropathy.

CD is an autoimmune disorder triggered by ingestion of gluten and results in an inflammatory enteropathy of the small intestine. Children with active CD have an increased risk of low bone density and fracture, likely because of vitamin and mineral malabsorption and chronic inflammation.[2] Numerous studies have shown that bone mineral density (BMD) measures improve fairly rapidly in patients with CD after treatment with a gluten-free diet. One such study found that children and adolescents with CD had complete recovery of BMD after 1 year of following the diet and that this was maintained over long-term follow-up.[3]

Given the known associations of both T1D and CD with osteopenia and fracture, Reilly and colleagues sought to determine whether persons with T1D and concomitant CD have a higher risk of fracture than patients with T1D alone. They used population-based T1D data from the Swedish National Patient Register along with nationwide histopathology data on CD. Because *International Classification of Disease* classification limitations, persons were classified as having T1D if diagnosed with diabetes by age 30 years. The researchers ultimately identified and analyzed data from 958 individuals with both T1D and CD along with 5 matched controls with T1D only per case.

Surprisingly, this study found that concomitant CD did not increase the risk of fractures in individuals with T1D (hazard ratio 0.77; 95% CI = 0.42–1.41). Of note, subjects were diagnosed with T1D at a median age of 9 years and CD at a median age of 12 years. They had follow-up data available for a median of 13 years (range 0–46). Duration of time with CD likewise did not affect fracture risk.

Although these results were unexpected given that both T1D and CD are independently associated with increased fracture risk compared with healthy populations, we can speculate on a number of reasons why the authors' hypothesis was not confirmed. The first is that the persons included in this study were diagnosed with T1D and CD at a young age. We know that childhood, particularly adolescence, is when the vast majority of bone mineral accrual occurs, and literature suggests that children who are diagnosed with CD at a younger age have better BMD recovery compared to older individuals. As such, the CD diagnosis in this study may have had a negligible impact on their ultimate fracture risk due to robust BMD recovery upon treatment with a gluten-free diet. The authors do not have data on adherence to this diet in their population but cite data from another chart review from their register that suggests adherence is likely overall quite good.

A second potential source of the unanticipated results in this study is that it seems that subjects with T1D in this population had routine screening for CD. Although the authors do not specifically give information on the screening rates or modalities used in their cohort, perhaps timely detection of CD through screening prevented the bone loss associated with long-standing enteropathy. A third reason for the negative results might be their length of follow-up. Median age at the end of the observation period was only 21 years, thus osteoporotic fractures occurring later in life are likely to have been missed.

Of note, this study also lacked BMD data. BMD measures would offer a more sensitive way to detect bone loss and/or failure to accrue bone than incident fractures. Of note, another study of teenagers with T1D diagnosed with CD after routine screening reported significantly decreased BMD z-scores in those children compared to teens with T1D and normal CD screens.[4] The authors might have found significantly lower BMD measures in subjects with both T1D and CD if that data were available. However, the clinical significance of such a finding in the setting of similar fracture rates is debatable.

This study has a number of limitations due to its use of a national registry, including lack of key information such as T1D glycemic control, compliance with gluten-free diet, calcium and vitamin D supplementation use, and laboratory markers of calcium metabolism and bone turnover. Also, it is a bit surprising that they only identified 17 fractures in their population of interest over a median follow-up period of 13 years. This fracture rate (~1.4 fractures per 1000 person-years) is much lower than that expected in a cohort followed through adolescence where much greater fracture rates are usually reported in healthy populations, with some studies reporting that 50% of all children will fracture at least one bone during childhood.[5] This calls into question the completeness of the fracture data ascertained by the register search, although it does not seem likely that this underreporting would differ between those with both T1D and CD and T1D alone.

Despite these limitations, this study contributes to the emerging recognition of bone disease as an additional long-term complication of T1D and highlights data from other reports that active CD is additionally deleterious for bone health. Optimizing nutritional and medical therapies during childhood for all children with T1D, especially those concomitantly affected by CD, will increase the likelihood that these at-risk children will safely experience active, fracture-free adult lives.

M. J. Schoelwer, MD

L. A. DiMeglio, MD, MPH

References

1. Kemink SG, Hermus AM, Swinkes LW, Lutterman JA, Smals AH. Osteopenia in insulin-dependent diabetes mellitus; prevalence and aspects of pathophysiology. *J Endocrinol Invest.* 2000;23:295-303.
2. Heikkila K, Pearce J, Maki M, Kaukinen K. Celiac disease and bone fractures: a systemic review and meta-analysis. *J Clin Endocrinol Metab.* 2015;100:25-34.
3. Mora S, Graziano B, Beccio S, et al. A prospective, longitudinal study of the long-term effect of treatment on bone density in children with celiac disease. *J Pediatr.* 2001;139:516-521.
4. Diniz-Santos DR, Brandao F, Adan L, Moreira A, Vicente EJ, Silva LR. Bone mineralization in young patients with type 1 diabetes mellitus and screening-identified evidence of celiac disease. *Dig Dis Sci.* 2008;53:1240-1245.
5. Jones IE, Williams SM, Dow N, Goulding A. How many children remain fracture-free during growth? A longitudinal study of children and adolescents participating in the Dunedin Multidisciplinary Health and Development Study. *Osteoporos Int.* 2002;13:990-995.

A Twin Study of Perthes Disease

Metcalfe D, Van Dijck S, Parsons N, et al (Harvard Med School, Boston, MA; Middlemore Hosp, Auckland, New Zealand; Univ of Southern Denmark, Odense; et al)

Pediatrics 137:e20153542, 2016

Background.—Legg-Calvé-Perthes disease (LCPD) is an idiopathic avascular necrosis of the femoral head. Its etiology is poorly understood, although previous studies have implicated low birth weight and possible genetic determinants. The aim of this study was to identify potential birth weight and genetic associations with LCPD.

Methods.—We extracted all twin pairs from the Danish Twin Registry (DTR) in which at least 1 individual had LCPD. The DTR captures every twin pair born alive in Denmark, and those with LCPD were identified by using health record linkage. Probanwise concordance was calculated to describe the likelihood that any given individual had LCPD if their co-twin was also diagnosed.

Results.—There were 81 twin pairs: 10 monozygotic, 51 dizygotic, and 20 unclassified (unknown zygosity [UZ]). There was no association between birth weight and being the affected co-twin. Four pairs (2 dizy-gotic and 2 UZ) were concordant for LCPD, which is greater than would be expected assuming no familial aggregation. There were no concordant monozygotic twin pairs. The overall probandwise concordance was 0.09 (95% confidence interval [CI]: 0.01−0.18): 0.00 for the monozygotic, 0.08 (95% CI: 0.00−0.18) for the dizygotic, and 0.18 (95% CI: 0.00−0.40) for the UZ twin pairs.

Conclusions.—This study found evidence of familial clustering in LCPD but did not show a genetic component. The absolute risk that a co-twin of an affected individual will develop LCPD is low, even in the case of monozygotic twin pairs.

▶ A century of research on Perthes disease (idiopathic avascular necrosis of the femoral head in children) has led to a better understanding of the pathophysiology, radiographic progression, and clinical outcomes but has brought us no closer to revealing its etiology. Both environmental and genetic factors have been proposed as causes of Perthes.[1] Indeed, some of the earliest descriptions of the condition include affected siblings, suggesting an inheritable trait.[2,3] Siblings, however, are exposed to the same environment, so familial clustering does not necessarily imply genetic causation.

Previous investigations of possible genetic factors for Perthes disease have explored several theories. Some studies have found an association between Perthes disease and thrombophilia due to factor V Leiden mutation or coagulation factor abnormalities, such as protein C and S deficiencies, producing local vascular occlusion, whereas other studies have not confirmed the findings. More recently a mutation in type II collagen alpha chain (COL2A1) has been identified in familial cases of bilateral Perthes disease from Asia[1] but the question of whether these cases truly represent Perthes disease and not a subtle form of skeletal dysplasia remains unresolved. So far Type II collagen mutation has not been reported in non-Asian population and not in unilateral cases of Perthes disease, which represent 85% to 90% of patients.

Twin studies provide an excellent opportunity to address the question of whether genetic factors play a major role in the etiology of Perthes disease. Comparison of monozygotic (nearly identical genetically) and dizygotic (about 50% genetically similar) twin pairs for concordant occurrence could help support or refute an underlying genetic basis for the disease. The present study is by far the largest of three twin studies of Perthes disease to date (81 twin pairs compared to 11 twin pairs previously), and the largest likely to be possible since the Danish Twin Registry is one of the largest and most detailed in existence. So, as definitively as can be stated from a twin study, there does not appear to be a genetic basis for Perthes disease.

This study, however, observed familial clustering, suggesting that environmental factors are likely to contribute to Perthes disease. Many environmental factors have been reported to be associated with Perthes disease over the years including socioeconomic deprivation, passive smoking exposure, hyperactivity, small stature, and geography. A recent study also suggests that in girls older than 10 years and involvement in high-demand activities such as competitive gymnastics may be a risk factor.[4] Another associated factor has been low birth weight. One of the previous twin studies found that it was always the lower birth weight twin who was one affected with Perthes disease.[5] The present, larger study did not support this observation.

In summary, the findings of this study do not support a genetic basis for Perthes disease using twin concordance methodology, although familial clustering of cases was observed suggesting that exposure to the same environmental factors plays a role. The current study analyzed data from a large, well-established twin registry and the findings are convincing. The impact of this study will be lasting because it is unlikely that a larger twin database with high-quality data will become available in the near future.

How can the findings be applied to pediatric practice? A natural question arises as to whether screening for Perthes disease in family members of an affected sibling or parent is warranted. Despite increased incidence of Perthes disease in family members of affected individuals, the absolute risk remains quite low, so radiographic screening is not warranted. However, because early detection and treatment may be effective in altering the natural history, families should be counseled to report symptoms of groin, thigh or knee pain, or signs of intermittent limp. This increased vigilance may be useful as the onset of Perthes disease is often insidious, subacute and episodic, and signs and symptoms may not be specific to the hip which can lead to delayed diagnosis.

Finally, has the study brought us any closer to understanding the etiology of Perthes disease? Yes, in a sense that the study convincingly sways us from searching for a single gene mutation as a cause of Perthes disease. The study supports the prevailing notion that the etiology of Perthes disease is multifactorial and that it may not even be a single disease but instead represents a final common pathway of interruption of the blood supply to the femoral head arising from the interaction of environmental factors with a variety of host factors (including some genetic patterns) that increase the patients' susceptibility. In time, we hope that an increasing number of these factors will be identified and effective treatments will be developed, shrinking the proportion of Perthes cases that truly fit the definition of "idiopathic."

S. R. Gilbert, MD

H. K. W. Kim, MD

References

1. Kim HK. Legg-Calve-Perthes disease: etiology, pathogenesis, and biology. *J Pediatr Orthop*. 2011;31:S141-S146.
2. Calvé J. On a particular form of pseudo-coxalgia associated with a characteristic deformity of the upper end of the femur: 1910. *Clin Orthop Relat Res*. 2006;451: 14-16.
3. Perthes G. The classic: on juvenile arthritis deformans. 1910. *Clin Orthop Relat Res*. 2012;470:2349-2368.
4. Larson AN, Kim HK, Herring JA. Female patients with late-onset Legg-Calvé-Perthes disease are frequently gymnasts: is there a mechanical etiology for this subset of patients? *J Pediatr Orthop*. 2013;33:811-815.
5. Lappin K, Kealey D, Cosgrove A, Graham K. Does low birthweight predispose to Perthes' disease? Perthes' disease in twins. *J Pediatr Orthop B*. 2003;12:307-310.

Safety of Botulinum Toxin Type A for Children With Nonambulatory Cerebral Palsy

Edwards P, Sakzewski L, Copeland L, et al (Lady Cilento Children's Hosp, Brisbane Australia; The Univ of Queensland, Brisbane, Australia)
Pediatrics 136:895-904, 2015

Objective.—To determine safety of intramuscular botulinum toxin A (BoNT-A) injections to reduce spasticity and improve care and comfort of nonambulatory children with cerebral palsy (CP).

Methods.—Nonambulatory children with CP were randomly allocated to receive either BoNT-A ($n = 23$) or sham procedure ($n = 18$) in Cycle 1. In Cycle 2, the BoNT-A group received a second episode of BoNT-A ($n = 20$) and sham group received their first episode of BoNT-A ($n = 17$). A pediatric rehabilitation specialist masked to group allocation graded each adverse event (AE) according to system, severity (mild, moderate, serious, sentinel) and causality (unlikely/unrelated; possible; probable/definite).

Results.—There was no difference for all moderate/serious AEs between the BoNT-A and sham/ control groups in either Cycle 1 (incident rate ratio $= 1.30$, 95% confidence interval $= 0.43-4.00$; $P = .64$) or Cycle 2 (incident rate ratio $= 0.72$, 95% confidence interval $= 0.30-1.75$; $P = .47$). In Cycle 2, 1 serious, 3 moderate (single-episode group), and 24 mild (single-episode group $n = 10$; 2 episode group $n = 14$) AEs were probably/definitely related to BoNT-A.

Conclusions.—Children receiving BoNT-A were at no greater risk of moderate/serious AEs compared with a sham control procedure. There was no increased risk of moderate/serious AEs between one and two episodes of BoNT-A.

▶ The safety of administering Botulinum toxin type A (BoNT-A) to children with nonambulatory cerebral palsy (CP) is investigated in this report. Caution has been urged in this population of children because of reports of respiratory compromise following injections. Naidu et al[1] studied the incidence of incontinence and respiratory events following BoNT-A injections and they reported 19 episodes of incontinence and 25 unplanned hospital admissions due to respiratory symptoms following 1980 injection episodes. Of relevance to this report is the finding of a strong association between the level of severity of CP and the occurrence of an unplanned hospital admission.

The Gross Motor Functional Classification System (GMFCS) was used in both articles to determine CP severity. It has 5 levels that go from "walks without limitations" (Level I), "walks with limitations (Level II), "walks using a hand-held mobility device" (Level III), "self-mobility with limitations such as using a powered mobility" (Level IV), to "transported in a manual wheelchair (Level V). The higher levels on the GMFCS correspond to more severe CP with presumably greater risk for respiratory problems and other adverse effects (AEs).

Lack of consistent definitions for what constitutes a relevant AE has resulted in quite a bit of variability in the incidence and type of AEs reported after treatment with BoNT-A. It was gratifying to read that these authors approached this issue by developing clear criteria for not only severity of reported AE but also the likelihood that the AE was related to the BoNT-A injection. Severity was graded from mild to sentinel (disability or death). In addition, the blinded reviewer was asked to evaluate "causality" using the categories "unlikely/unrelated," "possibly," and "probable/definite." This approach provides much needed clarity because this group of patients with CP have a high incidence of other health care concerns that could confound the interpretation of an AE following BoNT-A treatment.

The randomized double-blinded sham injection protocol that these authors have previously reported[2] provides a reasonable approach to the knotty problem of ethically investigating an invasive procedure using a control group in a group of children unable to give informed consent.

As with all studies that investigate the effects of clinical interventions, sample size issues are of concern. The authors provide a clear analysis of their calculations to take this into account. But still at issue is the fact that CP is not a homogenous disorder and that the plan of care for each child will need to be customized. Factors that are in play include the fragility of medical and neurological state, the magnitude of the positive benefit hoped for, and the long term plan in terms of whether repeated treatment every 3 to 6 months are worth it. Every time an injection with BoNT-A is given, an assessment of the benefits from the previous treatment should be reviewed to determine whether there was a meaningful change that led to either in improvement in a patient-centered goal such as comfort or decreased pain or a caregiver goal such as improvement in ease of dressing or bathing.

Within the group of nonambulatory CP, there are some children that appear to be more at risk for AEs than others. Those with gastrostomy tubes were 1.9 to 5.4 times more likely to have a moderate/severe AE. Interestingly, neither epilepsy nor hydrocephalus was associated with increased risk. The use of sedation in this group is another factor that could add to the risk of an AE. This study was not designed to separate out the effects of BoNT-A versus fentanyl when AEs were reported. Although fentanyl is considered a safe and effective analgesic, its role in those patients that had an AE cannot be ruled out. It's important to remember that this group of children has atypical brain structure that could result in unexpected responses to sedating medications.

These authors have done groundbreaking and important work on developing a research protocol that simulates injections. Without some form of control group, statements about the appropriate indications and effects of BoNT-A are suspect. Although not perfect, the paradigm that they have developed has sufficient safeguards built into it to satisfy the requirements of most institutional review boards.

At the end of the day, the decision to give BoNT-A to children with nonambulatory CP is a judgment call based on the practitioner and family's joint decision about treatment objectives, a thoughtful review of responses to previous treatments, and an careful assessment of the child's current medical stability.

Serial injections every 3 to 6 months without clear-cut benefit, runs the risk of exposure to potentially harmful AEs for little gain.

F. S. Pidcock, MD

References

1. Naidu K, Smith K, Sheedy M, Adair B, Yu X, Graham HK. Systemic adverse effects following botulinum toxin A therapy in children with cerebral palsy. *Dev Med Child Neurol.* 2010;52:139-144.
2. Thorley M, Donaghey S, Edwards P, et al. Evaluation of the effects of botulinum toxin A injections when used to improve ease of care and comfort in children with cerebral palsy who are non-ambulant: a double blind randomized controlled trial. *BMC Pediatr.* 2012;12:120.

17 Neonatology

Increasing Incidence of the Neonatal Abstinence Syndrome in U.S. Neonatal ICUs

Tolia VN, Patrick SW, Bennett MM, et al (Baylor Univ Med Ctr, Dallas, TX; Baylor Scott and White Health, Dallas, TX; Vanderbilt Univ School of Medicine, Nashville, TN; et al)

N Engl J Med 372:2118-2126, 2015

Background.—The incidence of the neonatal abstinence syndrome, a drug-withdrawal syndrome that most commonly occurs after in utero exposure to opioids, is known to have increased during the past decade. However, recent trends in the incidence of the syndrome and changes in demographic characteristics and hospital treatment of these infants have not been well characterized.

Methods.—Using multiple cross-sectional analyses and a deidentified data set, we analyzed data from infants with the neonatal abstinence syndrome from 2004 through 2013 in 299 neonatal intensive care units (NICUs) across the United States. We evaluated trends in incidence and health care utilization and changes in infant and maternal clinical characteristics.

Results.—Among 674,845 infants admitted to NICUs, we identified 10,327 with the neonatal abstinence syndrome. From 2004 through 2013, the rate of NICU admissions for the neonatal abstinence syndrome increased from 7 cases per 1000 admissions to 27 cases per 1000 admissions; the median length of stay increased from 13 days to 19 days ($P < 0.001$ for both trends). The total percentage of NICU days nationwide that were attributed to the neonatal abstinence syndrome increased from 0.6% to 4.0% ($P < 0.001$ for trend), with eight centers reporting that more than 20% of all NICU days were attributed to the care of these infants in 2013. Infants increasingly received pharmacotherapy (74% in 2004–2005 vs. 87% in 2012–2013, $P < 0.001$ for trend), with morphine the most commonly used drug (49% in 2004 vs. 72% in 2013, $P < 0.001$ for trend).

Conclusions.—From 2004 through 2013, the neonatal abstinence syndrome was responsible for a substantial and growing portion of resources dedicated to critically ill neonates in NICUs nationwide.

▶ Tolia et al demonstrate an absolute increase in the incidence of neonatal abstinence syndrome (NAS) in 2013 compared with 2004 in this publication. This observation consolidates the finding of Patrick and his associates, who initially observed a steep increase of NAS in the United States.[1]

NAS is not a new entity, having been identified in the mid-19th century as congenital morphinism in babies who were born to opioid-addicted mothers and who manifested signs of withdrawal. The incidence of congenital morphinism gradually increased with the abuse of heroin and morphine over time. The introduction of the hypodermic needle, along with commercial production of morphine and heroin, contributed to a further increase in congenital morphinism. Congenital morphinism was initially considered fatal, but it has been shown that babies with congenital morphinism can be saved with treatment.[2]

The incidence of NAS increased with the introduction of methadone for the treatment of opioid addiction, and escalated into an epidemic following the increased availability of opioid pain relievers. This situation worsened in the past 10 years, with addiction increasing along with easier access to heroin and morphine, lower prices, and the availability of newer prescription opioid analgesic medications. As demonstrated in this large and decade long study, this epidemic spread across the length and breadth of the United States, including rural America.

The incidence of NAS has been increasing not only in the United States, but also in Canada, Australia, and European countries, although heroin addiction is more common in Russia, Iran, and Afghanistan. In the United States, according to these authors, the incidence of NAS quadrupled from 2004 to 2013. NAS increased from 7 per 1000 admissions in 2004 to 27 per 1000 admissions in 2013. Interestingly, the rate of NAS is increasing more rapidly than the rate of opioid addiction. In some neonatal intensive care units (NICUs) in the United States, 20% to 40% of the beds are occupied with babies with NAS. If this trend continues at the same rate, some NICUs could have a census with 100% of infants with NAS within the next 10 to 15 years. This NAS increase is seen in every American state and affects all segments of the United States.[3]

The spectrum of substances associated with NAS has widened with time. Currently, NAS may be caused by the use or abuse of morphine, heroin, methadone, buprenorphine, or prescription opioid analgesics. NAS may also be caused by the use of antidepressants, anxiolytics, or other substances during pregnancy. The authors noted that 17% of NAS cases could be secondary to nonopioid medications, such as benzodiazepines and selective serotonin reuptake inhibitors. The epidemic of NAS has worsened further because of polysubstance abuse, including simultaneous use of multiple prescribed medications as well as concurrent use of both legal and illegal substances.

Although NAS affects all races, ethnicities, and regions, most studies have shown that a majority of babies are of Caucasian origin, and this study is no exception. In fact, during the study period, the percentage of Caucasian babies with NAS increased from 64% in 2004–2005 to 69% in 2008–2009 and to 76% in 2012–2013, while a decrease in incidence was seen among African American and Hispanic populations during the same time period. Although it is difficult to explain the increase of NAS in the Caucasian population specifically, the accessibility, affordability, and availability of these substances may be some of the factors that have contributed to this result. In addition, the majority of mothers are young and have low parity.

A majority of babies with NAS are born to mothers using methadone (31%, reflecting no change in the last 10 years), prescription pain relievers (24%, up from none 5 years ago), or buprenorphine (15%, up from 3% 5 years ago). Polydrug abuse has emerged as more a rule than an exception, although there is no mention of polydrug abuse in this article. Methadone dependence, prescription pain medication abuse, and polydrug use has all contributed to an increase in the incidence of NAS.

As the authors noted, in the past decade, neonates with NAS requiring medication to control symptoms increased not only in proportion (from 74% to 87%), but also the average duration of treatment (from 13 days to 19 days). Various causes for this increased incidence and severity include decreases in late preterm deliveries, increases in birth weight and gestation, and referrals from other hospitals. Increased use of morphine, decreased breastfeeding rates, and a decreased proportion of discharges on home medications may be additional reasons for prolonged hospital stays. Genetic factors, although not measured in this study, might also have played a role in the severity of NAS.

NAS is a treatable disease; however, as the authors mentioned, there are no standard pharmacological or nonpharmacological measures in the management of NAS. Nonpharmacological therapy has not received due recognition although this is less expensive, easily available, and usually less controversial. Nonpharmacological therapy needs to be initiated in all infants before starting pharmacological therapy. Nonpharmacological measures may even mitigate the need for pharmacological support. Optimal implementation of comprehensive nonpharmacological measures may not only decrease the need for medication but also the duration of treatment.

Breastfeeding for babies with NAS increased from 20% to only 35% in the past decade, compared with a breastfeeding rate of 80% among normal babies. Also there is no mention of duration of breastfeeding among these mothers. Breastfeeding increases maternal-infant bonding, increases maternal confidence, and encourages active maternal participation. In addition, breastfeeding decreases the length of hospital stay and the need for pharmacological treatment. Because of this range of benefits, breastfeeding should be encouraged unless the mother is using multiple medications or illegal substances such as morphine, heroin, and cocaine. Infections with hepatitis B, hepatitis C, and cytomegalovirus are not contraindications for breastfeeding.

There is wide variation in treatment protocols for NAS; many hospitals do not have a protocol. Also, the management of NAS differs across institutions and even in the same institution. Medications commonly used to treat NAS physiologically appear to be creating an in utero status and then weaning gradually in a controlled environment, buying time until the body is cleared of signs of opioid withdrawal. However, continuous administration of these drugs at the same time may not be completely beneficial to the baby, who has already sustained an insult in utero. There is much confusion regarding treatment options, the drug preferred, the adjunctive therapy added, time of initiation of medications, whether medication is required according to weight-based or symptom-based formulas, when escalation of medication is required, and lastly when to wean. Hence, there is an urgent need to have a uniform approach for the management of NAS.

Seventy-two percent of health care professionals report being comfortable prescribing morphine, compared with 49% a decade ago. Morphine has gained popularity because it is easy to use, has a short half-life, and has no alcohol content. In addition, the dose can be increased or decreased every 4 hours, if the baby's symptoms are not controlled as intended with the previous dose. Methadone use decreased to 19% because methadone has a long half-life, has 8% alcohol content, and is relatively difficult to titrate. Clonidine also gained some popularity as 9% of neonates were treated with this nonnarcotic, nonsedative, nonalcoholic medication; however, its longer half-life and theoretical risk of rebound hypertension are limiting factors. Buprenorphine also has a long half-life and high alcohol content, and is used in < 1% of cases. Larger studies are needed before the widespread usage of last 2 medications.

The Finnegan scoring system, introduced in 1975, continues to be popular and is used primarily for monitoring, titrating, and terminating the use of therapeutic agents for NAS. However, there is wide interobserver variation in scoring, as the majority of signs are subjective. Furthermore, different score patterns over time are used as criteria for determining different treatment options. Hence, there is a need for a shorter, simpler, and more objective scoring system for prompt and uniform management.

This extensive retrospective analysis further confirmed our experience in the field; however, the inclusion of neonates based on discharge diagnosis, and the lack of neonatal toxicology testing to confirm their diagnosis are limitations of the study. Furthermore, the inclusion of neonatal transfers and the exclusion of preterm neonates might have influenced the incidence of NAS. In addition, polydrug abuse was not commented on in this study; however, this article is well written, well edited, statistically sound, and numerically robust. It covers one of the most important public health problems of this decade and makes a valuable contribution to the literature.

P. Kocherlakota, MD

References

1. Patrick SW, Schumacher RE, Benneyworth BD, Krans EE, McAllister JM, Davis MM. Neonatal abstinence syndrome and associated health care expenditures: United States, 2000–2009. *JAMA*. 2012;307:1934-1940.
2. Kocherlakota P. Neonatal abstinence syndrome. *Pediatrics*. 2014;134:e547-e561.
3. Patrick SW, Davis MM, Lehman CU, Cooper WO. Increasing incidence and geographic distribution of neonatal abstinence syndrome: United States 2009 to 2012. *J Perinatol*. 2015;35:650-655.

A Cohort Comparison of Buprenorphine versus Methadone Treatment for Neonatal Abstinence Syndrome
Hall ES, Isemann BT, Wexelblatt SL, et al (Cincinnati Children's Hosp Med Ctr, OH; Univ of Cincinnati Med Ctr, OH)
J Pediatr 170:39-44, 2016

Objectives.—To compare the duration of opioid treatment and length of stay among infants treated for neonatal abstinence syndrome (NAS) by using a pilot buprenorphine vs conventional methadone treatment protocol.

Study Design.—This retrospective cohort analysis evaluated infants who received pharmacotherapy for NAS at 6 hospitals in Southwest Ohio from January 2012 through August 2014. A single neonatology provider group used a standardized methadone protocol across all 6 hospitals. However, at one of the sites, infants were managed with a buprenorphine protocol unless they had experienced chronic in utero exposure to methadone. Linear mixed models were used to calculate adjusted mean duration of opioid treatment and length of inpatient hospitalization with 95% CIs in infants treated with oral methadone compared with sublingual buprenorphine. The use of adjunct therapy was examined as a secondary outcome.

Results.—A total of 201 infants with NAS were treated with either buprenorphine (n = 38) or methadone (n = 163) after intrauterine exposure to short-acting opioids or buprenorphine. Buprenorphine therapy was associated with a shorter course of opioid treatment of 9.4 (CI 7.1-11.7) vs 14.0 (12.6-15.4) days ($P < .001$) and decreased hospital stay of 16.3 (13.7-18.9) vs 20.7 (19.1-22.2) days ($P < .001$) compared with methadone therapy. No difference was detected in the use of adjunct therapy (23.7% vs 25.8%, $P = .79$) between treatment groups.

Conclusion.—The choice of pharmacotherapeutic agent is an important determinant of hospital outcomes in infants with NAS. Sublingual buprenorphine may be superior to methadone for management of NAS in infants with select intrauterine opioid exposures (Tables 1 and 4).

▶ The explosion of the use of opioids in the United States at large had led to increases of exposure in pregnancy, resulting in a 5-fold increase neonatal abstinence syndrome (NAS) incidence. Nationally, 27 in 1000 neonatal intensive care unit (NICU) admissions are for NAS treatment, with regional variation and some centers are particularly hard hit by the epidemic.[1] Individual clinicians and health systems struggle with optimizing therapies given prolonged hospitalizations, increased costs, and detrimental effects on the mother—child dyad.

Supportive treatment is employed in all infants with in utero exposure to opioids. About half will require pharmacologic therapy to relieve symptoms and ensure proper weight gain. The current standard is the use of an opioid at a dose that controls symptoms and is subsequently slowly weaned. Morphine is the primary opioid in 85% of centers, with the remainder using methadone.[2]

The partial mu agonist buprenorphine has been investigated as a potential opioid in NAS due to a long half-life and well defined safety profile in adults. Interest for buprenorphine in NAS was also piqued by the MOTHER trial, in which maternal use of buprenorphine was associated with improved NAS outcomes. Reported use in infants thus far has been limited to small, open-label investigations.[3]

Hall and colleagues have described their experience with the use of buprenorphine in a treatment paradigm (Table 1). Buprenorphine treated infants had a 33% reduction in length of treatment compared to methadone (Table 4). Their observed effect size mirrors almost exactly the results demonstrated in the previously published phase 1, open label trial comparing buprenorphine to morphine.

TABLE 1.—Pilot Buprenorphine-Weaning Protocol

Initiation
   O Initiate protocol for infants with 3 consecutive Finnegan scores ≥8, or 2 consecutive Finnegan scores ≥12

	Buprenorphine Dose	Dosing Interval	Number of Doses
Step 1	4.4 µg/kg	Q8	3
Step 2	2.6 µg/kg	Q8	3
Step 3	1.7 µg/kg	Q8	3
Step 4	1.7 µg/kg	Q12	2
Step 5	1.7 µg/kg	Q24	1

Escalation
   O If average Finnegan scores >8 after 2 doses (9 h) increase dose by 0.8 µg/kg Q8 × 2 until Finnegan scores are 8 or below (5.2 × g/kg Q8 × 2, 6.0 µg/kg Q8 × 2, etc., max dose of 13 µg/kg Q8)
   O If average Finnegan scores <8, wean each day by 0.8 µg/kg until back to 4.4 µg/kg Q8 and advance to step 2

Weaning
   O Wean to next step if average Finnegan score is <8 for the past 24 hours.
   O If average Finnegan score is 8-12, do not wean
   O If average Finnegan score >12, go back one step on taper (backslide)
   O If average Finnegan score remains >12 for 48 h go back two steps on taper

Adjunct therapy
   O Consider adding phenobarbital if
      Infant at maximum buprenorphine dose of 39 µg/kg/day OR
      Unable to wean after 24-48 h

Discharge
   O Observe for 72 h from the last dose of step 5

Reprinted from Hall ES, Isemann BT, Wexelblatt SL, et al. A cohort comparison of buprenorphine versus methadone treatment for neonatal abstinence syndrome. *J Pediatr.* 2016;170:39-44, with permission Elsevier.

TABLE 4.—Adjusted Patient Outcomes Comparing Buprenorphine vs Methadone Treatment Groups Including Comparisons by in Utero Exposure

	Buprenorphine Treated	Methadone Treated	P Value
In utero exposure to short-acting opioids or buprenorphine, n = 201	n = 38	n = 163	
Days of opioid treatment, mean, (95% CI)	9.4 (7.1-11.7)	14.0 (12.6-15.4)	<.001
Length of stay, mean, (95% CI)	16.3 (13.7-18.9)	20.7 (19.1-22.2)	<.001
Received adjunct therapy	23.7%	25.8%	.79
In utero exposure to only short-acting opioids, n = 117	n = 23	n = 94	
Days of opioid treatment, mean, (95% CI)	7.0 (4.3-9.6)	11.8 (10.4-13.2)	.002
Length of stay, mean, (95% CI)	13.1 (10.2-16.2)	17.6 (16.0-19.2)	.004
Received adjunct therapy	8.7%	20.2%	.32
In utero exposure to buprenorphine +/− short-acting opioids, n = 84	n = 15	n = 69	
Days of opioid treatment, mean, (95% CI)	11.5 (7.6-15.4)	15.9 (13.9-17.9)	.04
Length of stay, mean, (95% CI)	18.1 (13.9-22.4)	22.9 (20.4-25.4)	.03
Received adjunct therapy	46.7%	33.3%	.33

Reprinted from Hall ES, Isemann BT, Wexelblatt SL, et al. A cohort comparison of buprenorphine versus methadone treatment for neonatal abstinence syndrome. *J Pediatr.* 2016;170:39-44, with permission Elsevier.

This similar finding in separate populations, study designs, and comparators give hints of a possible drug specific advantage over current therapies.

Interest in Hall's article stems from a desire to identify the best opioid for NAS. After years of practice largely driven by clinical observation, there are a number of recent published and ongoing studies comparing various regimens. A blinded, controlled investigation comparing buprenorphine to morphine will complete enrollment in mid-2016 (the B-BORN trial).[4] while a large multicenter trial comparing morphine and methadone (BABY trial) is ongoing.[5] The virtue of these blinded, controlled studies is the uniformity in populations, Finnegan scoring, and adherence to a protocol. The only difference is the drug used in the 2 groups.

What should not be lost in this search is that the choice of drug is only 1 of many factors that drive length of treatment. Indeed, the same team of investigators reported a 30% shorter duration of therapy in those centers which adhered to a strict treatment protocol compared with those without.[6] Interestingly, in this same study, the use of morphine or methadone was not associated with a difference in outcomes. Thus, although identifying the best drug is important, this is only one element in a comprehensive, uniform, and multidisciplinary team approach to NAS. Organizations such as the Vermont Oxford Network are a resource for health systems to share best practices in the treatment of NAS.

Practitioners investigating using buprenorphine in NAS should consider a few issues. First, the drug is administered sublingually and absorbed in the buccal mucosa within a minute or 2. The Hall group excluded use of buprenorphine to mothers taking methadone. Almost all the patients in the Kraft et al study had maternal methadone use. There is no evidence that any one opioid used in NAS is better or worse for specific in utero exposures. The buprenorphine formulation these studies contains 30% ethanol for solubility and stability of drug. Although many drugs used in the NICU contain ethanol, the absolute amount administered is small, and neonatal clearance is faster than in adults, some are concerned with the health effects of ethanol.

Although the formulations were the same, the initial dose, maximum dose, and specific titration protocols used by Hall and Kraft also differed. This highlights that the ideal titration regimen has not been established by any group for any of the commonly used medications. Here again the Cincinnati group are leaders in NAS therapeutics, as evidenced by their separate reporting of modern pharmacokinetic modeling methods to simulate an optimal regimen. A model of methadone exposure was used to generate a new dosing regimen associated with decreased length of stay.[7] A similar approach will be used with buprenorphine. The long half-life and safety margin of buprenorphine may eventually allow the rational dose design that would allow for less frequent, and perhaps even outpatient dosing for stabilized infants. The only caveat remains that while initial investigations suggest a specific efficacy advantage of buprenorphine, a much more comprehensive view will emerge following the publication of randomized, controlled clinical trial results.

W. K. Kraft, MD

References

1. Tolia VN, Patrick SW, Bennett MM, et al. Increasing incidence of the neonatal abstinence syndrome in U.S. neonatal ICUs. *N Engl J Med.* 2015;372:2118-2126.
2. Patrick SW, Schumacher RE, Horbar JD, et al. Improving care for neonatal abstinence syndrome. *Pediatrics.* 2016;137 http://dx.doi.org/10.1542/peds.2015−3835.
3. Kraft WK, Dysart K, Greenspan J, Gibson E, Kaltenbach K, Ehrlich M. Revised dose schema of sublingual buprenorphine in the treatment of the neonatal opioid abstinence syndrome. *Addiction.* 2011;106:574-580.
4. Blinded Trial of Buprenorphine or Morphine in the Treatment of the Neonatal Abstinence Syndrome. https://clinicaltrials.gov/ct2/show/NCT01452789?term =walter+kraft&rank=3 Accessed May 14, 2016.
5. Improving Outcomes in Neonatal Abstinence Syndrome. https://clinicaltrials.gov/ct2/show/NCT01958476?term=jonathan+davis&rank=1. Accessed May 14, 2016.
6. Hall ES, Wexelblatt SL, Crowley M, et al. OCHNAS consortium implementation of a neonatal abstinence syndrome weaning protocol: a multicenter cohort study. *Pediatrics.* 2015;136:e803-e810.
7. Hall ES, Meinzen-Derr J, Wexelblatt SL. Cohort analysis of a pharmacokinetic-modeled methadone weaning optimization for neonatal abstinence syndrome. *J Pediatr.* 2015;167:1221-1225.e1.

Randomized Trial of Late Surfactant Treatment in Ventilated Preterm Infants Receiving Inhaled Nitric Oxide

Ballard RA, for the TOLSURF Study Group (Univ of California San Francisco; et al)
J Pediatr 168:23-29, 2016

Objective.—To assess whether late surfactant treatment in extremely low gestational age (GA) newborn infants requiring ventilation at 7-14 days, who often have surfactant deficiency and dysfunction, safely improves survival without bronchopulmonary dysplasia (BPD).

Study Design.—Extremely low GA newborn infants (GA ≤28 0/7 weeks) who required mechanical ventilation at 7- 14 days were enrolled in a randomized, masked controlled trial at 25 US centers. All infants received inhaled nitric oxide and either surfactant (calfactant/Infasurf) or sham instillation every 1-3 days to a maximum of 5 doses while intubated. The primary outcome was survival at 36 weeks postmenstrual age (PMA) without BPD, as evaluated by physiological oxygen/flow reduction.

Results.—A total of 511 infants were enrolled between January 2010 and September 2013. There were no differences between the treated and control groups in mean birth weight (701 ± 164 g), GA (25.2 ± 1.2 weeks), percentage born at GA <26 weeks (70.6%), race, sex, severity of lung disease at enrollment, or comorbidities of prematurity. Survival without BPD did not differ between the treated and control groups at 36 weeks PMA (31.3% vs 31.7%; relative benefit, 0.98; 95% CI, 0.75-1.28; $P =.89$) or 40 weeks PMA (58.7% vs 54.1%; relative benefit, 1.08; 95% CI, 0.92-1.27; $P =.33$). There were no between-group differences in serious adverse events, comorbidities of prematurity, or severity of lung disease to 36 weeks.

Conclusion.—Late treatment with up to 5 doses of surfactant in ventilated premature infants receiving inhaled nitric oxide was well tolerated, but did not improve survival without BPD at 36 or 40 weeks. Pulmonary and neurodevelopmental assessments are ongoing.

Trial Registration.—ClinicalTrials.gov: NCT01022580.

▶ Improvements in obstetric and neonatal care have resulted in increasing survival of extremely preterm infants. However, serious sequelae such as bronchopulmonary dysplasia (BPD) remain one of the major morbidities associated with extremely preterm birth. More than 70% of surviving extremely low gestational age newborn (ELGAN) infants who require mechanical ventilation at 7 days of age develop BPD.[1,2] Furthermore, safe and effective postnatal therapies to reduce the likelihood of developing BPD are sorely lacking. In this large randomized multicenter study of ELGAN infants who required mechanical ventilation at 7 to 14 days of age, Ballard and colleagues assessed the effects of inhaled nitric oxide (iNO) alone versus a combination of iNO and surfactant on survival without bronchopulmonary dysplasia (BPD) at 36 weeks' postmenstrual age (PMA). The authors were unable to show a beneficial effect of combined iNO and surfactant therapy on their primary outcome of interest (ie, BPD-free survival at 36 weeks' PMA).

The pathophysiology of the "new" BPD so prevalent among ELGAN is strikingly different from the initial description by Northway[3] and is characterized by impaired alveolar and microvascular development and alterations in tone and reactivity of airway and vascular smooth muscle. Several factors have been implicated in the development of BPD, including structurally immature lungs, pulmonary surfactant dysfunction, perturbed intrauterine environment, oxidant stress, exposure to inflammation and infection, and genetic susceptibility. BPD is a multifactorial condition, rather than a single disease entity. Multiple and often coexisting pathological mechanisms and developmental processes influence the likelihood that an ELGAN will have an oxygen requirement at 36 weeks. Thus, it is likely that a multipronged approach will be needed to address this problem.

Here, the investigators sought to investigate a combination of therapies: iNO, which has previously been shown, at least in animal models and some human studies, to decrease the risk of BPD,[2,4] and exogenous surfactant, because surfactant deficiency/dysfunction has been reported in small studies of ventilated preterm infants after the first week of life.[5-7] The investigators should be congratulated for taking on the challenge of a multitherapy clinical trial in this vulnerable population of infants with persistent significant lung disease in the second week of life.

In this study, 511 infants < 28 weeks' gestational age (GA) who required mechanical ventilation at 7 to 14 days of age were treated with iNO and were randomized to receive either surfactant (Infasurf) or sham instillation every 24 to 72 hours for a maximum of 5 doses. The iNO protocol used in this study has previously been described by Ballard et al in their prior study of exogenous iNO therapy for the prevention of BPD in preterm infants.[2] Both study groups were comparable in most respects except for maternal age and education. There was no difference in survival without BPD at 36 or 40 weeks' PMA between the 2 groups. Furthermore, there was no difference in the days on mechanical ventilation before 36 weeks' PMA, days on supplemental oxygen, or rate of treatment with systemic steroids. Importantly, serious adverse events and comorbidities were comparable between the 2 groups. Follow-up of study participants with a focus on meaningful longer term outcomes such as pulmonary and neurodevelopmental morbidities is ongoing.

An intriguing, but not fully explored, aspect of the study findings is that nonwhite infants showed trends toward better outcomes in both treatment arms with 37% of nonwhite infants surviving without BPD compared with 24% of white infants. It would appear that the improved outcomes seen in nonwhite infants are primarily driven by iNO therapy and not surfactant. Previous studies of iNO alone for the prevention of BPD have shown similar trends, suggesting that nonwhite infants may respond differently to exogenous iNO compared with white infants.[2,4] It is also important to note that the current study was not powered to detect differences in subgroups of patients based on race/ethnicity. In this day of precision medicine, this intriguing finding must be further explored and validated. If the field of neonatology is to realize its promise of the right therapy at the right time for the right patient, it behooves all of us to pay more attention to racial/ethnic, developmental, and gender-based differences in the response to therapies.

M. Fuloria, MBBS

J. L. Aschner, MD

References

1. Laughon MM, Langer JC, Bose CL, et al. Eunice Kennedy Shriver National Institute of Child Health and Human Development Neonatal Research Network. Prediction of bronchopulmonary dysplasia by postnatal age in extremely premature infants. *Am J Respir Crit Care Med*. 2011;183:1715-1722.
2. Ballard RA, Truog WE, Cnaan A, et al. NO CLD Study Group. Inhaled nitric oxide in preterm infants undergoing mechanical ventilation. *N Engl J Med*. 2006;355:343-353.
3. Northway WH Jr, Rosan RC, Porter DY. Pulmonary disease following respirator therapy of hyaline-membrane disease. Bronchopulmonary dysplasia. *N Engl J Med*. 1967;276:357-368.
4. Schreiber MD, Gin-Mestan K, Marks JD, Huo D, Lee G, Srisuparp P. Inhaled nitric oxide in premature infants with the respiratory distress syndrome. *N Engl J Med*. 2003;349:2099-2107.
5. Merrill JD, Ballard RA, Cnaan A, et al. Dysfunction of pulmonary surfactant in chronically ventilated premature infants. *Pediatr Res*. 2004;56:918-926.
6. Merrill JD, Ballard PL, Courtney SE, et al. Pilot trial of late booster doses of surfactant for ventilated premature infants. *J Perinatol*. 2011;31:599-606.
7. Keller RL, Merrill JD, Black DM, et al. Late administration of surfactant replacement therapy increases surfactant protein-B content: a randomized pilot study. *Pediatr Res*. 2012;72:613-619.

Nonintubated Surfactant Application vs Conventional Therapy in Extremely Preterm Infants: A Randomized Clinical Trial

Kribs A, for the NINSAPP Trial Investigators (Children's Hosp Univ of Cologne, Germany; et al)
JAMA Pediatr 169:723-730, 2015

Importance.—Treatment of respiratory distress syndrome in premature infants with continuous positive airway pressure (CPAP) preserves surfactant and keeps the lung open but is insufficient in severe surfactant deficiency. Traditional surfactant administration is related to short periods of positive pressure ventilation and implies the risk of lung injury. CPAP with surfactant but without any positive pressure ventilation may work synergistically. This randomized trial investigated a less invasive surfactant application protocol (LISA).

Objective.—To test the hypothesis that LISA increases survival without bronchopulmonary dysplasia (BPD) at 36 weeks' gestational age in extremely preterm infants.

Design, Setting, and Participants.—The Nonintubated Surfactant Application trial was a multicenter, randomized, clinical, parallel-group study conducted between April 15, 2009, and March 25, 2012, in 13 level III neonatal intensive care units in Germany. The final follow-up date was June 21, 2012. Participants included 211 of 558 eligible (37.8%) spontaneously breathing preterm infants born between 23.0 and 26.8 weeks' gestational age with signs of respiratory distress syndrome. In an intention-to-treat design, infants were randomly assigned to receive surfactant either via a thin endotracheal catheter during CPAP-assisted spontaneous breathing (intervention group) or after conventional endotracheal intubation during mechanical ventilation (control group). Analysis was conducted from September 6, 2012, to June 20, 2013.

Intervention.—LISA via a thin catheter.

Main Outcomes and Measures.—Survival without BPD at 36 weeks' gestational age.

Results.—Of 211 infants who were randomized, 104 were randomized to the control group and 107 to the LISA group. Of the infants who received LISA, 72 (67.3%) survived without BPD compared with 61 (58.7%) of those in the control group. The reduction in absolute risk was 8.6% (95% CI, −5.0% to 21.9%; $P = .20$). Intervention group infants were less frequently intubated (80 infants [74.8%] vs 103 [99.0%]; $P < .001$) and required fewer days of mechanical ventilation. Significant reductions were seen in pneumothorax (5 of 105 intervention group infants [4.8%] vs 13 of 103 12.6%]; $P = .04$) and severe intraventricular hemorrhage (11 infants [10.3%] vs 23 [22.1%]; $P = .02$), and the combined survival without severe adverse events was increased in the intervention group (54 infants [50.5%] vs 37 [35.6%]; $P = .02$; absolute risk reduction, 14.9; 95% CI, 1.4 to 28.2).

Conclusions and Relevance.—LISA did not increase survival without BPD but was associated with increased survival without major complications.

Because major complications are related to lifelong disabilities, LISA may be a promising therapy for extremely preterm infants.

Trial Registration.—isrctn.org Identifier: ISRCTN64011614.

▶ "Nothing is more imminent than the impossible ... what we must always foresee is the unforeseen."—Victor Hugo, Les Miserables

Not so many years ago, the only notion more implausible than that of providing active management and respiratory support for preterm infants born at 23 weeks' gestation would have been the suggestion that this care could be provided without intubation soon after birth. And yet this may well be our way of the future for the extremely preterm infant, if we are to follow the pioneering approach of a team of German investigators led by Dr. Angela Kribs. Following on from previous work describing and evaluating a less invasive method of surfactant instillation by brief tracheal catheterization (the Cologne method), this group in 2015 published the results of an important clinical trial suggesting that avoidance of intubation in early life might be of benefit for extremely preterm infants, including those born on the cusp of viability.

The study of Kribs et al (the NINSAPP trial) compared application of continuous positive airway pressure (CPAP) and surfactant delivery via the Cologne method with the "standard" approach for preterm infants < 28 weeks' gestation, that of intubation in the delivery room, surfactant therapy and continued mechanical ventilation. Infants 23 to 26 weeks' gestation were included in the study if they exhibited features of respiratory distress syndrome and a modest oxygen requirement (FiO_2 > 0.30) in the first 2 hours of life. The interventions were applied in an unblinded manner, but protocols guided the clinicians in their management of both groups.

The primary outcome for the NINSAPP trial (survival without bronchopulmonary dysplasia [BPD]) did not differ in incidence between the study groups, but there were some significant differences in secondary outcomes suggesting a benefit of the less invasive approach. More infants survived without major complications (50% vs 36%), the rate of severe intraventricular haemorrhage was reduced (10% vs 22%), as was the pneumothorax rate (4.8 vs 13%), and the overall duration of mechanical ventilation.

The study is bold in several senses. It includes infants at 23 and 24 weeks' gestation, a patient group little studied in randomized trials in neonatology. Moreover, 1 of the randomization arms involved avoidance of intubation in the delivery room, which for many neonatologists represents a substantial departure from what would be considered standard practice in the most immature infants.

The intervention under study is at face value highly appealing, combining the quintessential lung-protective respiratory support technique (CPAP) with an innovative method of administering surfactant, which seems to result in excellent drug distribution and produces a prominent treatment effect. The approach does appear to have the potential to bear fruit, with reductions in rates of complications known to be associated with intubation and ventilation, including severe intracranial bleeding. It is noteworthy that this improvement occurred despite the fact that nearly half (47%) of the infants managed with CPAP and less-invasive surfactant did require intubation in the first 72 hours, and almost all of those born at 23 to 24 weeks' gestation required intubation at some time. The implication is that even a day or a few days during which the extremely preterm infant is spontaneously breathing on CPAP may be to their advantage in early life. Undoubtedly this is when the preterm lung is at its most vulnerable, whereas later, with further exposure to the rigors of an air-breathing existence, the lungs "harden up" and become less prone to ventilator-induced injury.

The study has some limitations. With just over 200 participants, it was under-powered to detect a clinically important difference (say, around 10%) in the rate of survival without BPD. The dose of porcine surfactant was not standardized, varying from 100 to 200 mg/kg, meaning that some infants in both groups received a dose that could be considered less than adequate. Finally, the study was not blinded, with the inevitable consequence that management of the infants after intervention may have been influenced by knowledge of the treatment group.

So what remains to be done to make the impossible become possible, and for tiny preterm infants to be managed on CPAP and, where necessary, less invasive surfactant therapy from the outset? First, it will require firm evidence of benefit from yet larger clinical trials in extremely preterm infants; although the method is appealing, it is not yet proven. Second, and assuming that short- and long-term benefits are established, there will need to be a wholesale change in philosophy on the part of all clinicians involved in the management of both the premature parturient and the newborn infant, to facilitate transition without the aid of an endotracheal tube. Finally, and as emphasized by the Cologne group and others, CPAP plus less invasive surfactant will need to be viewed as part of a package of delivery room care, which also potentially includes thermal stabilization, early caffeine therapy and maternal skin-to-skin contact. The approach can be foreseen and now must be pursued.

P. A. Dargaville, MD

Early Inhaled Budesonide for the Prevention of Bronchopulmonary Dysplasia
Bassler D, for the NEUROSIS Trial Group (Univ of Zurich, Switzerland; et al)
N Engl J Med 373:1497-1506, 2015

Background.—Systemic glucocorticoids reduce the incidence of bronchopulmonary dysplasia among extremely preterm infants, but they may compromise brain development. The effects of inhaled glucocorticoids on outcomes in these infants are unclear.

Methods.—We randomly assigned 863 infants (gestational age, 23 weeks 0 days to 27 weeks 6 days) to early (within 24 hours after birth) inhaled budesonide or placebo until they no longer required oxygen and positive-pressure support or until they reached a postmenstrual age of 32 weeks 0 days. The primary outcome was death or bronchopulmonary dysplasia, confirmed by means of standardized oxygen-saturation monitoring, at a postmenstrual age of 36 weeks.

Results.—A total of 175 of 437 infants assigned to budesonide for whom adequate data were available (40.0%), as compared with 194 of 419 infants assigned to placebo for whom adequate data were available (46.3%), died or had bronchopulmonary dysplasia (relative risk, stratified according to gestational age, 0.86; 95% confidence interval [CI], 0.75 to 1.00; $P = 0.05$). The incidence of bronchopulmonary dysplasia was 27.8% in the budesonide group versus 38.0% in the placebo group (relative risk, stratified according to gestational age, 0.74; 95% CI, 0.60 to 0.91; $P = 0.004$); death occurred in 16.9% and 13.6% of the patients, respectively (relative risk, stratified according to gestational age, 1.24; 95% CI, 0.91 to 1.69; $P = 0.17$). The proportion of infants who required surgical closure of a patent ductus arteriosus was lower in the budesonide group than in the placebo group (relative risk, stratified according to gestational age, 0.55; 95% CI, 0.36 to 0.83; $P = 0.004$), as was the proportion of infants who required reintubation (relative risk, stratified according to gestational age, 0.58; 95% CI, 0.35 to 0.96; $P = 0.03$). Rates of other neonatal illnesses and adverse events were similar in the two groups.

Conclusions.—Among extremely preterm infants, the incidence of bronchopulmonary dysplasia was lower among those who received early inhaled budesonide than among those who received placebo, but the advantage may have been gained at the expense of increased mortality. (Funded by the European Union and Chiesi Farmaceutici; ClinicalTrials. gov number, NCT01035190.)

▶ Postnatal corticosteroids to prevent or treat bronchopulmonary dysplasia (BPD) are one of the most controversial neonatal treatments with a checkered history that goes back more than 40 years. The report by Bassler et al conjures up thoughts such as, "what goes around comes around" and "déjà vu all over again"—for this trial and other recent large trials. These other articles are a report by Yeh et al[1] describing the addition of budesonide to surfactant treatment, a report from Baud et al[2] of low-dose hydrocortisone treatment for 10 days begun shortly after birth, and the National Institute of Child Health and Development (NICHD) Maternal-Fetal network trial reporting benefits of antenatal steroids for late preterm infants.[3]

I thought the postnatal steroid question was basically settled following the influential meta-regression analysis of the trials demonstrating benefit if the risk of BPD is high and neurodevelopmental harm if the risk of BPD is low in a given infant.[4] In general, the bias is to avoid early treatment. But the Bassler, Yeh,[1] and Baud[2] trials found decreases in BPD for very early treatments with steroids.

Let's evaluate these trials as we now have 3 new options for therapy to consider. The Bassler trial randomized infants on the first day of life to an inhaler containing budesonide that delivered 400 µg in 2 puffs every 12 hours for the first 14 days and 1 dose per day until infant was off oxygen or 32 weeks gestational age (GA) (Table 1). The dose and distribution of the steroid to the lungs was not known,[5] but systemic adsorption could be substantial. There was a 10.2% decrease in BPD but the competing outcome of death increased nonsignificantly

TABLE 1.—Comparisons of Three New Trials of Early Corticosteroids to Prevent BPD

	Bassler (1)	Yeh (2)	Baud (3)
Steroid	Budesonide – delivered dose unknown	Budesonide – 0.25 µg/kg	Hydrocortisone – 1 mg/kg/×7d and 0.5 mg/kg/×3d
Route	Aerosol – 2×/day until off oxygen or to 32 weeks	Mixed with surfactant	Infusion
Treatment initiation	Within 24 hr of birth	2 hr	16 h
Average BW/GA	800 g/26.1 weeks	909 g/26.7 weeks	840 g/26.5 weeks
Patients Randomized	863	265	266
% Received Antenatal steroid	90%	83%	92%
% Decrease in BPD	10.2%	21%	4%
Change in Death	Increased 3.3%	Decreased 3%	Decreased 5%
Other outcomes with steroid	Lower reintubation, less PDA ligation, less diuretic use	Fewer surfactant doses, Less PDA, lower inflammatory mediates in lung	More estubations by day 10, more late onset sepsis for infants <26 weeks
Neuro developmental Outcomes	—	No difference	—

by 3.3%. The secondary outcomes of lower intubation rate, less PDA, and less diuretic use were biologically plausible benefits from steroids that would be associated with less BPD.

The Yeh[1] trial has exploited observations in animal models that surfactant treatment can carry drugs to the distal lung and thus effectively target lung regions that may not receive aerosols and with less systemic exposure. The mixing of surfactant with budesonide for treatment of respiratory distress syndrome (RDS) was a very early exposure to steroid, which was repeated for the 34% of the treatment group that got a second dose of surfactant. Thus, the treatment resulted in a much shorter duration of steroid exposure than the nebulized steroid used by Bassler but with a qualitatively larger decrease in BPD of 21% and a 3% decrease in death.

The Baud[2] trial of 10 days of hydrocortisone infusion starting at 1 mg/kg at birth used a maintenance dose of hydrocortisone and not a high anti-inflammatory dose. For comparison, dexamethasone is 25 times more potent than hydrocortisone such that the dexamethasone equivalent dose would be 0.04 mg/kg. The combined primary outcome of survival without BPD was significant primarily because of a 5% increase in survival.

These 3 early treatment trials change the game as to when corticosteroids could be used to decrease BPD. Taken together, the results support mechanistic studies in animals demonstrating that the injury that progresses to BPD begins before or soon after birth.[6] The benefits from early treatments may be treatment of the relative adrenal insufficiency in many preterm infants plus anti-inflammatory effects of the steroid even at low doses. The infants in the trials were of similar size and gestational ages, and 83% to 92% of the infants had been exposed to antenatal steroids. Thus, this population differs from the postnatal steroid trials done before about 1994. We do not know how antennal steroid exposure might alter postnatal treatment responses.

A comment about the death differences in the trials seems appropriate. Mortality decreased for a 10-day hydrocortisone infusion and the budesonide in surfactant and treatment, but increased for the aerosol treatments continued for weeks. These are plausible outcomes given the more prolonged and perhaps higher exposure by nebulization. However, none of the differences in death rates were significant and thus may not be reproducible. Early steroid treatments—pick your strategy—are back on the table for decreasing BPD. But treatments for lung injury progressing toward BPD are also effective.[4] The surfactant plus budesonide strategy could be adapted for late treatments, as 2 recent trials demonstrated that surfactant treatments given after 10 to 14 days of age for respiratory failure were safe but not very effective.[7,8] Caution is warranted, however, as there are no follow-up data for 2 of the 3 early trials reviewed here. A report of a small trial of early treatment with hydrocortisone again raised concerns about neurodevelopment.[9] Very preterm infants may be exposed to antenatal steroids, early postnatal steroids followed by late postnatal steroids—a scary proposition.

A. H. Jobe, MD, PhD

References

1. Yeh TF, Chen CM, Wu SY, et al. Intratracheal administration of budesonide/surfactant to prevent bronchopulmonary dysplasia. *Am J Respir Crit Care Med.* 2016;193:86-95.
2. Baud O, Maury L, Lebail F, et al. PREMILOC trial study group. Effect of early low-dose hydrocortisone on survival without bronchopulmonary dysplasia in extremely preterm infants (PREMILOC): a double-blind, placebo-controlled, multicentre, randomised trial. *Lancet.* 2016;387:1827-1836.
3. Gyamfi-Bannerman C, Thom EA, Blackwell SC, et al. NICHD Maternal–Fetal Medicine Units Network. Antenatal betamethasone for women at risk for late preterm delivery. *N Engl J Med.* 2016;374:1311-1320.
4. Doyle LW, Halliday HL, Ehrenkranz RA, Davis PG, Sinclair JC. An update on the impact of postnatal systemic corticosteroids on mortality and cerebral palsy in preterm infants: effect modification by risk of bronchopulmonary dysplasia. *J Pediatr.* 2014;165:1258-1260.
5. Cole CH, Colton T, Shah BL, et al. Early inhaled glucocorticoid therapy to prevent bronchopulmonary dysplasia. *N Engl J Med.* 1999;340:1005-1010.
6. Jobe AH. Animal models, learning lessons to prevent and treat neonatal chronic lung disease. *Front Med (Lausanne).* 2015;2:49.
7. Ballard RA, Keller RL, Black DM, et al. TOLSURF Study Group. Randomized trial of late surfactant treatment in ventilated preterm infants receiving inhaled nitric oxide. *J Pediatr.* 2016;168:23-29.e4.
8. Hascoet JM, Picaud JC, Ligi I, et al. Late surfactant administration in very preterm neonates with prolonged respiratory distress and pulmonary outcome at 1 year of age: a randomized clinical trial. *JAMA Pediatr.* 2016;170:365-372.
9. Peltoniemi OM, Lano A, Yliherva A, Kari MA, Hallman M, Neonatal Hydrocortisone Working Group. Randomised trial of early neonatal hydrocortisone demonstrates potential undesired effects on neurodevelopment at preschool age. *Acta Paediatr.* 2016;105:159-164.

Endotracheal Intubation in Neonates: A Prospective Study of Adverse Safety Events in 162 Infants

Hatch LD, Grubb PH, Lea AS, et al (Vanderbilt Univ Med Ctr, Nashville, TN; Monroe Carell Jr Children's Hosp at Vanderbilt, Nashville, TN; et al)
J Pediatr 168:62-66, 2016

Objective.—To determine the rate of adverse events associated with endotracheal intubation in newborns and modifiable factors contributing to these events.

Study Design.—We conducted a prospective, observational study in a 100-bed, academic, level IV neonatal intensive care unit from September 2013 through June 2014. We collected data on intubations using standardized data collection instruments with validation by medical record review. Intubations in the delivery or operating rooms were excluded. The primary outcome was an intubation with any adverse event. Adverse events were defined and tracked prospectively as nonsevere or severe. We measured clinical variables including number of attempts to successful intubation and intubation urgency (elective, urgent, or emergent). We used logistic regression models to estimate the association of these variables with adverse events.

Results.—During the study period, 304 intubations occurred in 178 infants. Data were available for 273 intubations (90%) in 162 patients. Adverse events occurred in 107 (39%) intubations with nonsevere and severe events in 96 (35%) and 24 (8.8%) intubations, respectively. Increasing number of intubation attempts (OR 2.1, 95% CI, 1.6-2.6) and emergent intubations (OR 4.7, 95% CI, 1.7-13) were predictors of adverse events. The primary cause of emergent intubations was unplanned extubation (62%).

Conclusions.—Adverse events are common in the neonatal intensive care unit, occurring in 4 of 10 intubations. The odds of an adverse event doubled with increasing number of attempts and quadrupled in the emergent setting. Quality improvement efforts to address these factors are needed to improve patient safety (Table 1).

▶ "It's in!" the fellow declares triumphantly, as the colorimetric pedicap finally flashes bright yellow. You glance at the newborn's bedside monitor; the oxygen saturation is slowly rising above 40%. The nurse wipes bloody secretions from the infant's mouth—visible evidence of the local trauma induced by 3 intubation attempts.

The fellow records the procedure in her log: Procedure: Endotracheal Intubation. Result: Success.

Is this really success?

For years, neonatologists have studied success rates of neonatal intubation. We have tracked our trainees' declining proficiency in this skill and worried about the diminishing number of opportunities to teach this procedure. However, few studies have systematically reported adverse events during this high-risk procedure.

Hatch and colleagues' recent publication sheds important light on the prevalence of adverse events during neonatal intubation. The authors prospectively collected safety outcome data on 273 intubations in the Vanderbilt Neonatal Intensive Care Unit (NICU) (Appendix 1, pp. 1–2). They found a staggering 39% adverse event rate. Although most of these adverse events were deemed nonsevere, 9% of intubations were complicated by a severe adverse event, such as esophageal intubation with delayed recognition or cardiac arrest (Table 1).

Are these adverse events isolated to a single site? Likely not. In 2015, we published our experience of > 700 intubations performed in the Children's Hospital of Philadelphia (CHOP) NICU. Adverse events occurred in 22% of intubations studied.[1] Similar to Hatch et al, most of these events were nonsevere in nature; severe events occurred in 4% of intubations.

The rate of adverse events during neonatal intubation in both studies is unacceptably high. However, the differences in outcomes also suggest that some of these events may be preventable. For example, use of paralytic premedication was found to be protective against adverse events in the CHOP study. But

TABLE 1.—Intubation Associated Adverse Events by Severity (n = 273 Neonatal Intubation Encounters)

Nonsevere Events, n (%)		Severe Events, n (%)	
Any	96 (35)	Any	24 (8.8)
Esophageal intubation with immediate recognition	58 (21.4)	Hypotension receiving treatment*	10 (3.7)
Oral/airway bleeding	26 (9.5)	Transition to emergent	9 (3.3)
Difficult bag-mask ventilation	20 (7.3)	Chest compressions[†]	8 (2.9)
Mainstem bronchial intubation (confirmed by chest radiograph)	19 (7)	Code medications	2 (0.7)
Emesis	6 (2.2)	Pneumothorax	1 (0.4)
Chest wall rigidity[‡]	3 (1.1)	Direct airway trauma	1 (0.4)
		Death	1 (0.4)
		Esophageal intubation with delayed recognition	0

*Two infants were receiving treatment for hypotension prior to intubation but had escalation of treatment after intubation

[†]Four infants were receiving chest compressions at the time of the first intubation attempt that continued during the intubation attempts.

[‡]Two of 3 infants were treated with emergent intubation. No infant received pharmacologic treatment for chest wall rigidity.

Reprinted from Hatch LD, Grubb PH, Lea AS, et al. Endotracheal intubation in neonates: a prospective study of adverse safety events in 162 infants. *J Pediatr.* 2016;168:62-66, with permission Elsevier.

muscle relaxants were rarely used as premedication in the Vanderbilt cohort. These 2 studies also differ in terms of which adverse events were recorded and how they were defined, which may contribute to differences in outcomes. Both studies adapted adverse event definitions from the National Emergency Airway Registry for Children (NEAR4KIDS).[2] However, Hatch et al captured additional events thought to be applicable to neonates, such as chest wall rigidity. At CHOP we separately reported severe oxygen desaturations, which were deemed clinically relevant.

Large multisite neonatal studies, using standard definitions of neonatal-specific adverse events, would address some of these limitations. Further, a multicenter neonatal database would be a powerful tool for sites to benchmark their outcomes and identify best practices. A National Emergency Airway Registry for Neonates, NEAR4NEOS, is under development to fill this need.

Collecting and reporting safety events in a standardized fashion is only the first step in improving outcomes. Innovative interventions, such as video laryngoscopy, have been shown to improve the success of neonatal intubation.[3,4] Collaborations such as NEAR4NEOS may provide a robust setting for future clinical trials to determine whether these interventions also improve the safety of neonatal intubation.

In the meantime, I suggest we adjust our mental framework to consider the safety of intubation as a critical component of the procedure. In my mind, tracheal intubation without adverse events represents true success.

Appendix 1. Post-Intubation Provider Survey

Post-Intubation Provider Survey   **Patient Name**

First page to be filled out by senior provider supervising intubation course.*

Timing of Intubation (at beginning of procedure)*:	**Clinical Instability in 4 Hours Prior to Intubation:**
☐Emergent- see definition* ☐Urgent	☐CPR (chest compressions, epi)
☐Elective	☐Worsening Hypotension requiring therapy
	☐Greater than 2 spells requiring any intervention
Primary Reason for Intubation:	☐Worsening Hypoxia (↑ FIO2, ↑ INO or ↑ mean airway pressure)
☐Hypoxia ☐Code/Resuscitation	
☐Hypercarbia ☐Increased Work of Breathing	**Does the patient have craniofacial anomalies?** Yes/No
☐Apnea/Spells ☐Upper Airway Obstruction	
☐Surfactant ☐Pre-Surgical/Procedure/Transport	**Was patient able to be stabilized prior to intubation ?**
☐ET tube exchange ☐Self-extubation	(i.e. preoxygenation, effective bag-mask vent) yes/no
☐Other_____	

Premedication Practices

Opiates: ☐ Fentanyl ☐ Morphine ☐Dilaudid ☐Methadone ☐Remifentanil ☐Other_____

Sedatives: ☐Ativan ☐Versed ☐Phenobarbital ☐Pentobarbital ☐Other_____

Paralytic: ☐Vecuronium ☐Rocuronium ☐Cisatracurium ☐Succinylcholine ☐Other _____

Vagolytics: ☐Atropine ☐Robinul ☐Other_____

Other: ☐Propofol ☐Ketamine ☐ Etomidate ☐Other _____

☐No premedications used for intubation (Answer next question)

In the event no premedication was used, please provide reason:

☐Emergent/Code situation ☐No IV access ☐Upper Airway obstruction ☐Medications not readily available

☐Medications not needed ☐Concern for medication side effects (hypotension, apnea, etc.)

Other_____

Intubation Events- (Please check all boxes that occurred during intubation course)	
☐CPR- Chest compressions	☐CPR- medications (Epinephrine, Atropine)
☐Direct Airway Injury (i.e. Tracheal perforation)	☐Pneumothorax
☐Oral/Airway bleeding or trauma	☐Mainstem Bronchial Intubation
☐Rigid-chest syndrome (secondary to opiates)	☐Difficulty with bag-mask ventilation for any reason
☐Emesis	☐Hypoxia (Oxygen saturation less than 60)
☐Esophageal Intubation with desaturation prior to removal	☐Bradycardia (HR less than 60)
☐Esophageal Intubation with recognition prior to desaturation	☐Equipment needed not at bedside during procedure
☐Hypotension requiring treatment (IV fluids, ↑ BP meds)	☐Other_____
☐Pain/Agitation needing additional medications outside of the normal premedication sequence	
☐Transition from urgent/elective* intubation to emergent intubation* due to patient instability during procedure	

*Definitions:

Emergent Intubation- Establishment of airway necessary immediately due to physiologic instability. Vitals unable to stabilized until airway in place.

Urgent Intubation- Establishment of airway needed imminently (<4hrs) but time available for medication administration and pre-procedural patient stabilization.

Elective Intubation- Establishment of airway can begin at provider discretion due to patient stability.

Intubation Course-Course consists of one approach to secure an airway including one set of premedications. (Can involve multiple attempts)

Post-Intubation Provider Survey   **Patient Name**

If you attempted intubation, please fill out corresponding fields for each attempt.

Attempt 1

<u>Method</u>: ☐Oral ☐Nasal ☐Surgical/Tracheostomy <u>ET Tube Size</u>: ☐2.0 ☐2.5 ☐3.0 ☐3.5 ☐4.0   Cuffed/Uncuffed

<u>Equipment Used</u>: ☐Direct Laryngoscope ☐Video laryngoscope ☐Bronchoscopy ☐Other_____

<u>Blade Size</u>: ☐00 ☐0 ☐1   <u>Stylet Used</u>: ☐Yes ☐ No

<u>Current Clinical Role</u>:   ☐PGY-1 ☐PGY-2 ☐PGY-3 ☐1st yr Neo Fellow ☐2nd yr Neo Fellow ☐3rd yr Neo Fellow

                   ☐NNP ☐NICU Hospitalist ☐ Neo Attending ☐Other_____

<u>Prior neonatal intubation experience</u>: ☐<10 attempts at intubation ☐10-40 attempts ☐>40 attempts

<u>Was the attempt successful?</u> ☐ Yes ☐No

<u>If attempt was unsuccessful, what was reason?</u> (Check all that apply)

☐Cords not visualized ☐Patient decompensation prior to intubation ☐Cords visualized but ETT not able to be passed

☐Suctioning needed ☐Esophageal Intubation ☐Equipment failure ☐Other_____

Circle your view if able:

Grade1- Full Cords seen   Grade2- Partial Cords seen   Grade 3- Epiglottis seen only   Grade 4- Epiglottis not visible

Comments:

Attempt 2

<u>Method</u>: ☐Oral ☐Nasal ☐Surgical/Tracheostomy <u>ET Tube Size</u>: ☐2.0 ☐2.5 ☐3.0 ☐3.5 ☐4.0   Cuffed/Uncuffed

<u>Equipment Used</u>: ☐Direct Laryngoscope ☐Video laryngoscope ☐Bronchoscopy ☐Other_____

<u>Blade Size</u>: ☐00 ☐0 ☐1   <u>Stylet Used</u>: ☐Yes ☐ No

<u>Current Clinical Role</u>:   ☐PGY-1 ☐PGY-2 ☐PGY-3 ☐1st yr Neo Fellow ☐2nd yr Neo Fellow ☐3rd yr Neo Fellow

                   ☐NNP ☐NICU Hospitalist ☐ Neo Attending ☐Other_____

<u>Prior neonatal intubation experience</u>: ☐<10 attempts at intubation ☐10-40 attempts ☐>40 attempts

<u>Was the attempt successful?</u> ☐ Yes ☐No

<u>If attempt was unsuccessful, what was reason?</u> (Check all that apply)

☐Cords not visualized ☐Patient decompensation prior to intubation ☐Cords visualized but ETT not able to be passed

☐Suctioning needed ☐Esophageal Intubation ☐Equipment failure ☐Other_____

Circle your view if able:

Grade1- Full Cords seen   Grade2- Partial Cords seen   Grade 3- Epiglottis seen only   Grade 4- Epiglottis not visible

Comments:

---

*Definitions:

<u>Attempt</u>- Laryngoscope blade into and out of the mouth.

E. E. Foglia, MD

References

1. Foglia EE, Ades A, Napolitano N, Leffelman J, Nadkarni V, Nishisaki A. Factors associated with adverse events during tracheal intubation in the NICU. *Neonatology.* 2015;108:23-29.
2. Nishisaki A, Turner DA, Brown CA, Walls RM, Nadkarni VM, National Emergency Airway Registry for Children (NEAR4KIDS), Pediatric Acute Lung Injury and Sepsis Investigators (PALISI) Network. A national emergency airway registry

for children: landscape of tracheal intubation in 15 PICUs. *Crit Care Med.* 2013; 41:874-885.
3. O-Shea JE, Thio M, Kamlin CO, et al. Videolaryngoscopy to teach neonatal intubation: a randomized trial. *Pediatrics.* 2015;136:912-919.
4. Moussa A, Luangxay Y, Tremblay S, et al. Videolaryngoscope for teaching neonatal endotracheal intubation: a randomized controlled trial. *Pediatrics.* 2016;137: e20152156.

Neonatal Glycemia and Neurodevelopmental Outcomes at 2 Years

McKinlay CJD, for the CHYLD Study Group (Univ of Auckland, New Zealand; et al)
N Engl J Med 373:1507-1518, 2015

Background.—Neonatal hypoglycemia is common and can cause neurologic impairment, but evidence supporting thresholds for intervention is limited.

Methods.—We performed a prospective cohort study involving 528 neonates with a gestational age of at least 35 weeks who were considered to be at risk for hypoglycemia; all were treated to maintain a blood glucose concentration of at least 47 mg per deciliter (2.6 mmol per liter). We intermittently measured blood glucose for up to 7 days. We continuously monitored interstitial glucose concentrations, which were masked to clinical staff. Assessment at 2 years included Bayley Scales of Infant Development III and tests of executive and visual function.

Results.—Of 614 children, 528 were eligible, and 404 (77% of eligible children) were assessed; 216 children (53%) had neonatal hypoglycemia (blood glucose concentration, <47 mg per deciliter). Hypoglycemia, when treated to maintain a blood glucose concentration of at least 47 mg per deciliter, was not associated with an increased risk of the primary outcomes of neurosensory impairment (risk ratio, 0.95; 95% confidence interval [CI], 0.75 to 1.20; $P = 0.67$) and processing difficulty, defined as an executive-function score or motion coherence threshold that was more than 1.5 SD from the mean (risk ratio, 0.92; 95% CI, 0.56 to 1.51; $P = 0.74$). Risks were not increased among children with unrecognized hypoglycemia (a low interstitial glucose concentration only). The lowest blood glucose concentration, number of hypoglycemic episodes and events, and negative interstitial increment (area above the interstitial glucose concentration curve and below 47 mg per deciliter) also did not predict the outcome.

Conclusions.—In this cohort, neonatal hypoglycemia was not associated with an adverse neurologic outcome when treatment was provided to maintain a blood glucose concentration of at least 47 mg per deciliter. (Funded by the Eunice Kennedy Shriver National Institute of Child Health and Human Development and others.)

▶ The brain is uniquely dependent on glucose for oxidative metabolism and therefore is particularly vulnerable to hypoglycemic injury.[1] Management of low blood glucose concentrations in the newborn is aimed at avoiding hypoglycemic brain injury. One strategy commonly used to accomplish this is to screen asymptomatic newborn infants who are at risk for hypoglycemia and then treat identified low blood glucose concentrations before the infant becomes symptomatic. A further goal is to identify those newborns who may have a potential serious and recurrent disorder of hypoglycemia, such as congenital hyperinsulinemic hypoglycemia, fatty acid oxidation disorders, hypopituitarism, and glycogen storage diseases, so that brain injury can be prevented in these patients.[2]

Controversy about the impact of low glucose concentrations in newborn infants and their need for treatment exists because low blood glucose concentrations in newborns are extraordinarily common. This makes it difficult to discriminate between the minority of newborns who will have hypoglycemic brain injury from the vast majority of newborns in whom the low blood sugars are transient and without obvious adverse neurodevelopmental outcomes. There is little information to determine the glucose concentration threshold one should use for treatment and to determine the glucose concentration threshold and duration of hypoglycemia necessary to cause permanent neurological injury or to trigger an investigation into potential serious and recurrent disorders of hypoglycemia. Information of this type would have a positive impact on our ability to design safe and appropriate management strategies.

The newborns who are most commonly at risk for asymptomatic hypoglycemia are those born late preterm, those who are small for gestational age or intrauterine growth restricted (SGA/IUGR), those who are large for gestational age (LGA), or infants of diabetic mothers (IDM). These are the groups that McKinlay et al included in their prospective cohort study tracking 2-year neurodevelopmental outcomes of newborns with hypoglycemia defined as < 47 mg/dL (2.6 mmol/L) and treated to a goal glucose concentration equal to or greater than this value versus similarly at-risk newborns without hypoglycemia. They found that hypoglycemic newborns treated by their protocol with oral feeds, buccal dextrose gel, and/or intravenous dextrose had neurodevelopmental outcomes that were similar to those who never developed hypoglycemia. This assumes that the infants were screened in the first 48 hours before most feeds and treatment achieved or exceeded the target plasma glucose concentration of 47 mg/dL (2.6 mmol/L). This is the first outcomes-based evidence for the screening protocol that McKinlay et al employed and the practice of using ≥47 mg/dL (2.6 mmol/L) as a treatment goal.

This study did not, however, compare one management strategy or treatment threshold/goal versus another. Multiple studies from this research group have used a plasma glucose concentration of 47 mg/dL (2.6 mmol/L) as their threshold for diagnosis and treatment of neonatal hypoglycemia irrespective of age and a screening protocol that employs frequent measurements of blood glucose concentrations in the first 48 hours.[3-5] This is not a universally accepted diagnosis and treatment strategy or a definition of hypoglycemia.[6-9] To date, there are no outcomes-based data from randomized, controlled trials testing one strategy versus another to rationally choose among these and other recommendations for diagnosis and/or treatment of neonatal hypoglycemia. The variability among the diagnosis and treatment strategy recommendations among many publications that have not been based on randomized, controlled trials but on older literature reports reflects the need for further research to determine optimal approaches to diagnosing and preventing complications of neonatal hypoglycemia.[8,10] The high rates of neurodevelopmental delay at 2 years of age in the McKinlay et al study in both those newborns who experienced a hypoglycemic event (33%) and those who did not (36%) also should stimulate further research before one concludes that it was the treatment strategy that prevented hypoglycemia-induced neurodevelopmental delays.

An important feature of the McKinlay et al study is the use of Continuous Glucose Monitoring Sensors (CGMS) to monitor interstitial glucose concentrations. The data obtained from the CGMS system combined with their standard screening measurements and outcome data led to three important associative relationship observations. The first is that newborns who maintained plasma glucose concentrations greater than 54 mg/dL (3.0 mmol/L) had better outcomes than those newborns who did not. The second association was that if a newborn spent more time with glucose concentrations outside the range of 54 to 72 mg/dL (3.0 to 4.0 mmol/L) they had worse neurodevelopmental outcomes than those who spent more time within this range. These 2 associations should probably not change clinical practice. In fact, they are somewhat conflicting in the conclusions they might lead to. It is most likely that these associations simply show that sicker neonates have more unstable glucose concentrations and have worse 2-year neurodevelopmental outcomes. Based on these data, however, the possibility that increased glucose concentration variability, or slightly higher glucose concentrations themselves, caused worse neurodevelopmental outcomes cannot be excluded.

Third, the authors found that babies treated with dextrose for hypoglycemia who had a rapid increase in their blood and/or interstitial glucose concentrations after treatment had worse neurodevelopmental outcomes than those hypoglycemic newborns who did not have such a rapid rise in their glucose concentrations. Although the data are only associative, they call into question the traditional practice of treating an asymptomatic newborn with a low blood glucose concentration with a "mini-bolus" of intravenous dextrose (200 mg/kg over 5–10 minutes) followed by a continuous infusion of dextrose at a rate of 4 to 6 mg/kg/min. Hypoglycemic newborns treated with only a continuous dextrose infusion achieve glucose concentrations similar to those treated with the dextrose "mini-bolus" followed by the same continuous dextrose infusion rate within 20 to 30 minutes.[11] Given that no study has shown a benefit of the treatment of asymptomatic hypoglycemia, no matter how rapidly the glucose concentration is corrected, perhaps the alternative strategy of bypassing the "mini-bolus" and simply starting asymptomatic newborns who have persistently low glucose concentrations that are deemed necessary to treat intravenously on a continuous infusion of dextrose would be safer.

There are significant risks and benefits to any screening and treatment strategy for asymptomatic neonatal hypoglycemia. If a strategy is too aggressive, then risks of treatment increase, including a greater number of blood draws, use of formula supplementation that diminishes breastfeeding and maternal milk production, admission of the infant to the neonatal intensive care unit with separation from the mother, and use of intravenous catheters. These risks must be balanced against the potential harm due to asymptomatic hypoglycemia (if there is any), progression to symptomatic hypoglycemia, and delay in diagnosis and treatment of serious metabolic disorders. The study by McKinlay et al does not point to one strategy as superior to another. Furthermore, the observations in the McKinlay et al study cannot necessarily be extrapolated to symptomatic hypoglycemia or to different groups of newborn infants, such as more preterm infants, who were not included in the groups that McKinley, et al. studied, or those with recurrent low glucose concentrations. These patients also need to be studied further. But the study by McKinlay et al does provide some confidence that at least one screening and treatment protocol for asymptomatic glucose concentrations less than 47 mg/dL (2.6 mmol/L) leads to neurodevelopmental outcomes that are similar to at-risk newborns who did not experience a glucose concentrations < 47 mg/dL (2.6 mmol/L)

P. J. Rozance, MD

W. W. Hay, Jr, MD

References

1. Rozance PJ, Hay WW. Hypoglycemia in newborn infants: features associated with adverse outcomes. *Biol Neonate.* 2006;90:74-86.
2. Stanley CA, Rozance PJ, Thornton PS, et al. Re-evaluating "transitional neonatal hypoglycemia": mechanism and implications for management. *J Pediatr.* 2015; 166:1520-1525. 201.
3. Harris DL, Battin MR, Weston PJ, Harding JE. Continuous glucose monitoring in newborn babies at risk of hypoglycemia. *J Pediatr.* 2010;157:198-202.
4. Harris DL, Weston PJ, Harding JE. Incidence of neonatal hypoglycemia in babies identified as at risk. *J Pediatr.* 2012;161:787-791.
5. Harris DL, Weston PJ, Signal M, Chase JG, Harding JE. Dextrose gel for neonatal hypoglycaemia (the Sugar Babies Study): a randomised, double-blind, placebo-controlled trial. *Lancet.* 2013;382:2077-2083.
6. Boardman JP, Wusthoff CJ, Cowan FM. Hypoglycaemia and neonatal brain injury. *Arch Dis Child Educ Pract Ed.* 2015;98:2-6.
7. American Academy of Pediatrics Committee on Fetus and Newborn: routine evaluation of blood pressure, hematocrit, and glucose in newborns. *Pediatrics.* 1993;92:474-476.
8. Boluyt N, van KA, Offringa M. Neurodevelopment after neonatal hypoglycemia: a systematic review and design of an optimal future study. *Pediatrics.* 2006;117: 2231-2243.
9. Thornton PS, Stanley CA, De Leon DD, et al. Recommendations from the pediatric endocrine society for evaluation and management of persistent hypoglycemia in neonates, infants, and children. *J Pediatr.* 2006;167:238-245.
10. Hay WW Jr, Raju TN, Higgins RD, et al. Knowledge gaps and research needs for understanding and treating neonatal hypoglycemia: workshop report from Eunice Kennedy Shriver National Institute of Child Health and Human Development. *J Pediatr.* 2015;155:612-617.
11. Lilien LD, Pildes RS, Srinivasan G, Voora S, Yeh TF. Treatment of neonatal hypoglycemia with minibolus and intraveous glucose infusion. *J Pediatr.* 2009;97:295-298.

Neurodevelopmental Outcomes of Premature Infants Treated for Patent Ductus Arteriosus: A Population-Based Cohort Study

Janz-Robinson EM, behalf of the Neonatal Intensive Care Units Network (Canberra Hosp, Garran, Australian Capital Territory, Australia; et al)
J Pediatr 167:1025-1032, 2015

Objective.—To compare neurodevelopmental outcomes of extremely preterminfants diagnosed with patent ductus arteriosus (PDA) who were treated medically or surgically and those who were not diagnosed with PDA or who did not undergo treatment for PDA.

Study Design.—This retrospective population-based cohort study used data from a geographically defined area in New South Wales and the Australian Capital Territory served by a network of 10 neonatal intensive care units. Patients included all preterm infants born at <29 completed weeks of gestation between 1998 and 2004. Moderate/severe functional disability at 2-3 years corrected age was defined as developmental delay, cerebral palsy requiring aids, sensorineural or conductive deafness (requiring bilateral hearing aids or cochlear implant), or bilateral blindness (best visual acuity of <6/60).

Results.—Follow-up information at age 2-3 years was available for 1473 infants (74.8%). Compared with infants not diagnosed with a PDA or who did not receive PDA treatment for PDA, those with medically treated PDA (aOR, 1.622; 95% CI, 1.199-2.196) and those with surgically treated PDA (aOR, 2.001; 95% CI, 1.126-3.556) were at significantly greater risk for adverse neurodevelopmental outcomes at age 2-3 years.

Conclusion.—Our results demonstrate that treatment for PDA may be associated with a greater risk of adverse neurodevelopmental outcome at age 2-3 years. This was particularly so among infants born at <25 weeks gestation. These results may support permissive tolerance of PDAs; however, reasons for this association remain to be elucidated through carefully designed prospective trials (Fig 3).

▶ During fetal life, the ductus arteriosus connects the aorta to the main pulmonary artery shunting blood away from the developing lung. When a fetus is delivered prematurely, this normal part of fetal physiology becomes a pesky problem if it remains open after birth; blood flow reverses its direction through the patent ductus arteriosus (PDA) causing pulmonary edema. It seems natural then to just close the ductus either by medical or surgical means. However, as Janz-Robinson et al describe in their background, both of these treatments have important complications to consider. Despite hundreds of studies, the treatment of this tiny vessel continues to be a conundrum and spark controversy among neonatologists.

The large retrospective population-based study by Janz-Robinson et al is one of several that have investigated the association between PDA treatment and neurodevelopmental impairment (NDI). The authors compared infants who either did not have or were felt by their physicians not to require treatment of their PDA with those who were treated medically (with cyclooxygenase

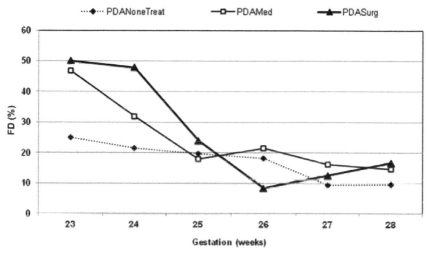

FIGURE 3.—GA-specific moderate-to-severe FD stratified by the 3 study groups: PDANoneTreat, n = 826; PDAMed, n = 569; PDASurg, n = 78. (Reprinted from Janz-Robinson EM, behalf of the Neonatal Intensive Care Units Network. Neurodevelopmental outcomes of premature infants treated for patent ductus arteriosus: a population-based cohort study. *J Pediatr.* 2015;167:1025-1032, with permission from Elsevier.)

inhibitors) or surgically (87% of the ligations occurred after failed medical treatment). They found that both medical treatment and surgical treatment of the PDA was associated with neurodevelopmental impairment at a corrected age of 2 to 3 years.

At this moment in time, no randomized controlled trials (RCTs) have been performed that can tell us whether surgical ligation plays a causative role in later NDI. The findings of Janz-Robinson et al are consistent with those of other cohort studies that have previously examined the relationship between surgery and NDI.[1-4]

Although there may be no RCTs that have examined the relationship between surgery and NDI, there are several RCTs and meta-analyses that have examined the relationship between the medical treatments used to close the PDA (cyclooxygenase inhibitors) and NDI.[5] These RCTs found that cyclooxygenase inhibitors, like indomethacin, either have no effect or a beneficial effect on neurodevelopment.[5] This is exactly the opposite of what Janz-Robinson et al reported.

So why then did Janz-Robinson et al find that infants who received medical treatment of a PDA have a higher incidence of functional disability at 2 to 3 years of age? Do their findings, as they conclude in the abstract, "support permissive tolerance of PDAs?" The answer to the latter question is no, and we will demonstrate how bias and residual confounding could result in a spurious association between PDA treatment and NDI/functional disability.

Selection bias is the main pitfall of most observational studies and the study of Janz-Robinson et al is no exception. To evaluate whether a medical treatment has detrimental effects, one would ideally want to identify infants who received treatment in an unbiased manner. In Janz-Robinson et al's study, infants received treatment because they were felt to "need it." Does needing PDA treatment carry with it certain biases? Of course it does! The most important factors that lead to NDI are the infant's degree of immaturity and severity of illness during the neonatal period. Many studies have shown that there is also a significant relationship between the variables that cause NDI (immaturity and illness severity), and the variables that Janz-Robinson et al were studying (the need for treatment of the PDA and its response to treatment). Therefore, not ensuring that the different PDA treatment groups are similar in their degree of immaturity and illness can confound the outcome of the analysis.

The authors used logistic regression to adjust for these confounders. They included several variables that are linked to maturity and illness: birth weight percentile, gestational age, antenatal steroid exposure, multiple birth, assisted conception, male sex, and outborn status. However, they failed to adjust for many of the more important variables known to be linked to maturity, illness, and NDI. In particular, they did not adjust for intraventricular hemorrhage (IVH), necrotizing enterocolitis (NEC), or bronchopulmonary dysplasia (BPD). IVH, NEC, and BPD are all strongly associated with NDI. Janz-Robertson et al argued that these important confounders were "on the casual pathway" between PDA treatment and functional disability and that including them in the multivariable analysis would obscure the relationship between PDA treatment and NDI.

Although observational studies have reported an association between "medical treatment of the PDA" and IVH, NEC, and BPD, prior RCTs and systemic reviews have found just the opposite—namely, that medical treatment of the PDA does not "cause" IVH, NEC, or BPD (in fact, indomethacin, when given before the onset of IVH, is actually protective against IVH).[5,6] In other words, the "need for PDA treatment" is really just a biomarker or surrogate variable for immaturity and illness severity—a biomarker that also identifies infants at risk for IVH, NEC, and BPD—just like other surrogate variables for immaturity and illness severity (eg, gestational age, birth weight, etc). Not adjusting for these important confounders (or other unspecified confounders, like differences in treatment practices) will result in residual confounding and lead to false conclusions about the associations between PDA treatment and NDI.

The randomized controlled trial is ubiquitously accepted as the gold standard of clinical research. It is not an uncommon scenario for the results of prior observational trials to be refuted by well-designed randomized controlled trials as we saw in this instance. Although the modern epidemiologist strives to conduct observational trials that are free of bias and residual confounding, it would be naive to think that even the best conducted observational trial could establish causation. Observational trials can only demonstrate associations between the predictor and the outcome studied.

So what can we learn from this study? The important finding in this study is the association between the need for PDA treatment (and its success or failure) and subsequent NDI. Even this association is limited by the gestational age of the infants studied. For infants at the limits of viability (23–24 weeks), the need for PDA treatment is strongly associated with NDI. At 25 to 28 weeks' gestation, however, there is little difference in functional disability between the treatment strategies (Fig 3). Instead of suggesting that PDA treatment causes neurodevelopmental impairment, this supports the idea that the need to intervene and treat a PDA is itself a marker of immaturity (and perhaps a better one than gestational age at 23 to 24 weeks) and can help identify infants at highest risk for neurodevelopmental impairment.

M. C. Liebowitz, MD

R. I. Clyman, MD

References

1. Wickremasinghe AC, Rogers EE, Piecuch RE, et al. Neurodevelopmental outcomes following two different treatment approaches (early ligation and selective ligation) for patent ductus arteriosus. *J Pediatr.* 2012;161:1065-1072.
2. Madan JC, Kendrick D, Hagadorn JI, Frantz ID, National Institute of Child Health and Human Development Neonatal Research Network. Patent ductus arteriosus therapy: impact on neonatal and 18-month outcome. *Pediatrics.* 2009;123: 674-681.
3. Bourgoin L, Cipierre C, Hauet Q, et al. Neurodevelopmental outcome at 2 years of age according to patent ductus arteriosus management in very preterm infants. *Neonatology.* 2016;109:139-146.
4. Kabra NS, Schmidt B, Roberts RS, Doyle LW, Papile L, Fanaroff A. Neurosensory impairment after surgical closure of patent ductus arterio- sus in extremely low birth weight infants: results from the Trial of Indomethacin Prophylaxis in Preterms. *J Pediatr.* 2007;150:229-234.
5. Fowlie PW, Davis PG, McGuire W. Prophylactic intravenous indomethacin for preventing mortality and morbidity in preterm infants. *Cochrane Database Syst Rev.* 2010;(7):CD000174.
6. Cooke L, Steer P, Woodgate P. Indomethacin for asymptomatic patent ductus arteriosus in preterm infants. *Cochrane Database Syst Rev.* 2003;(2):CD003745.

Stopping Parenteral Nutrition for 3 Hours Reduces False Positives in Newborn Screening

Tim-Aroon T, Harmon HM, Nock ML, et al (Univ Hosps Case Med Ctr, Cleveland, OH; Case Western Reserve Univ, Cleveland, OH)

J Pediatr 167:312-316, 2015

Objective.—To evaluate effects of holding parenteral nutrition (PN) for 3 hours prior to newborn screening (NBS) on false-positive NBS rate for amino acids (AAs) in very low birth weight (VLBW) infants (birth weight <1500 g).

Study Design.—We analyzed data from 12 567 consecutive births in 1 hospital between May 2010 and June 2013. VLBW infants were stratified into 3 groups: (1) infants without PN before NBS (no-PN group); (2) infants with early PN running at the time of NBS (early-PN group); and (3) infants with early-PN that were temporarily replaced by dextrose-containing intravenous fluid 3 hours prior to NBS (stop-PN group). We compared the false-positive rate for AA and cost effectiveness between the groups.

Results.—The false-positive rate for AA among 413 VLBW infants was significantly higher than infants with birth weight >1500 g (7.62% vs 0.05%; $P < .001$). There were no false-positive results for AA in the no-PN group. The false-positive rate for AA in the stop-PN group (2/65) was significantly lower than the early-PN group (29/245) (3.1% vs 11.8%; $P = .037$). The stop-PN group was more cost effective than early-PN group, saving $17.27 per infant screened ($5.53 vs $22.80) or $192.54 for each false-positive result for AA averted. Further reductions in inconclusive samples were also noted.

Conclusions.—VLBW and early-PN are significant factors for false-positive results for AA. Holding PN containing AAs for 3 hours before NBS collection is a practical and cost-effective method to significantly reduce the false-positive rate for AA in VLBW infants.

▶ There are several important findings reported by Tim-Aroon et al. First, and most importantly, very low birth weight (VLBW) and early implementation of parenteral nutrition influence the amino acid profiles used for screening newborns for inborn errors in metabolism. Second, the false-positive rate for screening can be reduced. Finally, intravenous amino acids can lead to high levels of specific analytes. Other studies show similar results and demonstrate the complexity of understanding the impact of immaturity, postnatal age, and intravenous nutrition (glucose, amino acids, and lipids) on metabolism and metabolic profiles.[1-3] As the authors discuss, reducing the false-positive rate by eliminating the confounding effect of intravenous nutrition has 2 important effects; it reduces the pain and stress caused by retesting and it decreases the cost of screening.

Most of the analytes used to diagnose inborn errors of metabolism change with postnatal age. The metabolism (and resultant metabolic profiles) of prematurely born infants are different from those of more mature infants. The most immature and fragile infants often require prolonged support with parenteral nutrition. The confounding effects of intravenous nutrition (amino acids and lipids) are independent of gestational age at birth and postnatal age.[4]

False-positive results, like false alarms, make us less vigilant—ie, "it is just the intravenous nutrition." False results (negative and positive), like any false alarms, increase stress and costs. Trying to explain to a parent why we are continuing to repeat a test is hard on the parent and the providers. False-negative results are equally important. Failure to diagnosis a real inborn error of metabolism would be rare but potentially devastating to the patient and his or her family. In any profiling, screening, or diagnostic test, there has to be a continuous effort, no matter how good the test, to push these false alarm rates toward zero.

Withholding intravenous amino acids for 3 hours is an effective strategy for reducing the false-positive rate and the associated stress (physical and mental). What is harder to know is if it is safe. Clinicians would be reluctant to withhold glucose for 3 hours in an infant who completely depended on intravenous nutrition. Withholding amino acids may be safe, but understanding the most effective and safest approach for reducing false-positive results is still undetermined. Other nutritional supplements also impact metabolic profiles and include intravenous lipids and L-carnitine. We believe the best approach will involve adjusting for these confounding variables: nutritional support, gestational age at birth, and postnatal age. Developing better algorithms that are gestational age/birth weight and nutritional support specific could reduce the false-positive rate and eliminate the need for withholding important nutritional support. Immature infants are often deficient in essential amino acids, lipids, and free carnitine, and withholding (even for a short period) key nutritional support in the most immature infants may not be prudent.

A more subtle but equally important finding is that VLBW infants more often have elevated levels of certain amino acids when they are on intravenous amino acids, and this occurs less often when amino acids are withheld for as little as 3 hours. These findings are reassuring; elevated levels do not persist when the amino acids are stopped. This finding is consistent with those of other studies that have shown a correlation between amino acid dose and increased amino acid levels.[5,6] What is much less clear is what levels (low and high) are safe.[4]

Nutrition is a dynamic interaction between what is provided (glucose/carbohydrates, protein/amino acids, lipids/fatty-acids/carnitine), how it is provided (intravenous or enteral), how it is used for energy and growth, and how each nutritional component is metabolized. Just as there are adverse events associated with drug—drug interactions that relate to metabolism, the potential for adverse side effects related to nutritional—nutritional interactions is also real. Just as both high and low values of glucose can cause injury, high and low values of amino acids and acylcarnitines may cause long-term morbidity. Investigations are needed to define what values are safe in premature infants. The authors are to be congratulated for adding important new information on how to better evaluate the metabolism of preterm/VLBW infants.

R. H. Clark, MD

D. Chace, PhD

References

1. Morris M, Fischer K, Leydiker K, Elliott L, Newby J, Abdenur JE. Reduction in newborn screening metabolic false-positive results following a new collection protocol. *Genet Med.* 2014;16:477-483.
2. Kalish BT, Le HD, Gura KM, Bistrian BR, Puder M. A metabolomic analysis of two intravenous lipid emulsions in a murine model. *PLoS One.* 2013;8:e59653.
3. Bulbul A, Okan F, Bulbul L, Nuhoglu A. Effect of low versus high early parenteral nutrition on plasma amino acid profiles in very low birth-weight infants. *J Matern Fetal Neonatal Med.* 2012;25:770-776.
4. Clark RH, Kelleher AS, Chace DH, Spitzer AR. Gestational age and age at sampling influence metabolic profiles in premature infants. *Pediatrics.* 2014;134: e37-e46.
5. Clark RH, Chace DH, Spitzer AR. Effects of two different doses of amino acid supplementation on growth and blood amino acid levels in premature neonates admitted to the neonatal intensive care unit: a randomized, controlled trial. *Pediatrics.* 2007;120:1286-1296.
6. Blanco CL, Gong AK, Schoolfield J, et al. Impact of early and high amino acid supplementation on ELBW infants at 2 years. *J Pediatr Gastroenterol Nutr.* 2012;54: 601-607.

Safety of Early High-Dose Recombinant Erythropoietin for Neuroprotection in Very Preterm Infants

Fauchère JC, on behalf of the Swiss Erythropoietin Neuroprotection Trial Group (Univ of Zurich, Switzerland; et al)

J Pediatr 167:52-57, 2015

Objective.—To investigate the safety and short term outcome of high dose recombinant human erythropoietin (rhEpo) given shortly after birth and subsequently over the first 2 days for neuroprotection to very preterm infants.

Study Design.—Randomized, double masked phase II trial. Preterm infants (gestational age 26 0/7-31 6/7 weeks) were given rhEpo ($n_t = 229$; 3000 U/kg body weight) or NaCl 0.9% ($n_c = 214$) intravenously at 3, 12-18, and 36-42 hours after birth.

Results.—There were no relevant differences between the groups for short-term outcomes such as mortality, retinopathy of prematurity, intraventricular hemorrhage, sepsis, necrotizing enterocolitis, and bronchopulmonary dysplasia. At day 7-10, we found significantly higher hematocrit values, reticulocyte, and white blood cell counts, and a lower platelet count in the rhEpo group.

Conclusions.—Early high-dose rhEpo administration to very premature infants is safe and causes no excess in mortality or major adverse events.

Trial Registration.—ClinicalTrials.gov: NCT00413946 (Table 2).

▶ Over the 25-plus years that neonatal erythropoietin (EPO) studies have been published, the message has cycled (in typical neonatology fashion) from "This might be great!" to "This IS great!" to "This might cause harm, don't use it!" to "No, really, it's great" to the current message in this publication: "We don't know yet how great it might be, but it certainly does not cause harm." What a roller-coaster ride.

Studies in the mid-1990s began exploring potential nonhematopoietic effects of erythropoiesis stimulating agents (ESAs) such as EPO and darbepoetin alfa (Darbe), a long-acting ESA, and a number of animal models provided evidence that higher ESA dosing might be the neuroprotective treatment neonatologists had been searching for to improve neurodevelopmental outcomes in preterm infants.[1] In January 2006, Fauchere and colleagues began enrolling preterm infants in a high-dose EPO study designed to evaluate neurodevelopmental outcomes at 2 years corrected age. The eligibility criteria were based on the Swiss Study Group's previous pilot study,[2] with 2 exceptions: infants 24 0/7 to 25 6/7 weeks were excluded, as were infants with grade III/IV intracranial hemorrhage. The resulting 443 preterm infants had an average weight greater than 1200 g and a gestational age greater than 29 weeks, somewhat larger than the micropremies on whom so many outcomes studies are focused. The ongoing PENUT (Preterm EPO Neuroprotection) Trial is evaluating preterm infants between 24 and 28 weeks' gestation,[3] and results of that trial will likely be more generalizable to the US neonatal intensive care unit (NICU) population of extremely low birth weight infants.

Similar to studies of oxygen use and retinopathy of prematurity (ROP) in which bronchopulmonary dysplasia (BPD) is always a related morbidity, EPO

TABLE 2.—Neonatal Morbidity According to Treatment

	Placebo		rhEpo		
	($n_c = 214$)	%	($n_t = 229$)	%	Difference, OR (CI 95%)
Death	12	5.6	12	5.2	OR 1.1 (0.5-2.5)
Survivors	202	94.4	217	94.8	OR 1.1 (0.5-2.5)
IVH grade 1-4 vs no IVH	41/214	21.1	43/229	18.8	OR 1.0 (0.6-1.6)
IVH with ventricular dilation (grade 3) vs no IVH	4/214	1.9	3/229	1.3	OR 0.7 (0.2-3.2)
Cerebral venous infarction (grade 4) vs no IVH	6/214	2.8	10/229	4.4	OR 1.6 (0.6-4.4)
Persisting periventricular echodensities (>7 d)	72/214	33.6	78/229	34.1	OR 1.0 (0.7-1.5)
Cystic PVL	3/214	1.4	4/229	1.7	OR 1.3 (0.3-5.7)
ROP grade 1-4 vs no ROP	19/191	9.9	20/212	9.4	OR 0.9 (0.5-1.8)
ROP grade 1 vs no ROP	8/191	4.2	6/212	2.8	OR 0.7 (0.2-2.0)
ROP grade 2 vs no ROP	6/191	3.1	12/212	5.7	OR 1.8 (0.7-4.9)
ROP grade 3 vs no ROP	5/191	2.6	2/212	0.9	OR 0.4 (0.1-1.9)
ROP grade 4	0/191	0	0/212	0	-
ROP plus disease vs no ROP	2/191	1.0	2/212	0.9	OR 0.9 (0.1-6.4)
ROP exam not assessed (death or no supplemental oxygen)	23/214	10.7	17/229	7.4	
Sepsis	29/214	13.6	31/229	13.5	OR 1.0 (0.6-1.7)
NEC	10/214	4.7	6/229	2.6	OR 0.6 (0.2-1.5)
PDA (treatment needed)	65/214	30.4	65/229	28.4	OR 0.9 (0.6-1.4)
PDA surgical ligation	10/214	4.7	4/229	1.7	OR 0.4 (0.1-1.2)
BPD (oxygen dependence at 36 0/7 wk PMA) vs no BPD	67/214	31.3	71/229	31.0	OR 1.0 (0.7-1.5)
BPD mild vs no BPD	40/214	18.7	43/229	18.8	OR 1.0 (0.6-1.6)
BPD moderate vs no BPD	21/214	9.8	18/229	7.9	OR 0.8 (0.4-1.6)
BPD severe vs no BPD	6/214	2.8	10/229	4.4	OR 1.6 (0.6-4.4)
Survivors without severe IVH, PVL, ROP	183/214	85.5	196/229	85.6	OR 1.0 (0.6-1.7)
Hemangioma	21/214	9.8	30/229	13.1	OR 1.4 (0.8-2.5)
Hematologic parameters					
Hematocrit at day 7-10 (%)	44.7		47.3		Diff −2.6 (−4.3 to −1.0)
Reticulocytes at day 7-10 (G/L)	80.4		372.5		Diff −292.2 (−334.6 to −249.6)
Platelet count at day 7-10 (G/L)	274.4		205.1		Diff 69.3 (41.2-97.5)
WBC count at day 7-10 (G/L)	13.4		19.4		Diff −6.0 (−8.1 to −3.9)

BPD, bronchopulmonary dysplasia; *NEC*, necrotizing enterocolitis; *PDA*, persistent ductus arteriosus.
The differences regarding the denominators for different variables are due to missing values.
Reprinted from Fauchère JC, on behalf of the Swiss Erythropoietin Neuroprotection Trial Group. Safety of early high-dose recombinant erythropoietin for neuroprotection in very preterm infants. *J Pediatr.* 2015;167:52-57, with permission from Elsevier.

investigators continue to focus on ROP outcomes when evaluating hematopoietic and nonhematopoietic effects of EPO in preterm infants (Table 2). This is primarily due to a Cochrane review in 2006[4] that mistakenly linked early EPO administration with an increased incidence of stage > 2 ROP. A corrected review was published in 2014,[5] but the damage was done. It may be possible in the near future to alter misperceptions with the addition of Fauchere's study and a recent EPO study performed by Zhu and colleagues in China.[6] When ROP outcomes from those 2 studies are included in the most recent counts (more than doubling the numbers reported in the 2014 review), the incidence of ROP in EPO-treated and placebo-treated infants is nearly identical: 119 of 988 (12.0%) of EPO-treated infants versus 128 of 959 (13.3%) of placebo-treated infants had ROP stage 3 or greater diagnosed during their hospital stay ($P = .414$).

This switch in focus from blood/transfusion effects to brain/neuroprotection effects has rejuvenated interest in the use of EPO in the NICU, resulting in a possible "comeback" for this important growth factor. But don't discount its hematopoietic properties when evaluating total impact on neurodevelopmental outcomes: in our recent ESA study,[7,8] we found a significant relationship between receiving 1 or more red cell transfusions and a worse cognitive outcome at 2 years of age in the placebo group, but not the ESA group.[9]

While we await the published results of the primary outcome, 2 papers based on magnetic resonance imaging of a subset of infants in Fauchere's study hint at possible structural neuroprotection. Leuchter and colleagues reported decreased white matter and gray matter infants in those infants receiving EPO compared with their placebo counterparts,[10] and O'Gorman and colleagues reported improved fractional anisotropy and white matter development in EPO-treated compared with placebo-treated infants.[11] Although the search for the elusive neonatal magic bullet of neuroprotection continues, ESAs nonetheless show great promise as neuroprotective agents in preterm infants.

R. K. Ohls, MD

References

1. Messier AM, Ohls RK. Neuroprotective effects of erythropoiesis-stimulating agents in term and preterm neonates. *Curr Opin Pediatr.* 2014;26:139-145.
2. Fauchere JC, Dame C, Vonthein R, et al. An approach to using recombinant erythropoietin for neuroprotection in very preterm infants. *Pediatrics.* 2008; 122:375-382.
3. Juul SE, Mayock D, Comstock BA, Heagerty PJ. Neuroprotective potential of erythropoietin in neonates; design of a randomized trial. *Matern Health Neonatol Perinatol.* 2015;1:27.
4. Ohlsson A, Aher SM. Early erythropoietin for preventing red blood cell transfusion in preterm and/or low birth weight infants. *Cochrane Database Syst Rev.* 2006;3:CD004863.
5. Ohlsson A, Aher SM. Early erythropoietin for preventing red blood cell transfusion in preterm and/or low birth weight infants. *Cochrane Database Syst Rev.* 2014;4:CD004863.
6. Song J, Sun H, Xu F, et al. Recombinant human erythropoietin improves neurological outcomes in very preterm infants. *Ann Neurol.* 2016;80:24-34.
7. Ohls RK, Kamath-Rayne BD, Christensen RD, et al. Cognitive outcomes of preterm infants randomized to darbepoetin, erythropoietin or placebo. *Pediatrics.* 2014;133:1023-1030.
8. Ohls RK, Christensen RD, Kamath-Rayne BD, et al. A randomized, masked, placebo controlled study of darbepoetin administered to preterm infants. *Pediatrics.* 2013;132:e119-e127.
9. Shah P, Cannon DC, Mani S, Lowe J, Ohls RK. Effect of blood transfusions on cognitive development in very low birth weight infants. *E-PAS.* 2015:1568.503.
10. Leuchter RH, Gui L, Poncet A, et al. Association between early administration of high-dose erythropoietin in preterm infants and brain MRI abnormality at term equivalent age. *JAMA.* 2014;312:817-824.
11. O'Gorman RL, Bucher HU, Held U, et al. Tract-based spatial statistics to assess the neuroprotective effect of early erythropoietin on white matter development in preterm infants. *Brain.* 2015;138:388-397.

Bifidobacterium breve BBG-001 in very preterm infants: a randomised controlled phase 3 trial

Costeloe K, on behalf of The Probiotics in Preterm Infants Study Collaborative Group (Barts and the London School of Medicine and Dentistry, UK; et al)
Lancet 387:649-660, 2016

Background.—Probiotics may reduce necrotising enterocolitis and late-onset sepsis after preterm birth. However, there has been concern about the rigour and generalisability of some trials and there is no agreement about whether or not they should be used routinely. We aimed to test the effectiveness of the probiotic *Bifidobacterium breve* BBG-001 to reduce necrotising enterocolitis, late-onset sepsis, and death in preterm infants.

Methods.—In this multicentre, randomised controlled phase 3 study (the PiPS trial), we recruited infants born between 23 and 30 weeks' gestational age within 48 h of birth from 24 hospitals in southeast England. Infants were randomly assigned (1:1) to probiotic or placebo via a minimisation algorithm randomisation programme. The probiotic intervention was *B breve* BBG-001 suspended in dilute elemental infant formula given enterally in a daily dose of 8·2 to 9·2 $\log_{10}$ CFU; the placebo was dilute infant formula alone. Clinicians and families were masked to allocation. The primary outcomes were necrotising enterocolitis (Bell stage 2 or 3), blood culture positive sepsis more than 72 h after birth; and death before discharge from hospital. All primary analyses were by intention to treat. This trial is registered with ISRCTN, number 05511098 and EudraCT, number 2006-003445-17.

Findings.—Between July 1, 2010, and July 31, 2013, 1315 infants were recruited; of whom 654 were allocated to probiotic and 661 to placebo. Five infants had consent withdrawn after randomisation, thus 650 were analysed in the probiotic group and 660 in the placebo group. Rates of the primary outcomes did not differ significantly between the probiotic and placebo groups. 61 infants (9%) in the probiotic group had necrotising enterocolitis compared with 66 (10%) in the placebo group (adjusted risk ratio 0·93 (95% CI 0·68—1·27); 73 (11%) infants in the probiotics group had sepsis compared with 77 (12%) in the placebo group (0·97 (0·73—1·29); and 54 (8%) deaths occurred before discharge home in the probiotic group compared with 56 (9%) in the placebo group (0·93 [0·67—1·30]). No probiotic-associated adverse events were reported.

Interpretation.—There is no evidence of benefit for this intervention in this population; this result does not support the routine use of *B breve* BBG-001 for prevention of necrotising enterocolitis and late-onset sepsis in very preterm infants.

▶ Necrotizing enterocolitis (NEC) remains an important cause of mortality and long-term morbidity in preterm infants. Since early descriptions of the disease more than 50 years ago, little has been learned about the pathogenesis of this common problem. As a direct result of the lack of knowledge about the disease, efforts either to prevent or treat NEC have generally been disappointing (with the exception of promoting the use of human breast milk). Over the last 2 decades, the incidence of the disease in the United States has increased, mortality rates have remained unchanged, and a growing body of literature has clearly documented the long-term neurocognitive complications seen commonly in those that survive.

A major development in the last decade has been the massive effort devoted to studying the human microbiome, which is the term for the surprisingly complex consortia of microbes living in the gut and elsewhere in the human body. The clinical relevance of the microbiome seemingly spans from intestinal disease to immune disorders to central nervous system conditions, and particular attention has been paid to establishment of a healthy microbiome in the newborn period. Efforts to study the microbiome have been catalyzed by advances in molecular techniques for the culture-independent analysis of microbes with corresponding bioinformatics approaches. Together, these factors have generated great enthusiasm to revisit the old hypothesis that aberrant communities of gut bacteria are at least partly to blame for the pathogenesis of NEC. In the last several years, several reports were published documenting patterns of dysbiosis associated with onset of NEC, although admittedly the observed patterns of disordered colonization have varied from study to study.

Assuming that the research community can agree that NEC is associated with aberrant patterns of colonization, significant questions remain about how this knowledge might be leveraged to improve clinical outcomes. In other fields, therapies to manipulate the microbiome have included fecal transplantation and dietary interventions, but these are not practical in preterm newborns. For this reason, many investigators have studied whether prophylactic administration of probiotic strains of bacteria improves outcomes in preterm infants at risk for NEC. The ProPrems trial was a large randomized clinical trial that showed the efficacy of probiotics in reducing the incidence of NEC,[1] and a recent Cochrane database review of the existing literature concluded that prophylactic administration should be incorporated into standard care of preterm infants to reduce the incidence of NEC.[2] Nevertheless, major issues remain about the efficacy and safety of probiotics. Some of the confusion stems from the fact that probiotics have historically been regarded as a nutritional supplement and, thus, have been immune from the regulatory scrutiny afforded to pharmaceuticals. Moreover, the medical community has not agreed on which organisms to use and at what dose. Finally, lingering concerns remain about the safety of probiotic administration owing to scattered reports about bacteremia following probiotic administration and also a single high-profile case of fungal contamination of a particular probiotic preparation.

Against this background, there was considerable anticipation surrounding the results of the PiPS trial. It is difficult to imagine a better execution of a well-powered, randomized, blinded, placebo-controlled intervention in preterm infants. In this study, 1315 preterm infants from 24 hospitals in the United Kingdom were randomly assigned to receive a daily dose of either *Bifidobacterium breve* BBG-001 diluted in infant formula or a placebo. The study drug was packaged in an amber bottle, thus, blinding care providers and family members. Clinical information was recorded meticulously and the investigators used polymerase chain reaction and conventional culture to determine whether *B breve* could be seen in subsequently collected fecal samples. Primary outcomes were advanced NEC, sepsis, and death.

Unfortunately, administration of the study drug did not confer any demonstrable health benefits. In the probiotic group, 9% of infants had Bell's stage 2 or 3 NEC, 11% had sepsis, and 8% died before discharge from the hospital. In the placebo group, 10% had NEC, 12% had sepsis, and 9% died before hospital discharge. The lack of benefit persisted in subgroup analyses (eg, specific gestational ages). Microbiological evaluation found that fecal samples from most (but not all) infants in the study group contained *B breve*, proving that the exogenously delivered strain survived gastrointestinal transit into the distal gut. Interestingly, however, fecal samples from many infants in the control arm also contained *B breve*, leading the authors to theorize that cross-contamination of subjects in the control arm with the study group masked therapeutic effects of the drug itself. There were no evident safety concerns related to *B breve* administration.

The negative results of this flawlessly executed PiPS trial leave us with 2 possible take-home messages. It may be that the benefits of probiotic administration in preterm infants simply do not outweigh the risks. However, it is equally possible that some probiotics are efficacious, whereas other strains are not, such as the particular strain selected by the PiPS investigators. Regrettably, these investigators selected a probiotic strain that had not previously been studied as a supplement in preterm infants. As a result, after waiting many years for the design and rollout of this clinical trial, we are now back where we started, lacking enough safety and efficacy data to incorporate probiotics into the care of preterm infants.

M. J. Morowitz, MD, FACS

References

1. Jacobs SE, Tobin JM, Opie GF, et al. Probiotic effects on late-onset sepsis in very preterm infants: a randomized controlled trial. *Pediatrics*. 2013;132:1055-1062.
2. AlFaleh K, Anabrees J. Probiotics for prevention of necrotizing enterocolitis in preterm infants. *Cochrane Database Syst Rev*. 2014;(4):CD005496.

18 Neurology

Acute Flaccid Myelitis of Unknown Etiology in California, 2012-2015
Van Haren K, Ayscue P, Waubant E, et al (Stanford Univ School of Medicine, CA; US Ctrs for Disease Control and Prevention, Atlanta, GA, Univ of California; et al)
JAMA 314:2663-2671, 2015

Importance.—There has been limited surveillance for acute flaccid paralysis in North America since the regional eradication of poliovirus. In 2012, the California Department of Public Health received several reports of acute flaccid paralysis cases of unknown etiology.

Objective.—To quantify disease incidence and identify potential etiologies of acute flaccid paralysis cases with evidence of spinal motor neuron injury.

Design, Setting, and Participants.—Case series of acute flaccid paralysis in patients with radiological or neurophysiological findings suggestive of spinal motor neuron involvement reported to the California Department of Public Health with symptom onset between June 2012 and July 2015. Patients meeting diagnostic criteria for other acute flaccid paralysis etiologies were excluded. Cerebrospinal fluid, serum samples, nasopharyngeal swab specimens, and stool specimens were submitted to the state laboratory for infectious agent testing.

Main Outcomes and Measures.—Case incidence and infectious agent association.

Results.—Fifty-nine cases were identified. Median age was 9 years (interquartile range [IQR], 4-14 years; 50 of the cases were younger than 21 years). Symptoms that preceded or were concurrent included respiratory or gastrointestinal illness (n = 54), fever (n = 47), and limb myalgia (n = 41). Fifty-six patients had T2 hyperintensity of spinal gray matter on magnetic resonance imaging and 43 patients had cerebrospinal fluid pleocytosis. During the course of the initial hospitalization, 42 patients received intravenous steroids; 43, intravenous immunoglobulin; and 13, plasma exchange; or a combination of these treatments. Among 45 patients with follow-up data, 38 had persistent weakness at a median follow-up of 9 months (IQR, 3-12 months). Two patients, both immunocompromised adults, died within 60 days of symptom onset. Enteroviruses were the most frequently detected pathogen in either nasopharynx swab specimens, stool specimens, serum samples (15 of 45 patients tested).

No pathogens were isolated from the cerebrospinal fluid. The incidence of reported cases was significantly higher during a national enterovirus D68 outbreak occurring from August 2014 through January 2015 (0.16 cases per 100 000 person-years) compared with other monitoring periods (0.028 cases per 100 000 person-years; $P < .001$).

Conclusions and Relevance.—In this series of patients identified in California from June 2012 through July 2015, clinical manifestations indicated a rare but distinct syndrome of acute flaccid paralysis with evidence of spinal motor neuron involvement. The etiology remains undetermined, most patients were children and young adults, and motor weakness was prolonged (Fig 1, Table 2).

▶ In the early 1900s the United States was subject to an epidemic of an acute flaccid myelitis, known as *infantile paralysis*, which we now associate with poliomyelitis. As widespread as this early epidemic was, polio was eradicated in the United States as well as most of the world through strict vaccination efforts. The last reported case of poliomyelitis in the United States was in 1979. Despite this dramatic decline and eventual eradication of this potentially devastating disorder, occasionally other enteroviral infections have been associated with a similar clinical syndrome.

Since 2012, the California Department of Public Health has noted the reappearance of an acute flaccid myelitis that has primarily similar affects as polio in children and adolescents. Van Haren et al report 59 patients identified in California from June 2012 through July 2015, with clinical manifestations of an acute flaccid paralysis and evidence of spinal motor neuron involvement. What distinguishes these cases from polio, however, is the lack of a unifying etiology. Of the 59 patients, 45 had specimens submitted for viral detection. Fifteen had an enterovirus species detected in at least 1 specimen source (eg, nasopharyngeal swab, serum sample, stool swab), and enterovirus D68 was found in 9 patients. No viral pathogens were isolated from the cerebrospinal fluid in any of the tested patients.

Clinically, the median age of the affected patients was 9 years, and 50 of the patients were younger than 21 years. The syndrome was often seen with an associated respiratory or gastrointestinal illness with fever and limb myalgia. Symptoms included limb weakness in all patients with an interesting predominance for upper-extremity involvement (73%) versus lower-extremity involvement. Also frequently seen were myalgias, headache, and neurogenic bowel or bladder dysfunction (Table 2). Spinal MRI on 56 patients was abnormal with T2 hyperintensity of the spinal gray matter (Fig 1). Forty-three patients had cerebrospinal fluid pleocytosis.

Given the clinical presentation with patient age, associated prodromal illness, and weakness, differential diagnosis should include Guillain-Barre, acute transverse myelitis, tick paralysis and poliomyelitis, or similar infectious myelitis. While the authors do not comment on the presence or absence of deep tendon reflexes, the MRI data are quite convincing that the primary neuro-anatomic area of involvement is the spinal gray matter. This finding strongly supports a

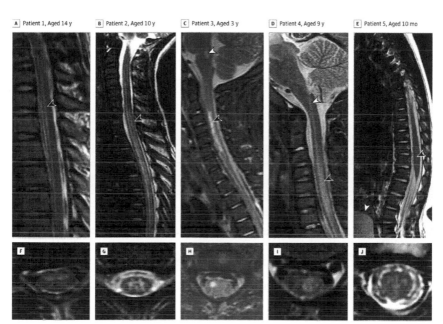

FIGURE 1.—Sagittal and Axial Magnetic Resonance Imaging (MRI) of the Spinal Cord From Representative Patients in This Case Series. Spinal cord MRI typically revealed longitudinally extensive (>3 vertebral bodies) T2 hyperintense lesions affecting spinal gray matter with relative sparing of adjacent white matter (A-J), although various accompanying radiological features were also observed. In some patients, lesions traversed the entire cord with a stable, symmetric appearance (arrowhead in A), whereas other patients demonstrated patchy, asymmetric lesions affecting discrete segments of the cord (arrowheads in B and C). In other patients, subtler lesions (white arrowhead in D) were observed adjacent to more severely affected segments manifesting cord edema (black arrowhead in D). Brainstem lesions were occasionally observed (white arrowheads in C and D) and often correlated with cranial nerve weakness. Although certain lesions appeared to affect dorsal as well as ventral gray matter, the lesions were typically more prominent within the ventral gray matter (G and J), consistent with the location of the spinal motor neurons. Axial sequences revealed spinal lesions that included a "snake eyes" or "owl eyes" appearance highlighting the bilateral ventral horns (F and J), increased T2 signal highlighting the majority of the spinal gray matter (G), unilateral lesions of the ventral horns (H and I), lesions affecting both spinal gray matter and adjacent white matter (I). A distended bladder was observed (white arrowhead in part E) in association with edematous lesions of the conus (black arrowhead in E) in a child with lower limb paralysis. Brainstem and cord lesions are consistent with descriptions of similar cases reported in Colorado in 2014.[21] The black arrowheads in the sagittal images (A-E) demarcate the approximate anatomic level of the associated axial images (F-J, respectively). (Reprinted from Van Haren K, Ayscue P, Waubant E, et al. Acute flaccid myelitis of unknown etiology in California, 2012-2015. *JAMA.* 2015;314:2663-2671, with permission from American Medical Association.)

diagnosis of a poliolike myelitis and makes Guillain-Barre, tick paralysis, and acute transverse myelitis unlikely.

Because poliomyelitis was a highly contagious infection, any regional grouping or clustering of cases is of utmost concern. The hope is that we are not re-entering another epidemic of a crippling childhood disease. The failure to find a unifying pathologic agent does not argue against the infectious nature of this disorder, it just suggests that multiple pathogens may be involved, and we still need to treat this as a potentially contagious disease. Interestingly, despite being a presumed infectious disease, most of the reported patients received

TABLE 2.—Symptoms and Clinical Features of Acute Flaccid Myelitis Cases of Unknown Etiology in California, June 2012 Through July 2015

	Total Cases (N = 59)[a]
Prodromal symptoms[b]	
Concurrent or prodromal illness	54 (92)
Fever >38°C	47 (80)
Respiratory symptoms	42 (71)
Gastrointestinal symptoms	38 (64)
Rash	6 (10)
Neurological symptoms	
Limb weakness or paralysis	59 (100)
Upper limbs affected	43 (73)
1 limb affected	5 (9)
2 or 3 limbs affected	25 (42)
4 limbs affected	29 (49)
Limb myalgia	41 (69)
Headache at onset of neurological symptoms	29 (49)
Sensory deficit on neurological examination	26 (44)
Neurogenic bowel or bladder	30 (51)
Focal paresthesia	21 (36)
Stiff neck	20 (34)
Respiratory insufficiency requiring intubation	20 (34)
Cranial neuropathy	16 (27)
Altered mental status	13 (22)
Hospital course	
Received intravenous immunoglobulin	43 (73)
Received intravenous steroids	42 (71)
Received plasmapheresis	13 (22)
Diagnostic Studies	
Cerebrospinal fluid	(n = 58)
Pleocytosis (white blood cell count >5/μL)	43 (74)
Protein elevation (>45 mg/dL)	28 (48)
White blood cell count, median (IQR), /μL	41 (5-99)
Protein level, median (IQR), mg/dL	44 (29-70)
Neuroimaging of brain	(n = 48)
No supratentorial lesions	33 (69)
Sinus or mastoid inflammation	9 (19)
Type of lesion	
Subcortical white matter	9 (19)
Cortical gray matter	6 (12)
Thalamic	4 (8)
Caudate	2 (4)
Cerebellar	2 (4)
Neuroimaging of spine	
T2 hyperintensity of spinal gray matter	56 (95)
Lesion >3 vertebral lengths	53 (90)
Spinal cord edema	29 (49)
Spinal gray matter lesion enhancement	23 (39)
Spinal nerve root enhancement	12 (20)
Nerve root thickening or clumping	6 (10)
Paraspinal muscle edema or enhancement	6 (10)

Abbreviation: IQR, interquartile range.
[a]Data are expressed as No. (%) unless otherwise indicated.
[b]Onset within 31-day period prior to limb weakness.
Reprinted from Van Haren K, Ayscue P, Waubant E, et al. Acute flaccid myelitis of unknown etiology in California, 2012-2015. *JAMA.* 2015;314:2663-2671, with permission from American Medical Association.

some form of immune modulation therapy with intravenous steroids, intravenous immunoglobulin, plasmapheresis, or a combination of these treatments. This topic is of interest, as immune modulation could potentially be contraindicated. The authors did report that 2 adult immunocompromised patients died with this disorder. In terms of outcome, of the 45 reported patients with follow-up data, 38 had persistent weakness at a median follow-up of 9 months.

The significance of this report is to remind us that while poliomyelitis may have been eradicated in the United States 37 years ago, similar syndromes mediated by other pathogens exist. The susceptible population appears to remain those younger than 21 years of age, and the outcome is not dissimilar to what was seen with poliomyelitis. The question of regional host susceptibility with genetic vulnerability to potentially less potent viral agents remains a possible explanation for the appearance of this clinical entity so similar to poliomyelitis. Continued surveillance is necessary to thwart any potential future widespread occurrences.

T. K. Koch, MD

Clinical Risk Score for Persistent Postconcussion Symptoms Among Children With Acute Concussion in the ED

Zemek R, for the Pediatric Emergency Research Canada (PERC) Concussion Team (Univ of Ottawa, Canada; et al)
JAMA 315:1014-1025, 2016

Importance.—Approximately one-third of children experiencing acute concussion experience ongoing somatic, cognitive, and psychological or behavioral symptoms, referred to as persistent postconcussion symptoms (PPCS). However, validated and pragmatic tools enabling clinicians to identify patients at risk for PPCS do not exist.

Objective.—To derive and validate a clinical risk score for PPCS among children presenting to the emergency department.

Design, Setting, and Participants.—Prospective, multicenter cohort study (Predicting and Preventing Postconcussive Problems in Pediatrics [5P]) enrolled young patients (aged 5-<18 years) who presented within 48 hours of an acute head injury at 1 of 9 pediatric emergency departments within the Pediatric Emergency Research Canada (PERC) network from August 2013 through September 2014 (derivation cohort) and from October 2014 through June 2015 (validation cohort). Participants completed follow-up 28 days after the injury.

Exposures.—All eligible patients had concussions consistent with the Zurich consensus diagnostic criteria.

Main Outcomes and Measures.—The primary outcome was PPCS risk score at 28 days, which was defined as 3 or more new or worsening symptoms using the patient-reported Postconcussion Symptom Inventory compared with recalled state of being prior to the injury.

Results.—In total, 3063 patients (median age, 12.0 years [interquartile range, 9.2-14.6 years]; 1205 [39.3%] girls) were enrolled (n = 2006 in the derivation cohort; n = 1057 in the validation cohort) and 2584 of whom (n = 1701 [85%] in the derivation cohort; n = 883 [84%] in the validation cohort) completed follow-up at 28 days after the injury. Persistent postconcussion symptoms were present in 801 patients (31.0%) (n = 510 [30.0%] in the derivation cohort and n = 291 [33.0%] in the validation cohort). The 12-point PPCS risk score model for the derivation cohort included the variables of female sex, age of 13 years or older, physician-diagnosed migraine history, prior concussion with symptoms lasting longer than 1 week, headache, sensitivity to noise, fatigue, answering questions slowly, and 4 or more errors on the Balance Error Scoring System tandem stance. The area under the curve was 0.71 (95% CI, 0.69-0.74) for the derivation cohort and 0.68 (95% CI, 0.65-0.72) for the validation cohort.

Conclusions and Relevance.—A clinical risk score developed among children presenting to the emergency department with concussion and head injury within the previous 48 hours had modest discrimination to stratify PPCS risk at 28 days. Before this score is adopted in clinical practice, further research is needed for external validation, assessment of accuracy in an office setting, and determination of clinical utility.

▶ "Concentrate and ask again" says the Magic Eight Ball, which can be a typical feeling among health care providers attempting to predict concussion recovery in kids. "When you've seen one concussion, you've seen one concussion" is a commonly agreed-upon statement among specialty practitioners accustomed to caring for kids slow to recover from such an injury. This reflects the knowledge that many factors contribute to prolonged recovery from concussion, and determining the best advice, management and intervention for a given child is every bit as much of an art as it is a science (maybe even more art!).

And yet, from the primary care perspective, experience dictates that the vast majority of kids with concussions recover fully over the course of days to weeks. This observation is supported by multiple prospective studies.[1,2] Furthermore, 1 strong, evidence-based intervention that reduces the likelihood of prolonged post-concussion symptoms/postconcussion syndrome is cognitive restructuring, a brief counseling intervention that provides education, reassurance and assistance with activity management. If you have difficulty with the psychological term "cognitive restructuring," then think about this as "anticipatory guidance," a term with which all pediatric providers are familiar and should be comfortable. When parents take a newborn baby home from the hospital, we explain what to expect. When a child gets a vaccination, we explain what to expect. It only makes sense for health care providers to also provide credible information to parents and patients after something as worrisome as a brain injury. Provision of accurate and balanced cognitive restructuring may reduce the likelihood for developing chronic postconcussion symptoms by as much as 15% to 20% in controlled studies.[3,4] If this treatment was a medication, we'd all be prescribing it!

So how does a health care provider initially seeing a concussion patient provide the proper level of reassurance, anticipatory guidance, and vigilance to ensure optimal recovery without over- or underplaying the significance of the injury? How can we avoid the seemingly random Magic Eight Ball method of predicting concussion outcomes? How can we target the appropriate interventions and monitoring toward the patients most likely to benefit?

First steps first. After a concussion diagnosis is determined, it is important to provide clear and correct information about concussions to parents and their children. Explanation of concussion as a brain injury, emphasizing the importance of avoiding premature return to contact risk, explaining the common symptoms and reassuring everyone that the majority recover over time with proper management are essential. There are multiple good online resources that provide educational material, videos, handouts and other types of unbiased information for practitioners and families, including the Center for Disease Control and Prevention (http://www.cdc.gov/headsup/index.html), the American Academy of Pediatrics (http://pediatrics.aappublications.org/content/126/3/597 and other documents online), and the American Academy of Neurology (https://www.aan.com/concussion).

Who should provide return to school and return to play information? This is almost always next (after diagnosis and initial education and reassurance), and there is some argument to be made that detailed return to school/play information is really beyond the scope of the acute care provider (emergency room or urgent care). At the same time, information provided in the acute setting is often extremely important to the family. They hang on every word—from the diagnosis of concussion versus traumatic brain injury, to advice about preventing future injuries, to when and where is the appropriate follow-up, to how many days it will take for their child to recover. So the brief acute care visit can provide an extremely important initial opportunity to manage this injury effectively.

Here is where the Predicting and Preventing Postconcussive Problems in Pediatrics [5P] study can provide evidence-based guidance for the acute health care provider.[5] Using a prospective, multicenter cohort study, they derived a clinically useful prediction tool for persistent symptoms at 4 weeks post-injury and validated it in a separate cohort. By scoring 9 clinical characteristics, a health care provider may be able to stratify acute concussion/mild TBI patients into low-risk (4.1%—11.8% likelihood of symptoms at 4 weeks), medium risk (16.4%—47.6%), and high-risk (57.1%—80.8%) groups. Although it has its limitations, this prediction model offered a statistically significant improvement over physician judgment. It is important to recognize that this 5P prediction rule doesn't address every risk factor known for persistent symptoms but nonetheless provides a potentially useful tool for the initial assessment.

So, back to our question about predicting concussion outcome and providing anticipatory guidance. The acute care provider would ideally provide reassurance, education, and counseling for prevention of repeat injuries. Without being too prescriptive, general information about returning to school and non-contact activity may be provided, with a goal of allowing the follow-up physician considerable flexibility to manage the injured child's recovery as the longitudinal course of symptoms becomes clearer. Using the 5P score to estimate likelihood for prolonged symptoms may be helpful, but the provider must also be cautious about the nocebo effect; if the patient is told that he or she is sure to have difficulties in recovery, it can become a self-fulfilling prophecy. Perhaps the most prudent use of this score is to help decide on the degree of follow-up, with patients at higher risk for prolonged symptoms being given earlier or more frequent contact with postconcussion care providers. With this new 5P data, coupled with prudent and effective information provided at the initial medical contact, we can improve on the Magic Eight Ball's response and say "Outlook good" for our youth concussion patients.

C. C. Giza, MD

References

1. Barlow KM, Crawford S, Stevenson A, Sandhu SS, Belanger F, Dewey D. Epidemiology of postconcussion syndrome in pediatric mild traumatic brain injury. *Pediatrics.* 2010;126:e374-e381.
2. McCrea M, Guskiewicz K, Randolph C, et al. Incidence, clinical course, and predictors of prolonged recovery time following sport-related concussion in high school and college athletes. *J Int Neuropsychol Soc.* 2013;19:22-33.
3. Mittenberg W, Canyock EM, Condit D, Patton C. Treatment of post-concussion syndrome following mild head injury. *J Clin Exp Neuropsychol.* 2001;23:829-836.
4. Ponsford J, Willmott C, Rothwell A, et al. Impact of early intervention on outcome after mild traumatic brain injury in children. *Pediatrics.* 2001;108:1297-1303.
5. Zemek R, Barrowman N, Freedman SB, et al. Clinical risk score for persistent postconcussion symptoms among children with acute concussion in the ED. *JAMA.* 2016;315:1014-1025.

Physical Maturity and Concussion Symptom Duration among Adolescent Ice Hockey Players
Kriz PK, Stein C, Kent J, et al (Brown Univ, Providence, RI; Boston Children's Hosp, Boston, MA; South Shore Hosp, Weymouth, MA)
J Pediatr 171:234-239, 2016

Objective.—To investigate the association between physical maturity and risk of prolonged concussion symptoms in adolescent ice hockey players.

Study Design.—Prospective cohort study of 145 patients ages 13-18 years with concussion referred to 3 hospital-affiliated sports medicine clinics between September 1, 2012 and March 31, 2015. Concussion evaluations included Post Concussive Symptom Score, neurologic examination, and postinjury computerized neurocognitive testing. Pubertal development at initial visit was assessed by the Pubertal Developmental Scale. Duration of concussion symptoms (days) was the main outcome. Statistical comparisons were conducted using Student t test, Wilcoxon rank sum, and logistic regression.

Results.—Mean symptom duration was 44.5 ± 48.7 days. Nearly one-half (48.3%) of all players enrolled had prolonged concussion symptoms (≥28 days); most (86.9%) had symptom resolution by 90 days. Among males, less physically mature adolescents took longer to recover than more physically mature players (54.5 days vs 33.4 days; $P = .004$). "Early" Pubertal Category Score was the strongest predictor of prolonged symptoms (OR = 4.29, 95% CI 1.24-14.85; $P = .021$) among males.

Among females, heavier weight increased the odds of experiencing pro-longed symptoms (OR 1.07, 95% CI 1.00-1.14; $P = .039$).

Conclusions.—Among adolescent ice hockey players, early-pubertal stage is independently associated with longer recovery from concussion in males, and heavier weight is associated with longer concussion recovery in females. Until further studies determine valid physical maturity indica-tors, peripubertal collision sport athletes should compete in leagues grouped by relative age and be discouraged from "playing up" on varsity teams (Fig 2, Table 2).

▶ There is a general consensus in the concussion community that children take longer to recover from concussions than adults. The 4th Consensus Statement on Concussion in Sport recommends a more conservative approach to return to play in childhood and adolescence. It notes the different physiological response and longer recovery after concussion for children, as well as specific risks (eg, diffuse cerebral swelling).[1]

In most competitive sports, stratification of competition is usually age-based. There has been little thought or research into different criteria other than age to

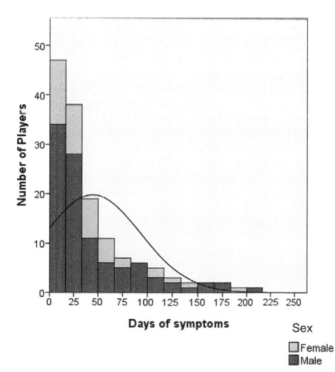

FIGURE 2.—Duration of concussion symptoms among adolescent male and female ice hockey players, scholastic seasons 2012-2013 through 2014-2015. One U14 female player experienced symptoms for 324 days. (Reprinted from Kriz PK, Stein C, Kent J, et al. Physical maturity and concussion symptom duration among adolescent ice hockey players. *J Pediatr.* 2016;171:234-239, with permission from Elsevier.)

TABLE 2.—Adolescent Male Subgroup: Independent Effect of Potential Predictor Variables on Odds of Persistent Concussive Symptoms for More Than 28 Days

Potential Predictor Variables	aOR (95% CI)	P Value
Age (y)	1.32 (0.61-2.88)	.484
Weight (lbs)	0.96 (0.93-0.99)	.008
Height (in)	1.14 (0.95-1.37)	.155
Pubertal Category Score (early vs late)	4.29 (1.24-14.85)	.021
PCSS	1.04 (1.01-1.06)	.003
Defense/goalie vs center/wing	0.49 (0.16-1.51)	.214
10th-12th grade vs 7th-9th grade	1.50 (0.17-13.69)	.718

Reprinted from Kriz PK, Stein C, Kent J, et al. Physical maturity and concussion symptom duration among adolescent ice hockey players. *J Pediatr.* 2016;171:234-239, with permission from Elsevier.

stratify athletes into different competitive groups. Due to high costs and equipment restraints, youth ice hockey leagues sometimes do not even use age stratification. It is not uncommon for younger, less physically mature hockey players to compete with more mature athletes who are faster and stronger.

Concussions remain the most common injury in youth ice hockey—more than 15% from age 9 to 16 years old and almost 25% in boy's high school leagues.[2,3] Body checking, in which a player drives the shoulder, upper arm, hip, and elbow into an opponent, remains a legal maneuver for male adolescents participating in youth and high school hockey. Kriz et al took a novel approach in looking at physical maturity, rather than just age, as a marker in adolescent ice hockey players and examining the risk of prolonged concussion symptoms. The authors conducted a prospective study with 145 high school ice hockey players (101 boys and 44 girls) aged 13 to 18 years, seen at 3 outpatient concussion clinics to investigate the association between physical maturation and risk of prolonged concussion symptoms.

Demographic, anthropometric, and injury data were collected during the initial evaluation. The Pubertal Development Scale, involving a self-assessment questionnaire of 5 items of physical development (growth in height, body hair, skin changes, facial hair, and voice changes for boys; breast development and menses for girls), was used to measure physical maturity dividing players into either "early" or "late." The Post Concussion Symptom Score (PCSS) and ImPACT computerized neurocognitive testing was done at initial and follow-up appointment to measure concussion symptoms, severity, and duration. Duration of concussion symptoms was the primary outcome variable measured, and a concussion was considered prolonged if symptoms lasted more than 28 days.

The authors concluded that there is an increased risk for prolonged concussion signs and symptoms among all adolescent ice hockey players. Notably, nearly 50% of this cohort suffered from prolonged concussion sign and symptom duration, and the mean time for full symptom recovery was 45 days (Fig 2). Compared with previous reports (football and soccer), where nearly all athletes recovered in 28 days, these athletes on average suffered concussion signs and symptoms an additional 20 days.[4] As the authors noted, this may be more an attribute of study design because the focus was on specialty sports medicine clinics with more than one-third (36.6%) presenting > 21 days from injury. Because there is a general paucity of research looking at concussion risk and symptoms in ice hockey, further studies are needed to determine whether the prolonged recovery time noted in this study is reflective of a sport medicine clinic selection bias or other factors involved in youth ice hockey.

The adolescent ice hockey cohort was grouped by pubertal development and gender. In the male cohort, early-pubertal stage was associated with longer concussion sign and symptom duration. Heavier weight in male players was associated with a decreased risk of prolonged symptoms (Table 2). This suggests that stratification by physical maturity or weight rather than just age may be beneficial for male youth ice hockey leagues. Interestingly, in the female cohort, heavier weight but not physical maturity was associated with risk of prolonged symptoms.

The conflicting findings between male and female ice hockey players should be further investigated to confirm whether there are gender-specific differences in concussion risk. Of note, this study only had 5 female players in the early pubertal category. The finding of heavier weight associated with increased risk of prolonged symptoms in females but decreased risk in males needs to be further investigated. The study was also limited in that only 44.1% of adolescent players enrolled within 10 days of their injury. This approach may select for a more involved group of concussed athletes requiring referral to a sports medicine clinic. Additionally, the Pubertal Development Scale, which was used at the primary indicator of physical maturity, has limited studies on validity when self-administered and needs further research.

The American Academy of Pediatrics recommends expanding nonchecking ice hockey programs for boys 15 years and older and restricting body checking to the highest competition levels starting no earlier than age 15. This study challenges this recent opinion in that 65% of freshman versus 27% of sophomores were in early stages of pubertal development and none were postpubertal. The findings also support concerns within the youth athletic community that adolescents might have longer recoveries from concussions than adults.

Medical professionals should educate athletes, parents, and coaches on the inherent risk of "playing up" with more mature players. Similar studies can be done in high school football and boys' lacrosse, 2 other collision sports that commonly permit underclassmen to compete in varsity teams with more physically mature players. Medical professionals can work with youth hockey organizations to advocate for the option of nonchecking divisions for players who are in the earlier stages of pubertal development or who are undersized. This study can also help providers educate youth ice hockey players and parents about how long they might be symptomatic after a concussion.

M. Kapadia, MD, MSc

References

1. McCrory P, Meeuwisse WH, Aubry M, et al. Consensus statement on concussion in sport: the 4th International Conference on Concussion in Sport held in Zurich, November 2012. *Br J Sports Med*. 2013;47:250-258.

2. Emery CA, Meeuwisse WH. Injury rates, risk factors, and mechanisms of injury in minor hockey. *Am J Sports Med.* 2006;34:1960-1969.
3. Roberts WO, Brust JD, Leonard B. Youth ice hockey tournament injuries: rates and patterns compared to season play. *Med Sci Sports Exerc.* 1999;31:46-51.
4. Collins M, Lovell M, Iverson GL, Ide T, Maroon J. Examining concussion rates and return to play in high school football players wearing newer helmet technology: a three-year prospective cohort study. *Neurosurgery.* 2006;58:275-286.

Frequency of Pediatric Migraine With Aura in a Clinic-Based Sample

Genizi J, Khourieh Matar A, Zelnik N, et al (Bnai Zion Med Ctr, Haifa, Israel; Carmel Med Ctr, Haifa, Israel; et al)
Headache 56:113-117, 2016

Objective.—To assess the prevalence and risk factors for pediatric migraine with aura (MWA) among patients presenting to pediatric neurology clinics.

Background.—Headache is a common complaint among children, and the prevalence of migraine is about 8%. Up to one third of adults with migraine report experiencing aura; however, the exact percentage in children is unknown.

Methods.—Medical records of children presenting with headache to three pediatric neurology clinics in Haifa in the last 5 years were retrospectively reviewed. Inclusion criteria were a diagnosis of migraine headache at 5-18 years of age.

Results.—Of 260 children (140 female) who had migraine, 26.2% experienced aura. MWA was more common among females compared to males (32.6% vs 18.9%, $P < .01$) and among older children (OR: 2.50, 95% CI: 1.20-5.20; $P < .01$). Among those who experienced aura, visual aura was more common in females than males (66.7% vs 33.3%, $P < .04$). Family history of migraine was strongly related to MWA ($P < .02$): the odds of MWA were 2.46 times greater in children who had a family history of migraine. (OR: 2.46, 95% CI: 1.08-5.62; $P < .03$).

Conclusions.—MWA is as common in children as in adults. Aura is more common in older children. Children who have MWA are more likely to have a family history of migraine.

▶ In our experience at our pediatric headache center, migrainous sensory or visual complaints are relatively common in children with migraine but not necessarily indicative of aura. Careful history taking is needed to delineate and properly classify the symptoms. An often-useful strategy used in our clinic for visual symptoms is to have the child or adolescent draw what they see. The clinician may find the patient's drawing clarifying diagnostically; however, if a child is unable to draw his or her visual symptoms, it does not necessarily indicate lack of visual aura.

Migraine is a complex disorder of the brain with identifiable phases. The first phase—the premonitory phase—precedes the headache and is characterized by a broad spectrum of possible symptoms such as fatigue, neck discomfort, irritability, food cravings, light and sound sensitivity, and increased yawning. The subset of migraineurs who have migraine with aura may then go on to develop aura symptoms before or during the headache. The headache phase is characterized by throbbing head pain, movement sensitivity, light and sound sensitivity, and nausea/vomiting. Symptoms that may have begun in the premonitory phase, such as photophobia, phonophobia, and neck pain, may also play prominently in the headache phase. Difficulty concentrating, blurry vision, and vertigo are also common features during the headache phase. Finally, once the headache has resolved, many migraineurs may experience a postdromal phase characterized by fatigue and mental fogginess.

Aura is a particularly fascinating aspect of migraine, although by no means a required feature. Migraine aura is thought to be due to cortical spreading depression—a wave of depolarization that spreads across the involved cortex at the relatively slow rate of 2—5 mm/min.[1] A key feature for recognizing aura, therefore, is that the symptoms spread or progress over minutes, for example, do the visual spots grow? Does the tingling sensation start in the fingers and progress up the hand and arm over minutes? If the child is describing just a little flash of light for a couple seconds when they stand up, that's not aura.

Even for pediatric migraine specialists, accurate differentiation of migraine with visual aura versus migraine associated visual disturbances versus premonitory symptoms may be challenging in younger patients, particularly in the first visit. Many children, as one would expect, are not critically analyzing and documenting the characterization and duration of their symptoms as they are experiencing them.

Genizi et al found migraine equally likely to affect boys and girls up to the age of 12, but in older children, females were more often affected (62% vs 38%, $P = .03$). Twenty six percent of their patients who were retrospectively identified to have migraine also had aura per International Criteria for Headache Disorders (ICHD) II criteria. This observation is in line with a recent retrospective review of 495 Italian children in which 29.7% had migraine with aura.[2] It is also similar to the frequency found in adults in that approximately a third of adult migraineurs have aura.[3]

Sixty-five percent of those with migraine with aura (MWA) in Genizi et al were reported to have visual aura. In the aforementioned Italian study, visual aura occurred in 87.1% of those with aura. Genizi et al reported children with visual aura were older (13 vs 11 years, $P < .001$), and older children were 2.5 times more likely to have aura than younger children (odds ratio 2.5, 95% confidence interval: 1.20—5.20; $P < .01$).

The authors thoughtfully discuss possible mechanisms for the lower frequency of migraine aura in prepubertal children. The authors state that brain maturation, particularly in the pain processing centers, may not yet be complete in younger children. This brain immaturity may be involved in the heterogeneity of migraine features in younger children as the pathophysiologic mechanisms of migraine, and migraine aura, may not yet be fully developed. The fact that features of migraine may differ somewhat over the course of brain development is recognized in the ICHD 3b diagnostic criteria for migraine in children; it is noted that headache is most often bilateral rather than unilateral in pediatric migraine, and the duration can be as short as 2 hours as opposed to adult requirements of at least 4 hours' duration.[4] Our experience in our pediatric headache program has also demonstrated that as children grow and develop, their migraine phenotype also evolves.

This article strengthens the known epidemiologic patterns seen in pediatric migraine, namely, that about a quarter of pediatric migraineurs will have aura. Pediatricians therefore should remember that the majority of children with migraine will not have aura, and therefore they should not be dissuaded from diagnosing migraine due to absence of aura.

W. Qubty, MD

A. Gelfand, MD

References

1. Leao AA. Spreading depression of activity in cerebral cortex. *J Neurophysiol.* 1944;7:359-390.
2. Tarasco V, Grasso G, Versace A, et al. Epidemiological and clinical features of migraine in the pediatric population of Northern Italy. *Cephalalgia.* 2016;36: 510-517.
3. Russell MB, Rasmussen BK, Fenger K, Olesen J. Migraine without aura and migraine with aura are distinct clinical entities: a study of four hundred and eighty-four male and female migraineurs from the general population. *Cephalalgia.* 1996;16:239-245.
4. Headache Classification Committee of the International Headache Society. The International Classification of Headache Disorders, 3rd edition (beta version). *Cephalalgia.* 2013;33:629-808.

Incidence of Dravet Syndrome in a US Population
Wu YW, Sullivan J, McDaniel SS, et al (Univ of California, San Francisco; Univ of Michigan, Ann Arbor)
Pediatrics 136:e1310-e1315, 2015

Objective.—De novo mutations of the gene sodium channel 1α (*SCN1A*) are the major cause of Dravet syndrome, an infantile epileptic encephalopathy. US incidence of DS has been estimated at 1 in 40 000, but no US epidemiologic studies have been performed since the advent of genetic testing.

Methods.—In a retrospective, population-based cohort of all infants born at Kaiser Permanente Northern California during 2007—2010, we electronically identified patients who received ≥2 seizure diagnoses before age 12 months and who were also prescribed anticonvulsants at 24 months. A child neurologist reviewed records to identify infants who met 4 of 5 criteria for clinical Dravet syndrome: normal development before seizure onset; ≥2 seizures before age 12 months; myoclonic, hemiclonic, or generalized tonic-clonic seizures; ≥2 seizures lasting >10 minutes; and refractory seizures after age 2 years. *SCN1A* gene sequencing was performed as part of routine clinical care.

Results.—Eight infants met the study criteria for clinical Dravet syndrome, yielding an incidence of 1 per 15 700. Six of these infants (incidence of 1 per 20 900) had a de novo *SCN1A* missense mutation that is likely to be pathogenic. One infant had an inherited *SCN1A* variant that is unlikely to be pathogenic. All 8 experienced febrile seizures, and 6 had prolonged seizures lasting >10 minutes by age 1 year.

Conclusions.—Dravet syndrome due to an *SCN1A* mutation is twice as common in the United States as previously thought. Genetic testing should be considered in children with ≥2 prolonged febrile seizures by 1 year of age.

▶ Major advances have taken place in the understanding of the genetic mechanisms that underlie epilepsy, and the majority of previously termed "idiopathic" epilepsies are now considered genetic. Dravet syndrome has been a model for genetic epilepsies, and *SCN1A* has become one of the most relevant epilepsy genes today. Mutations in the gene encoding the alpha-1 subunit of the voltage gated sodium channel (*SCN1A*) are associated with several epilepsy syndromes, ranging from relatively mild phenotypes found in families with genetic epilepsy with febrile seizures plus (GEFS+) to the severe infantile-onset epilepsy, Dravet syndrome.

Despite these recent major advances, many neurologists and pediatricians do not regard genetic testing as contributing to patient care. This view should be challenged, particularly in light of Wu et al's new findings highlighting that Dravet syndrome appears to be more common than previously thought: the incidence of children with clinical Dravet syndrome in Northern California was 1 in 15 700. Seventy-five percent of these carried a *SCN1A* mutation, which is equivalent to an incidence of 1 per 20 900 when only *SCN1A* mutation–positive cases are considered. The authors emphasize how important it is to make an early diagnosis, particularly in the very young children to inform treatment.

Seizures in Dravet syndrome are usually refractory to standard antiepileptic medication, and from the second year of life, affected children develop an epileptic encephalopathy resulting in cognitive, behavioral, and motor impairment. Children often have recurrent episodes of status epilepticus that may be life threatening, and the incidence of sudden unexpected death in epilepsy is significantly higher in Dravet syndrome compared with other epilepsy syndromes.[1,2]

Successful medical intervention is important in improving the quality of life in children and their families. Randomized controlled trials have shown that certain combinations of medication can improve seizure control in Dravet syndrome,[3] and aggressive focused therapy should be commenced as soon as possible.[4]

The clinical diagnosis of Dravet syndrome is based on recognition of seizure types, clinical course, and electroencephalogram features. The diagnosis is usually not made until 2 to 4 years of age, even by experienced clinicians. Most children present to general pediatricians in emergency departments where it may be difficult to make a distinction between the first seizures in Dravet syndrome and "milder" epilepsy phenotypes. Because of the complexities in making an electroclinical diagnosis of Dravet syndrome and with the potential to improve seizure control and implications for family counseling, molecular genetic testing can aid clinicians in making an early diagnosis of Dravet syndrome.[5]

Although Dravet syndrome is rare, Wu et al show that its incidence is significantly higher than previously thought. The evidence suggests that early intervention can achieve better outcomes and the authors rightly conclude that genetic testing should be considered in children presenting with 2 or more prolonged febrile seizures by 1 year of age.

Being able to make a genetic diagnosis in Dravet syndrome has significant positive implications for patients. The benefits include a better informed antiepileptic drug (AED) choice, sparing of further unnecessary investigations and improved access to additional therapies such as physiotherapy, occupational therapy and speech and language therapy. Furthermore, the confirmation of a diagnosis gives parents "an answer" and allows them to adjust their goals for the future.[5] Any child with Dravet syndrome should be treated with AEDs shown to be efficacious in this syndrome,[3] and the use of lamotrigine and/or carbamazepine is discouraged to avoid seizure exacerbation.

The ability to offer genetic counseling is one of the recognized advantages of genetic testing, and knowledge of an underlying genetic diagnosis is associated with relief and positive adjustment enabling parents to readjust their goals and expectations. Knowing that a condition is likely or unlikely to be inherited allows families to make informed reproductive choices.

Despite the advances of genetic testing, Dravet syndrome remains a clinical diagnosis. Any child with a typical clinical presentation of Dravet syndrome, irrespective of mutation status (25% are *SCN1A* mutation negative), should have access to appropriate therapies. Finally, whenever faced with a young child or infant with prolonged febrile seizures, think of Dravet syndrome—test early and treat early.

A. Brunklaus, MD(Res)

References

1. Dravet C, Bureau M, Oguni H, et al. Severe myoclonic epilepsy in infancy (Dravet syndrome). In: Roger J, Bureau M, Dravet C, Genton P, Tassinari CA, Wolf P, eds. *Epileptic Syndromes in Infancy, Childhood and Adolescence.* London: John Libbey; 2005:89-113.
2. Sakauchi M, Oguni H, Kato I, et al. Mortality in Dravet syndrome: search for risk factors in Japanese patients. *Epilepsia.* 2011;52:50-54.
3. Chiron C, Marchand MC, Tran A, et al. Stiripentol in severe myoclonic epilepsy in infancy: a randomised placebo-controlled syndrome-dedicated trial. STICLO study group. *Lancet.* 2000;356:1638-1642.
4. Mullen SA, Scheffer IE. Translational research in epilepsy genetics: sodium channels in man to interneuronopathy in mouse. *Arch Neurol.* 2009;66:21-26.
5. Brunklaus A, Dorris L, Ellis R, et al. The clinical utility of an SCN1A genetic diagnosis in infantile-onset epilepsy. *Dev Med Child Neurol.* 2013;55:154-161.

19 Newborn

A Randomized Trial of Phototherapy with Filtered Sunlight in African Neonates

Slusher TM, Olusanya BO, Vreman HJ, et al (Univ of Minnesota, in Minneapolis; Ctr for Healthy Start Initiative, Lagos, Nigeria; Stanford Univ, CA; et al)
N Engl J Med 373:1115-1124, 2015

Background.—Sequelae of severe neonatal hyperbilirubinemia constitute a substantial disease burden in areas where effective conventional phototherapy is unavailable. We previously found that the use of filtered sunlight for the purpose of phototherapy is a safe and efficacious method for reducing total bilirubin. However, its relative safety and efficacy as compared with conventional phototherapy are unknown.

Methods.—We conducted a randomized, controlled noninferiority trial in which filtered sunlight was compared with conventional phototherapy for the treatment of hyperbilirubinemia in term and late-preterm neonates in a large, urban Nigerian maternity hospital. The primary end point was efficacy, which was defined as a rate of increase in total serum bilirubin of less than 0.2 mg per deciliter per hour for infants up to 72 hours of age or a decrease in total serum bilirubin for infants older than 72 hours of age who received at least 5 hours of phototherapy; we prespecified a noninferiority margin of 10% for the difference in efficacy rates between groups. The need for an exchange transfusion was a secondary end point. We also assessed safety, which was defined as the absence of the need to withdraw therapy because of hyperthermia, hypothermia, dehydration, or sunburn.

Results.—We enrolled 447 infants and randomly assigned 224 to filtered sunlight and 223 to conventional phototherapy. Filtered sunlight was efficacious on 93% of treatment days that could be evaluated, as compared with 90% for conventional phototherapy, and had a higher mean level of irradiance (40 vs. 17 μW per square centimeter per nanometer, $P < 0.001$). Temperatures higher than 38.0°C occurred in 5% of the infants receiving filtered sunlight and in 1% of those receiving conventional phototherapy ($P < 0.001$), but no infant met the criteria for withdrawal from the study for reasons of safety or required an exchange transfusion.

Conclusions.—Filtered sunlight was noninferior to conventional phototherapy for the treatment of neonatal hyperbilirubinemia and did not result in any study withdrawals for reasons of safety. (Funded by the Thrasher Research Fund, Salt Lake City, and the National Center for

Advancing Translational Sciences of the National Institutes of Health; Clinical Trials.gov number, NCT01434810.) (Fig 2).

▶ Neonatal jaundice and kernicterus are significant public health problems in developing countries, especially Africa, due to a combination of diminished capacity for diagnosis and treatment of hyperbilirubinemia and higher prevalence of comorbidities such as infection, undiagnosed and untreated Rh incompatibility, and glucose-6-phosphate dehydrogenase (G6PD) deficiency. The trial reported by Slusher et al follows years of dedicated effort to develop a low-cost, feasible option for phototherapy in these countries.

The phototherapy units they developed use 2 types of filters (film similar to that used for tinting glass windows in motor vehicles), which screen out almost all harmful ultraviolet light while letting 2 levels of blue light through. The different filters allow infants to be moved from one unit to the other depending on the level of cloud cover. The phototherapy tents are large enough to allow mothers to breastfeed their babies inside and to allow health workers to monitor temperatures and supply moistened towels as needed to keep the babies cool.

The design of this study, a randomized, unblinded noninferiority trial, is suitable for the research question. The article indicates that subjects were eligible for inclusion if their total serum bilirubin (TSB) was "3 mg per deciliter lower than the guideline recommended by the American Academy of Pediatrics (AAP)," but one must go to the supplemental material online to find out that they used the AAP's "high-risk" threshold for all infants, even though most of the babies were born at term. The inclusion based on a TSB 3 mg/dL below the high-risk threshold "was as a safety precaution, since filtered sun-light had not been used for this purpose previously and hemolysis resulting from a deficiency of glucose-6-phosphate dehydrogenase or from blood-group incompatibilities is common in Nigeria." Indeed, among included infants who were tested, 35% were G6PD deficient, 45% had ABO incompatibility with their mother, and 8% Rh incompatibility.

However, providing this wide margin of safety meant that many included subjects probably did not need phototherapy; indeed, there were no subjects with TSB levels > 15 mg/dL. The AAP's high-risk phototherapy treatment threshold is about 3 mg/dL above the line between low and low-intermediate risk zones in Fig 2 of the guideline,[1] the so-called Bhutani nomogram. Thus, infants in this study whose TSB levels were 3 mg/dL below that line presumably had TSB levels in that low-intermediate risk zone.

The efficacy end point, a rate of rise of total serum bilirubin (TSB) < 0.2 mg/dL/hour for infants up to 72 hours old and a drop in TSB for infants < 72 hours old, would likely have been achieved in many infants even without phototherapy. For infants in that low-intermediate risk zone the expected rise in TSB between 24 and 72 hours is about 6 or 7 mg/dL, or about 0.125 to 0.15 mg/dL/hour. Thus, the 90% success rate with conventional phototherapy, even though it provides much less light than the intensive phototherapy currently recommended by the AAP, is not surprising. Similarly, we know that blue light reduces TSB levels and that infants in the filtered sunlight group were exposed to more of it, so I have

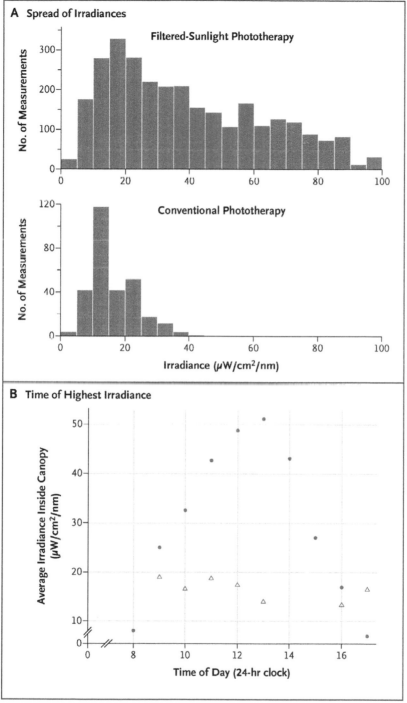

FIGURE 2.—Spread of irradiances and time of highest irradiance for filtered-sunlight phototherapy versus conventional phototherapy. Panel A shows the measured canopy irradiances for infants assigned to filtered-sunlight phototherapy (upper graph) and conventional phototherapy (lower graph). Panel B shows the average canopy irradiance as a function of time of day for all treatment days for filtered-sunlight phototherapy (circles) and conventional phototherapy (triangles). (Reprinted from Slusher TM, Olusanya BO, Vreman HJ, et al. A randomized trial of phototherapy with filtered sunlight in African neonates. *N Engl J Med.* 2015;373:1115-1124, with permission from Massachusetts Medical Society.)

little doubt that the authors' conclusion that efficacy of filtered sunlight is non-inferior to that of conventional phototherapy is correct.

Given the predictability of the efficacy outcome, perhaps the most important results of this study relate to safety. Although temperatures > 38° C occurred more often in the filtered sunlight group, they were uncommon and none of the infants needed to withdraw from the study for safety reasons. At least under the closely monitored conditions of this randomized trial, filtered sunlight appears to be at least as effective as conventional phototherapy, similarly safe, and to have many advantages in areas related to cost, reliability, and feasibility.

Several important questions remain before this new technology is widely disseminated, however. Chief among these is the question of when and to whom it should be applied. As the authors point out, no subjects in the current study had TSB levels close to those at which kernicterus occurs or exchange transfusions are indicated. If phototherapy is to be done with a goal of preventing either of these outcomes, it will be important to do additional studies not only to demonstrate its efficacy at high bilirubin levels, but also to develop risk prediction models that will allow us to estimate numbers needed to treat to prevent one exchange transfusion or 1 kernicterus case. These studies are needed to develop guidelines to avoid diversion of scarce resources to jaundice treatment in infants or settings in which the expected benefit is small. In the meantime, the authors are to be congratulated on this important milestone.

T. B. Newman, MD, MPH

Reference

1. American Academy of Pediatrics. Subcommittee on Hyperbilirubinemia. Management of hyperbilirubinemia in the newborn infant 35 or more weeks of gestation. *Pediatrics*. 2004;114:297-316.

Bilirubin Concentrations in Jaundiced Neonates with Conjunctival Icterus

Azzuqa A, Watchko JF (Univ of Pittsburgh School of Medicine, PA)
J Pediatr 167:840-844, 2015

Objectives.—To assess the total serum bilirubin (TSB) levels at which conjunctival icterus is observed in neonates of ≥34 weeks gestation during the first week of life.

Study Design.—Two convenience samples of neonates were examined for conjunctival icterus within 4 hours of TSB measurements. A concurrent assessment of cephalopedal cutaneous icterus was performed and the TSB characterized using the Bhutani hour-specific risk zone nomogram.

Results.—Two hundred forty neonates were studied of which 76 had conjunctival icterus. Conjunctival icterus was always accompanied by cutaneous jaundice to at least the chest and more often than not a TSB >14.9 mg/dL (255 umol/L) consistently in the 76th%-95th% to >95th% range on the Bhutani nomogram. Only a few infants with TSB in the range of 10-14.9 mg/dL (171-255 umol/L) had conjunctival icterus.

Conclusions.—Conjunctival icterus was observed in a subset of jaundiced neonates and associated with elevated hour-specific TSB levels frequently >95th% on the Bhutani nomogram. Conjunctival icterus is a sign of clinically relevant hyperbilirubinemia that merits a TSB measurement and evaluation of the infant (Fig 2).

▶ Neonatal jaundice has been a subject of discussion in the medical literature for centuries. As early as 1724, Johann Juncker drew a distinction between "true jaundice" and "the icteric tinge which may be observed in infants, immediately after birth."[1] A lot has changed with respect to the recognition and management of jaundice in the past 300 years, and yet those of us who see newborns in clinical practice still wrestle with the same essential question. Which infants have jaundice in excess of that which is physiologic?

Pediatricians have long observed that newborns primarily manifest jaundice via discoloration of the skin. Clinical experience tells us, and this study confirms, that while conjunctival icterus is present in some infants, it is never the *first* sign of hyperbilirubinemia, the way it is in older children. As the authors point out, the classic description of head-to-toe neonatal jaundice progression published by Kramer[2] doesn't even mention the appearance of the conjunctiva. Interesting!

The temptation in our current era of universal hyperbilirubinemia screening via serum or transcutaneous bilirubin measurements is to rely so heavily on these objective data that we almost disregard the appearance of the baby. But unless we are routinely making repeated serial measurements, we are still faced with the problem of how to decide which babies are jaundiced enough to need follow-up testing.

Thankfully, this study reminds us that a careful physical examination of the entire baby can still provide helpful information. By collecting some data on the relationship between total serum bilirubin (TSB) levels and conjunctival icterus, Azzuqa and Watchko have finally given us an evidence-based reason to believe the widely accepted notion that infants with yellow eyes generally have jaundice that is "worse" than those without. The presence of a strong

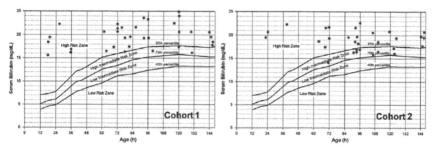

FIGURE 2.—Plot of TSB levels in infants with conjunctival icterus as a function of hour-specific percentile risk zone on the Bhutani nomogram in cohort 1 and cohort 2. *Represents an individual neonate with conjunctival icterus; those in cohort 2 represent concordant exams. (Reprinted from Azzuqa A, Watchko JF. Bilirubin concentrations in jaundiced neonates with conjunctival icterus. *J Pediatr.* 2015;167:840-844, with permission from Elsevier.)

correlation between conjunctival icterus and TSB levels > 75th percentile on the Bhutani nomogram (Fig 2) makes this finding useful in clinical practice, with a couple of notable exceptions: First, because conjunctival icterus was primarily noted when the TSB level was in the midteens or older, this finding would likely be absent in very young babies (< 48 hours old) even if the TSB level was well above the 95th percentile. Second, because some babies without any conjunctival icterus had TSB levels as high as 20 or 21, we must not let the absence of conjunctival icterus deter us from further evaluation when other information suggests it is justified.

The study by Maisels et al mentioned in this article also finds a general connection between higher bilirubin levels and the presence of conjunctival icterus.[3] In contrast to Azzuqa and Watchko, Maisels et al made transcutaneous bilirubin (TcB) measurements on an outpatient cohort of infants 3 to 10 days old and found conjunctival icterus present in 17% of infants with TcB levels < 10 mg/dL and 73% of infants with levels 10.0 to 14.9 mg/dL. Obviously, conjunctival icterus was not a useful indicator of significant hyperbilirubinemia in their patients because most babies with moderately elevated bilirubin levels exhibited it. I do think it is worth noting that these assessments were made in infants coming to the clinic for any reason, even if jaundice was not a clinical concern. It makes me wonder if conjunctival icterus has a somewhat different time course for appearance and resolution than dermal icterus does. Might it be that conjunctival icterus is a late-to-appear and last-to-disappear sign?

Just as the benefits (and pitfalls) of using a visual assessment for jaundice have been debated,[4-7] I'm sure the same will be true of the visual assessment of conjunctival icterus. There is bound to be some disagreement on the utility of this clinical sign. After all, the recognition of physical findings is dependent on the eye of the observer, something inextricably influenced by experience, history, and suboptimal room lighting.

At least we now know that the yellow discoloration we see in the whites of the eyes is most correctly referred to as "conjunctival icterus," not "scleral icterus." As someone who has frequently used the more popular (but incorrect) term, I've made a note of it.

J. L. Aby, MD

References

1. Gartner LM. Neonatal jaundice a selected retrospective. In: Smith GF, Vidyasagar D, eds. Historical Review and Recent Advances in Neonatal and Perinatal Medicine. 1980. http://www.neonatology.org.
2. Kramer LI. Advancement of dermal icterus in the jaundiced newborn. *Amer J Dis Child.* 1969;118:454-458.
3. Maisels MJ, Coffey MP, Gendelman B, et al. Diagnosing jaundice by eye — outpatient assessment of conjunctival icterus in the newborn. *J Pediatr.* 2016;172: 212-214.e1.
4. Manzar S. Cephalo-caudal progression of jaundice: a reliable, non-invasive clinical method to assess the degree of neonatal hyperbilirubinemia. *J Trop Pediatr.* 1999; 45:312-313.
5. Riskin A, Tamir A, Kugelman A, Hemo M, Bader D. Is visual assessment of jaundice reliable as a screening tool to detect significant neonatal hyperbilirubinemia? *J Pediatr.* 2008;152:782-787.

6. Kaplan M, Shchors I, Algur N, Bromiker R, Schimmel MS, Hammerman C. Visual Screening versus transcutaneous bilirubinometry for predischarge jaundice assessment. *Acta Paediatr.* 2008;97:759-763.

7. Keren R, Tremont K, Luan X, Cnaan A. Visual assessment of jaundice in term and late preterm infants. *Arch Dis Child. Fetal Neo Ed.* 2009;94:F317-F322.

Effect of Ursodeoxycholic Acid on Indirect Hyperbilirubinemia in Neonates Treated With Phototherapy

Honar N, Ghashghaei Saadi E, Saki F, et al (Shiraz Univ of Med Sciences, Iran)
J Pediatr Gastroenterol Nutr 62.97-100, 2016

Background.—Hyperbilirubinemia is a common neonatal problem. The present study aimed to investigate the effect of ursodeoxycholic acid in reducing indirect hyperbilirubinemia of infants under phototherapy.

Methods.—This double-blind randomized clinical trial was conducted on neonates with jaundice, who had received phototherapy in the hospitals affiliated with the Shiraz University of Medical Sciences in 2013. A total of 80 neonates were enrolled in the study and were randomly divided into 2 groups. The intervention group (n=40) with indirect hyperbilirubinemia received 10 mg $\cdot$ kg^{-1} $\cdot$ day^{-1} divided every 12 hours Ursobil (capsule 300 mg) in addition to phototherapy, whereas the control group (n = 40) received only phototherapy. Total bilirubin levels were measured every 12 hours until reaching <10 mg/dL, and then phototherapy was disrupted. The duration of phototherapy was measured. The 2 groups were compared regarding total bilirubin levels at different time points and duration of phototherapy using the generalized estimating equation (GEE) test.

Results.—The mean of total bilirubin in the intervention group was 12 ± 1.6, 10 ± 1.1, and 9.8 ± 0.2 mg/dL 12, 24, and 48 hours after the beginning of phototherapy, respectively. On the contrary, these measures were 14.4 ± 1.3, 12.5 ± 1.4, and 10.1 ± 1.1 mg/dL in the control group, respectively, (P<0.05). The mean time required for phototherapy to decrease the bilirubin level to <10 mg/dL was 15.5 ± 6 and 44.6 ± 13.3 hours in the case and the control group, respectively, (P = 0.001).

Conclusions.—Ursodeoxycholic acid had additive effect with phototherapy in neonates with indirect hyperbilirubinemia. This drug also reduced the time period needed for phototherapy and, consequently, decreased the hospitalization period (Fig 1).

▶ Phototherapy converts indirect bilirubin to isomers that can be excreted in the bile or urine without the need for conjugation. The ability of phototherapy to decrease the serum bilirubin level depends both on the rate of formation of these isomers as well as the rapidity with which they can be cleared. Ursodeoxycholic acid (UDCA) is known to stimulate bile flow and lowers conjugated bilirubin levels in various cholestatic conditions; therefore, it seems reasonable to expect that an agent that increases bile flow might also help to decrease indirect serum bilirubin levels in infants who are receiving phototherapy. Although

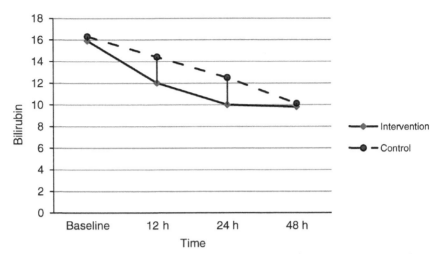

FIGURE 1.—Results of GEE analysis of the total bilirubin levels in the case and control groups during therapy. GEE=generalized estimating equation. (Reprinted from Honar N, Ghashghaei Saadi E, Saki F, et al. Effect of ursodeoxycholic acid on indirect hyperbilirubinemia in neonates treated with phototherapy. *J Pediatr Gastroenterol Nutr.* 2016;62:97-100, with permission from European Society for Pediatric Gastroenterology, Hepatology, and Nutrition and North American Society for Pediatric Gastroenterology, Hepatology, and Nutrition.)

not previously studied in infants in a controlled fashion, the use of UDCA has been recommended as a means of optimizing bile flow in infants and children with Crigler-Najjar disease who are receiving phototherapy in response to an exacerbation of their hyperbilirubinemia.[1] In this study, Honar and colleagues randomly assigned 80 jaundiced infants who were receiving phototherapy for the treatment of their nonhemolytic hyperbilirubinemia to receive, in addition, either UDCA (study group) or a placebo (controls). When the study group was compared with the controls, the bilirubin levels at 12, 24, and 48 hours after initiation of phototherapy were significantly lower (Fig 1), and the time required for phototherapy to reduce the bilirubin to a level less than 10 mg/dL was, on average, 29 hours less. The strengths of the study included the randomized, controlled, study design and the blinding of the participating clinicians.

One might question, however, the need for phototherapy in infants who were, on average, more than 3 ï¿½ days old and, in the absence of hemolytic disease, would not have met the American Academy of Pediatrics guidelines for the use of phototherapy. Although both groups received similar phototherapy treatment, none received what would be considered intensive phototherapy, nor do we have any measurements of the irradiance delivered to these infants. The mean duration of phototherapy in the study group was 15.5 ± 6 hours, which is a duration of phototherapy that is very similar to that provided to 3- to 5-day old infants readmitted to our institution with significantly higher bilirubin levels. We do, of course, provide intensive phototherapy with an irradiance of at least 30 ï¿½W/cmï¿½/nm above and a fiber optic light-emitting diode blanket below the infant, and we discontinue phototherapy when the bilirubin level is less than 14 mg/dL. Nevertheless, the use of more irradiance delivered to a greater surface area can achieve results that are similar to those obtained in the UDCA infants in this study.

On the other hand, because UDCA is a drug that is well tolerated and has a good safety profile, its use might well be considered in limited-resource countries where both equipment and electricity are not readily available. In this situation, either supplementing phototherapy with UDCA or using UDCA to avoid the need for phototherapy is an intervention that certainly deserves consideration.[2]

Although phototherapy has long been considered safe, detailed, long-term follow-up studies of infants who have received phototherapy are limited, and numerous short-term adverse effects of this therapy are well documented.[3] But we also need considerably more data on the use and safety of UDCA in the newborn before we can consider its wider use as a means of preventing or treating hyperbilirubinemia.

M. J. Maisels, MB, BCh, DSc

References

1. Strauss KA, Robinson DL, Vreman HJ, Puffenberger EG, Hart G, Morton DH. Management of hyperbilirubinemia and prevention of kernicterus in 20 patients with Crigler-Najjar disease. *Eur J Pediatr.* 2006;165:306-319.
2. Slusher TM, Olusanya BO, Vreman HJ, et al. A randomized trial of phototherapy with filtered sunlight in African neonates. *New Eng J Med.* 2015;373:1115-1124.
3. Maisels MJ. Sister Jean Ward, phototherapy, and jaundice: a unique human and photochemical interaction. *J Perinatol.* 2015;35:671-675.

Respiratory Rate During the First 24 Hours of Life in Healthy Term Infants

Tveiten L, Diep LM, Halvorsen T, et al (Innlandet Hosp Trust, Elverum, Norway; Oslo Univ Hosp, Norway; Univ of Bergen, Norway)
Pediatrics 137:e20152326, 2016

Background and Objective.—Abnormal respiratory rate (RR) is a key symptom of disease in the abstract newborn. The aim of this study was to establish the reference range for RR during the first 24 hours of life in healthy infants born at term.

Methods.—Infants were included at the hospital postnatal ward when time permitted. During sleep or a defined quiet state, RR was counted at 2, 4, 8, 16, and 24 hours by placing the bell of a stethoscope in front of the nostrils and mouth for 60 seconds. Data on maternal health, pregnancies, and births were obtained from medical records and the Medical Birth Registry of Norway.

Results.—The study included 953 infants. Median RRs were 46 breaths/minute at 2 hours, thereafter 42 to 44 breaths/minute. The 95th percentile was 65 breaths/minute at 2 hours, thereafter 58 to 60 breaths/minute. The fifth percentile was 30 to 32 breaths/minute. Within these limits, the intra-individual variation was wide. The overall mean RR was 5.2 (95% confidence interval [CI], 4.7 to 5.7, $P < .001$) breaths/minute higher while awake than during sleep, 3.1 (95% CI, 1.5 to 4.8, $P < .001$) breaths/minute higher after heavy meconium staining of the amniotic fluid, and 1.6 (95% CI, 0.8 to 2.4, $P < .001$) breaths/minute higher in boys than girls. RR did not differ for infants born after vaginal versus cesarean deliveries.

Conclusions.—The RR percentiles established from this study allow for a scientifically based use of RR when assessing newborn infants born at term.

▶ Observant parents and pediatricians alike will attest to the fact that watching a newborn baby breathe, while fascinating, may be anxiety provoking. This is particularly true during rapid eye movement (REM) sleep when irregular breathing, bursts of rapid breathing, and even brief pauses in breathing may occur. Parents give a sigh of relief when they are told by their pediatrician that their healthy newborn simply has a normal condition that they will outgrow called, "periodic breathing."[1]

Normal breathing among newborns has often been defined by experts as a respiratory rate (RR) of 30 to 60 breaths/minute.[2-4] Is there enough evidence to say that breathing < 30 breaths/minute is too slow and defines "bradypnea," or that breathing > 60 breaths/minute is too fast and defines "tachypnea" for a newborn? Unfortunately, the evidence in the published literature is limited. One recent systematic review showed a range of 26 to 68 breaths/minute (1st to 99th percentile) among normal newborns.[5] A 2015 retrospective chart review study showed a range of 20 to 60 breaths/minute (1st to 99th percentile) and 25 to 51 breaths/minute (5th to 95th percentile) among 0— to less than 3 months old seen in an emergency department setting.[6] Similarly, a 2013 cross-sectional study showed a range of 22 to 76 breaths/minute (1st to 99th percentile) and 27 to 62 breaths/minute (5th to 95th percentile) among hospitalized 0 to less than < 3-month-olds.[7]

Tveitan and colleagues note that scientific studies are needed to determine a reference range for the RR of healthy newborns. Their study of 953 full-term newborns is a welcomed addition to the literature. In this study, they were careful to measure the RR over 60 seconds at 2, 4, 8, 16, and 24 hours when the newborn was quiet or asleep. Respiratory rates were measured by stethoscopic auscultation at the nose/mouth so as not to disturb the newborn. This publication provides clear tables demonstrating proposed reference ranges for newborn RRs. The results demonstrated a mean RR that was 5.2 breaths/minute (95% confidence interval [CI]: 4.7—5.7) higher among awake newborns when compared with that of sleeping newborns, and 3.1 breaths/minute (95% CI: 1.5—4.8) higher for newborns with heavy meconium staining of the amniotic fluid when compared with that of newborns without such staining. Based on the figures provided, there is an apparent slowing in RR by 4 hours of life (mean 43.1 breaths/minute) when compared with 2 hours (47.3 breaths/minute) of life. The reference ranges provided are similar to those reported in studies noted above. At 24 hours of life, the RR range was from 28 to 70 breaths/minute (1st to 99th percentile) and 31 to 59 breaths/minute (5th to 95th percentile).

Returning to the question of what constitutes bradypnea and tachypnea for a newborn, based on the current literature, it seems that a RR of 25 to

60 breaths/minute is well within the normal range. Respiratory rates below and above this range should raise the index of suspicion for illness. For newborns with bradypnea, clinicians should consider underlying causes of respiratory depression including various forms of shock, hypotonia, hypermagnesemia, central nervous system depression from drugs, spinal cord injury, hypothermia, hypothyroidism, and metabolic disease.[8] As was the case for a recent newborn in our region, the clinician should carefully assess the bradypneic newborn and be prepared to intubate if respiratory depression worsens or the newborn becomes apneic. For newborns with tachypnea, clinicians should consider underlying disorders such as sepsis, pneumonia, meconium aspiration syndrome, respiratory distress syndrome, pneumothorax, congenital heart disease, delayed transition, transient tachypnea of the newborn and metabolic disease.[9] Appropriate laboratory and radiographic studies should be performed. Again, the clinician should monitor and be prepared for worsening respiratory distress and respiratory failure.

The 2016 study by Iveiten et al is a well-designed, prospective study of a large number of healthy newborns with RRs measured over a full minute during a quiet state or while asleep. The well-presented data provide further evidence to support previously established norms for newborn RRs. There are limitations to this study, however, in that the results are based on a single site with a study population that consisted of largely nonsmoking, married, Caucasian (93.5%) mothers and their newborns. Also, breastfeeding rates in Norway are among the highest in the world, with 97% of newborns breastfeeding at one month of life.[10] To expand our understanding of the range of normal respiratory rates, it will be important to see if similar results are found in more diverse samples of newborns around the world.

E. K. Chung, MD, MPH

D. Walmsley, DO

References

1. Kelly DH, Carley DW, Shannon DC. Periodic breathing. *Ann N Y Acad Sci.* 1988; 533:301-304.
2. Harriet Lane Service (Johns Hopkins Hospital), Flerlage J, Engorn B. *The Harriet Lane Handbook: A Manual for Pediatric House Officers.* 20th ed. Philadelphia, PA: Saunders/Elsevier; 2015.
3. Fletcher MA. *Physical Diagnosis in Neonatology.*. Philadelphia, PA: Lippincott-Raven; 1998.
4. Kliegman R, Stanton B, St Geme JW, Schor NF, Behrman RE. *Nelson Textbook of Pediatrics.* 20th ed. Philadelphia, PA: Elsevier; 2016.
5. Fleming S, Thompson M, Stevens R, et al. Normal ranges of heart rate and respiratory rate in children from birth to 18 years of age: a systematic review of observational studies. *Lancet.* 2011;377:1011-1018.
6. O'Leary F, Hayen A, Lockie F, Peat J. Defining normal ranges and centiles for heart and respiratory rates in infants and children: a cross-sectional study of patients attending an Australian tertiary hospital paediatric emergency department. *Arch Dis Child.* 2015;100:733-737.
7. Bonafide CP, Brady PW, Keren R, Conway PH, Marsolo K, Daymont C. Development of heart and respiratory rate percentile curves for hospitalized children. *Pediatrics.* 2013;131:e1150-1157.

8. Perlman M. Diagnosing and managing neonatal respiratory depression. *Can Fam Physician.* 1985;31:1019-1023.

9. Hermansen CL, Mahajan A. Newborn respiratory distress. *Am Fam Physician.* 2015;92:994-1002.

10. Haggkvist AP, Brantsaeter AL, Grjibovski AM, Helsing E, Meltzer HM, Haugen M. Prevalence of breast-feeding in the Norwegian Mother and Child Cohort Study and health service-related correlates of cessation of full breast-feeding. *Public Health Nutr.* 2010;13:2076-2086.

Late Diagnosis of Coarctation Despite Prenatal Ultrasound and Postnatal Pulse Oximetry

Lannering K, Bartos M, Mellander M (Queen Silvia Children's Hosp at the Sahlgrenska Univ Hosp, Gothenburg, Sweden)
Pediatrics 136:e406-e412, 2015

Objectives.—To determine what contribution prenatal ultrasound screening and neonatal pulse oximetry screening (POS) make to the timely diagnosis of neonatal coarctation of the aorta (CoA).

Methods.—We identified infants and fetuses diagnosed with isolated CoA in our referral area between 2003 and 2012 who died without surgery, underwent surgical repair before 2 months of age, or were terminated after a prenatal diagnosis. Clinical data were collected from hospital charts.

Results.—Only 3 of the 90 cases were diagnosed prenatally. Two of the 3 were born alive and in 1 case the couple opted for termination of pregnancy. Nineteen of the remaining 87 cases were born in units that used POS (hand and foot) and 4 of 19 screened positive. Of the remaining 83 cases, 46 were discharged undiagnosed (7 after nondiagnostic echocardiography), including 9 with a murmur and weak femoral pulses and 8 with a murmur and normal pulses. One was diagnosed postmortem after dying at home, and 22 of the remaining 45 discharged infants were in circulatory failure on readmission. Five of the patients who were not discharged died without surgery and undiagnosed CoA was the most probable cause of death in 2 of these patients.

Conclusions.—The contribution of prenatal ultrasound screening and postnatal POS to the timely diagnosis of CoA was low. Careful physical examination of all newborns therefore continues to play a fundamental role in detecting this life-threatening cardiac defect, and better screening methods need to be developed.

▶ Newborn infants are precious, beautiful, fragile, and unpredictable. Many diseases—infectious, metabolic, cardiac—may be subtle in their clinical presentations until quite late. Over a few short hours, neonates may deteriorate from a picture of cherubic health to acute, life-threatening illness. Hence, the development of screening tests, tools, and algorithms that give pediatricians a fighting chance at diagnosing a serious neonatal disease while still early in its course and therefore better amenable to treatment and to the best long-term outcomes.

Among the critical congenital heart defects (CCHD, which includes ductal-dependent defects), coarctation of the aorta (CoA) is among the most common to go undetected, and for undiagnosed newborns discharged home, it can lead to dire consequences. Numerous studies have demonstrated this diagnostic gap, concisely reviewed in this article. In the current era, we increasingly rely on prenatal ultrasound and neonatal pulse oximetry. Both strategies continue to evolve: the most recent guidelines for screening prenatal ultrasound mandate visualization of both outflow tracts in addition to the so-called 4-chamber view,[1] and pulse oximetry in the newborn nursery has steadily gained widespread acceptance as a standard to screen for CCHD.[2,3]

This population-based study originating from Sweden analyzes the contributions of prenatal ultrasound and postnatal pulse oximetry to timely diagnosis of neonatal CoA. Unique to this study are data on weak or absent femoral pulses, data that are not generally published in other studies. We thus have a more complete picture of the Swedish process. Unfortunately, the results confirm that CoA remains underdiagnosed before hospital discharge. The fault lies not necessarily in the screening strategies—CoA will continue to elude some efforts—but in how newborn babies are followed and what the threshold of clinical concern should be. These Swedish data indicate that our threshold for clinical suspicion should be quite low indeed.

Certain study details may preclude generalization of these pessimistic results. Importantly, the study is limited by the evolution of screening strategies throughout the study period; not all babies were recipients of the current standards of care. Prenatal detection rates of CoA can be extremely robust at some high-level centers (see Johnson et al[4]); although few centers can match that level, the Swedish prenatal detection rate (3 of 90 cases, or 3.3%) seems exceptionally low (see Mouledoux et al[5] for more typical prenatal detection rates). After routine hospital discharge from the nursery (age >12–24 hours), Sweden's policy for routine newborn outpatient follow-up is at 4 to 6 weeks of age, which is a considerably longer period than here in the United States or that recommended by the World Health Organization.[6] Moreover, it is not clear why patients with equivocal echocardiograms were not monitored for an additional time period as the patent arterial duct closed. Indeed, the system in Sweden appears to differ from those in other developed countries in that "pediatricians" perform echocardiograms in outlying hospitals; their level of training and experience is not known from this study, but we would not expect their level of expertise to be as high as would be at a tertiary care center with pediatric cardiology consultants. Finally, one wonders why some babies in this cohort with weak or absent lower extremity pulses should ever be discharged from hospital without a thorough cardiac evaluation.

We are left to wonder how to improve detection rates of CoA in the newborn infant. Additional strategies include serial prenatal ultrasounds (including one later in gestation), with a low threshold for concern with chamber and outflow tract disproportion.[7,8] And what about blood pressure screening in the newborn nursery? Fuhgeddaboudit.[9,10]

Take-away lessons from this article include the following: (1) Obstetrical ultrasound screening for cardiac defects can still be improved, and minimum standards need to be raised across the board. (2) One should not feel too comfortable with pulse oximetry screening for detecting CoA. (3) "Echocardiography" of newborns may not be performed universally according to standards set by pediatric cardiologists and may also be equivocal in the presence of a patent arterial duct, so caution must still be maintained. (4) Close outpatient follow-up after hospital discharge of the newborn should help decrease delayed diagnosis of CoA and reduce morbidity and mortality.

"Feel the pulses" is the single most important lesson I try to impart to our students and residents. Newborn physical examination is not perfect, but no single screening process is entirely adequate. The pediatrician or general practitioner therefore still needs to bring the entire armamentarium—which, yes, includes physical examination and clinical judgment—to reduce the morbidity associated with delayed diagnosis of CoA.

C. K. L. Phoon, MPhil, MD

References

1. American Institute of Ultrasound in Medicine. AIUM practice guideline for the performance of obstetric ultrasound examinations. *J Ultrasound Med.* 2013;32: 1083-1101.
2. Mahle WT, Newburger JW, Matherne GP, et al. Role of pulse oximetry in examining newborns for congenital heart disease: a scientific statement from the AHA and AAP. *Pediatrics.* 2009;124:823-836.
3. Fillipps DJ, Bucciarelli RL. Cardiac evaluation of the newborn. *Pediatr Clin N Am.* 2015;62:471-489.
4. Johnson LC, Lieberman E, O'Leary E, Geggel RL. Prenatal and newborn screening for critical congenital heart disease: Findings from a nursery. *Pediatrics.* 2014; 134:916-922.
5. Mouledoux JH, Walsh WF. Evaluating the diagnostic gap: Statewide incidence of undiagnosed critical congenital heart disease before newborn screening with pulse oximetry. *Pediatr Cardiol.* 2013;34:1680-1686.
6. World Health Organization (WHO). *WHO Recommendations on Postnatal Care of the Mother and Newborn.* Geneva, Switzerland: World Health Organization (WHO); 2013, https://www.guideline.gov/content.aspx?id=47900. Accessed April 28, 2016.
7. Durand I, Deverriere G, Thill C, et al. Prental detection of coarctation of the aorta in a non-selected population: A prospective analysis of 10 years of experience. *Pediatr Cardiol.* 2015;36:1248-1254.
8. Matsui H, Mellander M, Roughton M, Jicinska H, Gardiner HM. Morphological and physiological predictors of fetal aortic coarctation. *Circulation.* 2008;118: 1793-1801.
9. Boelke KL, Hokanson JS. Blood pressure screening for critical congenital heart disease in neonates. *Pediatr Cardiol.* 2014;35:1349-1355.
10. Patankar N, Fernandes N, Kumar K, Manja V, Lakshminrusimha S. Does measurement of four-limb blood pressures at birth improve detection of aortic arch anomalies? *J Perinatol.* 2016;36:376-380.

Planned Out-of-Hospital Birth and Birth Outcomes

Snowden JM, Tilden EL, Snyder J, et al (Oregon Health and Science Univ, Portland; et al)
N Engl J Med 373:2642-2453, 2015

Background.—The frequency of planned out-of-hospital birth in the United States has increased in recent years. The value of studies assessing the perinatal risks of planned out-of-hospital birth versus hospital birth has been limited by cases in which transfer to a hospital is required and a birth that was initially planned as an out-of-hospital birth is misclassified as a hospital birth.

Methods.—We performed a population-based, retrospective cohort study of all births that occurred in Oregon during 2012 and 2013 using data from newly revised Oregon birth certificates that allowed for the disaggregation of hospital births into the categories of planned in hospital births and planned out-of-hospital births that took place in the hospital after a woman's intrapartum transfer to the hospital. We assessed perinatal morbidity and mortality, maternal morbidity, and obstetrical procedures according to the planned birth setting (out of hospital vs. hospital).

Results.—Planned out-of-hospital birth was associated with a higher rate of perinatal death than was planned in-hospital birth (3.9 vs. 1.8 deaths per 1000 deliveries, *P* = 0.003; odds ratio after adjustment for maternal characteristics and medical conditions, 2.43; 95% confidence interval [CI], 1.37 to 4.30; adjusted risk difference, 1.52 deaths per 1000 births; 95% CI, 0.51 to 2.54). The odds for neonatal seizure were higher and the odds for admission to a neonatal intensive care unit lower with planned out-of-hospital births than with planned in-hospital birth. Planned out-of-hospital birth was also strongly associated with unassisted vaginal delivery (93.8%, vs. 71.9% with planned in-hospital births; *P* < 0.001) and with decreased odds for obstetrical procedures.

Conclusions.—Perinatal mortality was higher with planned out-of-hospital birth than with planned in-hospital birth, but the absolute risk of death was low in both settings. (Funded by the Eunice Kennedy Shriver National Institute of Child Health and Human Development.)

▶ All births involve risk; home births probably incur more. In his recent piece, Snowden has added his voice to the choir, while rectifying a recurring methodologic flaw in other work by distinguishing births based on their intended location. His article adds to an increasingly robust literature that, while balancing those risks with benefits, has fairly consistently, albeit not uniformly, demonstrated that, given the current standards for home deliveries in the United States, some small number of newborns will be harmed because of their parents' choice of birth venue. Importantly, despite that fact, more and more women, and more educated women, are choosing to deliver at home. The key question, then, is whether these data represent the final nail in the coffin of home births, or should they be the start of a dialogue about risks, rights, and ways forward? I believe the latter approach is more reasoned and more respectful of individuals' values and life choices.

In the first instance, although risk is involved in home births, the degree of risk is unclear with excess perinatal mortality apparently in the range of 1 or 2 per 1000 (indeed, in this article it was 1.52 per thousand) and, with reasonable safeguards, would undoubtedly (as reflected in European cohorts) be lower. Differences in findings between studies are due in part to methodologic differences (eg, do investigators count all out-of-hospital births as home births or only planned births, as did the Snowden study? are confounders adequately considered, what outcomes are used?), and in part to differences in policy and practice between locales assessed.

Snowden's work is based on births in Oregon, and Oregon at the time of the study was sui generis, not merely because of the weather and the food trucks, but also because unlicensed/unregulated midwives practiced there. Beyond that, the higher mortality rates in the United States compared with some European countries may relate to the fact that the United States, as a whole, is sui generis, in part because of its geography (great distances between homes and back-up hospitals in many regions) and demography (women may be older and heavier), and partly because of the approach of its guilds. Countries that have achieved better home birth results have usually had midwifes and obstetricians working pari passu in developing and implementing guidelines, and in integrating care.

However, even with a perfected home birth system, all risks cannot be eliminated. Any experienced obstetrician or midwife knows that although there are often auguries of obstetrical disaster that allow for safe transit to hospitals, there are also calamities that occur without warning and that require an immediate, in situ response if a child is to be salvaged intact. If one accepts the harsh reality that there is some irreducible level of risk, what then? Should home births be banned. Do potential harms outweigh any amount of family-perceived good? There are 2 arguments against any attempts to ban: the need to value patient values and the futility of demanding a zero-risk perinatal universe.

Informed consent includes considerations of medical facts and patient values. The process is not merely an anodyne balancing of biologic benefits and burdens. With values involved, the weighing can be as grave as deciding whether a life with impairment is worth living, or as solipsistic as whether the surgical pain associated with cosmetic surgery is worth the anticipated increase in self-esteem. Although physicians can bring medical values (beneficence, truth telling) into the process, it is not for them to unilaterally determine whether the patient's own values are insufficient to tip the scales. Physicians have the right to refuse to participate if they think the biologic risk overwhelms a potential value-based benefit (eg, they could refuse to perform a tuboplasty if in vitro fertilization is readily available and affordable), they should be loath to do so if the balance is anywhere close to equipoise and the values deeply held.

And in a world in which risks can never be reduced to zero, women cannot have options foreclosed merely because their choice entails some increased relative risk. A walk in the rain increases the relative risk of getting struck by lightning, a left turn has a 3-fold risk of a motor vehicle collision relative to a right turn. If the sole goal of the 9 months of gestation were to minimize risk, pregnant women would not only be denied access to bars, but to Shake Shack and Godiva chocolates as well. Trials of labor encumber a risk not dissimilar to that reported in many studies of home births; a risk obstetrical organizations believe is reasonable. Life with minimal risk is life in a bubble.

Given these realities, the way forward is fairly straightforward: make hospital births more accommodating, make home births safer. Models for the latter are easily found across the pond. The Royal College of Obstetricians and Gynecologists and the Royal College of Midwifery have jointly crafted and published guidelines for safe home births and their outcomes speak to the success of the endeavor. As they said in their joint statement on home births, "There is ample evidence showing that labouring at home increases a woman's likelihood of a birth that is both satisfying and safe."[1] Those words and their Colleges' deeds make a fitting mission statement for their American cousins.

H. Minkoff, MD

S. Karakash, MD

Reference

1. Royal College of Obstetricians and Gynaecologists/Royal College of Midwives Joint statement No. 2. 2007. http://www.rsfq.qc.ca/pdf/recherches/UK_Homebirth_Statement.pdf. Accessed March 29, 2016.

Relationship Between Cesarean Delivery Rate and Maternal and Neonatal Mortality

Molina G, Weiser TG, Lipsitz SR, et al (Harvard T.H. Chan School of Public Health, Boston, MA; Stanford Univ, CA; et al)
JAMA 314:2263-2270, 2015

Importance.—Based on older analyses, the World Health Organization (WHO) recommends that cesarean delivery rates should not exceed 10 to 15 per 100 live births to optimize maternal and neonatal outcomes.

Objectives.—To estimate the contemporary relationship between national levels of cesarean delivery and maternal and neonatal mortality.

Design, Setting, and Participants.—Cross-sectional, ecological study estimating annual cesarean delivery rates from data collected during 2005 to 2012 for all 194 WHO member states. The year of analysis was 2012. Cesarean delivery rates were available for 54 countries for 2012. For the 118 countries for which 2012 data were not available, the 2012 cesarean delivery rate was imputed from other years. For the 22 countries for which no cesarean rate data were available, the rate was imputed from total health expenditure per capita, fertility rate, life expectancy, percent of urban population, and geographic region.

Exposures.—Cesarean delivery rate.

Main Outcomes and Measures.—The relationship between population-level cesarean delivery rate and maternal mortality ratios (maternal death from pregnancy related causes during pregnancy or up to 42 days postpartum per 100 000 live births) or neonatal mortality rates (neonatal mortality before age 28 days per 1000 live births).

Results.—The estimated number of cesarean deliveries in 2012 was 22.9 million (95% CI, 22.5 million to 23.2 million). At a country-level, cesarean delivery rate estimates up to 19.1 per 100 live births (95% CI, 16.3 to 21.9) and 19.4 per 100 live births (95% CI, 18.6 to 20.3) were inversely correlated with maternal mortality ratio (adjusted slope coefficient, −10.1; 95% CI, −16.8 to −3.4; $P = .003$) and neonatal mortality rate (adjusted slope coefficient, −0.8; 95% CI, −1.1 to −0.5; $P < .001$), respectively (adjusted for total health expenditure per capita, population, percent of urban population, fertility rate, and region). Higher cesarean delivery rates were not correlated with maternal or neonatal mortality at a country level. A sensitivity analysis including only 76 countries with the highest-quality cesarean delivery rate information had a similar result: cesarean delivery rates greater than 6.9 to 20.1 per 100 live births were inversely correlated with the maternal mortality ratio (slope coefficient, −21.3; 95% CI, −32.2 to −10.5, $P < .001$). Cesarean delivery rates of 12.6 to 24.0 per 100 live births were inversely correlated with neonatal mortality (slope coefficient, −1.4; 95%CI, −2.3 to −0.4; $P = .004$).

Conclusions and Relevance.—National cesarean delivery rates of up to approximately 19 per 100 live births were associated with lower maternal or neonatal mortality among WHO member states. Previously recommended national target rates for cesarean deliveries may be too low.

▶ Summarizing the 1985 World Health Organization (WHO) summit, "Appropriate Technology for Birth,"[1] countries with the lowest perinatal mortality rates had cesarean delivery rates of less than 10%. Using these data, the authors concluded that "there is no justification for any region to have a rate higher than 10–15%." Since that time, this rate has been the WHO target.

The authors of this new, exciting study set out to reexamine this question with a much larger, more contemporary dataset. They found a higher rate of up to 19 cesarean deliveries per 100 live births was associated with lower maternal and neonatal mortality. The study was an impressive undertaking that involved combing data from databases from the 194 WHO states. The large numbers and inclusion of maternal mortality in addition to perinatal mortality is certainly a move toward better scientific accuracy; however, I am left wondering if, on a population level, this is the appropriate question to ask and the correct outcome to examine on a population level.

Examining perinatal mortality rates alone across a few countries does not seem to be the best way of determining the optimal cesarean delivery rate. Adding maternal mortality as an outcome of interest makes sense; however, to say that the optimal rate can be determined by these 2 factors alone is a great oversimplification of a complex problem. In addition to mortality, there are so many other important maternal and perinatal morbidities that should be given weight.

Maternal and neonatal mortality are much more common in the developing world, but even in that context, they are far less common than maternal and neonatal morbidities. For example, prolonged obstructed labor is associated with higher rates of urinary fistula formation. In addition, cesarean deliveries can have intra- and postoperative complications, and these rates rise with each subsequent cesarean delivery. The rate of placenta accrete is on the rise and can result in massive transfusions, hysterectomies, and prolonged hospitalizations. On the neonatal side, there are advantages to performing cesarean deliveries for fetal distress and malpresentation, and new emerging data demonstrate differences in the newborn gut microbial environment in babies delivered by cesarean that may negatively affect health later in life. These are only few of the many important maternal and neonatal outcomes that deserve consideration.

The decision to perform a cesarean delivery is influenced by so many factors that vary greatly on a population, country, city, hospital, and even provider. There are logistical issues, cultural preferences, medical-legal pressures—to name a few—that intersect in many places and ways. These complex intersections likely explain in part why the cesarean delivery rate is a low as 10 per 100 live births in some countries and greater than 80 per 100 live births in others.

To say that all countries, cities, and hospitals should target the same rate is unrealistic and perhaps not appropriate. The question we need to work on answering is what mode of delivery will provide the best outcome for an individual mother and baby given a certain set of circumstances. No one would argue that the cesarean rate is too high in some parts of the world and too low in others. However determining the optimal rate is far less important than determining how countries should get there and precisely which women will benefit from cesarean delivery in which settings. Cesarean or no? This is the difficult decision clinicians are faced with daily, and we need better evidence to guide us.

S. N. Bernstein, MD

Reference

1. World Health Organization. Appropriate technology for birth. *Lancet.* 1985;24: 436-437.

Leukocyte Telomere Length in Newborns: Implications for the Role of Telomeres in Human Disease

Factor-Litvak P, Susser E, Kezios K, et al (Columbia Univ, NY; et al)
Pediatrics 137:e20153927, 2016

Background and Objective.—In adults, leukocyte telomere length (LTL) is variable, familial, and longer in women and in offspring conceived by older fathers. Although short LTL is associated with atherosclerotic cardiovascular disease, long LTL is associated with major cancers. The prevailing notion is that LTL is a "telomeric clock, " whose movement (expressed in LTL attrition) reflects the pace of aging. Accordingly, individuals with short LTL are considered to be biologically older than their peers. Recent studies suggest that LTL is largely determined before adulthood. We examined whether factors that largely characterize LTL in adults also influence LTL in newborns.

Methods.—LTL was measured in blood samples from 490 newborns and their parents.

Results.—LTL (mean ± SD) was longer (9.50 ± 0.70 kb) in newborns than in their mothers (7.92 ± 0.67 kb) and fathers (7.70 ± 0.71 kb) (both $P < .0001$); there was no difference in the variance of LTL among the 3 groups. Newborn LTL correlated more strongly with age-adjusted LTL in mothers ($r = 0.47$; $P < .01$) than in fathers ($r = 0.36$; $P < .01$) (P for interaction = .02). Newborn LTL was longer by 0.144 kb in girls than in boys ($P = .02$), and LTL was longer by 0.175 kb in mothers than in fathers ($P < .0001$). For each 1-year increase in father's age, newborn LTL increased by 0.016 kb (95% confidence interval: 0.04 to 0.28) ($P = .0086$).

Conclusions.—The large LTL variation across newborns challenges the telomeric clock model. Having inherently short or long LTL may be largely determined at birth, anteceding by decades disease manifestation in adults.

▶ The study by Factor-Litvak et al on leukocyte telomere length, tested in a large group of newborns (n = 490) and their parents, represents the first comprehensive examination of telomere length at birth in relation to parental telomere length. Although some findings from this study confirm previous studies with children and adults including longer telomeres in females[1] and longer telomeres for the newborns of older fathers and heritability of length with mothers,[2] Factor-Litvak et al's findings challenge the notion of telomere length as biological clock.

Factor-Litvak et al found a similar variance in leukocyte telomere length in newborns compared with mothers and fathers. They conclude that because there is already a large variation of telomere length present at birth, predisposition for disease, including chronic disease such as atherosclerosis and diabetes mellitus, as well as certain cancers is less determined by environmental and other exposures in adulthood than leukocyte telomere length at birth.

The study population where telomere length was investigated was from a larger, well-characterized parent study, the Nulliparous Pregnancy Study Monitoring Mothers-to-be (NuMoM2b study), a prospective cohort study of 10 000 nulliparous women with singleton gestations. Among these, a smaller number (n = 944) were asked to participate in the leukocyte telomere length study.

Although the authors do not challenge the notion that accumulated exposures to oxidative stress may result in accelerated attrition in adulthood leading to increased risk for chronic disease, they do argue that the significant variance present at birth, a range of newborn telomere birth lengths of approximately 4 kilobases, is much larger than the impact of adult environmental exposures that may impact disease.

The study by Factor-Litvak et al is the largest study of telomere length in newborns and makes a significant contribution to telomere science, underscoring the importance of prenatal and early life studies. Smaller studies have suggested that various adverse exposures in pregnancy including prenatal stress can have significant impacts on telomere length at birth (approximately 1.5–2 kilobases)[3] and that adverse birth outcomes such as preterm birth can be associated with shorter telomere length in adulthood.[4] Studies with mice have found that longer telomere length at birth is associated with overall resistance to disease later in life, again suggesting the need to better understand risk factors for shorter telomere length at birth.[5]

Meanwhile, however, there is evidence suggesting that recent adverse life advents or hardship in adulthood are associated with increased adult telomere attrition, whereas childhood ones are not.[6,7] Furthermore, accelerated telomere attrition in adulthood is associated with risk of incident cardiovascular events,[8] and risk factors for greater attrition include exposures in adulthood such as active smoking and features of the metabolic syndrome.[9]

These findings from adult studies, however, need to be placed in context. In the years since the discovery of telomeres and the Nobel Prize awarded for that discovery in 2009, there have been fewer longitudinal studies of telomere length attrition than cross-sectional ones. For some of these longitudinal studies, the strongest predictor of rate of telomere attrition is telomere length at baseline, possibly attesting to the importance of exposures at birth or early in childhood that set the stage for lifelong health.[10] For other studies, short telomere length is associated with incident disease such as insulin resistance diabetes mellitus; however, it is not clear when during the life span the shortening occurred.[11,12] Further comprehensive studies from birth are needed to untangle how exposures in utero versus those in early childhood and thereafter impact telomere length dynamics and risk for disease. Factor-Litvak et al's important study should be followed by others using a longitudinal study design of telomere length dynamics in relation to human health from birth through older age.

J. M. Wojcicki, PhD, MPH

References

1. Wojcicki JM, Olveda R, Heyman MB, et al. Cord blood telomere length in Latino infants: relation with maternal education and infant sex. *J Perinatol.* 2016;36: 235-241.
2. Broer L, Codd V, Nyholt DR, et al. Meta-analysis of telomere length in 19,713 subjects reveals high heritability, stronger maternal inheritance and a paternal age effect. *Eur J Hum Genet.* 2013;21:1163-1168.
3. Marchetto NM, Glynn RA, Ferry ML, et al. Prenatal stress and newborn telomere length. *Am J Obstet Gynecol.* 2016;215:94.e1-8.
4. Smeets CC, Codd V, Samani NJ, Hokken-Koelega AC. Leukocyte telomere length in young adults birth preterm: support for accelerated biological ageing. *PLoS One.* 2015;10:e0143951.
5. Ilmonen P, Kotraschal A, Penn DJ. Telomere attrition due to infection. *PLoS One.* 2008;3:e2143.
6. Van Ockenburg SL, Bos EH, de Jonge P, van der Harst P, Gans ROB, Rosmalen JGM. Stressful life events and leukocyte telomere attrition in adulthood: a prospective population-based cohort study. *Psychol Med.* 2015;45: 2975-2984.
7. Epel ES, Blackburn EH, Lin J, et al. Accelerated telomere shortening in response to life stress. *Proc Natl Acad Sci U S A.* 2004;101:17312-17315.
8. Baragetti A, Palmen J, Garlaschelli K, et al. Telomere shortening over 6 years is associated with increased subclinical carotid vascular damage and worse cardiovascular prognosis in the general population. *J Intern Med.* 2015;277:478-487.

9. Huzen J, Wong LS, van Veldhuisen DJ, et al. Telomere length loss due to smoking and metabolic traits. *J Intern Med.* 2014;275:155-163.
10. Weischer M, Bojesen SE, Nordestgaard BG. Telomere shortening unrelated to smoking body weight, physical activity and alcohol intake: 4,576 general population individuals with repeat measurements 10 years apart. *PLoS Genetics.* 2014;10:e1004191.
11. Verhulst S, Dalgård C, Labat C, et al. A short leucocyte telomere length is associated with development of insulin resistance. *Diabetologia.* 2016;59:1258-1265.
12. Willeit P, Raschenberg J, Heydon EE, et al. Leucocyte telomere length and risk of type 2 diabetes mellitus: new prospective cohort study and literature-based meta-analysis. *PLoS One.* 2014;9:e112483.

Crib Bumpers Continue to Cause Infant Deaths: A Need for a New Preventive Approach

Scheers NJ, Woodard DW, Thach BT (BDS Data Analytics, Alexandria, VA; US Dept of Labor, Dallas, TX; Washington Univ, St Louis, MO)
J Pediatr 169:93-97.e1, 2016

Objectives.—To assess whether clutter (comforters, blankets, pillows, toys) caused bumper deaths and provide an analysis of bumper-related incidents/injuries and their causal mechanisms.

Study Design.—Bumper-related deaths (January 1, 1985, to October 31, 2012) and incidents/injuries (January 1, 1990, to October 31, 2012) were identified from the US Consumer Product Safety Commission (CPSC) databases and classified by mechanism. Statistical analyses include mean age, 95% CIs, χ^2 test for trend, and ANOVA with a paired-comparisons information-criterion post hoc test for age differences among injury mechanisms.

Results.—There were 3 times more bumper deaths reported in the last 7 years than the 3 previous time periods ($\chi^2_{(3)} = 13.5$, $P \le .01$). This could be attributable to increased reporting by the states, diagnostic shift, or both, or possibly a true increase in deaths. Bumpers caused 48 suffocations, 67% by a bumper alone, not clutter, and 33% by wedgings between a bumper and another object. The number of CPSC-reported deaths was compared with those from the National Center for the Review and Prevention of Child Deaths, 2008-2011; the latter reported substantially more deaths than CPSC, increasing the total to 77 deaths. Injury mechanisms showed significant differences by age ($F_{4,120} = 3.2$, $P < .001$) and were caused by design, construction, and quality control problems. Eleven injuries were apparent life-threatening events.

Conclusion.—The effectiveness of public health recommendations, industry voluntary standard requirements, and the benefits of crib bumper use were not supported by the data. Study limitations include an undercount of CPSC reported deaths, lack of denominator information, and voluntary incident reports (Fig 1).

▶ How many deaths from crib bumpers are too many before the Consumer Products Safety Commission (CPSC) formally bans them? This is a reasonable

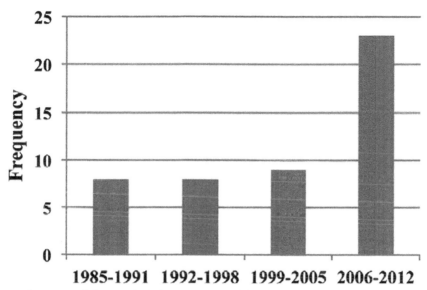

FIGURE 1.—Crib bumper deaths by year. (Reprinted from Scheers NJ, Woodard DW, Thach BT. Crib bumpers continue to cause infant deaths: a need for a new preventive approach. *J Pediatr.* 2016;169:93-97.e1, with permission from Elsevier.)

question to ask. A product that serves no purpose other than decoration has now been shown to be directly responsible for 48 deaths between 1985 and 2012. Although this number may not seem like a lot, the fact that the rate over the most recent 6 years is 3 times higher than any previous 6-year interval is concerning (Fig 1). Additionally, given the wide variation in reporting to the CPSC and still prevalent lack of standardized death scene investigation and reporting, it is likely that the total number of crib bumper related deaths is even higher.

In addition to deaths, Scheer et al also report on 146 nonfatal bumper injuries, which are classified by 2 mechanisms as near-suffocation or limb entrapment. Eleven of the near-suffocation events were significant enough to be brought to the hospital as an apparent life threatening event. Younger children were more likely to experience near-suffocation, while older infants were more likely to be injured by falls or limb entrapment injuries. Based on these reports and cases reported to the National Center for Child Death Review, the American Academy of Pediatrics recommends against the use of crib bumpers.[1] A few locales and 1 state (Maryland) have banned the sale of crib bumpers.[2]

What have we learned in the past few decades about sudden unexpected infant deaths (SUID)? The biggest take-home is that the sleep environment matters. The original "Back to Sleep" recommendation lead to a significant drop in sudden infant death syndrome (SIDS) deaths from 1992 to 2001 of 120 of 100 000 live births to 56 of 100 000.[1] Unfortunately, the rate of decline of

SIDS cases has leveled off, and the overall SUID rate has remained stable as the number of Unexplained or Accidental Suffocation in Bed cases have increased. The shift in nomenclature has come with the improved and more standardized infant death investigation protocols and Child Fatality Review Processes from the National Center for Child Death Review and the Centers for Disease Control. The "Back to Sleep" message from the Eunice Kennedy Shriver National Institute for Child Health and Human Development was recently rebranded the "Safe to Sleep" campaign,[3] which focuses more on the infant sleep environment.

A more complete safety message to parents supplements the original "back to sleep" message: children should be placed Alone, on their Back, and in a Crib (or bassinette). Creating the safest sleep environment reduces the risk of asphyxiation, rebreathing, and SIDS. The "triple risk model" best explains the potential pathogenesis of SIDS and includes the convergence of environmental stressors, in a vulnerable infant, during a critical developmental period.[4] Since specific tests for infant vulnerability do not exist, the most modifiable risk factors are the environmental stressors. In addition to removing tobacco smoke exposure, the immediate sleeping environment is the most modifiable risk factor.

As noted in the American Academy of Pediatrics safe sleep policy, having infants sleep on soft mattresses or adult mattresses (with or without other occupants), exposing sleeping infants to crib bumpers and other soft objects, placing sleeping infants on couches (with or without an adult), and placing infants to sleep prone are all associated with an increased risk of SUID.[1] Clearly, educating parents is one approach to reducing the SUID risk of infants. Comprehensive nursery educational programs have been shown to improve self-reported sleep practices.[5] Although one-on-one education might show promise, policy changes potentially can make a much greater impact. I would wholeheartedly concur with the authors of this article who call on the CPSC to ban the sale of crib bumpers nationally.

S. D. Krugman, MD, MS

References

1. American Academy of Pediatrics. Technical report: SIDS and other sleep related deaths: expansion of recommendations for a safe sleeping environment. *Pediatrics.* 2011;128:e1341-e1367.
2. Code of Maryland. Title 10–11-07. Prohibition of sale of baby bumper pads. 2013. http://www.dsd.state.md.us/comar/comarhtml/10/10.11.07.03.htm. Accessed March 23, 2016.
3. https://www.nichd.nih.gov/sts/Pages/default.aspx. Accessed March 23, 2016.
4. Filiano JJ, Kinney HC. A perspective on neuropathologic findings in victims of the sudden infant death syndrome: the triple-risk model. *Biol Neonate.* 1994;65:194-197.
5. Goodstein MH, Bell T, Krugman SD. Improving infant sleep safety through a comprehensive hospital-based program. *Clin Pediatr.* 2015;54:212-221.

Unsafe from the Start: Serious Misuse of Car Safety Seats at Newborn Discharge

Hoffman BD, Gallardo AR, Carlson KF (Oregon Health and Science Univ, Portland)
J Pediatr 171:48-54, 2016

Objective.—To estimate prevalence of car safety seat (CSS) misuse for newborns on hospital discharge; and to identify potential risk and protective factors for CSS misuse.

Study Design.—We randomly sampled 291 mother—baby dyads from the newborn unit of an academic health center. Participants completed a survey and designated someone (themselves or another caregiver) to position their newborn in the CSS and install the CSS in their vehicle. Certified child passenger safety technicians assessed positioning and installation using nationally standardized criteria. To examine factors associated with CSS misuse, we used logistic regression to compute ORs and 95% CIs.

Results.—A total of 291 families (81% of those eligible) participated. Nearly all (95%) CSSs were misused, with 1 or more errors in positioning (86%) and/or installation (77%). Serious CSS misuse occurred for 91% of all infants. Frequent misuses included harness and chest clip errors, incorrect recline angle, and seat belt/lower anchor use errors. Families with mothers of color (OR, 6.3; 95% CI, 1.8-21.6), non-English language (OR, 4.9; 95% CI, 1.1-21.2), Medicaid (OR, 10.3; 95% CI, 2.4-44.4), or lower educational level (OR, 4.5; 95% CI, 1.7-12.4) were more likely to misuse CSSs. However, families that worked with a child passenger safety technician before delivery were significantly less likely to misuse their CSSs (OR, 0.1; 95% CI, 0.0-0.4).

Conclusion.—Nearly all parents of newborn infants misused CSSs. Resources should be devoted to ensuring families with newborns leave the hospital correctly using their CSS (Tables 1 and 3).

▶ Car safety seats (CSSs) aren't controversial. Every state requires that infants be restrained in CSSs because they save lives. In the United States in 2012, there were 1168 traffic fatalities among children 0 to 14 years old. CSSs are found to decrease mortality rates in cars by 71% for infants and by 54% for toddlers.[1] This finding is in addition to the reduction in serious injuries and hospitalizations. But CSSs aren't easy to use. As a new mother and pediatric resident, I made at least 3 errors when I first put my son in our CSS. And it turns out, I'm not alone. In fact, according to this new study by Hoffman et al, CSSs are almost impossible to use correctly.

The authors studied CSS misuse among mother-baby dyads at discharge from the newborn nursery of an academic medical center. They found serious CSS misuse in 91% of families. This number is astronomical. Almost no one is using their CSSs correctly! This rate is somewhat higher than the rates of CSS misuse found in 2 prior similar studies of newborns at hospital discharge (85% and 78%)[2,3] and the overall CSS critical misuse rate of 72.6% found

TABLE 1.—Misuse Categories and Types of CSS Misuse

Critical Misuse*	Serious Misuse†	Any Misuse†
• Age/weight inappropriateness of CSS • Harness strap not used • Improper harness belt paths/slots • Improper use of locking clip to seat belt • Improper vehicle seat belt paths/slots • Incorrect seat direction • Incorrect location of CSS • Loose harness straps • Loose vehicle seat belt • Unbuckled harness strap • Unbuckled vehicle seat belt • Visible damage to CSS	Includes all critical misuses plus: • Harness retainer clip not used • Harness retainer clip too high or too low for infant • Improper lower anchor paths/slots • Loose lower anchor webbing • Unbuckled lower anchors • Incorrect recline angle of CSS	Includes all critical and serious misuses plus: • Harness belt twisted • Use of nonregulated products, or thick clothing • Lower anchors used with vehicle seat belt contrary to manufacturer guidelines • Vehicle seat belt webbing twisted • Incorrect use of CSS lock-offs • Locking clip used unnecessarily • CSS handle in incorrect position for car travel • Incorrect spacing between CSS and vehicle seat contrary to manufacturer guidelines

Reprinted from Hoffman BD, Gallardo AR, Carlson KF. Unsafe from the start: serious misuse of car safety seats at newborn discharge. *J Pediatr.* 2016;171:48-54, with permission from Elsevier.
Editor's Note: Please refer to original journal article for full references.
*US Department of Transportation, National Highway Traffic Safety Administration: Misuse of child restraints, 2004, p 32.[15]
†Safe Kids Worldwide, National Child Passenger Certification Program.[14]

TABLE 3.—Types and Frequencies of CSS Errors Among 291 Newborn Families

Type of Error	Frequency, n (%)
Positioning errors*	
Harness too loose	201 (69)
Harness retainer clip too low	103 (35)
Incorrect harness slot	91 (31)
Nonregulated product used	62 (21)
Buckle strap too far from baby	50 (17)
Caregiver unable to adjust harness	51 (17)
Harness webbing twisted	33 (11)
Caregiver unable to connect buckle	32 (11)
Installation errors*	
>1-inch motion of CSS	128 (44)
Incorrect recline angle	118 (41)
Seatbelt retractor not locked†	74 (53)
CSS contacts front seat	59 (20)
CSS too loosely attached to lower anchorsz	47 (31)
Seatbelt and lower anchors used together	39 (14)
Incorrect seatbelt path†	32 (23)
Lower anchors used in middle seat‡	25 (16)

Reprinted from Hoffman BD, Gallardo AR, Carlson KF. Unsafe from the start: serious misuse of car safety seats at newborn discharge. *J Pediatr.* 2016;171:48-54, with permission from Elsevier.
*Categories are not mutually exclusive.
†Percentages calculated among families that used vehicle seatbelts.
‡Percentages calculated among families that used lower anchors.

in a 2004 study conducted by the National Highway Traffic Safety Administration.[4] The higher rate of CSS misuse in this study is likely attributable to the additional errors that the authors included in their definition of serious misuse compared with the prior studies (Table 1).

The authors chose to include incorrect recline angle, lower anchor misuse, and incorrect retainer clip positioning in their definition of serious misuse, because their experience and available data show that these errors place restrained children at increased risk. But whatever the exact number, all of these studies found a CSS misuse rate that is incredibly high and represents an enormous missed opportunity. These are children whose caregivers have already obtained a CSS—we just need to help them use it correctly.

The authors make 2 additional important contributions to the dialogue around this issue, both of which should inform the development of future interventions. First, they found that the participants who had worked with a certified child passenger safety technician (CPST) prior to delivery were one-tenth as likely to make serious errors. However, 77% of these families still made 1 or more serious errors, especially in the positioning of their infants (Table 3). Clearly working with a CPST prior to delivery is helpful, but it is not sufficient to adequately address the issue of CSS misuse. Second, the authors found that nonwhite, non—English-speaking, and Medicaid-insured families were at increased risk of CSS misuse. Future interventions should be designed to reach these more vulnerable populations so that they are not at increased risk of motor vehicle injuries.

Clear recommendations about the safe transportation of newborns at hospital discharge already exist. The American Academy of Pediatrics (AAP) published a policy statement in 1999 recommending that child passenger safety educational materials be provided to families prior to discharge from the newborn nursery, in addition to hands-on teaching.[5] More recently, in 2015, the National Highway Traffic Safety Administration, in conjunction with the AAP and other invested groups, published a set of recommendations for child passenger safety discharge policies that apply to children of all ages at the time of hospital discharge, not just newborns.[6] The group recommended comprehensive child passenger safety policies and that hospitals work closely with CPSTs to develop and implement these policies. More research is needed to determine the extent to which hospitals are implementing such policies and which interventions are most effective.

In addition to the development of robust child passenger safety policies by hospitals, there are immediate, practical steps that individual practitioners can take to address this issue. At a minimum, it is important that providers in hospitals and clinics provide accurate, up-to-date information and educational materials about child passenger safety. The AAP provides helpful resources for families and providers, including a 1-hour training video for providers (http://www2.aap.org/sections/ipp/CPSCurriculum.cfm) created by Dr. Hoffman, the lead author of this article. In addition, providers must be able to direct their patients to CPST resources in the community. This is easier said than done. For example, the San Francisco Fire Department historically provided CSS checks at neighborhood fire stations, but they no longer provide this service. Now the only place to obtain a free CSS check with a CPST in San Francisco is at the California Highway Patrol, but these are by appointment only, which can take weeks to make. There are also for-profit businesses in San Francisco that charge at least $125 for a single CSS check, but this is often prohibitively expensive for families. To find car seat inspection locations in your own community, visit www.seatcheck.org.

Hoffman et al have highlighted the critical and pervasive issue of CSS misuse. They also evaluated the risk for CSS misuse, which has important implications for future interventions. I look forward to future research that will identify effective (and affordable) interventions to decrease CSS misuse. In the meantime, many resources exist to support pediatric providers who wish to address this issue. Given that most of our patients will travel to and from our hospitals and clinics in motor vehicles, it is important to treat every encounter as an opportunity to ensure that our patients get home safely.

T. Clark, MD

References

1. National Highway Traffic Safety Administration, National Center for Statistics and Analysis. Traffic safety facts, 2012 data. http://www-nrd/nhtsa.dot.gov/pubs/812011.pdf. Accessed April 25, 2016.
2. Rogers SC, Gallo K, Saleheen H, Lapidus G. Wishful thinking: safe transportation of newborns at hospital discharge. *J Trauma Acute Care Surg.* 2012;73: S262-S266.
3. Tessier K. Effectiveness of hands-on education for correct child restraint use by parents. *Accid Anal Prev.* 2010;42:1041-1047.
4. National Highway Transportation Safety Administration. *Results of the National Child Restraint Use Special Study* (Publication no. DOT HS 812 142). Washington, DC: National Highway Traffic Safety Administration; 2015, http://www-nrd.nhtsa.dot.gov/Pubs/812142.pdf. Accessed April 25, 2016.
5. Bull M, Agran P, Laraque D, et al. American Academy of Pediatrics, Committee on Injury and Poison Prevention. Safe Transportation of newborns at hospital discharge. *Pediatrics.* 1999;104:986-987.
6. National Highway Transportation Safety Administration.. *Hospital discharge recommendations for safe transportation of children: best practice recommendations developed by an expert working group convened by the National Highway Traffic Safety Administration* (Publication no. DOT HS 812 106). Washington, DC: National Highway Traffic Safety Administration; 2015, http://www.nhtsa.gov/staticfiles/nti/pdf/812106_HospitalDischrgeRecSafeTransChildren.pdf. Accessed April 25, 2016.

Complications following circumcision: Presentations to the emergency department

Gold G, Young S, O'Brien M, et al (Royal Children's Hosp Melbourne, Victoria, Australia; Univ of Melbourne, Victoria, Australia; et al)
J Paediatr Child Health 51:1158-1163, 2015

Background.—Circumcision is the most common surgical procedure performed on boys in Australia. Patient presentations to the emergency department (ED) following circumcision are common; however, no Australian research has investigated acute care presentations.

Objectives.—To identify reasons for presentation to the ED after circumcision and determine whether the setting (community vs. hospital) in which the procedure had been performed has any bearing on the sequelae seen.

Methods.—Retrospective chart review of children presenting with circumcision related problems to the Royal Children's Hospital, Melbourne, Australia, between 2012 and 2014. Descriptive and χ^2 analysis included sequelae of community- versus hospital-performed procedures.

Results.—Over a 29-month period, we identified 167 children with a circumcision-related ED presentation. Mean age was 3 years. A percentage of 54.5 had been performed for non-medical, 29.9% for medical reasons and 14.4% for reasons unknown. When location was known ($n = 152$), 60.5% were performed in the community and 39.5% in hospital. Reasons for presentation were: bleeding (53.9%), pain (38.3%), swelling (37.1%), redness (25.7%), decreased urine output (13.8%), fever (7.2%) and pus (6%). 29.9% were diagnosed as normal healing post circumcision. Patients were admitted in 39.1% versus 15% ($P = 0.001$) and re-operated in 18.5% versus 1.7% ($P = 0.001$) after community- versus hospital-operated circumcisions.

Conclusions.—A range of reasons cause patients to seek help in the ED following a circumcision. Parents would have profited from better explanation of post-circumcision appearance of the penis. ED presentations after community-performed procedures required more re-operations than after hospital-performed circumcisions.

▶ Circumcision (especially neonatal) is the most common surgical procedure performed in young males, although there are wide variations regionally in prevalence, mostly driven by cultural, religious, ethical, and/or social customs and beliefs. In the United States, for example, rates vary from about 40% in the west to about 80% in the central states[1] with a mean of about 60% overall. In contrast, in Australia, 10% to 20% of newborn males are circumcised for what might be considered nonclinical reasons.[2]

Controversies regarding the relative medical benefits versus complications of the procedure have led leading medical organizations to develop policy and guideline statements. In Australia, the Royal Australasian College of Physicians Division of Paediatrics and Child Health has determined routine male circumcision to be medically unnecessary, although respect for parental choice is encouraged.[2] As government funding for routine nontherapeutic circumcision performed within public hospitals was discontinued, the procedure became more commonly performed in outpatient clinics, specialists offices, and perhaps nonmedical facilities such as private homes and less frequently performed within the major pediatric hospitals, including the Royal Children's Hospital in Melbourne.

Gold et al performed a retrospective study to explore the impact of moving circumcisions outside the hospital setting on postprocedure emergency department (ED) presentations and the identifiable complications in males 0 to 18 years of age. Limitations of the study include its retrospective design as well as the lack of reliable data on the total pool of circumcisions, level of training and type of provider performing the procedure, type of device used, data on patients who may have presented with complications to a non-ED facility, and data on any pre-procedure information parents may have received regarding healing and complications. Nevertheless, the study adds useful data to the literature on complications and, in particular, seeks to address the question of the safety impact of a change in setting from in-hospital to the less controllable outside community.

Within the study period of 2012 to 2014, 1478 patients presented with concerns. Of the 141 patients, representing 167 ED complaints, 55% had a circumcision performed for nonmedical indications. For approximately 60% of the patients, the procedure was done within the community setting. Similar to previous studies, the major complaints were bleeding, pain, and swelling, followed by redness, decreased urine output, pus, and fever. Most (119) did not require hospital admission and were discharged from the ED, but of those who were admitted, 39.1% came from community-performed circumcisions versus 15% ($P = .001$) of those from the hospital setting, with 18.5% versus 1.7% ($P = .0001$) requiring operative intervention, respectively. About 80% of the circumcisions done in the community setting were for routine nonclinical reasons, whereas 80% of those done in the hospital were of older age and done for medical indications and should have been at higher risk for postsurgical complications. Despite the study limitations and overall small numbers of readmissions, ongoing surveillance would probably be prudent to determine whether this concerning trend is confirmed.

More interesting, Gold et al found that about 30% of the ED presentation complaints were determined to be simply the natural healing postprocedure process of which parents were unaware. As suggested by the authors, an opportunity to impact a reduction in unnecessary ED visits, reduction of the associated costs and use of resources as well as alleviate undo parental anxiety was identified. Instituting effective parental education, explaining the expected posthealing process and penile appearance, is likely to achieve tangible benefits.

Nelson et al from the Department of Urology, Children's Boston Hospital, developed a visual tool for parents to aid in their understanding of postcircumcision healing.[3] They used actual photographs compiled within an atlas to demonstrate the sequence of healing and included descriptions of complications. The atlas was well received by parents, served to decrease anxiety, and resulted in a significant decrease in postsurgical phone calls without an increase in delayed recognition of complications. Actual ED visits, however, were not assessed.

Technological advances are allowing more procedures to move from in-hospital settings to outpatient settings, leaving parents with the responsibility of monitoring their children's recovery at home. By providing enhanced education, parents can become effective partners in the care of their children if they are able to distinguish the normal healing and recovery process versus complications requiring ED or acute care clinic visits postprocedure (not just circumcisions). As Gold et al suggests, educating or improving the instructions given to parents about the most common surgical procedure performed in children, circumcision, would be a reasonable and cost-effective place to start.

C. A. Miller, MD

References

1. Owings M, et al. Trends in Circumcision for Male Newborns in U.S. Hospitals: 1979–2010. http://www.cdc.gov/nchs/data/hestat/circumcision_2013/Circumcision_2013.htm.
2. The Royal Australasian College of Physicians. Circumcision of infant males. 2010. p. 1-28.
3. Nelson CP, Rosoklija I, Grant R, Retik AB. Development and implementation of a photographic atlas for parental instruction and guidance after outpatient penile surgery. *J Pediatr Urol.* 2012;8:521-526.

20 Nutrition

Routine Amoxicillin for Uncomplicated Severe Acute Malnutrition in Children
Isanaka S, Langendorf C, Berthé F, et al (Médecins sans Frontières Operational Ctr Paris, France)
N Engl J Med 374:444-453, 2016

Background.—High-quality evidence supporting a community-based treatment protocol for children with severe acute malnutrition, including routine antibiotic use at admission to a nutritional treatment program, remains limited. In view of the costs and consequences of emerging resistance associated with routine antibiotic use, more evidence is required to support this practice.

Methods.—In a double-blind, placebo-controlled trial in Niger, we randomly assigned children who were 6 to 59 months of age and had uncomplicated severe acute malnutrition to receive amoxicillin or placebo for 7 days. The primary outcome was nutritional recovery at or before week 8.

Results.—A total of 2412 children underwent randomization, and 2399 children were included in the analysis. Nutritional recovery occurred in 65.9% of children in the amoxicillin group (790 of 1199) and in 62.7% of children in the placebo group (752 of 1200). There was no significant difference in the likelihood of nutritional recovery (risk ratio for amoxicillin vs. placebo, 1.05; 95% confidence interval [CI], 0.99 to 1.12; $P = 0.10$). In secondary analyses, amoxicillin decreased the risk of transfer to inpatient care by 14% (26.4% in the amoxicillin group vs. 30.7% in the placebo group; risk ratio, 0.86; 95% CI, 0.76 to 0.98; $P = 0.02$).

Conclusions.—We found no benefit of routine antibiotic use with respect to nutritional recovery from uncomplicated severe acute malnutrition in Niger. In regions with adequate infrastructure for surveillance and management of complications, health care facilities could consider eliminating the routine use of antibiotics in protocols for the treatment of uncomplicated severe acute malnutrition. (Funded by Médecins sans Frontières Operational Center Paris; ClinicalTrials.gov number, NCT01613547.)

▶ The proof may not always be in the pudding but rather in the population. This notable study by Isanaka et al has the potential to change practice on a global level and contributes further to our knowledge of uncomplicated severe acute malnutrition in children.

The World Health Organization has long recommended empiric antibiotic therapy for all children hospitalized for severe acute malnutrition (SAM). As

SAM therapy has progressively moved from inpatient wards to outpatient clinics, the need for antibiotic therapy has been questioned. In 2013, a randomized, double-blind, placebo-controlled trial among 2767 Malawian children showed that nutritional recovery and mortality were improved with the incorporation of antibiotics (either amoxicillin or cefdinir, compared with placebo) into protocols for uncomplicated SAM.[1] Subsequently, community-based protocols were developed worldwide in locations where SAM was prevalent despite a lack of generalizable, high-grade data. The 2013 Malawian trial, albeit groundbreaking in its outcomes, examined a unique population of children with a high prevalence of human immunodeficiency virus (HIV) exposure and infection (~18% of mothers tested were HIV positive) and kwashiorkor (~70% of children).

In contrast, Isanaka and colleagues randomized 2412 children from Madarounfa, Niger with SAM (defined as a weight-for-height z score of less than −3, a mid-upper-arm circumference of less than 115 mm, or both) to either amoxicillin or placebo. This trial, which is only the second randomized controlled trial to examine the routine use of antibiotics in community-based malnutrition programs, is novel in that it is more readily generalizable with only 1 child of the 2412 randomized with confirmed HIV infection. Moreover, malnutrition was predominately due to marasmus rather than kwashiorkor because those with bipedal edema were excluded. There was no difference in the primary outcome between study arms, with 65.9% of children in the amoxicillin group and 62.7% in the placebo group experiencing nutritional recovery (risk ratio for amoxicillin vs placebo, 1.05; 95% confidence interval, 0.99 to 1.12; $P = .10$). The authors therefore conclude that there is no benefit to routine antibiotic use for uncomplicated SAM—quite the game-changer!

The routine use of antibiotics does not come without risk (economically or medically), especially when provided on such a large scale. According to the annual 2014 medical report in Madarounfa, Niger, an alarming 15% of all antibiotic use in children under 5 years of age was attributed to SAM treatment protocols. Furthermore, even though the overall prevalence of bacterial gastroenteritis, bacteremia, and bacteriuria was low, antibiotic resistance is a tangible threat with many of the bacteria isolates from children at admission to the nutritional program showing resistance to amoxicillin and amoxicillin-clavulanate. In such a high-risk population who may need frequent access to antibiotics for life-threatening infections, preventing antibiotic resistance is paramount.

Even though the Isanaka paper found no difference in nutritional recovery at 8 weeks between the amoxicillin and placebo groups, there were some improved outcomes that came from the addition of amoxicillin to the "170 kcal per kilogram per day Plumpy'Nut (Nutriset)" and "routine medicine" cocktail. The children in the amoxicillin group had a statistically significant shorter nutritional recovery by 2 days, and there was a decreased risk of transfer to inpatient care. Despite this, it is still not enough to support the continued prescription of large-scale antibiotic regimens in uncomplicated SAM.

This doesn't mean that antibiotic therapy is not exceedingly advantageous in certain subgroups of children with malnutrition, such as those with HIV, severe gastrointestinal mucosal disease, marasmic kwashiorkor, or kwashiorkor alone. Rather, the study supports the notion that we need to find which population of patients would benefit from broad-spectrum antibiotic regimens in the treatment of uncomplicated SAM. For now, children with uncomplicated SAM treated as outpatients do not seem to benefit from empiric antibiotics.

As a scientific community, we still have much to learn about not only the relationship between the type of nutritional therapy provided and the gastrointestinal microbiome in patients with SAM but also the effects that broad-spectrum antibiotics may have on both. Subramanian et al report that there is significant microbiota immaturity in severe malnutrition and that microbiota maturity indices perhaps represent a way to categorize malnutrition.[2] Understanding the gut microbiome in patients with malnutrition may help direct therapy in the near future. Without a better understanding in today's world, it is hard to know just what role antibiotics should and do play in the malnourished state.

This revolutionary "negative" study may again shift the paradigm of nutritional recovery in outpatient community-based malnutrition programs worldwide. The resources saved from more appropriate antibiotic allocation and stewardship can be used to improve the "infrastructure for surveillance and management of complications" in countries such as Niger and beyond.

A. N. Carey, MD
C. Duggan, MD, MPH

References

1. Trehan I, Goldbach HS, LaGrone LN, et al. Antibiotics as part of the management of severe acute malnutrition. *N Engl J Med.* 2013;368:425-435.
2. Subramanian S, Huq S, Yatsunenko T, et al. Persistent gut microbiota immaturity in malnourished Bangladeshi children. *Nature.* 2014;510:417-421.

Racial and Ethnic Disparities in Dietary Intake among California Children
Guerrero AD, Chung PJ (David Geffen School of Medicine at Univ of California, Los Angeles)
J Acad Nutr Diet 116:439-448, 2016

Background.—The prevalence of childhood obesity among racial and ethnic minority groups is high. Multiple factors affect the development of childhood obesity, including dietary practices.

Objective.—To examine the racial and ethnic differences in reported dietary practices among the largest minority groups of California children.

Methods.—Data from the 2007 and 2009 California Health Interview Survey were analyzed using multivariate regression with survey weights to examine how race, ethnicity, sociodemographic characteristics, and child factors were associated with specific dietary practices.

Results.—The sample included 15,902 children aged 2 to 11 years. In multivariate regressions, substantial differences in fruit juice, fruit, vegetable, sugar-sweetened beverages, sweets, and fast-food consumption were found among the major racial and ethnic groups of children. Asians regardless of interview language were more likely than whites to have low vegetable intake consumption (Asians English interview odds ratio [OR] 1.20,

95% CI 1.01 to 1.43; Asians non-English-interview OR 2.09, 95% CI 1.23 to 3.57) and low fruit consumption (Asians English interview OR 1.69, 95% CI 1.41 to 2.03; Asians non-English interview OR 3.04, 95% CI 2.00 to 4.6). Latinos regardless of interview language were also more likely than whites to have high fruit juice (Latinos English interview OR 1.54, 95% CI 1.28 to 1.84 and Latinos non-English interview OR 1.29, 95% CI 1.02 to 1.62) and fast-food consumption (Latinos English interview OR 1.74, 95% CI 1.46 to 2.08 and Latinos non-English interview OR 1.48, 95% CI 1.16 to 1.91); but Latinos were less likely than whites to consume sweets (Latinos English interview OR 0.81, 95% CI 0.66 to 0.99 and Latinos non-English interview OR 0.56, 95% CI 1.16 to 1.91).

Conclusions.—Significant racial and ethnic differences exist in the dietary practices of California children. Increased fruit and vegetable consumption appears to be associated with parent education but not income. Our findings suggest that anticipatory guidance and dietary counseling might benefit from tailoring to specific ethnic groups to potentially address disparities in overweight and obesity (Table 3).

▶ The prevalence of obesity in the United States in both children and adults is staggering. To help prevent and treat this issue, clinicians need to understand the behaviors that lead to obesity as well as who is at greatest risk for these behaviors. In 2007, an expert committee released guidelines for practitioners on childhood obesity prevention and treatment.[1] These guidelines recommended screening in clinical settings for high-risk lifestyle behaviors, including unhealthy dietary practices such as consumption of sugar-sweetened beverages and fruit juices, inadequate intake of fruit and vegetables, intake of energy-dense foods, and frequency of eating out. Because racial and ethnic disparities exist in both the prevalence of obesity and its associated comorbidities, particular attention is warranted on how these dietary practices vary by race and ethnicity.

This study offers an evaluation of the specific dietary practices recommended in the expert committee guidelines on obesity. California is racially and ethnically highly diverse, thus making it an excellent site for evaluating differences among various racial and ethnic groups. The authors used a large population-based sample of children across California from 4 racial/ethnic groups: Asians, Latinos, African Americans, and whites. This is the first published study evaluating the prevalence of all of the behaviors across all of these racial/ethnic groups. The differences the authors found offer a starting point for increasing provider awareness of the risk children in certain racial/ethnic groups have for these dietary behaviors.

Children from the different racial and ethnic groups varied in their likelihood of having any one of the poor dietary habits (Table 3). Asian children were found to be at higher risk, compared to white children, for inadequate fruit and vegetable intake, but not for sugar-sweetened beverage, fruit juice, or sweet intake. African American children had a higher risk for sugar-sweetened beverage and fruit juice intake compared with white children. Latino children, on the other hand, had increased odds of nearly all of the dietary practices—inadequate vegetable intake, sugar-sweetened beverage and juice intake, and weekly fast-food intake.

TABLE 3.—Adjusted Odds Ratios (95% CI) of Child Dietary Practices by Race/Ethnicity and Language of Children Aged 2 to 11 Years: California Health Interview Survey 2007 and 2009[a] (N = 15,902)

Characteristic	Fruit (<2 Servings Yesterday)	Vegetables (<2 Servings Yesterday)	Sugar-Sweetened Beverages (≥1 Servings Yesterday)	Fruit Juice (≥2 Servings Yesterday)	Sweets (≥1 Servings Yesterday)	Fast Food (≥1 Servings Last Week)
	adjusted odds ratio (95% CI)					
Child race/ethnicity (reference category: white)						
Latino (English interview)	1.00 (0.85-1.19)	1.51 (1.28-1.79)*	1.75 (1.47-2.09)*	1.54 (1.28-1.84)*	0.81 (0.66-0.99)*	1.74 (1.46-2.08)*
Latino (non-English interview)	0.95 (0.77-1.19)	1.47 (1.17-1.86)*	1.34 (1.03-1.75)*	1.29 (1.02-1.62)*	0.56 (0.44-0.72)*	1.48 (1.16-1.91)*
African American	1.11 (0.86-1.43)	1.26 (0.99-1.61)	1.48 (1.13-1.93)*	1.61 (1.25-2.08)*	0.82 (0.63-1.07)	1.15 (0.89-1.48)
Asian (English interview)	1.69 (1.41-2.03)*	1.20 (1.01-1.43)*	1.14 (0.96-1.38)	0.99 (0.80-1.24)	0.85 (0.69-1.02)	1.22 (1.03-1.46)*
Asian (non-English interview)	3.04 (2.00-4.62)*	2.09 (1.23-3.57)*	0.69 (0.39-1.21)	0.77 (0.48-1.24)	0.91 (0.56-1.47)	0.91 (0.45-1.81)
Caregiver education (reference category: <high school degree)						
High school graduate	0.81 (0.63-1.05)	0.85 (0.67-1.07)	1.12 (0.87-1.47)	1.01 (0.82-1.26)	1.23 (0.97-1.55)	1.63 (1.31-2.00)*
At least some college	0.71 (0.54-0.93)*	0.68 (0.54-0.87)*	0.87 (0.65-1.14)	0.93 (0.75-1.15)	1.26 (0.99-1.59)	1.63 (1.27-2.08)*
Bachelor's degree	0.72 (0.53-0.95)*	0.69 (0.55-0.87)*	0.85 (0.65-1.16)	0.71 (0.56-0.89)*	1.25 (0.97-1.63)	1.51 (1.21-1.89)*
Master's degree or higher	0.49 (0.36-0.67)*	0.56 (0.44-0.72)*	0.68 (0.50-0.93)*	0.63 (0.48-0.83)*	1.28 (0.97-1.70)	1.10 (0.87-1.39)
Income (referent: ≥500% FPT[b])						
0%-99% FPT	1.02 (0.81-1.27)	1.00 (0.78-1.28)	1.32 (1.06-1.65)*	1.76 (1.42-2.19)*	0.78 (0.63-0.97)*	0.88 (0.69-1.10)
100%-199% FPT	1.06 (0.88-1.29)	0.88 (0.75-1.06)	1.41 (1.15-1.70)*	1.47 (1.21-1.77)*	0.98 (0.79-1.19)	1.06 (0.87-1.28)
200%-299% FPT	1.14 (0.95-1.37)	0.90 (0.75-1.08)	1.38 (1.16-1.65)*	1.17 (0.94-1.46)	0.83 (0.70-0.99)*	1.29 (1.08-1.56)*
300%-399% FPT	1.16 (0.97-1.38)	0.99 (0.85-1.15)	1.04 (0.86-1.24)	1.28 (1.03-1.59)*	0.92 (0.76-1.09)	1.43 (1.19-1.72)*
400%-499% FPT	1.13 (0.93-1.37)	0.99 (0.78-1.28)	1.14 (0.97-1.34)	1.07 (0.86-1.32)	0.89 (0.75-1.07)	1.34 (1.12-1.61)*
Physician assessed child's nutrition at last visit						
Yes	0.85 (0.75-0.95)*	0.80 (0.68-0.92)*	0.87 (0.76-1.01)	0.97 (0.84-1.12)	1.04 (0.92-1.18)	0.97 (0.87-1.09)

[a]Analyses adjusted for child age, child sex, child body mass index, single-parent household status, household size, geography, caregiver age, and caregiver sex, and survey year.
[b]FPT = federal poverty threshold.
*P < 0.05. Boldface text indicates odds ratios found to be statistically significant at the P = 0.05 value.
Reprinted from Guerrero AD, Chung PJ, Racial and ethnic disparities in dietary intake among California children. *J Acad Nutr Diet.* 2016;116:439-448, with permission from the Academy of Nutrition and Dietetics.

Yet they had a lower risk for excess sweet intake. There were clear differences in dietary practices across racial/ethnic groups.

The authors are to be commended for evaluating dietary practices of Asians and Latinos separately by language of interview, as a proxy for acculturation. Given the relationship of acculturation with dietary practices, this is a real strength of this study. Interestingly, English-speaking Asians, but not non-English-speaking Asians, were found to have higher odds of weekly fast-food intake compared with white children. This adds to the growing pool of evidence on the negative impact of acculturation on dietary practices. However, both English-speaking and non-English-speaking Latinos had similar odds of having each dietary practice. Recognizing subgroups within racial and ethnic groups is important; both Latinos and Asians are not homogenous populations. More work is needed to further understand the process of acculturation and its impact on dietary practices.

Findings were also presented on the relationship of caregiver education and income with these dietary practices. The relationships varied in such a way to suggest that the relationships are complex. For example, higher education levels, but not income, were protective against inadequate fruit and vegetable intake. From a clinical standpoint, there was no clear message other than that these relationships vary.

Not surprisingly, these dietary practices were common among all children. In all groups, more than half of children consumed fast food on a weekly basis. More than half of the children also had inadequate daily vegetable intake (< 2 servings the day before) and excessive intake of sweets (≥1 serving the day before). Regardless of the racial/ethnic group, these higher risk dietary practices are extremely common, emphasizing the need to screen widely across all groups of children for these practices.

Other factors related to dietary intake need to be considered in dietary counseling. For example, accessibility to supermarkets is known to influence dietary intake.[2] Parental perceptions of a healthy weight, which vary by racial/ethnic group, have also been shown to be related to dietary intake.[3,4] Moreover, parental feeding practices, which may vary by racial/ethnic group, are known to be related to child dietary intake.[5,6] Providers must consider individual-, family-, and community-level factors when counseling families. This, of course, includes consideration of the influence of culture on diet-related beliefs and behaviors.

This study has important limitations. The main limitation is the measure of dietary practices by parent report using 1 item for each practice. Parents determined what defined a serving of different items, which of course introduces error. Furthermore, although Asians and Latinos were evaluated separately by language spoken, they were still evaluated as large groups, despite clear evidence suggesting differences in health behaviors among racial and ethnic subgroups. Additionally, the language spoken is a crude measure of acculturation. The use of better measures is needed to more fully understand these relationships and their mechanisms.

The care families receive in clinical settings is important to addressing the obesity epidemic. Unhealthy dietary practices are common across all children emphasizing the importance of dietary screening and counseling by providers. The racial/ethnic and sociodemographic differences noted in this study can help providers recognize the different risks for these dietary practices for children in different groups, hence offering a starting point for counseling on these topics in the clinical setting.

D. A. Thompson, MD, MPH

References

1. Barlow SE, Expert Committee. Expert committee recommendations regarding the prevention, assessment, and treatment of child and adolescent overweight and obesity: summary report. *Pediatrics*. 2007;120:S164-S192.
2. Moore LV, Diez Roux AV, Nettleton JA, Jacobs DR. Associations of the local food environment with diet quality—a comparison of assessments based on surveys and geographic information systems: the multi-ethnic study of atherosclerosis. *Am. J. Epidemiol*. 2008;167:917-924.
3. Musaad SM, Donovan SM, Fiese BH. Parental perception of child weight in the first two years-of-life: a potential link between infant feeding and preschoolers' diet. *Appetite*. 2015;91:90-100.
4. Hernandez RG, Garcia J, Thompson DA. Racial-ethnic differences in parental body image perceptions of preschoolers: implications for engaging minority parents in weight-related discussions. *Clin Pediatr (Phila)*. 2015;54:1293-1296.
5. Orlet Fisher J, Mitchell DC, Wright HS, Birch LL. Parental influences on young girls' fruit and vegetable, micronutrient, and fat intakes. *J Am Diet Assoc*. 2002; 102:58-64.
6. Zhou N, Cheah CS, Van Hook J, Thompson DA, Jones SS. A cultural understanding of Chinese immigrant mothers' feeding practices. A qualitative study. *Appetite*. 2015;87:160-167.

Effect of sibling birth on BMI trajectory in the first 6 years of life
Mosli RH, Kaciroti N, Corwyn RF, et al (King Abdulaziz Univ, Jeddah, Saudi Arabia; Univ of Michigan, Ann Arbor; Univ of Arkansas at Little Rock, Little Rock; et al)
Pediatrics 137:e20152456, 2016

Background and Objective.—This study examined the longitudinal association between birth of a sibling and changes in body mass index z-score (BMIz) trajectory during the first 6 years of life.

Methods.—Children ($n = 697$) were recruited across 10 sites in the United States at the time of birth. Sibship composition was assessed every 3 months. Anthropometry was completed when the child was age 15 months, 24 months, 36 months, 54 months, and in first grade. Children were classified based on the timing of their sibling's birth. A piecewise quadratic regression model adjusted for potential confounders examined the association of the birth of a sibling with subsequent BMIz trajectory.

Results.—Children whose sibling was born when they were 24 to 36 months or 36 to 54 months old, compared with children who did not experience the birth of a sibling by first grade, had a lower subsequent BMIz trajectory and a significantly lower BMIz at first grade (0.27 vs 0.51, P value = 0.04 and 0.26 vs 0.51, P value = 0.03, respectively). Children who did not experience the birth of a sibling by the time they were in first grade had 2.94 greater odds of obesity (*P* value = 0.046) at first grade compared with children who experienced the birth of a sibling when they were between 36 to 54 months old.

Conclusions.—A birth of a sibling when the child is 24 to 54 months old is associated with a healthier BMIz trajectory. Identifying the underlying mechanism of association can help inform intervention programs.

▶ Beginning with Sir Francis Galton's English Men of Science published in 1874, researchers have examined relationships between siblings and outcomes related to health, achievement, behavior, and intelligence.[1-3] Interest in this topic is germane to the United States, where the majority of parents have more than 1 child,[4] and the birth of a sibling has potentially dramatic effects on family dynamics in both the short- and long-term. In the short-term, older siblings are commonly already experiencing their own rapid development, and an addition to the family has the potential to affect numerous health, behavior, and developmental domains.

For example, interesting associations between birth order, presence or absence of siblings, and weight status have been discovered for more than 50 years. Studies from diverse cultures are generally consistent in describing within-family differences in weight status: firstborn children have a higher prevalence of obesity than their younger siblings. Early research revealed that although birth weight increased with birth order, by age 3 years, firstborn children were significantly heavier than later born children.[5] A European study from the 1970s then found evidence that only children had higher rates of obesity than firstborn children with siblings[6] even as they approached adulthood.[7] Contemporary data from Japanese middle school students are similar.[8]

Three recent studies describing diverse populations (African American,[9] Italian,[10] German[11]) and more sophisticated methodology all found that being either firstborn or an only child increased obesity risk. For example, Stettler et al examined an African American cohort and found only 3 variables collected at birth were associated with young adult adiposity: firstborn status, female sex, and maternal pre-pregnancy body mass index (BMI).[9] Being firstborn had the strongest association with an odds ratio (OR) of 4.0 (95% confidence interval [CI], 1.4–11.2). One further 2012 study of 12 000 children from 8 European countries found firstborn children without siblings were more likely to be overweight (OR 1.52, 95% CI 1.34–1.72) at age 2 to 9 years than peers with siblings.[12] Also, the longer firstborns remained an only child before birth of a sibling, the stronger the association with overweight.

The study by Mosli et al adds to this interesting literature by demonstrating that body mass index (BMI) trajectories differ for older siblings based upon the timing of their new younger siblings birth. Specifically, experiencing the birth of a sibling between ages 24 and 54 months was associated with a healthier BMI trajectory through entry into first grade than those who remained the youngest family member. These results come from data from the National Institute of Health and Human Development Study of Early Child Care and Youth Development, a study of 1364 families recruited in 1991 across 10 sites in the United States. Although the data in the publication did not describe the entire family composition or the role of birth order, the significant protective effect on obesity at entry into first grade among those experiencing the birth of a sibling when they were 36 to 54 months old is particularly noteworthy.

The reasons for the associations among sibling birth, birth order, and weight status are unclear and may only be uncovered by prospectively designed studies to evaluate these questions. Mosli et al proposed that changes in parenting practices may occur that affect the older sibling's rate of weight gain or alternatively that the child adapts into a leadership role that contributes to healthier weight status. Regardless of the mechanism, it is clear that parenting behavior differs between siblings.[13]

Unfortunately, surprisingly little is known about how parenting of infants and toddlers differs between children in the same family, which individual or family level characteristics influence these differences particularly with regard to obesity-related behaviors and how parenting of an individual child differs once a new sibling is born. It is clear that parenting behavior changes between first and subsequent children as parental knowledge and experience increases as demonstrated by the simple example of a reduced number of physician visits with increasing birth order.[14] How the birth of a new child modifies the parenting approaches to the older siblings is a question that requires further exploration.

I. Paul, MD, MSc

References

1. Galton F. *English Men of Science: Their Nature and Nurture*. London: Macmillan & Co; 1874.
2. Greenwood M Jr, Yule GU. On the determination of size of family and of the distribution of characters in order of birth from samples taken through members of the sibships. *J Roy Stat Soc*. 1914;77:179-199.
3. Gini C. Superiority of the eldest. *J Hered*. 1915;37:37-39.
4. Cohort Fertility Tables. http://www.cdc.gov/nchs/nvss/cohort_fertility_tables.htm. Accessed May 10, 2016.
5. Lowe CR, Gibson JR. Weight at third birthday related to birth weight, duration of gestation, and birth order. *Br J Prev Soc Med*. 1953;7:78-82.
6. Jacoby A, Altman DG, Cook J, Holland WW, Elliott A. Influence of some social and environmental factors on the nutrient intake and nutritional status of schoolchildren. *Br J Prev Soc Med*. 1975;29:116-120.
7. Ravelli GP, Belmont L. Obesity in nineteen-year-old men: family size and birth order associations. *Am J Epidemiol*. 1979;109:66-70.
8. Wang H, Sekine M, Chen X, Kanayama H, Yamagami T, Kagamimori S. Sib-size, birth order and risk of overweight in junior high school students in Japan: results of the Toyama Birth Cohort Study. *Prev Med*. 2007;44:45-51.
9. Stettler N, Tershakovec AM, Zemel BS, et al. Early risk factors for increased adiposity: a cohort study of African American subjects followed from birth to young adulthood. *Am J Clin Nutr*. 2000;72:378-383.
10. Celi F, Bini V, De Giorgi G, et al. Epidemiology of overweight and obesity among school children and adolescents in three provinces of central Italy, 1993–2001: study of potential influencing variables. *Eur J Clin Nutr*. 2003;57:1045-1051.
11. Karaolis-Danckert N, Buyken AE, Kulig M, et al. How pre- and postnatal risk factors modify the effect of rapid weight gain in infancy and early childhood on subsequent fat mass development: results from the Multicenter Allergy Study 90. *Am J Clin Nutr*. 2008;87:1356-1364.
12. Hunsberger M, Formisano A, Reisch LA, et al. Overweight singletons compared to children with siblings: the IDEFICS study. *Nutr Diabetes*. 2012;2:e35.

13. Kaley F, Reid V, Flynn E. Investigating the biographic, social and temperamental correlates of young infants' sleeping, crying and feeding routines. *Infant Behav Dev.* 2012;35:596-605.
14. Tessler R. Birth order, family size, and children's use of physician services. *Health Serv Res.* 1980;15:55-62.

Early Life Growth Trajectories in Cystic Fibrosis are Associated with Pulmonary Function at Age 6 Years

Sanders DB, Fink A, Mayer-Hamblett N, et al (Univ of Wisconsin School of Medicine and Public Health, Madison; Cystic Fibrosis Foundation, Bethesda, MD; Univ of Washington, Seattle; et al)
J Pediatr 167:1081-1088, 2015

Objective.—To determine whether severity of lung disease at age 6 years is associated with changes in nutritional status before age 6 within individual children with cystic fibrosis (CF).

Study Design.—Children with CF born between 1994 and 2005 and followed in the CF Foundation Patient Registry from age ≤2 through 7 years were assessed according to changes in annualized weight-for-length (WFL) percentiles between ages 0 and 2 years and body mass index (BMI) percentiles between ages 2 and 6 years. The association between growth trajectories before age 6 and forced expiratory volume in 1 second (FEV_1)% predicted at age 6-7 years was evaluated using multivariable linear regression.

Results.—A total of 6805 subjects met inclusion criteria. Children with annualized WFL-BMI always >50th percentile (N = 1323 [19%]) had the highest adjusted mean (95% CI) FEV_1 at 6-7 years (101.8 [100.1, 103.5]). FEV_1 at 6-7 years for children whose WFL-BMI increased >10 percentile points by age 6 years was 98.3 (96.6, 100.0). This was statistically significantly higher than FEV_1 for children whose WFL-BMI was stable (94.4 [92.6, 96.2]) or decreased >10 percentile points (92.9 [91.1, 94.8]). Among children whose WFL-BMI increased >10 percentile points, achieving and maintaining WFL-BMI >50th percentile at younger ages was associated with significantly higher FEV_1 at 6- 7 years.

Conclusions.—Within-patient changes in nutritional status in the first 6 years of life are significantly associated with FEV_1 at age 6-7 years. The establishment of a clear relationship between early childhood growth measurements and later lung function suggests that early nutritional interventions may impact on eventual lung health (Fig 3).

▶ It seems intuitive: better nutrition leads to better growth, which leads to healthier children with better lung function. In the pre—newborn screen days, children with cystic fibrosis (CF) commonly were diagnosed because of growth failure. Today most children with CF are diagnosed before they have obvious respiratory symptoms and before they have any growth abnormalities.[1]

We know the "high-achieving" CF centers use higher enzyme doses, more nutritional supplements, and more tube feedings than "low-achieving" centers.[2]

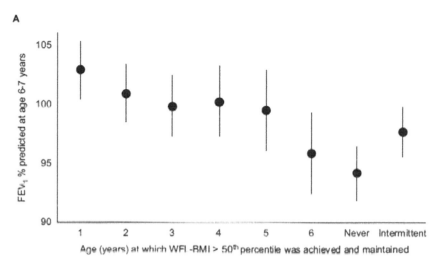

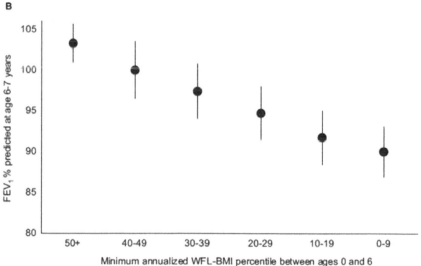

FIGURE 3.—Mean FEV_1% predicted at ages 6-7 years associated with **A**, age at which subjects whose WFL-BMI increased >10 percentile points first reached and maintained WFL-BMI >50th percentile and **B**, the lowest annualized WFL-BMI percentile for subjects whose WFL-BMI decreased >10 percentile points. The *vertical bars* represent the 95% CIs. (Reprinted from Sanders DB, Fink A, Mayer-Hamblett N, et al. Early life growth trajectories in cystic fibrosis are associated with pulmonary function at age 6 years. *J Pediatr.* 2015;167:1081-1088, with permission from Elsevier.)

In 2009, the CF Foundation (CFF) recommended children maintain at least the 50th percentile for weight-for length (WFL) or body mass index (BMI).[3] However, there is limited evidence to support an association between growth in early childhood and later lung health for individual patients. Previous studies have described associations between growth indices at one point in time in early childhood and lung function later in childhood, but they have not looked at growth over time in early childhood and whether improvements in growth over time can lead to improved lung function or whether the timing of changes is important.[4,5] In this study, Sanders et al[6] provide important evidence to support the hypothesis that good nutrition is critical to good pulmonary outcomes in children with CF.

Sanders et al[6] followed the growth and spirometry of children diagnosed with CF before age 2 years. They evaluated the association between these different growth trajectories and the forced expiratory volume in 1 second (FEV_1) percent predicted at 6 to 7 years. Sanders et al found that those children with WFL-BMI that was always above the 50th percentile (that is, the children who were meeting the CFF goal) had the best FEV_1 at age 6 to 7 years. Those with increasing WFL-BMI had the next best FEV_1, followed by those who were stable and those with decreasing WFL-BMI over time (Fig 3). Interestingly, they also found that the sooner the nutritional deficit is corrected, the better the pulmonary outcome and the more severe the growth failure at one point during the study, the worse the pulmonary outcome. Together these data suggest a significant relationship between early childhood growth and later lung function.

This study has several limitations. First, this is an observational study and does not prove that improved nutrition actually caused the improved lung function. Moreover, early acquisition of resistant bacteria or an isolated severe lung infection may have lasting ill effects on growth. Unfortunately, the only lung function parameter followed was the FEV_1. Although FEV_1 is an important marker,[7] it might have been interesting to look at other more sensitive signs of early lung disease such as lung clearance index or computed tomography scans, or to look at clinically relevant outcomes such as frequency of pulmonary exacerbations. In addition, although the differences between the groups were statistically significant, they were small, and all of the FEV_1 were in the normal range. This study may suffer to some extent from selection bias. For example, not all Class I, II, and III mutations are similarly severe, as assumed by the authors. Some even present with pancreatic sufficiency, a marker of generally milder CF, and those with intrinsically milder CF may have self-selected to the healthiest group. Lastly, the study may not be generalizable to the children with CF born today because children in this study were born before widespread newborn screening and had low rates of some standard pulmonary treatments, such as Pulmozyme, inhaled tobramycin, and chronic azithromycin. This cohort was diagnosed before age 2 years based on clinical symptoms, so it may represent a more severely affected group of patients than those diagnosed by newborn screening who have few symptoms early in life.

Despite these limitations, this is an important article that lends strong support to the CF Foundation recommendation to keep WFL-BMI above the 50th percentile. Importantly, it also shows us that the earlier we achieve this goal, the greater the benefit for lung function. However, reversing nutritional failure in CF is difficult. Families with CF face many challenges on a daily basis, and the frequent food battles are particularly difficult. This study provides CF families another good reason to keep fighting the good fight.

D. Nielson, MD

E. Gibb, MD

References

1. Dijk FN, McKay K, Barzi F, Gaskin KJ, Fitzgerald DA. Improved survival in cystic fibrosis patients diagnosed by newborn screening compared to a historical cohort from the same centre. *Arch Dis Child.* 2011;96:1118-1123.
2. Johnson C, Butler SM, Konstan MW, Morgan W, Wohl ME. Factors influencing outcomes in cystic fibrosis: a center-based analysis. *Chest.* 2003;123:20-27.
3. Borowitz D, Robinson KA, Rosenfeld M, et al. Cystic fibrosis foundation evidence-based guidelines for management of infants with cystic fibrosis. *J Pediatr.* 2009;155: S73-S93.
4. Konstan M, Butler S, Wohl M, et al. Growth and nutritional indexes in early life predict pulmonary function in cystic fibrosis. *J Pediatr.* 2003;142:624-630.
5. Yen EH, Quinton H, Borowitz D. Better nutritional status in early childhood is associated with improved clinical outcomes and survival in patients with cystic fibrosis. *J Pediatr.* 2013;162:530-535.e1.
6. Sanders DB, Emerson J, Ren CL, Schechter MS, Gibson RL, Morgan W, Rosenfeld MEPIC Study Group. Early childhood risk factors for decreased FEV1 at age six to seven years in young children with cystic Fibrosis. *Ann Am Thorac Soc.* 2015;12:1170-1176.
7. Corey M, Edwards L, Levison H, Knowles M. Longitudinal analysis of pulmonary function decline in patients with cystic fibrosis. *J Pediatr.* 1997;131:809-814.

Types of Infant Formulas Consumed in the United States

Rossen LM, Simon AE, Herrick KA (Ctrs for Disease Control and Prevention, Hyattsville, MD)
Clin Pediatr 55:278-285, 2016

We examined consumption of different types of infant formula (eg, cow's milk, soy, gentle/lactose-reduced, and specialty) and regular milk among a nationally representative sample of 1864 infants, 0 to 12 months old, from the National Health and Nutrition Examination Survey, 2003-2010. Among the 81% of infants who were fed formula or regular milk, 69% consumed cow's milk formula, 12% consumed soy formula, 5% consumed gentle/lactose-reduced formulas, 6% consumed specialty formulas, and 13% consumed regular milk products. There were differences by household education and income in the percentage of infants consuming cow's milk formula and regular milk products. The majority of infants in the United States who were fed formula or regular milk consumed cow's milk formula (69%), with lower percentages receiving soy, specialty, gentle/sensitive, or lactose-free/reduced formulas. Contrary to national recommendations, 13% of infants younger than 1 year consumed regular milk, and the percentage varied by household education and income levels (Tables 2 and 3).

▶ All experts and the American Academy of Pediatrics agree that human breast milk is the ideal feed for infants exclusively up to 6 months of age and should be the primary beverage through the first year of life. Although we have recently seen an increase in the number of infants leaving the hospital after delivery who are breastfeeding, the percentage of infants who continue to be breastfed dwindles quickly after discharge. We, as health care professionals caring for infants,

TABLE 2.—Percentage of Infants 0 to 12 Months Old Consuming Different Types of Formula or Regular Milk, NHANES 2003-2010, by Family Income-to-Poverty Ratio (IPR)[a]

	Overall (Unweighted n = 1587)	IPR ≤185% (Unweighted n = 1004)[b]	IPR >185% (Unweighted n = 474)[b]
Cow's milk formula	68.9 (65.1-72.5)	72.4 (68.5-76.3)	64.9 (59.5-70.2)[c]
Soy-based	11.6 (9.6-14.0)	8.3 (6.1-10.4)	15.8 (11.9-19.6)[c]
Specialty	6.3 (4.9-8.1)	6.5 (4.3-8.9)	6.0 (3.5-8.5)
Gentle/lactose-reduced	5.4 (3.6-7.8)	3.8 (2.4-5.1)	7.3 (3.1-11.4)
Regular milk (not formula)	12.6 (10.3-15.3)	14.4 (12.4-16.4)	10.9 (8.1-13.6)[c]

[a]Data are presented as percentage (95% confidence interval). Percentages in each column do not sum to 100 because children may consume more than one type of formula. Percentages are adjusted for age (in months) of the child.
[b]Sample sizes for these variables are based on the 1478 infants without missing data on IPR.
[c]Indicates significant difference from reference group, IPR ≤185%, P < .05.
Reprinted from Rossen LM, Simon AE, Herrick KA. Types of infant formulas consumed in the United States. *Clin Pediatr.* 2016;55:278-285, with permission from The Author(s).

TABLE 3.—Percentage of Infants 0 to 12 Months Old Consuming Different Types of Formula or Regular Milk, NHANES 2003-2010, by Household Education Level[a]

	<High School (Unweighted n = 543)[b]	High School/GED (Unweighted n = 412)[b]	Some College+ (Unweighted n = 563)[b]
Cow's milk formula	72.8 (67.9-77.8)	68.2 (61.3-75.1)	65.3 (60.4-70.1)[c]
Soy-based	8.2 (4.6-11.7)	11.8 (7.6-15.9)	13.9 (10.7-17.1)[c]
Specialty	5.5 (2.9-8.0)	7.3 (3.6-11.0)	6.4 (4.1-8.6)
Gentle/lactose-reduced	2.4 (1.2-3.7)	4.4 (1.9-6.8)	8.4 (4.4-12.5)[c]
Regular milk (not formula)	15.3 (12.5-18.1)	12.2 (8.9-15.6)	11.6 (9.0-14.1)[c]

[a]Data are presented as percentage (95% confidence interval). Percentages in each column do not sum to 100 because children may consume more than one type of formula. Percentages are adjusted for age (in months) of the child.
[b]Sample sizes for these variables are based on the 1518 infants without missing data.
[c]Indicates significant difference from reference group, <high school, P < .05.
Reprinted from Rossen LM, Simon AE, Herrick KA. Types of infant formulas consumed in the United States. *Clin Pediatr.* 2016;55:278-285, with permission from The Author(s).

should do what we can to alter that trend, but we must also be aware of what those non-breastfeeding infants are ingesting.

This paper by Rossen et al reviews National Health and Nutrition Examination Survey (NHANES) data from 2003 to 2010 to elucidate what these children are drinking. The data reveal that the majority (69%) of non-breastfeeding infants receive cow's milk formula but that more educated and wealthier families are more likely to give their infants non—cow's milk formulas (ie, soy formulas and so-called gentle formulas) (Table 2). In addition, those infants from families in lower income groups and lower educational levels are more likely to receive regular milk products not specifically designed for infants, a practice that contravenes expert recommendations (Table 3).

Many parents and pediatricians attribute various problematic infant behaviors to formula intolerance. Although in many cases a formula change may, in fact, alleviate those symptoms, formulas are often changed with little rationale. When the symptomology does not resolve, multiple formula changes ensue, often leading to an extensively hydrolyzed or amino acid—based formula that is substantially more expensive. Despite no improvement, those more expensive formulas are routinely continued.

Companies that produce infant formula products have provided us with a variety of formulas, and this number continues to grow. There are a variety of formulas that differ in the content of macro and micronutrients. In addition, parents can choose among organic and generic formulas. Furthermore, the formula industry is consistently tweaking its routine formulas in attempt to mimic human milk more closely than their competitors and then tout their own specific product as the ideal feed for formula fed infants.

The Rossen et al article offers us some insight into the rough proportion of families offering their infants various types of formulas. The NHANES data do not appear to mirror the demographics in the United States. It underestimates the number of Caucasians and oversamples the number of Mexican Americans. Given these considerations, it would appear to underestimate the number of infants ingesting non—cow milk formulas. In addition, the formula categories are very broad, particularly the specialized formulas and the gentle formulas. I can understand the limitations of this kind of study given the limited number of families interviewed and the wide variety of formulas that are available to them; however, more information would be instructive.

Infant formulas are regulated by federal law, which mandates upper and lower limits of nutrients; all are safe, but evidence-based rationales for various formulas are rarely available. Nevertheless, families often change formulas in many instances at the recommendation of their pediatrician. It would be helpful to know why these changes are instituted. Are they initiated by the family or the pediatrician? What are the symptoms that engender the changes? How are the choices made? How often does a change result in improvement? Is the improvement, when it occurs, due to the formula change, a placebo effect, or coincidental with the change?

It would also be helpful to have some evidence that these changes make clinical sense. Clearly patients with documented protein hypersensitivity or gastroesophageal reflux have been shown to improve with a formula change, but where is the evidence for a 19-calorie-per-ounce formula, a partially hydrolyzed formula, or a lactose-reduced formula? Where is evidence that no long-term harm is caused by these changes?

The Rossen article does reflect that some infants are ingesting regular milk products earlier than has been recommended and so points out an issue that pediatricians should address. Overall, however, it essentially indirectly points out how much more we need to know about the feeding choices available to families with infants.

A. Jelin, MD

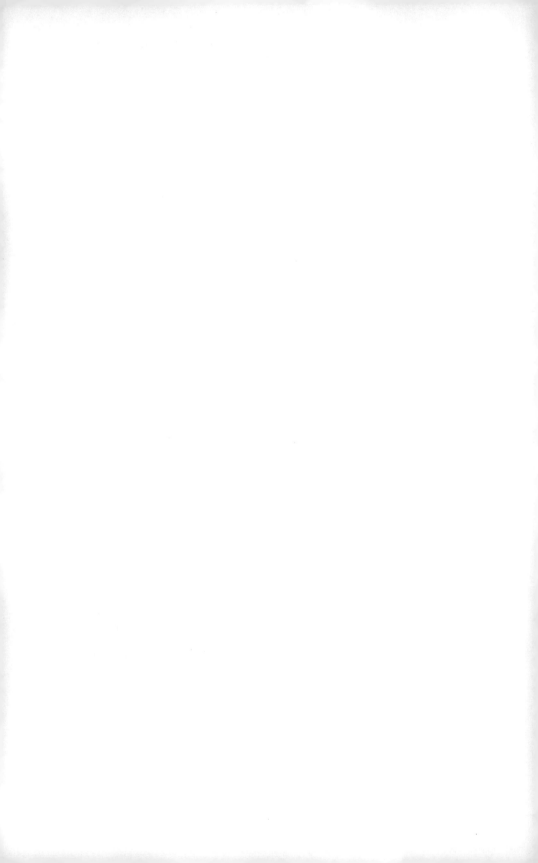

21 Oncology

Predictors of Malignancy in Children with Thyroid Nodules

Mussa A, De Andrea M, Motta M, et al (Univ of Torino, Italy; Azienda Ospedaliera Ordine Mauriziano, Torino, Italy; Azienda Ospedaliera Ordine Mauriziano di Torino, Italy; et al)

J Pediatr 167:886-892.e1, 2015

Objective.—To evaluate the diagnostic accuracy of clinical, laboratory, and ultrasound (US) imaging characteristics of thyroid nodules in assessing the likelihood of malignancy.

Study Design.—Data from 184 children and adolescents with thyroid nodules were evaluated and compared with respective cytologic/histologic outcomes. A regression model was designed to assess the predictors associated with malignancy and to calculate ORs.

Results.—Twenty-nine malignant neoplasms (25 papillary, 1 medullary, 3 Hurtle-cell carcinomas), 8 follicular adenomas, and 147 goitrous nodules (92 based on cytology, 55 on follow-up) were diagnosed. Fine-needle aspiration biopsy diagnostic accuracy, sensitivity, and specificity were 91%, 100%, and 88%, respectively. Male sex, compression symptoms, palpable lymphopathy, thyroid stimulating hormone concentration, microcalcifications, indistinct margins, hypoechoic US pattern, pathologic lymph node alterations, and increased intranodular vascularization were associated with malignancy. Regular margins, mixed echoic pattern, and peripheral-only vascularization were associated with benignity. During follow-up, nodule growth was associated with malignant disease, especially with levothyroxine therapy. A multivariate analysis confirmed that microcalcifications, hypoechoic pattern, intranodular vascularization, lymph node alterations, and thyroid stimulating hormone concentration were independent predictors of malignant outcome. For each predictor, we provide sensitivity, specificity, and positive/negative predictive values.

Conclusions.—Clinical, laboratory, and US features of nodules can be used as predictors of malignancy in children. Although none has diagnostic accuracy as high as that of fine-needle aspiration biopsy, these predictors should be considered in deciding the diagnostic approach of children with thyroid nodules.

▶ The most common complaint I hear from my patients and families diagnosed with thyroid nodules are that they are "rare," and the most common comment I hear from my thyroid cancer patients is that thyroid cancer is the "good cancer" because everyone survives the disease. Just typing the sentence makes me look over my shoulder in paranoia to ensure that a patient or family member isn't within eyesight. The reality is that in practice the use of these descriptive is isolating for the patient, and the qualifications of "rare" and "good" are often used to decrease the priority of investing in clinical and research efforts to better understand and improve our approach to evaluation and care. Other diseases have suffered from a similar approach, but for each, there are certain articles that take us one step forward in addressing shortfalls in care. The article by Mussa et al is one of these articles, and there are several important take-away messages worth reviewing.[1]

The first issue to extinguish is that thyroid nodules are not rare. Within the United States it is estimated that up 1%, or 750 000 children and adolescents, may have a nodule palpable on physical exam and an even higher number based on incidental discovery during nonthyroid head and neck imaging. The risk of developing a thyroid nodule is based on multiple factors, including geographic location, iodine status, age, gender, and family history with an increased incidence with advancing age (puberty > prepuberty), female gender, and a family history of thyroid nodules and thyroid cancer. Previous exposure to radiation, either secondary to the treatment of a nonthyroid malignancy or potentially from repeat exposure from diagnostic imaging, as well as a personal history of autoimmune thyroid disease, are also associated with an increased risk for developing a nodule and thyroid cancer. When a thyroid nodule is diagnosed in a pediatric patient, there is a 4- to 5-fold higher risk of malignancy compared with adults (20%–25% vs 5%–10%, respectively), and for unknown reasons, across all ages of patients (children and adults), the rate of newly diagnosed patients with differentiated thyroid cancer is increasing faster than any other form of malignancy both within the United States and internationally.

Current data for the United States shows that thyroid cancer is the second most common malignancy diagnosed in adolescent girls between 15 and 19 years of age. For pediatric patients diagnosed with thyroid cancer, up to 70% will have metastasis to cervical lymph nodes and up to 15% of patients with extensive lymph node metastasis will have thyroid cancer that has spread to the lungs. Although few children die from thyroid cancer, the surgical and medical complication rate is high, as is the risk of recurrent disease, both factors that are expressed over a longer period of time when compared with an adult patient.

The 3 most significant improvements to the evaluation and care of patients with thyroid nodules and thyroid cancer happened more than 50 years ago: the incorporation of radioactive iodine (RAI) to treat hyperthyroidism and thyroid cancer (circa 1946), fine needle aspiration (FNA) to aid in preoperative diagnosis (circa 1952), and ultrasound (US) scanning of the thyroid gland (circa 1967). The timing of discovery is likely serendipitous but does reflect our continued efforts to develop tools that allow for stratification of therapy in an effort to ensure excellent outcome while reducing the risk of complications of therapy These issues are of critical importance for a child, especially for a disease that has low disease-specific mortality.

So how are we doing 70 years after the incorporation of RAI into clinical practice? Well, it depends on your optimism; are you a glass-half-full or a glass-half-empty sort of provider? The reality is that we're getting there, in small steps, but we are heading in the right direction. As of 2016, we now have specific guidelines for the management of pediatric patients with thyroid nodules and thyroid cancer (www.thyroid.org),[2] the majority of patients undergo US evaluation, an increasing number of patients have FNA before surgery, and there are attempts to identify patients that may not benefit from extensive surgery or from radioiodine therapy. At the same time, we continue to be woefully behind in many areas; there are few high-volume pediatric thyroid centers in the country, there is exceedingly limited investment to discovering the molecular landscape of pediatric thyroid cancer that would lead to improved diagnosis as well as treatment options for patients with progressive, nonresponsive disease, and there is limited access to high-volume thyroid surgeons who operate in a pediatric environment ("high volume" is defined as a surgeon performing > 30 thyroid surgeries per year).

Where does the study by Mussa et al fit in? Well, this is one of the more extensive and thoughtful evaluations of US in pediatric patients to date designed to identify US features of thyroid nodules that are predictive for malignancy. To no surprise, there is crossover between adult and pediatric data for several US features (the presence of microcalcifications); however, there are also several features that were not comparable secondary to differences in study design (Table)

Although the authors thoughtfully identify several limitations in the concluding paragraphs of the article, the most significant strength and limitation in regard to extrapolating the data to many centers is not discussed: a standardized protocol to ensure complete US evaluation of a thyroid nodule(s) as well as the expertise required to interpret thyroid US images. For anyone who regularly cares for pediatric patients with thyroid disease on a near daily basis, we are reminded of the disparity in the quality and completeness of thyroid US exams despite the fact that there are guidelines sponsored by the American Institute of Ultrasound Medicine (AIUM) that define the required training as well as performance and reporting of the exam. The AIUM guidelines are age indeterminate and were developed in conjunction with the American College of Radiology (ACR), the Society of Radiologists in US, and the Society of Pediatric Radiology.

What do we need to do to improve care? To start, we need to follow published standards of care and continuously review outcomes so that recommendations evolve based on updated data. Patients should not be referred from a primary care provider to a surgeon; they should be referred to an endocrinologist. The pediatric endocrinologist (pediatric thyroidologist) should review the images (not just the report) to ensure the US study was complete and then decide whether FNA is warranted. The FNA should be performed using conscious sedation, using US guidance with bedside confirmation of sample adequacy and read by a thyroid cytopathologist. The endocrinologist should then review the US and FNA data, decide whether surgery is indicated, and refer the patient to a high-volume thyroid surgeon with a recommended surgical approach. Postoperatively, the endocrinologist/thyroidologist decides on the surveillance plan as well as whether radioiodine therapy is warranted for thyroid cancer patients.

The only path to accomplish these standards is to regionalize care to high-volume pediatric thyroid centers, a critical and necessary next step in the evolution to improve our approach to caring for pediatric patients with thyroid nodules and thyroid cancer.

Low-disease specific mortality is a wonderful place to start, but we have a long way to go to decrease avoidable medical and surgical complications.

TABLE.—Review of US Features to Predict Malignancy in Thyroid Nodules From Three Systematic Review Articles (2 Adult and 1 Pediatric) Compared to Mussa et al. (1)

Subject	Nodules Examined	Frequency of Cancer	Nodule Feature	Specificity for Malignancy
Adult systematic review and meta-analysis[3]	12,786	not reported	Microcalcifications	88%
			Infiltrative margins	83%
			Taller than wide*	97%
			Hypoechoic pattern	62%
			Intranodular blood flow	78%
			Suspicious lymph nodes	not reported
			TSH	not reported
Adult systematic review and meta-analysis[4]	17,151	20% (PTC 84%)	Microcalcifications	81%
			Infiltrative margins	79%
			Taller than wide	93%
			Hypoechoic pattern	56%
			Intranodular blood flow	53%
			Suspicious lymph nodes	not reported
			TSH	not reported
Pediatric systematic review and meta-analysis[5]	750	27% (PTC 87%)	Microcalcifications	92%
			Infiltrative margins	93%
			Taller than wide	76%
			Hypoechoic pattern	68%
			Intranodular blood flow	73%
			Suspicious lymph nodes	86%
			TSH	not reported
Current Study (1)	147	20% (PTC 86%)	Microcalcifications	97%
			Infiltrative margins	76%
			Taller than wide	not reported
			Hypoechoic pattern	56%
			Intranodular blood flow	86%
			Suspicious lymph nodes	96%
			TSH	50%

Editor's Note: Please refer to original journal article for full references.

Although the article by Mussa et al is excellent, it is troubling to realize that we are still discussing US features that may predict malignancy 50 years after this tool was introduced into practice. As the authors conclude, there are several US features that are consistent with malignancy; however, "none has [a] diagnostic accuracy as high as that of fine-needle aspiration biopsy." In other words, data from the US should be used to select patients for FNA but cannot be relied on for surgical planning. Thus, with rare exception (the appropriate use of "rare"), all patients should have a FNA before going to the operating room.

As we embark on the era after the publication of the first pediatric management guidelines for thyroid nodules and differentiated thyroid cancer, it is time for our community to master the 50-plus—year-old technologies of thyroid US and FNA to ensure that all pediatric patients receive complete and accurate preoperative evaluation and that surgical and medical care is provided in high-volume pediatric thyroid centers in an effort to ensure optimal outcome and reduce avoidable complications. It's the right thing to do for our patients and the only path that will allow us to move on to the more challenging aspects of defining the molecular landscape of pediatric thyroid nodules and thyroid cancer so that we can improve our ability to identify malignant disease when the results of FNA are indeterminate (25%—30% of FNA results) and to develop an individualized approach to using systemic treatment options for patients with progressive, nonresponsive disease.

As long as they go forward, even small steps will eventually lead to improved patient care.

A. J. Bauer, MD

References

1. Francis GL, Waguespack SG, Bauer AJ, et al. American Thyroid Association Guidelines Task Force. Management guidelines for children with thyroid nodules and differentiated thyroid cancer. *Thyroid.* 2015;25:716-759.
2. Remonti LR, Kramer CK, Leitão CB, Pinto LC, Gross JL. Thyroid ultrasound features and risk of carcinoma: a systematic review and meta-analysis of observational studies. *Thyroid.* 2015;25:538-550.
3. Brito JP, Gionfriddo MR, Al Nofal A, et al. The accuracy of thyroid nodule ultrasound to predict thyroid cancer: systematic review and meta-analysis. *J Clin Endocrinol Metab.* 2014;99:1253-1263.
4. Al Nofal A, Gionfriddo MR, Javed A, et al. Accuracy of thyroid nodule sonography for the detection of thyroid cancer in children: systematic review and meta-analysis. *Clin Endocrinol (Oxf).* 2016;84:423-430.

Comparative Toxicity by Sex Among Children Treated for Acute Lymphoblastic Leukemia: A Report From the Children's Oncology Group

Meeske KA, Ji L, Freyer DR, et al (Children's Hosp Los Angeles, CA; Univ of Southern California, Los Angeles, CA; et al)
Pediatr Blood Cancer 62:2140-2149, 2015

Background.—Epidemiologic studies find sex-based differences in incidence, survival, and long-term outcomes for children with cancer. The purpose of this study was to determine whether male and female patients differ with regard to acute treatment-related toxicities.

Procedures.—We reviewed data collected on the Children's cancer group (CCG) high-risk acute lymphoblastic leukemia (ALL-HR) study (CCG-1961), and compared male and female patients' toxicity incidence and related variables in the first four phases of treatment. Similar analyses were performed with standard-risk ALL (ALL-SR) patients enrolled in CCG-1991.

Results.—Among ALL-HR patients, females had significantly more hospital days, delays in therapy, grade 3 or 4 toxicities (e.g., gastrointestinal, liver), and supportive care interventions (e.g., transfusions, intravenous antibiotics) than males. Females were significantly more likely to have died of treatment-related causes than males (Hazard ratio=2.8, 95% CI = 1.5−5.3, P = 0.002). Five months after beginning treatment, the cumulative incidence of treatment-related deaths was 2.6% for females and 1.2% for males. Similar disparities were found among ALL-SR patients, with females experiencing significantly more hospital days and treatment-related toxicities than males.

Conclusions.—This study complements cancer survivorship studies that also report an increase in treatment-related late effects among females. Risk profiles appear to be different for male and female patients, with females having greater risk of developing both acute and long-term treatment-related toxicities. The underlying biological mechanisms for these sex differences are poorly understood and warrant further study in order to determine how sex-based outcome disparities can be addressed in future clinical trials and practice.

▶ The dramatic improvement in survival of childhood acute lymphoblastic leukemia (ALL) observed over the last 40 years is one of the most significant advances achieved in pediatric medicine.[1] However, both acute and long-term therapy-related toxicity remain major contributors to morbidity and mortality.[2] Unfortunately, predicting which patients will experience acute toxicities caused by cancer-directed therapy is a major challenge.

Significant proportions of children with ALL will develop systemic infection due to immunosuppression from cytotoxic therapy, pancreatitis attributable to asparaginase administration, osteonecrosis associated with glucocorticoid exposure, or peripheral neuropathy attributable to vincristine, among others. Many of these complications will result in permanent deficits that will persist across their life span; thus, the importance of prediction and prevention of toxicities, where possible. Close monitoring and aggressive supportive care have led to significant improvement in some of these complications. However, with few exceptions, we are unable to accurately predict toxicity, and thus we cannot prospectively adjust therapy for the minority who will develop severe morbidity.

Sex is important! It is well established that female survivors of childhood cancer are at increased risk for multiple late-onset complications, relative to males.[3] Meeske et al evaluated outcomes for a large number of patients enrolled on 2 concurrent randomized trials for treatment of ALL to determine whether females may also have more acute treatment related toxicities than males. Robust demographic, anthropomorphic, clinical, therapeutic, and adverse events data allowed them to evaluate toxicity, while adjusting for many potential confounders. Evaluation of major outcomes including incidence of grade 3/4 toxicity, number of hospital days, need for supportive care interventions, and mortality clearly demonstrated that females have an increased risk of acute treatment-related complications. These results are consistent with previous reports from the Nordic Society of Pediatric Hematology and UK Oncology and Medical Research Council citing increased treatment related mortality for females with ALL.[4,5]

Because the magnitude of these sex-based differences in rates of toxicities is relatively small, these data should not result in immediate changes to current, standard ALL therapeutic regimens for females. There are, however, 2 important benefits from the data presented in this article:

1. The conclusions should refine our pretherapy counseling for families and children with ALL. During the informed consent process before induction of therapy, patients and parents deserve answers based on objective data about risks from therapy. Of course, they want to know the chance of cure, but they also want to know the anticipated and potential adverse effects of therapy. Although there will always be large uncertainty, this article informs caregivers about sex-based differences in toxicity that are important for educating patients and families about general risk of therapy related adverse events.

2. The findings should encourage further inquiry regarding the underlying biological mechanisms that increase risk for toxicity among females. Exploring the question of "why" could identify biologic markers that allow more precise risk prediction. The authors discuss potential explanations for the increased risk of treatment related toxicity for females such as sex-based differences in immune response, drug clearance, gastrointestinal toxicities, and distribution of body fat. Although this line of broad conjecture is academically interesting, genetic investigation may provide a more precise understanding. Recent successes in "personalized" therapy for patients with ALL, based on genetic and molecular characterization, have focused on identifying the small groups of patients at very high risk of toxicity, rather and large groups with small absolute increased risk. We must be exceptionally selective about any group for which we alter established primary therapies because therapy adjustment could increase leukemia relapse rates.

A successful model of clinically actionable risk prediction is the identification of patients at high risk of severe toxicity from 6-mercaptopurine (6MP). It is now well established that rare patients who are homozygous for a risk allele within the TPMT gene are likely to have severe, even fatal, immunosuppression if given a standard dose of 6MP. In many treatment protocols, these patients are now identified prospectively and given a dose of 6MP reduced by 90%. This dose reduction leads to dramatically improved toxicity profiles without compromising leukemia eradication. Another high-risk allele for 6-mercaptopurine sensitivity has been discovered within a different gene, *NUDT15*.[6] Efforts are ongoing to include this as part of patient evaluation in some clinical trials. Similar research is striving to find sensitive and specific biomarkers that predict acute osteonecrosis, pancreatitis cardiotoxicity, venous thromboembolism, and peripheral neuropathy so that we may consider therapy adjustment in a small group of high risk patients.[7] Although an association of isolated single nucleotide poylmorphisms with certain toxicity classes is important, this will only explain a minority of the toxicity burden. A developing method of pathway analysis to associate genotype with outcomes in leukemia patients may also hold promise in the context of toxicity prediction.[8]

This article contributes to a growing body of pediatric leukemia research examining acute and chronic treatment related adverse effects by demonstrating that females are at increased risk of acute toxicity. This result needs further exploration though future clinical and biological research in order to identify a subgroup a females who are truly high-risk. Only then will researchers developing clinical trials for ALL have the opportunity (and the burden) to carefully weigh potential benefits vs harms of decreasing or otherwise altering therapy for the appropriate subgroup of patients.

T. B. Alexander, MD, MPH

G. T. Armstrong, MD, MSCE

References

1. Pui CH, Yang JJ, Hunger SP, et al. Childhood acute lymphoblastic leukemia: progress through collaboration. *J Clin Oncol.* 2015;33:2938-2948.
2. Armstrong GT, Chen Y, Yasui Y, et al. Reduction in late mortality among 5-year survivors of childhood cancer. *N Engl J Med.* 2016;374:833-842.
3. Armstrong GT, Sklar CA, Hudson MM, Robison LL. Long-term health status among survivors of childhood cancer: does sex matter? *J Clin Oncol.* 2007;25:4477-4489.
4. Lund B, Asberg A, Heyman M, et al. Risk factors for treatment related mortality in childhood acute lymphoblastic leukaemia. *Pediatr Blood Cancer.* 2011;56:551-559.
5. Wheeler K, Chessells JM, Bailey CC, Richards SM. Treatment related deaths during induction and in first remission in acute lymphoblastic leukaemia: MRC UKALL X. *Arch Dis Child.* 1996;74:101-107.
6. Moriyama T, Nishii R, Perez-Andreu V, et al. NUDT15 polymorphisms alter thiopurine metabolism and hematopoietic toxicity. *Nat Genet.* 2016;48:367-373.
7. Moriyama T, Relling MV, Yang JJ. Inherited genetic variation in childhood acute lymphoblastic leukemia. *Blood.* 2015;125:3988-3995.
8. Wesolowska-Andersen A, Borst L, Dalgaard MD, et al. Genomic profiling of thousands of candidate polymorphisms predicts risk of relapse in 778 Danish and German childhood acute lymphoblastic leukemia patients. *Leukemia.* 2015;29: 297-303.

Integrative Clinical Sequencing in the Management of Refractory or Relapsed Cancer in Youth

Mody RJ, Wu Y-M, Lonigro RJ, et al (Univ of Michigan, Ann Arbor; et al)
JAMA 314:913-925, 2015

Importance.—Cancer is caused by a diverse array of somatic and germline genomic aberrations. Advances in genomic sequencing technologies have improved the ability to detect these molecular aberrations with greater sensitivity. However, integrating them into clinical management in an individualized manner has proven challenging.

Objective.—To evaluate the use of integrative clinical sequencing and genetic counseling in the assessment and treatment of children and young adults with cancer.

Design, Setting, and Participants.—Single-site, observational, consecutive case series (May 2012-October 2014) involving 102 children and young adults (mean age, 10.6 years; median age, 11.5 years, range, 0-22 years) with relapsed, refractory, or rare cancer.

Exposures.—Participants underwent integrative clinical exome (tumor and germline DNA) and transcriptome (tumor RNA) sequencing and genetic counseling. Results were discussed by a precision medicine tumor board, which made recommendations to families and their physicians.

Main Outcomes and Measures.—Proportion of patients with potentially actionable findings, results of clinical actions based on integrative clinical sequencing, and estimated proportion of patients or their families at risk of future cancer.

Results.—Of the 104 screened patients, 102 enrolled with 91 (89%) having adequate tumor tissue to complete sequencing. Only the 91 patients were included in all calculations, including 28 (31%) with hematological malignancies and 63 (69%) with solid tumors. Forty-two patients (46%) had actionable findings that changed their cancer management: 15 of 28 (54%) with hematological malignancies and 27 of 63 (43%) with solid tumors. Individualized actions were taken in 23 of the 91 (25%) based on actionable integrative clinical sequencing findings, including change in treatment for 14 patients (15%) and genetic counseling for future risk for 9 patients (10%). Nine of 91 (10%) of the personalized clinical interventions resulted in ongoing partial clinical remission of 8 to 16 months or helped sustain complete clinical remission of 6 to 21 months. All 9 patients and families with actionable incidental genetic findings agreed to genetic counseling and screening.

Conclusions and Relevance.—In this single-center case series involving young patients with relapsed or refractory cancer, incorporation of integrative clinical sequencing data into clinical management was feasible, revealed potentially actionable findings in 46% of patients, and was associated with change in treatment and family genetic counseling for a small proportion of patients. The lack of a control group limited assessing whether better clinical outcomes resulted from this approach than outcomes that would have occurred with standard care.

▶ On January 20, 2015, President Obama announced the Precision Medicine Initiative, a program aimed at accelerating biomedical research in precision (sometimes called *personalized*) medicine. With an investment of $215 million, this program had the goal of using cutting edge genomic technologies to develop new treatments that are both patient centered and patient specific. New drugs developed in this program, for example, would not be intended for all patients with a particular disorder; rather, such medications would be directed toward patients who are expected to benefit from them most, based on factors such as the disorder's genomic underpinnings, the patient's metabolic profile, and the complex interplay between the 2. Given the natural linkage between precision medicine and cancer research, $70 million was ear marked particularly for the National Cancer Institute to support research into the genomic drivers of cancer and the development of personalized cancer treatments.

While precision cancer medicine has been an area of active research ever since the development of such genomically targeted treatments like imatinib and trastuzumab, the Precision Medicine Initiative officially heralds the arrival of the era of precision cancer medicine. Targeted therapies have reached the clinic for several adult cancer subtypes, and there is a great amount of optimism about the role of precision cancer medicine in adult cancer care. In pediatric oncology, however, the jury is still out. Prior to the recent study by Mody et al, no evidence was available on the use of genomic sequencing in children with cancer. This work represents the first systematic analysis of the feasibility of the integration of genomic tumor sequencing into pediatric clinical care.

In their report, Mody et al describe the first prospective case series of 102 pediatric and young adult subjects with relapsed, refractory, or rare pediatric cancers. They report potentially actionable findings in 46% of participants (with actionable defined as genomic alterations that could lead to a change in patient management: diagnosis, prognosis, treatment, counseling, or identification of a possible cancer predisposition syndrome). Clinical action was taken for 25% of subjects, with 10% showing some degree of clinical response. Germline findings were discovered in an additional 10% of subjects, leading to further counseling and screening for a possible familial cancer predisposition syndrome. As an early-phase feasibility trial, however, no data are available at this time regarding long-term survival of enrolled subjects or about how the integration of genomic sequencing into clinical care may impact patient outcomes.

Without question, these findings are interesting and promising. At the least, they show that there is a role for genomic sequencing in the care of pediatric cancer patients. Several other reports of similar work at other institutions have since been published, and many more pediatric cancer centers are working to integrate genomic sequencing into clinical care. We must take care, however, to proceed with guarded optimism. The lay press often grasps onto early results such as these, leading to widely circulated reports with grandiose conclusions along the lines of, "we are finally on the verge of ridding humanity of the diseases that have plagued it."[1]

Combining this with the inherent complexity of genomic technologies can lead to both misunderstanding and unrealistic optimism among patients and families. Prior work suggests that one-third of individuals have significant misperceptions about personal genomics[2] and that nearly two-thirds of adult cancer patients have the mistaken belief that genomic sequencing would greatly improve the treatment of their cancer.[3] It is the responsibility of the medical profession to ensure that these false impressions are minimized, thereby ensuring that patients and surrogates are accurately informed of the true risks and benefits of potential treatments and interventions.

Medicine is not without cautionary tales of the cart being put before the horse. Perhaps the most extraordinary of these centers around the use of bone marrow transplantation for breast cancer.[4] Bone marrow transplantation was still in its relative infancy in the late 1980s, but early data seemed to show that it was better than any other available treatment for advanced breast cancer, a disease with few effective treatments at that time. No controlled trials had yet been performed, and the public began clamoring to make transplantation readily accessible, even outside of a clinical trial. The medical community was similarly enthusiastic, and over the next decade, thousands of women with breast cancer received bone marrow transplants. By 2000, however, the definitive randomized trial results were in: bone marrow transplantation provided no survival benefit to patients but did cause increased treatment-related toxicity and mortality. Thousands of women had undergone a risky and nonbeneficial treatment because the medical profession had jumped the gun.

The risks inherent in bone marrow transplantation greatly outweigh those of undergoing genomic sequencing, but the message is similar. Extreme care is necessary when new technologies arise with unproven safety and efficacy. The future is now for precision medicine, and it is likely that genomics will yield great benefit for many future pediatric patients. The work by Mody and colleagues may prove to be one of the first steps toward the realization of personalized medicine in pediatrics, but for now, we must be sure to explain to patients and families both the promise of this new technology as well as its limits.

J. M. Marron, MD

References

1. Wadhwa V. *The Triumph of Genomic Medicine Is Just Beginning.* Washington Post; 2014.
2. Gollust SE, Gordon ES, Zayac C, et al. Motivations and perceptions of early adopters of personalized genomics: perspectives from research participants. *Public Health Genomics.* 2012;15:22-30.
3. Blanchette PS, Spreafico A, Miller FA, et al. Genomic testing in cancer: patient knowledge, attitudes, and expectations. *Cancer.* 2014;120:3066-3073.
4. Welch HG, Mogielnicki J. Presumed benefit: lessons from the American experience with marrow transplantation for breast cancer. *BMJ.* 2002;324:1088-1092.

22 Ophthalmology

Effect of Time Spent Outdoors at School on the Development of Myopia Among Children in China: A Randomized Clinical Trial

He M, Xiang F, Zeng Y, et al (Sun Yat-sen Univ, Guangzhou, China; et al)
JAMA 314.1142-1148, 2015

Importance.—Myopia has reached epidemic levels in parts of East and Southeast Asia. However, there is no effective intervention to prevent the development of myopia.

Objective.—To assess the efficacy of increasing time spent outdoors at school in preventing incident myopia.

Design, Setting, and Participants.—Cluster randomized trial of children in grade 1 from 12 primary schools in Guangzhou, China, conducted between October 2010 and October 2013.

Interventions.—For 6 intervention schools (n = 952 students), 1 additional 40-minute class of outdoor activities was added to each school day, and parents were encouraged to engage their children in outdoor activities after school hours, especially during weekends and holidays. Children and parents in the 6 control schools (n = 951 students) continued their usual pattern of activity.

Main Outcomes and Measures.—The primary outcome measure was the 3-year cumulative incidence rate of myopia (defined using the Refractive Error Study in Children spherical equivalent refractive error standard of ≤−0.5 diopters [D]) among the students without established myopia at baseline. Secondary outcome measures were changes in spherical equivalent refraction and axial length among all students, analyzed using mixed linear models and intention-to-treat principles. Data from the right eyes were used for the analysis.

Results.—There were 952 children in the intervention group and 951 in the control group with a mean (SD) age of 6.6 (0.34) years. The cumulative incidence rate of myopia was 30.4% in the intervention group (259 incident cases among 853 eligible participants) and 39.5% (287 incident cases among 726 eligible participants) in the control group (difference of −9.1% [95% CI, −14.1% to −4.1%]; P < .001). There was also a significant difference in the 3-year change in spherical equivalent refraction for the intervention group (−1.42 D) compared with the control group (−1.59 D) (difference of 0.17 D [95% CI, 0.01 to 0.33 D]; P = .04). Elongation of axial length was not significantly different between the intervention group (0.95 mm) and the control group (0.98 mm) (difference of −0.03 mm [95% CI, −0.07 to 0.003 mm]; P = .07).

Conclusions and Relevance.—Among 6-year-old children in Guangzhou, China, the addition of 40 minutes of outdoor activity at school compared with usual activity resulted in a reduced incidence rate of myopia over the next 3 years. Further studies are needed to assess long-term follow-up of these children and the generalizability of these findings.

Trial Registration.—clinicaltrials.gov Identifier: NCT00848900.

▶ Of all of the imaginable reasons to promote time outdoors for young children, who would have guessed myopia prevention? Myopia seems to be growing in prevalence and can be an important health problem. Untreated myopia can impair educational outcomes, and long-term, significant myopia can lead to retinal detachment. This study builds on prior observational work regarding the relationship between outdoor activity and decreased myopia and starts to build the argument that there is a causal relationship.

The scientist and the skeptic in me wants to know what the mechanism is. Is there a growth factor released by the retina in response to sunlight—or not released indoors—that effects the axial length of the eye? Does the extra time spent outdoors somehow lead to changes in the shape of the eye related to greater pupil constriction? More basic science research is needed. More trials are also needed to evaluate what the right "dose" of the outdoors is or how best to "deliver" the outdoors to young children. I also wonder how long the intervention is required. Is there regression, so that the benefit does not last even with continued outdoor activity or does the benefit fade away if individuals have less outdoor exposure?

Truthfully, however, I would rather not precisely understand the mechanism. I like the idea of having another reason to promote outdoors time for children, and I think it is great that I am able to use this study by He et al as another argument with local school leaders. Wouldn't it be terrible if a pharmaceutical company figured out what the underlying mechanism is and developed a myopia prevention pill to replace the outdoor time?

One of the important strengths of this study is that the subjects received standardized eye exams. No information is provided about the care of those who were subsequently identified with myopia. In the United States, we have a major problem providing both follow-up after an abnormal screen and ensuring that those with myopia receive and use corrective lenses and have timely repeat evaluations. As fascinating as myopia primary prevention is, we should not lose focus on these key components of care.

Still, I am excited about being able to advocate for the outdoors. Forty minutes of outdoor activity might be difficult, given all of the material that children even in early elementary school are expected to learn. However, one of the key points is that the outdoor time doesn't have to be doing vigorous activity. Creative teachers could take advantage of this time. It is depressing to think that we might not be able to afford 40 minutes of outdoors time daily. Certainly some schools would have problems due to weather, pollution, safety, insufficient staff to monitor the children, or simply lack of access. These barriers all have policy solutions that should be pursued.

It should be recognized that the relationship between the outdoors and visual health seems to have been known for quite a long time. As Theodore Roosevelt once said, "The lack of power to take joy in outdoor nature is as real a misfortune as the lack of power to take joy in books."[1]

A. R. Kemper, MD, MPH, MS

Reference

1. Roosevelt T. The people of the pacific coast. *The Outlook*. 1911;49:159-162.

Evaluation of Temporal Association Between Vaccinations and Retinal Hemorrhage in Children

Binenbaum G, Christian CW, Guttmann K, et al (The Children's Hosp of Philadelphia, Pennsylvania: et al)
JAMA Ophthalmol 133:1261-1265, 2015

Importance.—Vaccinations have been proposed as a cause of retinal hemorrhage in children, primarily as part of a defense strategy in high-stakes abusive head trauma cases. If vaccination injections cause retinal hemorrhage, this consideration would affect the evaluation of children for suspected child abuse.

Objectives.—To describe the prevalence and causes of retinal hemorrhage among infants and young children in an outpatient ophthalmology clinic and to test the hypothesis that, if vaccination injections cause retinal hemorrhage, then retinal hemorrhage would be seen frequently and be temporally associated with immunization.

Design, Setting, and Participants.—Retrospective cohort study between June 1, 2009, and August 30, 2012, at The Children's Hospital of Philadelphia pediatric ophthalmology clinics among 5177 children 1 to 23 months old undergoing a dilated fundus examination as an outpatient for any reason. Children with intraocular surgery or active retinal neovascularization were excluded from the study.

Main Outcomes and Measures.—The prevalence and causes of retinal hemorrhage, as well as the temporal association between vaccination injection within 7, 14, or 21 days preceding examination and retinal hemorrhage.

Results.—Among 7675 outpatient fundus examinations, 9 of 5177 children had retinal hemorrhage for a prevalence of 0.17% (95% CI, 0.09%-0.33%). All 9 had abusive head trauma diagnosable with nonocular findings. Among a subset of 2210 children who had complete immunization records and underwent 3425 fundoscopic examinations, 163 children had an eye examination within 7 days of vaccination, 323 within 14 days, and 494 within 21 days. No children had retinal hemorrhage within 7 days of vaccination, 1 child had hemorrhage within 14 days, and no additional child had hemorrhage within 21 days. There was no temporal association between vaccination injection and retinal hemorrhage in the prior 7 days (P > .99), 14 days (P = .33), or 21 days (P = .46).

Conclusions and Relevance.—Retinal hemorrhage was rare among out-patients younger than 2 years. Considering both immediate and delayed effects, no temporal association existed between vaccination injection and retinal hemorrhage. Vaccination injections should not be considered a potential cause of retinal hemorrhage in children, and this unsupported theory should not be accepted clinically or in legal proceedings. Ophthalmologists noting incidental retinal hemorrhage on an outpatient examination should consider a child abuse evaluation in the absence of other known ocular or medical disease.

▶ Abusive head trauma (AHT) remains a sad reality in pediatric inpatient services across the country and around the world. Despite the long history of medical recognition of this entity, its existence has been a source of great debate and controversy in courtrooms and the literature. Arguments against AHT have focused on the purported lack of animal or biofidelic models to support the concept of shaking as a cause of subdural hematomas (SDH) and retinal hemorrhages (RH), 2 findings present in many infant and young child victims.

The clinical and epidemiologic evidence for AHT, however, is compelling.[1,2] Multiple studies have documented the rarity of these findings in minor accidental falls often alleged to be the cause.[3] Additionally a study of confessions of convicted perpetrators demonstrated very similar mechanisms of injury, including shaking, leading to a common pattern of injuries in victims, including retinal hemorrhages.[4]

Despite their high incidence in cases clearly representing AHT (eg, infants with SDH, hypoxic ischemic brain injury, rib and long bone fractures), in the courtroom, retinal hemorrhages remain one of the more controversial findings in cases of AHT. Extensive research including large series of clinical cases, post-mortem studies, and various models (animal, mechanical, computer simulations) support the concept of vitreoretinal traction as a result of shaking as the mechanism leading to RH.[5] In the past decade, it has become increasingly apparent that too numerous to count, multilayered RHs involving both the posterior pole and the periphery of the retina (where interestingly the vitreous is most tightly adherent to the retina) are more specific for a shaking injury then a few RHs limited to the intraretinal layer in the posterior poles.[6] Although the latter pattern has been seen in accidental head injury, this still remains an uncommon finding and should raise serious concerns for child abuse.

Vaccinations, among other nonabusive mechanisms, have been raised as possible causes of RH. The hypothesized mechanism by which vaccinations may cause RH states that vaccinations cause raised histamine levels, which can result in lowering of vitamin C levels. Despite the tenuousness of this theory, that vitamin C levels in the bloodstream normally vary widely, and that RH have not been frequently reported in actual cases of scurvy, this theory has been raised in court.

The authors of this article developed a very creative study to test the vaccine theory by reviewing a large number of dilated eye exams of infants and children in the age range we typically see AHT (1–23 months of age). The authors appropriately eliminated patients with conditions known to be associated with intraocular hemorrhage. All the infants were examined by pediatric ophthalmologists for a variety of reasons in an outpatient clinic setting associated with a children's hospital with a long experience in the evaluation of AHT cases. To add to the inclusiveness of the study, the authors included 9 infants and children receiving outpatient eye exams after a recent hospitalization for AHT. A total of 5177 young patients underwent 7675 fundus exams.

As noted by the authors, vaccination rates for infants and children in their catchment area are quite high. Thus, if the vaccine theory is correct, they should have found patients with RHs. To further test the alleged vaccine mechanism, a subgroup of 2210 patients with known vaccine records were further divided into 3 groups based on time from the last vaccination(s) to the eye exam. In this group, the potential for early or delayed effects were able to be determined.

The results of the study demonstrate clear and compelling evidence that vaccinations do not cause RH. Of the 5177 patients examined, the finding of RH was rare and associated only with a recent prior hospitalization for AHT. No evidence for an early or delayed effect of vaccines was found in the subset of patients with known vaccine visits.

This study is important in a number of ways. It is obviously not possible to develop a study that tests the effects of shaking directly on infants and children. We are thus left looking for other ways to verify that shaking is injurious to a young patient's brain and eyes. In addition, well-designed clinical studies can eliminate various nonabusive theories to explain the findings of AHT by actually observing for temporally associated findings (eg, presence of RH after multiply witnessed short falls). This large study effectively eliminates vaccines, whether given singly or in combination at the same patient visit, as a cause of RH. As well, given the number of examinations, this study documents the rarity of retinal hemorrhages in a large group of infants and children. This reinforces the belief that the detection of RH in any child under 2 years of age, regardless of whether the RH are few in number and limited to the posterior pole or numerous, multilayered, and extending to the periphery, is very uncommon and should raise significant concerns for child abuse.

The only patients in this study found to have RH were those with a known recent hospitalization for AHT. This is not to say that RH is by itself diagnostic of abuse. There is a differential diagnosis for RH (eg, coagulopathies, glutaric aciduria type 1, leukemia) that must be considered and appropriate evaluations performed. Additionally, in this age range, a skeletal survey and computed tomography or magnetic resonance imaging of the head should be performed.

K. P. Coulter, MD

References

1. Feldman KW, Bethel R, Shugerman RP, et al. The cause of infant and toddler subdural hemorrhage: a prospective study. *Pediatrics*. 2001;108:636-646.
2. Duhaime AC, Alario AJ, Lewander WJ, et al. Head injury in very young children: mechanisms, injury types, and ophthalmological findings in 100 hospitalized patients younger than 2 years of age. *Pediatrics*. 1992;90:179-185.
3. Reece RM, Sege R. Childhood head injuries: accidental or inflicted? *Arch Pediatr Adolesc Med*. 2000;154:11-15.
4. Starling SP, Patel S, Burke BL, et al. Analysis of perpetrator admissions to inflicted traumatic brain injury in children. *Arch Pediatr Adolesc Med*. 2004;158:454-458.

5. Levin AV. Retinal haemorrhage and child abuse. In: London: Churchill Livingstone; 2000:151-219.
6. Morad Y, Kim YM, Armstrong DC, et al. Correlation between retinal abnormalities and intracranial abnormalities in the shaken baby syndrome. *Am J Ophthalmol.* 2002;134:354-359.

Safety of Retinopathy of Prematurity Examination and Imaging in Premature Infants

Wade KC, on behalf of the e-Retinopathy of Prematurity Study Cooperative Group (Children's Hosp of Philadelphia, PA; et al)
J Pediatr 167:994-1000, 2015

Objectives.—To describe adverse events (AEs) and noteworthy clinical or ocular findings associated with retinopathy of prematurity (ROP) evaluation procedures.

Study Design.—Descriptive analysis of predefined AEs and noteworthy findings reported in a prospective observational cohort study of infants <1251 g birth weight who had ROP study visits consisting of both binocular indirect ophthalmoscopy (BIO) and digital retinal imaging. We compared infant characteristics during ROP visits with and without AEs. We compared respiratory support, nutrition, and number of apnea, bradycardia, or hypoxia events 12 hours before and after ROP visits.

Results.—A total of 1257 infants, mean birth weight 802 g, had 4263 BIO and 4048 imaging sessions (total 8311 procedures). No serious AEs were related to ROP visits. Sixty-five AEs were reported among 61 infants for an AE rate of 4.9% infants (61/1257) or 0.8% total procedures (65/8311 BIO + imaging). Most AEs were due to apnea, bradycardia, and/or hypoxia (68%), tachycardia (16%), or emesis (8%). At ROP visit, infants with AEs, compared with those without, were more likely to be on mechanical ventilation (26% vs 12%, P =.04) even after adjustment for weight and postmenstrual age. Noteworthy clinical findings were reported during 8% BIO and 15% imaging examinations. Respiratory and nutrition support were not significantly different before and after ROP evaluations.

Conclusions.—Retinal imaging by nonphysicians combined with BIO was safe. Noteworthy clinical findings occurred during both procedures. Ventilator support was a risk factor for AEs. Monitoring rates of AEs and noteworthy findings are important to the safe implementation of ROP imaging protocols.

Trial Registration.—Clinicaltrials.gov: NCT01264276 (Table 2).

▶ Every day thousands of examinations for retinopathy of prematurity (ROP) are performed. Each exam carries potential risk for the infant's well-being. Therefore, the report by Wade and colleagues is reassuring both in its findings that side effects were uncommon (Table 2) and that adverse events were transient. In this review, I walk through the examination and describe points in the exam process when problems can arise and what those problems may be.

TABLE 2.—Description of AEs During or Shortly After ROP Study Visits (n = 65 AEs)

AEs During ROP Evaluation (n = 59)	n Events (%)
Apnea, bradycardia, and/or hypoxia	42 (71%)
Tachycardia	9 (15%)
Emesis	5 (8%)
Epistaxis	1 (2%)
Arrhythmia (bradycardia)	1 (2%)
Retinal hemorrhage	1 (2%)
AEs after ROP evaluations (n = 6)	**n events (%) and associated clinical circumstances**
Apnea, bradycardia, and hypoxia events	4 (67%)
Required bag mask positive pressure ventilation and increased respiratory support	1 attributable to water droplets from CPAP device, resolved
	2 attributable to opiates and ROP laser surgery, resolved with intubation
	1 attributable to GBS sepsis, resolved with intubation and antibiotics
Feeding intolerance	1 (17%)
Required intravenous fluids and antibiotics	Infant with emesis and abdominal distention. Stopped feeds, started antibiotics, symptoms resolved. Resumed full enteral feeds within 24 hours. No evidence NEC.
Respiratory insufficiency	1 (17%)
Required increased mode of respiratory support	Increased respiratory distress that resolved with change in respiratory support from nasalcannula to CPAP attributable to chronic lung disease and recent weaning off CPAP.

NEC, necrotizing enterocolitis; GBS, Group B Streptococcus.
Reprinted from Wade KC, on behalf of the e-Retinopathy of Prematurity Study Cooperative Group. Safety of retinopathy of prematurity examination and imaging in premature infants. *J Pediatr.* 2015;167:994-1000, with permission from Elsevier.

Exams start with a call from the ophthalmologist/examiner asking that the nursery staff dilate the pupils of infants who need an examination. In some centers, this is a predetermined time, but in most, the call occurs at the examiner's discretion. Failure to follow the order for dilation can result in unnecessary delays in the examination and constitutes a serious breach in the care of the infant. Consequently, a system must be in place to ensure compliance with dilating drop orders. In most nurseries, compliance is assured by communicating with a charge nurse or neonatologist.

The dilating drops required for examination with a camera or indirect binocular ophthalmoscope (IBO) may have side effects. The most widely used drop is a mixture of 0.2% cyclopentolate and 0.5% neo-synephrine. Usually the drops are administered at brief (5-minute) intervals at least twice an hour before the exam.

Although the current dilating mixture is very safe, stronger drops may be required when dilation is poor and may have serious side effects. For example, 2.5% neo-synephrine (or higher concentrations) may cause increases in blood pressure and heart rate. Stronger anticholinergics are especially fraught with potential side effects. The most common of these are changes in heart rate and respiratory rate, but ileus can occur and can be severe enough to mimic the findings in necrotizing enterocolitis. Neonatal staff should be alert to these possible complications. In infants with an inflammatory component to their ROP, the use of topical steroids may be indicated. These drops carry the potential for causing elevated pressure (glaucoma) and cataracts if used for a prolonged period of time.

Next, usually about an hour after administration of drops, the eyes of the infant are examined. Most examiners use a lid speculum, and some may depress the sclera with a blunt metal rod. Topical anesthesia is used in most situations but often does little to blunt the vagal response elicited by this aspect of the exam. Some infants are sedated (eg, with morphine) before the examination. Even so, interruptions and prolongation of the examination often ensue. The report by Wade et al shows that those infants on respiratory support are at highest risk for apnea, bradycardia, and emesis, usually as a result of the exam. Interestingly, IBO and camera diagnosis both show similar rates of adverse events. This is not surprising because commonly used cameras involve contact and pressure on the eye.

The examiner then makes notes, draws his or her findings, and submits these for electronic uploading or charting. Another pitfall in the examination process can occur at this stage: failure to communicate with the neonatal staff and family the findings of the exam and the timing of the next examination.

This brief summary should inform decisions about eye examinations in the nursery. Such a seemingly innocuous procedure, the ROP exam, is not without its possible problems. Fortunately, the problems are uncommon and virtually never lead to permanent harm to the infants. The choice of dilating drop is important. Strong anticholinergic agents should be avoided unless absolutely necessary and infants on such drops (eg, atropine, cyclopentolate) should be monitored with possible systemic absorptions problems in mind. The use of an eye speculum is not always necessary. Most exams of premature infants' eyes are screening exams. The posterior pole of the retina can often be visualized without a speculum or scleral depressor. Plus disease is usually the sign that an infant requires treatment. Plus disease (ie, an amount of dilation and tortuosity of retinal vessels in the posterior pole consistent with published photos) can be visualized without instruments on the eye. Eyedrops and eye manipulation may have effects that last several hours. Consequently, the infant should be under surveillance with this in mind after the examination. Most importantly, a system for logging exams, results of exams, and follow-up planning should be in place.

W. V. Good, MD

23 Pediatric Surgery

Effect of Reduction in the Use of Computed Tomography on Clinical Outcomes of Appendicitis

Bachur RG, Levy JA, Callahan MJ, et al (Harvard Med School, Boston, MA)
JAMA Pediatr 169:755-760, 2015

Importance.—Advanced diagnostic imaging is commonly used in the evaluation of suspected appendicitis in children. Despite its inferior diagnostic performance, ultrasonography (US) is now preferred to computed tomography (CT) owing to concerns about ionizing radiation exposure. With changes in imaging modalities, the influence on outcomes should be assessed.

Objectives.—To review trends in the use of US and CT for children with appendicitis and to investigate simultaneous changes in the proportions of negative appendectomy, appendiceal perforation, and emergency department (ED) revisits.

Design, Setting, and Participants.—We reviewed the Pediatric Health Information System administrative database for children who presented to the ED with the diagnosis of appendicitis or who underwent an appendectomy in 35 US pediatric institutions from January 1, 2010, through December 31, 2013.

Main Outcomes and Measures.—We studied the use of US and CT for trends and their association with negative appendectomy, appendiceal perforation, and 3-day ED revisits.

Results.—Our investigation included 52 153 children with appendicitis. Use of US increased 46% (from 24.0% in 2010 to 35.3% in 2013; absolute difference, 11.3%; adjusted test for linear trend, $P = .02$), whereas use of CT decreased 48% (from 21.4% in 2010 to 11.6% in 2013; absolute difference, -9.8%; adjusted test for linear trend, $P < .001$). The proportion of negative appendectomy declined during the 4-year study period from 4.7% in 2010 to 3.6% in 2013 (test for linear trend, $P = .002$), whereas the proportion of perforations (32.3% in 2010 to 31.9% in 2013) and ED revisits (5.6% in 2010 and 2013) did not change (adjusted tests for linear trend, $P = .64$ and $P = .84$, respectively).

Conclusions and Relevance.—Among children with suspected appendicitis, the use of US imaging has increased substantially as the use of CT has declined. Despite the increased reliance on the diagnostically inferior US, important condition-specific quality measures, including the frequency of appendiceal perforation and ED revisits, remained stable, and the proportion of negative appendectomy declined slightly.

▶ After hundreds of years, appendicitis remains the surgeon's quintessential diagnostic dilemma. A literature search on pediatric appendicitis finds 2657 articles published in the last 20 years, 425 of which discuss the use of CT scanning. Yet, despite these hundreds and hundreds of studies on the evaluation of a patient with suspected appendicitis, we remain confused about best practice. The article in the *Journal of the American Medical Association Pediatrics* by Dr Bachur and his colleagues uses an administrative database to review the changes in outcomes over a 4-year period during which CT scan use in the diagnosis of appendicitis declined and that of ultrasound scan increased in the 35 pediatric institutions submitting data. This article reports that CT scan use decreased from 21% to 12% from 2010 to 2013, with a concomitant increase in ultrasound use from 24% to 35%, leaving about 50% of patients each year who had no imaging at all. During this interval, there was no change in the rate of perforation, which remained at 32%. A small decrease in the rate of negative appendectomy from 4.7% to 3.1% was also noted, which the authors comment may have been influenced by increased experience with ultrasound scan or perhaps the use of increased serial examination in the emergency department. Interestingly, a concurrent article reported that 99.7% of patients evaluated for appendicitis had preoperative imaging during a similar period (> 50% had CT scans), with a perforation rate of 22% and a similar negative appendectomy rate of 4.6%.[1] Clearly, even to this day, there remains a variety of practice patterns in the diagnosis of appendicitis but little difference in the measured outcomes, driving home the main message of Dr Bachur's article: as we have known for a while, CT scanning really isn't the end-all in diagnosis of appendicitis. So how then do we approach this long-standing diagnostic conundrum?

To determine how better to improve our diagnostic protocol for patients with appendicitis, first we need to rethink what outcomes to measure. I suggest that the rate of perforation is unlikely to change based on the use of or the type of diagnostic imaging, as most patients with a perforated appendix already have it when they present to the emergency department. If there are enough patients with perforating appendices while in our emergency rooms to measure a difference, then we should close our doors and send our patients somewhere that is doing a better job. So let's drop that as a measure. Measurement of negative appendectomy rate is clearly important. Back in 2003, Stephen and colleagues[2] found that CT scanning does not have better accuracy at diagnosing appendicitis than a good history, physical, and laboratory evaluation in most patients. Dr Bachur's report reiterates this as more than 50% of patients in this study underwent no imaging at all. I think it reasonable to demand that patients with suspected appendicitis be evaluated by an experienced clinician before an imaging study is ordered to determine a pretest probability of appendicitis. That way we can avoid unnecessary testing for most of these patients. Exposure to ionizing radiation should surely be avoided when possible; therefore, measuring the rate of CT scanning as an outcome seems prudent as well.

The real issue then becomes what to do with the populations in which there is a genuine diagnostic dilemma, such as adolescent females, those patients with atypical history and inconsistent examination, and those with unexpected laboratory values. For these patients, we need to come up with a better diagnostic protocol that can give us the pretest probability of appendicitis. The literature is full of clinical diagnostic tools: the Alvarado and Pediatric Appendicitis Scores, the use of C-reactive protein, white blood cell count and left shift, bilirubin, and various others in evaluation of appendicitis. Shogilev and colleagues[3] nicely review many of the laboratory markers that have discriminatory potential in the evaluation of appendicitis. Recently, several studies found the utility of incorporating imaging studies and clinical decision-support tools along with ultrasound scan to improve diagnostic accuracy and also limit the number of CT scans used for diagnosis.[4] What we need now is incorporation of this vast collection of data into the creation of a decision support protocol that incorporates our best bedside skills as physicians, proven useful laboratory evaluations, and calculated stepwise application of imaging studies to maximize our diagnostic accuracy and minimize the harm of unnecessary tests, radiation, and surgery. Once created, the protocol will need validation and then dissemination to all providers that care for pediatric patients in the emergency setting. Appendicitis has been with us for a very long time, and it remains one of the most common reasons for abdominal surgery. It's time we figure out how best to manage it.

C. M. Kelleher, MD

References

1. Kotagal M, Richards MK, Flum DR, et al. Use and accuracy of diagnostic imaging in the evaluation of pediatric appendicitis. *J Pediatr Surg*. 2015;50:642-646.
2. Stephen A, Segev DL, Ryan DP, et al. Diagnosis of acute appendicitis in a pediatric population: to CT or not to CT. *J Pediatr Surg*. 2003;38:367-371.
3. Shogilev DJ, Duus N, Odom SR, Shapiro NI. Diagnosing appendicitis: evidence-based review of the diagnostic approach in 2014. *West J Emerg Med*. 2014;15:859-871.
4. Srinivasan A, Servaes S, Peña A, Darge K. Utility of CT after sonography for suspected appendicitis in children: integration of a clinical scoring system with a staged imaging protocol. *Emerg Radiol*. 2015;22:31-42.

In-hospital Surgical Delay Does Not Increase the Risk for Perforated Appendicitis in Children: A Single-center Retrospective Cohort Study
Almström M, Svensson JF, Patkova B, et al (Karolinska Univ Hosp, Stockholm, Sweden)
Ann Surg 2016 [Epub ahead of print]

Objective.—To investigate the correlation between in-hospital surgical delay before appendectomy for suspected appendicitis and the finding of perforated appendicitis in children.

Methods.—All children undergoing acute appendectomy for suspected acute appendicitis at Karolinska University Hospital, Stockholm, Sweden from 2006 to 2013 were reviewed for the exposure of surgical delay.

Primary endpoint was the histopathologic finding of perforated appendicitis. The main explanatory variable was in-hospital surgical delay, using surgery within 12 hours as reference. Secondary endpoints were postoperative wound infection, intra-abdominal abscess, reoperation, length of hospital stay, and readmission. To adjust for selection bias, a logistic regression model was created to estimate odds ratios for the main outcome measures. Missing data were replaced using multiple imputation.

Results.—The study comprised 2756 children operated for acute appendicitis. Six hundred sixty-one (24.0%) had a histopathologic diagnosis of perforated appendicitis. In the multivariate logistic regression analysis, increased time to surgery was not associated with increased risk of histopathologic perforation. There was no association between the timing of surgery and postoperative wound infection, intra-abdominal abscess, reoperation, or readmission.

Conclusions.—In-hospital delay of acute appendectomy in children was not associated with an increased rate of histopathologic perforation. Timing of surgery was not an independent risk factor for postoperative complications. The results were not dependent on the magnitude of the surgical delay. The findings are analogous with previous findings in adults and may aid the utilization of available hospital- and operative resources.

▶ Appendicitis is one of the most common surgical emergencies in adults and children.[1] While the presenting signs and symptoms of appendicitis have remained unchanged for many decades, refinements in its evaluation and treatment have been the subject of considerable interest in the last 10 to 20 years. Treatment of suspected appendicitis with antibiotics alone, the emergence of CT and ultrasonography for diagnosis, and the initial nonoperative therapy for perforated appendicitis with or without interval appendectomy have introduced additional complexity to the management of appendicitis that was not present previously. While appendicitis is the classic condition causing the acute abdomen, there has also been a change in the urgency with which suspected cases of appendicitis are treated. Appendicitis has become "urgent" rather than "emergent."

This report by Almstrom et al seeks to assess the impact of surgical delay on outcomes of uncomplicated appendicitis in children. Two European studies from the mid-1990s suggested that surgical delay had no statistically adverse impact on perforation rate or postoperative complications. [2,3] The authors of this study cite previous work with conflicting results and, therefore, aimed to better understand the impact of delay in this cohort study. All children who underwent appendectomy for suspected acute appendicitis over a 7-year period were included, and the effect of surgical delay on the main outcome, histopathologic evidence of appendiceal perforation, was assessed. The impact of this delay on postoperative complications was also quantified. The study began with 2888 children 0 to 15 years of age. After excluding patients who had a negative appendectomy and those with incomplete pathology data, the final study population was 2756. Univariate analysis showed that younger children, night-time surgery, higher temperature, and elevation of C-reactive protein (CRP) and white blood count (WBC) were associated with perforated appendicitis, not a surprising finding. Female sex was also associated with perforation, but the reason for this is less clear. Assessing the population from another point of view, surgical delay correlated statistically with older age, daytime operation, lower temperature, and lower CRP and WBC. In the authors' adjusted multivariate logistic regression analysis, no statistical association between surgical delay and perforation was noted and no association with postoperative complications was seen.

This study adds solid and well-analyzed data to support the safety of a reasonable surgical delay on the important outcomes in children with suspected appendicitis. The patient sample is of significant size for a single institution and, most importantly, the authors have controlled for bias and other confounders to isolate surgical delay as a risk factor. A careful review of the article reveals several notable findings worthy of comment. First, the authors considered surgical delay only if surgery occurred more than 12 hours after admission to the emergency department. In hospitals in which surgery is delayed to the following morning for cases admitted overnight, many of these cases (presumably performed before the 12-hour mark) would not have been considered delayed when using the criteria in this study. On the other end of the spectrum, the study shows that nearly 18% of cases were delayed by more than 24 hours and that the longest delays (> 36 hours) were associated with a perforation rate (19.1%) lower than what was seen in patients undergoing surgery within 24 hours of presentation. Second, the article cites a reference by Carr[4] to support their definition of perforation, and it is implied that microscopic findings on slides were used to distinguish between perforated and nonperforated appendicitis. Other definitions of perforated appendicitis exist, and one commonly used definition, namely, a visible hole in the appendix or a spilled fecalith in the abdomen, was proposed by St Peter et al in 2008.[5] Furthermore, the authors do not mention whether the attending pathologist was blinded to, and therefore unbiased by, the operative findings when rendering a pathologic opinion. Finally, this study provides us with the incidence of perforation (24%) in cases of appendicitis in children and the negative appendectomy rate (3.8%) that can be expected when modern imaging modalities are used for diagnosis.

Based on the current study, which adds incrementally to a growing body of evidence, it appears that surgical delay in performing an appendectomy for suspected appendicitis in children is safe and does not result in an increased incidence of perforation or other complications. While it has become increasingly clear that emergent or night-time surgery for appendicitis in children is not medically necessary, further information regarding the costs associated with surgical delay as well as the effect of surgical delay on patient satisfaction are needed to fully appreciate the overall impact of this management strategy.

R. A. Cowles, MD

References

1. Bhangu A, Søreide K, Di Saverio S, et al. Acute appendicitis: modern understanding of pathogenesis, diagnosis, and management. *Lancet.* 2015;386:1278-1287.
2. Surana R, Quinn F, Puri P. Is it necessary to perform appendicectomy in the middle of the night in children? *BMJ.* 1993;306:1168.

3. Walker SJ, West CR, Colmer MR. Acute appendicitis: does removal of a normal appendix matter, what is the value of diagnostic accuracy and is surgical delay important? *Ann R Coll Surg Engl.* 1995;77:358-363.

4. Carr NJ. The pathology of acute appendicitis. *Ann Diagn Pathol.* 2000;4:46-58.

5. St Peter SD, Sharp SW, Holcomb GW 3rd, Ostlie DJ. An evidence-based definition for perforated appendicitis derived from a prospective randomized trial. *J Pediatr Surg.* 2008;43:2242-2245.

A Clinical Tool for the Prediction of Venous Thromboembolism in Pediatric Trauma Patients

Connelly CR, Laird A, Barton JS, et al (Oregon Health & Science Univ, Portland; Univ of Texas, Houston)
JAMA Surg 151:50-57, 2016

Importance.—Although rare, the incidence of venous thromboembolism (VTE) in pediatric trauma patients is increasing, and the consequences of VTE in children are significant. Studies have demonstrated increasing VTE risk in older pediatric trauma patients and improved VTE rates with institutional interventions. While national evidence-based guidelines for VTE screening and prevention are in place for adults, none exist for pediatric patients, to our knowledge.

Objectives.—To develop a risk prediction calculator for VTE in children admitted to the hospital after traumatic injury to assist efforts in developing screening and prophylaxis guidelines for this population.

Design, Setting, and Participants.—Retrospective review of 536 423 pediatric patients 0 to 17 years old using the National Trauma Data Bank from January 1, 2007, to December 31, 2012. Five mixed-effects logistic regression models of varying complexity were fit on a training data set. Model validity was determined by comparison of the area under the receiver operating characteristic curve (AUROC) for the training and validation data sets from the original model fit. A clinical tool to predict the risk of VTE based on individual patient clinical characteristics was developed from the optimal model.

Main Outcome and Measure.—Diagnosis of VTE during hospital admission.

Results.—Venous thromboembolism was diagnosed in 1141 of 536 423 children (overall rate, 0.2%). The AUROCs in the training data set were high (range, 0.873-0.946) for each model, with minimal AUROC attenuation in the validation data set. A prediction tool was developed from a model that achieved a balance of high performance (AUROCs, 0.945 and 0.932 in the training and validation data sets, respectively; $P = .048$) and parsimony. Points are assigned to each variable considered (Glasgow Coma Scale score, age, sex, intensive care unit admission, intubation, transfusion of blood products, central venous catheter placement, presence of pelvic or lower extremity fractures, and major surgery), and the points total is converted to a VTE risk score. The predicted risk of VTE ranged from 0.0% to 14.4%.

Conclusions and Relevance.—We developed a simple clinical tool to predict the risk of developing VTE in pediatric trauma patients. It is based on a model created using a large national database and was internally validated. The clinical tool requires external validation but provides an initial step toward the development of the specific VTE protocols for pediatric trauma patients.

▶ Connelly and coworkers provide a comprehensive risk prediction analysis of venous thromboembolism (VTE) in children suffering pediatric trauma. They rightfully considered that the Glasgow Coma Score is most strongly associated with risk but also found important contributions owing to the variables of age category and intensive care unit (ICU) admission. These 3 variables together constitute their "model 3." Other variables considered are either not independently predictive, do not add appreciably to prediction, or are of low incidence in the study population. These other variables include the presence of diabetes mellitus, malignancy, a (preexisting) bleeding disorder, and obesity and are similar to the array of variables used in other current studies of VTE in pediatric trauma.

Unfortunately, the analysis and scoring system are not as useful as one might at first believe. The area under the receiver operating characteristic curve is 0.932 in model 3. Yet the low incidence (0.2%) of VTE as identified in the National Trauma Data Bank (NTDB), together with the retrospective use of ICD-9 codes, gives a false impression that this scoring system is accurate and reliable, when it is not. The very rarity of VTE, as defined here, in the pediatric age group biases the outcome prediction in favor of accuracy, as a negative prediction alone would be accurate 99.8% of the time. Moreover, the VTE rate is certainly underestimated, both by underreporting inherent in the NTDB and by a nonrecognition of clinically silent VTE. In one recent prospective pediatric clinical investigation,[1] VTE was found in 18% of 93 consecutive children admitted to a pediatric intensive care unit with, as is common, placement of a central venous catheter. So as not to miss asymptomatic VTE, radiographic surveillance (Doppler ultrasound scan) was performed. Such VTE can still contribute to death and morbidity, as clinical symptoms can be obscured by the multiple acute events that occur early on in the ICU setting, and as such VTE can become clinically important during longer hospital stays or even following hospital discharge.

The study, further, can justifiably omit in the final model, a preexisting bleeding disorder but might have included the acquired bleeding diathesis that often accompanies trauma: uncontrolled bleeding still contributes to 30% to 40% of trauma deaths in the United States each year.[2] This bleeding diathesis is secondary to acidosis, hypoxia, or hypothermia, which are known to adversely affect platelet function and clotting reactions.[3] Conceivably, the presence of a significant hypocoagulability may have a negative influence on VTE risk. On the other hand, the study of Connelly et al shows that for those few who have a preexisting bleeding disorder, there is an increased incidence of VTE.

The study does not address the question as to whether any, and how many, patients died shortly after hospital admission, as had such patients survived longer, VTE would have undoubtedly developed in some. In this regard, the studies cited above show that the mean time to identification of a VTE in the ICU setting is about 7 days, with some VTEs not becoming apparent for up to 30 days.

Nonetheless, the proposed scoring system is a major step forward and provides a framework within which other and more relevant pediatric variables may be included and with which other analyses may be compared. For example, the Children's Hospital Hospital-Acquired Database (CHAT) project,[4] recently funded by the Hemostasis and Thrombosis Research Society of North America, seeks to study and identify 53 candidate risk factors for pediatric hospital-acquired VTE and to create a risk-scoring assessment tool. Bedside devices to assess clotting and platelet function in real time, more sensitive than the d-dimer or ACT, can also help. Such devices include rotational thromboelastometry (ROTEM) and microfluidic flow devices to assess platelet function.[5] Finally, while VTE is less common in children than in adults, an ability to predict VTE and thereby provide earlier treatment in children has the potential to preserve and improve the quality of up to 60 to 80 or more years of life.

E. Grabowski, MD

References

1. Beck C, Dubois J, Grignon A, Lacroix J, Michele D. Incidence and risk factors of catheter-related deep venous thrombosis in a pediatric intensive care unit: a prospective study. *J Pediatr.* 1998;133:237-241.
2. Kauvar DS, Wade CE. The epidemiology and modern management of traumatic hemorrhage: US and international perspectives. *Crit Care.* 2005;9:S1-S9.
3. Wolberg A, Meng ZH, Monroe DM, Hoffman M. A systematic evaluation of the effect of temperature on coagulation enzyme activity and platelet function. *J Trauma.* 2003;55:886-891.
4. Mahajerin A, Branchford BR, Amankwah EK, et al. Hospital-associated venous thromboembolism in pediatrics: a systematic review and meta-analysis of risk factors and risk-assessment models. *Haematologica.* 2015;100:1045-1050.
5. Grabowski EF, Curran MA, Van Cott EM. Assessment of a cohort of primarily pediatric patients with a presumptive diagnosis of type 1 von Willebrand disease with a novel high shear rate, non-citrated blood flow device. *Thromb Res.* 2012;129:e18-e24.

Bladder Function After Fetal Surgery for Myelomeningocele
Brock JW III, for the MOMS Investigators (Vanderbilt Univ Med Ctr, Nashville, TN; et al)
Pediatrics 136:e906-e913, 2015

Background.—A substudy of the Management of Myelomeningocele Study evaluating urological outcomes was conducted.

Methods.—Pregnant women diagnosed with fetal myelomeningocele were randomly assigned to either prenatal or standard postnatal surgical repair. The substudy included patients randomly assigned after April 18, 2005. The primary outcome was defined in their children as death or the need for clean intermittent catheterization (CIC) by 30 months of age characterized by prespecified criteria. Secondary outcomes included bladder and kidney abnormalities observed by urodynamics and renal/bladder ultrasound at 12 and 30 months, which were analyzed as repeated measures.

Results.—Of the 115 women enrolled in the substudy, the primary outcome occurred in 52% of children in the prenatal surgery group and 66% in the postnatal surgery group (relative risk [RR]: 0.78; 95% confidence interval [CI]: 0.57—1.07). Actual rates of CIC use were 38% and 51% in the prenatal and postnatal surgery groups, respectively (RR: 0.74; 95% CI: 0.48—1.12). Prenatal surgery resulted in less trabeculation (RR: 0.39; 95% CI: 0.19—0.79) and fewer cases of open bladder neck on urodynamics (RR: 0.61; 95% CI: 0.40—0.92) after adjustment by child's gender and lesion level. The difference in trabeculation was confirmed by ultrasound.

Conclusions.—Prenatal surgery did not significantly reduce the need for CIC by 30 months of age but was associated with less bladder trabeculation and open bladder neck. The implications of these findings are unclear now, but support the need for long-term urologic follow-up of patients with myelomeningocele regardless of type of surgical repair.

▶ The Management of Myelomeningocele Study (MOMS) trial had its origins at a national pediatric neurosurgical meeting. An ultimatum was laid down that either a randomized, controlled trial be performed, or everyone was going to start performing prenatal myelomeningocele closure, thereby losing the opportunity to show a benefit for this new procedure. The MOMS trial found that prenatal myelomeningocele repair decreased the rate of ventriculoperitoneal shunting and improved mental and motor function at 30 months.[1] Unfortunately, urologists did not see an improvement in bladder function in the children who underwent prenatal closure compared with postnatal closure.[2-4] Because the patients selected for the MOMS trial were the lowest-risk group, this finding was disappointing. One possible explanation was that urologists taking care of these children, who are spread out all across the United States, used varying criteria in choosing when to institute clean intermittent catheterization (CIC). In this follow-up study, the investigators used strict criteria applied by an independent committee of urologists blinded to treatment group to review the records and determine if the use of CIC was warranted and also to review the results of urodynamic studies. At 30-month follow-up, there was no difference in the proportion of patients in the prenatal and postnatal groups who had hydronephrosis or who were using CIC. There was a glimmer of hope in that the patients who underwent prenatal closure were more likely to have a closed bladder neck, although there was no difference in bladder leak point pressure, a marker for urinary continence.

For a parent with a child with spina bifida, the management of the bladder and bowel are lifelong issues that eventually need to be managed by the child when he or she is capable of performing CIC and taking anticholinergic medications and polyethylene glycol on a schedule. One of the major goals of preemptive management of bladder dysfunction is to prevent severe bladder deterioration that would require intestinal augmentation of the bladder. Unfortunately, the tendency is for bladder function to deteriorate during adolescence because of tethered cord and patient noncompliance with CIC and anticholinergic medication.[5] So although it was encouraging to see that there was no worsening in hydronephrosis and bladder function between 12 and 30 months, the riskiest period remains many years in the future. It will be interesting to see if the prenatal group has better executive function and is more compliant as adolescents with medical therapy and performing CIC on themselves. The warning in the concluding paragraph that "it is imperative to continue to monitor all children with myelomeningocele from birth no matter how the spinal defect was closed" is a wise reminder that prenatal surgery is only one part of a lifelong effort to maintain renal and bladder health.

H.-Y. Wu, MD

References

1. Adzick NS, Thom EA, Spong CY, et al. A randomized trial of prenatal versus postnatal repair of myelomeningocele. *N Engl J Med.* 2011;364:993-1004.
2. Holmes NM, Nguyen HT, Harrison MR, et al. Fetal intervention for myelomeningocele: effect on postnatal bladder function. *J Urol.* 2001;186:2383-2386.
3. Clayton DB, Tanaka ST, Trusler L, et al. Long-term urological impact of fetal myelomeningocele closure. *J Urol.* 2011;186:1581-1585.
4. Lee NG, Gomez P, Uberoi V, et al. In utero closure of myelomeningocele does not improve lower urinary tract function. *J Urol.* 2012;188:1567-1571.
5. Woodhouse CRJ. Myelomeningocele in young adults. *BJU International.* 2005;95:223-230.

Feeding Post-Pyloromyotomy: A Meta-analysis
Sullivan KJ, for the Canadian Association of Paediatric Surgeons Evidence-Based Resource (Children's Hosp of Eastern Ontario, Ottawa, Ontario, Canada)
Pediatrics 137:e20152550, 2016

Context.—Postoperative emesis is common after pyloromyotomy. Although postoperative feeding is likely to be an influencing factor, there is no consensus on optimal feeding.

Objective.—To compare the effect of feeding regimens on clinical outcomes of infants after pyloromyotomy.

Data Sources.—Cumulative Index to Nursing and Allied Health Literature, The Cochrane Central Register of Controlled Trials, Embase, and Medline.

Study Selection.—Two reviewers independently assessed studies for inclusion based on a priori inclusion criteria.

Data Extraction.—Data were extracted on methodological quality, general study and intervention characteristics, and clinical outcomes.

Results.—Fourteen studies were included. Ad libitum feeding was associated with significantly shorter length of stay (LOS) when compared with structured feeding (mean difference [MD] -4.66; 95% confidence interval [CI], -8.38 to -0.95; $P = .01$). Although gradual feeding significantly decreased emesis episodes (MD −1.70; 95% CI, −2.17 to −1.23; $P < .00001$), rapid feeding led to significantly shorter LOS (MD 22.05; 95% CI, 2.18 to 41.93; $P = .03$). Late feeding resulted in a significant decrease in number of patients with emesis (odds ratio 3.13; 95% CI, 2.26 to 4.35; $P < .00001$).

Limitations.—Exclusion of non-English studies, lack of randomized controlled trials, insufficient number of studies to perform publication bias or subgroup analysis for potential predictors of emesis.

Conclusions.—Ad libitum feeding is recommended for patients after pyloromyotomy as it leads to decreased LOS. If physicians still prefer structured feeding, early rapid feeds are recommended as they should lead to a reduced LOS.

▶ Surgical dogma is slow to change. The first successful pyloromyotomy was performed by Fredet in 1908. In 1912, Ramstedt simplified the procedure and described what would become the classic surgical approach for the treatment of pyloric stenosis. This was the first revolution in the care of infants with this condition, and the treatment remained largely unchanged for 80 years. Historically, feedings were held for some time postoperatively. Today, many or most surgeons still wait at least 4 to 6 hours to allow for the return of normal gastric peristalsis. The data to support this practice are lacking and based primarily on old literature.[1,2]

The next major change in the care of patients with pyloric stenosis occurred when Alain put a scope in the abdomen in 1991. This was the first application of laparoscopic surgery to a pediatric-specific illness. Although initially controversial, this technique has since been widely adopted. It is unclear whether the decrease in perioperative complications is attributable to surgical technique or rather to other advances in the care of hospitalized infants since the early 1990s. Regardless, within 20 years of Alain's first laparoscopic pyloromyotomy, the technique became the preferred approach of many pediatric surgeons.

Along with improved cosmesis, early studies found that laparoscopic pyloromyotomy was associated with less postoperative emesis and lower pain scores.[3] Is it possible that minimally invasive surgeons began to feed patients earlier than their colleagues did to show a benefit of a laparoscopic approach over open surgery? After all, surgeons have for many years promoted laparoscopic surgery as less painful with an opportunity for decreased medication use, decreased length of hospital stay, and a quicker return to work. Surgical complications are uncommon after pyloromyotomy regardless of approach, and narcotic pain medication is often not necessary. These infants may not be in a hurry to get back to the workforce, but careful study can find differences in length of hospital stay, time needed to reach full feedings, and incidence or frequency of emesis. In what is classic "anything you can do I can do better" fashion, proponents of open surgery began to accelerate feeding schedules. Eventually, factors such as preoperative electrolyte derangement,[4] resuscitation, or patient weight[5] were correlated with lengthened stay rather than operative technique.

In this article by Sullivan et al, 14 carefully chosen studies were systematically reviewed in an attempt to answer the divisive question of optimal feeding schedule after pyloromyotomy. Meta-analysis led to conclusions that ad libitum and early feeding are favored, whether open or laparoscopic pyloromyotomy is performed. A late feeding regimen, defined as initiating feedings more than 4 hours after surgery, significantly decreases the odds of emesis but may prolong hospitalization unless feedings are advanced rapidly. There was no significant difference in perioperative complications attributed to the rate or volume of feedings. Emesis after discharge and the need for readmission were nearly identical in all groups.

The authors point out that while typically benign, vomiting does increase patient discomfort, length of stay, and parental anxiety. This last point is crucial. One needs to manage parental expectations by explaining that vomiting is not unusual postoperatively, although it should be less forceful and less frequent than the preoperative vomiting. The authors do an excellent job interpreting data extracted from a heterogeneous group of studies. The results clearly show what many have presumed for years. Early feeding after pyloromyotomy may lead to more emesis, but it also leads to quicker discharge home. Slower feeding schedules may diminish the amount of vomiting episodes, but they prolong hospitalization. Presented with the evidence, I suspect that some pediatric surgeons will adjust their practice. As surgical dogma is slow to change, I suspect that many others will not.

J. T. Aidlen, MD

References

1. Schärli AF, Leditschke JF. Gastric motility after pyloromyotomy in infants. Areappraissal of postoperative feeding. *Surgery*. 1968;64:1133-1137.
2. Faber H, Davis JH. Gastric peristalsis after pyloromyotomy in infants: with special reference to postoperative care of pyloric stenosis. *JAMA*. 1940;114:847-850.
3. St Peter SD, Holcomb GW, Calkins CM, et al. Open versus laparoscopic pyloromyotomy for pyloric stenosis: a prospective, randomized trial. *Ann Surg*. 2006; 244:363-370.
4. St Peter SD, Tsao K, Sharp SW, Holcomb GW, Ostlie DJ. Predictors of emesis and time to goal intake after pyloromyotomy: analysis from a prospective trial. *J Pediatr Surg*. 2008;43:2038-2041.
5. Lee SL, Stark RS. Can patient factors predict early discharge after pyloromyotomy. *Perm J*. 2011;15:44-46.

Randomized Controlled Trial of Laparoscopic and Open Nissen Fundoplication in Children
Fyhn TJ, Knatten CK, Edwin B, et al (Univ of Oslo, Norway; et al)
Ann Surg 261:1061-1067, 2015

Objective.—The aim was to compare recurrence of gastroesophageal reflux disease (GERD) in children randomized to laparoscopic (LF) or open Nissen fundoplication (OF).

Background.—LF is considered superior to OF by most pediatric surgeons even though this has not been shown in any randomized controlled trial in children.

Methods.—Patients referred for fundoplication between 2003 and 2009 were eligible for inclusion in this 2-center, unstratified, randomized, parallel-group study conducted in Norway. The main outcome measure was recurrence of GERD, which was defined as GERD combined with a reflux index greater than 4 on pH monitoring and/or gastroesophageal reflux and/or herniated wrap on upper gastrointestinal (UGI) contrast study. Only experienced laparoscopic surgeons performed the LF. Postoperative follow-up included 24-hour pH monitoring, UGI contrast study, and a clinical examination at 6 months and phone interviews after 1, 2, and 4 years.

Results.—Eighty-seven children were included and randomized to either LF (n = 44) or OF (n − 43).Median age was 4.7 years (0.2−15.4) in the LF group and 3.7 years (0.2−14.2) in the OF group. Twenty-three patients in both groups were neurologically impaired. Median follow-up time was 4.0 years (0.3−8.9). Significantly more patients undergoing LF (37%) experienced recurrence of GERD compared to those undergoing OF (7%); risk ratio for recurrence in the LF group was 5.2 (95% confidence interval: 1.6−16.6) (*P* = 0.001).

Conclusions.—Children operated with LF have a higher recurrence rate of GERD than those operated with OF.

▶ Given the high prevalence of pathologic gastroesophageal reflux disease (GERD) in children, fundoplication has long been a common operation in pediatric surgery. The advent of laparoscopic fundoplication in the early 1990s was quickly embraced by pediatric surgeons. Like many technological innovations in surgery, minimally invasive surgery for GERD was widely adopted well before any objective evidence supporting its superiority to traditional open fundoplication. In 2009, 16 years after the first laparoscopic fundoplication was reported in a child, the American Pediatric Surgical Association (APSA) published a position paper on the procedure, noting the lack of any randomized controlled study comparing laparoscopic to open antireflux operations.[1]

For adult patients, multiple prospective randomized controlled trials comparing open and laparoscopic fundoplication have demonstrated equivalent treatment outcomes between the 2 approaches,[2] with a more recent study suggesting superiority for the laparoscopic approach.[3] However, results with this operation in adults cannot be translated to children. Unlike in adults, comorbid conditions are common in children needing fundoplication. These comorbidities include neurologic impairment, chronic respiratory disease, retching, spasticity, seizure disorder, presence of ventriculo-peritoneal shunt, history of esophageal atresia or congenital diaphragmatic hernia, or need for a gastrostomy tube. The presence of any of these conditions increases the likelihood of complications, including higher risk of recurrence, after the operation.

Until the current study, the vast majority of data comparing open and laparoscopic fundoplication came from retrospective studies, most of which reported the superiority of the laparoscopic approach. Those retrospective studies, however, are highly confounded because children undergoing open surgery tended to have more comorbidities and therefore higher complication rates, including recurrence of GERD. Two randomized control trials were previously reported, showing no significant difference in complication rates or recurrent reflux, but these studies were limited by a short follow-up of only 30 days[4] or a small cohort of only 39 subjects.[5]

Dr Fyhn and colleagues should be commended for performing this randomized controlled trial with long-term follow-up comparing open and laparoscopic fundoplication in children. In this prospective, 2-center, block-randomized, parallel-group study, the authors followed 87 children up to 15 years of age for a median of 4 years after their Nissen fundoplication. The primary endpoint, recurrence of GERD, was defined as the presence of both "troublesome symptoms" and either a reflux index > 4 by 24-hour pH probe or a herniated wrap on upper gastrointestinal series. Although target enrollment could not be achieved due to a slower recruitment than anticipated, the results are still quite compelling. The authors found that recurrent reflux occurred in only 7% of subjects after open fundoplication and in 37% of subjects after laparoscopic fundoplication, for a risk ratio of recurrence of 5.2 and a higher rate of redo fundoplication in the laparoscopic group.

We can only hypothesize why laparoscopic fundoplication was associated with such an increased risk of recurrent GERD in this study. As the authors suggest, maybe the development of adhesions following the open procedure decreases the risk of recurrence in that group. Regardless, the results are provocative and suggest that additional long-term randomized trials are needed. The broader lesson we should learn is that it is not reasonable for surgeons to adopt widely a new, unproven technique, only to wait 22 years for a study to suggest that it is inferior to the operation that it largely supplanted. A more prudent approach might serve our patients better.

A. M. Goldstein, MD

References

1. Kane TD, Brown MF, Chen MK. Position paper on laparoscopic antireflux operations in infants and children for gastroesophageal reflux disease. *J Pediatr Surg.* 2009;44:1034-1040.
2. Peters MJ, Mukhtar A, Yunus RM, et al. Meta-analysis of randomized clinical trials comparing open and laparoscopic anti-reflux surgery. *Am J Gastroenterol.* 2009;104:1548-1561.
3. Salminen P, Hurme S, Ovaska J. Fifteen-year outcome of laparoscopic and open Nissen fundoplication: a randomized clinical trial. *Ann Thorac Surg.* 2012;93: 228-233.
4. Knatten CK, Fyhn TJ, Edwin B, et al. Thirty-day outcome in children randomized to open and laparoscopic Nissen fundopolication. *J Pediatr Surg.* 2012;47: 1990-1996.
5. Pacilli M, Eaton S, McHoney M, et al. Four year follow-up of a randomised controlled trial comparing open and laparoscopic Nissen fundoplication in children. *Arch Dis Child.* 2014;99:516-521.

Implementation of pediatric cervical spine clearance guidelines at a combined trauma center: Twelve-month impact

Rosati SF, Maarouf R, Wolfe L, et al (Virginia Commonwealth Univ Health System, Richmond)
J Trauma Acute Care Surg 78:1117-1121, 2015

Background.—Pediatric cervical spine clearance guidelines should reduce computed tomography (CT) usage in combined pediatric and adult trauma centers biased by adult CT clearance.

Methods.—Cervical spine clearance under age 15 years was compared 12 months before (128 patients) and after (105 patients) guideline implementation, emphasizing National Emergency X Radiography Utilization Study (NEXUS) criteria when appropriate.

Results.—CT scans in patients clearable by NEXUS criteria decreased 23% ($p = .01$) and decreased by 16% in cases where radiography other than CT was indicated by guidelines ($p = 0.01$).

Conclusion.—Guideline implementation can have an immediate effect in decreasing pediatric cervical spine CT usage and should improve across time.

Level of Evidence.—Care management study, level IV.

▶ Cervical spine injuries (CSI) occur in less than 2% of seriously injured children. Despite this low incidence, many clinicians place emphasis on radiographic imaging to exclude CSI. While the benefits of imaging in pediatric trauma evaluation are well described, it is generally believed that the practice of liberal imaging presents considerable risks to the patient and should be applied judiciously, especially in small children with rapidly growing and metabolically active tissues. In recent years, many investigators have raised concerns about the liberal use of plain radiographs, CT scan, and MRI in children with reference to imaging-related short- and long-term morbidity, resource consumption, and cost. The increased risk of fatal and nonfatal cancers associated with CT-related radiation has gained attention from physicians and consumers. In fact, both the US Food and Drug Administration (FDA) Center for Devices and Radiological Health and the National Cancer Institute published guidelines designed to limit unnecessary imaging in children. Although proponents of liberal imaging argue that a single missed CSI may cost more than multiple diagnostic tests, the use of non–evidence-based testing contributes to suboptimal clinical practice and to potential risk. It has been particularly difficult to overcome the urge to scan in institutions in which children are frequently evaluated by adult specialty providers, even though missed injuries are exceedingly rare.

Two seminal studies (NEXUS and Canadian Cervical Spine Rules)[1,2] used clinical criteria (neurological deficit, cervical spine tenderness, intoxication, decreased mental status, and distracting injuries) to rule out CSI in adults without the need for imaging. These criteria have been applied to pediatric patients in a study by Viccellio and colleagues[3] that evaluated 3065 blunt trauma patients younger than 18 years of age and identified 603 (19.6%) low-risk patients in whom imaging could have been avoided. In another retrospective review of

206 pediatric patients less than 16 years of age, Jaffe and colleagues[4] suggested that the absence of 8 clinical criteria (neck pain; neck tenderness; abnormality of reflexes, strength, or sensation; direct trauma to the neck; limitation of neck mobility; and abnormal mental status) enabled a clinician to detect CSI in children with a sensitivity of 98% and a specificity of 54%. In 2007, our group evaluated a clinical decision tool to determine if even the youngest patients (younger than 3 years) could be cleared without imaging. In this multicenter retrospective study evaluating more than 20 000 infants and toddlers, we found that CT imaging was disproportionately performed at non—free-standing pediatric specialty hospitals. We also found that 3 simple clinical predictors (Glasgow Coma Score [GCS], age, and mechanism of injury) could be used to obviate the need for cervical spine imaging in more than two-thirds of patients regardless of where they presented.[5]

The authors of the reviewed report implemented a similar clinical guidelines strategy emphasizing the use of physical examination and NEXUS criteria to clear the cervical spine in injured children presenting to their level I combined (adult and pediatric) trauma center. The primary outcome measure was the use of CT scans in children younger than 15 years. They compared the use of CT scans for cervical spine clearance 12 months before and after implementation of these guidelines. A total of 233 children were evaluated during the 2-year period (128 before and 105 after). For children clearable by NEXUS criteria, the implementation guidelines had an immediate effect, decreasing CT use by 23%. Importantly, there were no missed injuries. These results offer even more evidence that much of the imaging that is done to clear the c-spine in a child is unnecessary and that the clinical evaluation of pediatric trauma patients with suspected c-spine injury is very effective in predicting who will benefit from cross-sectional imaging. Most importantly, the investigators prospectively show that simple clinical criteria, like GCS, used in concert with the physical examination, can safely predict CSI in children, reducing the dependence on imaging for many patients, including the very young, even when the child is evaluated in a combined (adult and pediatric) trauma center.

P. T. Masiakos

References

1. Hoffman JR, Wolfson AB, Todd K, Mower WR. Selective cervical spine radiography in blunt trauma: methodology of the National Emergency X-Radiography Study (NEXUS). *Ann Emerg Med.* 1998;32:461-469.
2. Steill IG, Wells GA, Vandemheen KL, et al. The Canadian C-Spine rule for radiography in alert and stable trauma patients. *JAMA.* 2001;286:1841-1848.
3. Viccellio P, Simon H, Pressman BD, Shah MN, Mower WR, Hoffman JR. A prospective multicenter study of cervical spine injury in children. *Pediatrics.* 2001;108:E20.
4. Jaffe DM, Binns H, Radkowski MA, Barthel MJ, Engelhard HH. 3rd. Developing a clinical algorithm for early management of cervical spine injury in child trauma victims. *Ann Emerg Med.* 1987;16:270-276.
5. Pieretti-Vanmarcke R, Velmahos GC, Nance ML, et al. Clinical clearance of the cervical spine in blunt trauma patients younger than 3 years: a multi-center study of the american association for the surgery of trauma. *J Trauma.* 2009;67: 543-549.

Weight Loss and Health Status 3 Years after Bariatric Surgery in Adolescents

Inge TH, for the Teen-LABS Consortium (Cincinnati Children's Hosp Med Ctr, OH; et al)

N Engl J Med 374:113-123, 2016

Background.—Bariatric surgery is increasingly considered for the treatment of adolescents with severe obesity, but few prospective adolescent-specific studies examining the efficacy and safety of weight-loss surgery are available to support clinical decision making.

Methods.—We prospectively enrolled 242 adolescents undergoing weight-loss surgery at five U.S. centers. Patients undergoing Roux-en-Y gastric bypass (161 participants) or sleeve gastrectomy (67) were included in the analysis. Changes in body weight, coexisting conditions, cardiometabolic risk factors, and weight related quality of life and postoperative complications were evaluated through 3 years after the procedure.

Results.—The mean (±SD) baseline age of the participants was 17 ± 1.6 years, and the mean body-mass index (the weight in kilograms divided by the square of the height in meters) was 53; 75% of the participants were female, and 72% were white. At 3 years after the procedure, the mean weight had decreased by 27% (95% confidence interval [CI], 25 to 29) in the total cohort, by 28% (95% CI, 25 to 30) among participants who underwent gastric bypass, and by 26% (95% CI, 22 to 30) among those who underwent sleeve gastrectomy. By 3 years after the procedure, remission of type 2 diabetes occurred in 95% (95% CI, 85 to 100) of participants who had had the condition at baseline, remission of abnormal kidney function occurred in 86% (95% CI, 72 to 100), remission of prediabetes in 76% (95% CI, 56 to 97), remission of elevated blood pressure in 74% (95% CI, 64 to 84), and remission of dyslipidemia in 66% (95% CI, 57 to 74). Weight-related quality of life also improved significantly. However, at 3 years after the bariatric procedure, hypoferritinemia was found in 57% (95% CI, 50 to 65) of the participants, and 13% (95% CI, 9 to 18) of the participants had undergone one or more additional intraabdominal procedures.

Conclusions.—In this multicenter, prospective study of bariatric surgery in adolescents, we found significant improvements in weight, cardiometabolic health, and weight-related quality of life at 3 years after the procedure. Risks associated with surgery included specific micronutrient deficiencies and the need for additional abdominal procedures. (Funded by the National Institute of Diabetes and Digestive and Kidney Diseases and others; Teen-LABS ClinicalTrials.gov number, NCT00474318.)

▶ Primary care pediatricians are perfectly positioned to appreciate the onset of severe obesity in patients far in advance of other health care providers. As such, they represent the ideal resource for information and guidance about appropriate avenues for the treatment of obesity, including surgery. While weight-loss surgery for adults has grown rapidly in recent decades, many pediatricians are reluctant to recommend this option for adolescents, favoring instead a program of monitored weight management, even when such programs ultimately prove unsuccessful. In a survey performed in 2007,[1] nearly half of respondents indicated they would never refer a pediatric patient for weight-loss surgery, and almost as many agreed that 18 years was the minimum age at which they would consider a bariatric consult. Although the motivation behind this thinking remains unclear, the perceived risks of performing these operations in teenagers and the lack of long-term data to guide clinical decision making may contribute to this reluctance. The article by Inge et al advances this discussion and provides important insights to assist pediatric providers to identify those patients that may benefit most from surgical treatment.

This is the first prospective multicenter study to look at long-term outcomes of bariatric surgery in adolescents. The study offers a large sample size and rigorous standardized methods for data collection to obtain follow-up in what most will acknowledge is a difficult population with which to follow up. In addition to analyzing changes in body weight, coexisting conditions, and cardio-metabolic risk factors, the study emphasizes quality-of-life issues and follows significant outcomes that are often overlooked, including reoperation and micronutrient deficiencies. The authors report significant and sustained improvements in weight, associated comorbidities, and quality of life. Surprisingly, the outcome of this head-to-head comparison of gastric bypass and sleeve gastrectomy found near equal weight loss and equally good clinical outcomes 3 years after surgery (46% and 48%, respectively). This finding is important, as most adult studies show fewer complications at 5 years in patients who undergo the sleeve as opposed to the gastric bypass, including the need for reoperation and micronutrient deficiency.

Severe obesity remains an important health issue for adolescents, and weight-loss surgery is the only treatment that offers the significant promise of long-term sustained weight loss. This study again shows the problem with delays in referral—patients in this study had an average body mass index (BMI) of 53 (weight, 149 kg) at baseline and a BMI of 38 (weight, 108 kg) 3 years after surgery. The problem with referring patients who already have a BMI greater than 45 is that they are unlikely to ever attain a normal weight, as body weight loss after bariatric surgery is relatively fixed at 30%. Therefore, patients who are referred earlier are more likely to reach and maintain a healthy weight long term. Furthermore, adolescents who suffer from severe comorbidities like diabetes and hypertension clearly derive greater benefit from weight loss surgery than adults. Type II diabetes resolves in 95% of adolescents with either operation compared with only 50% to 80% in adults, whereas hypertension resolves in 80% of adolescents and only 40% of adults. These findings suggest that adolescents undergoing weight loss surgery have a much greater opportunity to mitigate the progression of the cardio-metabolic consequences of obesity. Wouldn't it make more sense to effectively treat patients with morbid obesity earlier in the course of their disease rather than wait for irreversible cardio-metabolic disease to set in?

The study is not without limitations. It does not fit into the category of a randomized, controlled clinical trial, and there was no comparison of expected outcomes between weight-loss surgery and nonsurgical treatment. Having this information would be important, as it appears to account in some measure for the reluctance to refer among pediatricians. Also, a substantial number of patients required other abdominal operations after their bariatric procedure. Further analysis of these complications and comorbid outcomes, to determine if they were a consequence of the surgery or other inherent risk factors, would also be useful, but the sample sizes were too small to draw meaningful statistical conclusions.

The obvious oversight in this discussion is the failure to view obesity as a killer. Many studies found improved life expectancy in adult patients undergoing weight-loss surgery. The 2 most cited are the Swedish Obesity Study and a study from Canada published in 2004, in which a control cohort was matched to a weight-loss surgery group. In this 2-cohort study, the reduction in risk of mortality 5 years after weight-loss surgery was 89%.[2] There is reason to believe that years of exposure to the state of obesity may be similar to years of exposure to smoking. If this is the case, then early weight-loss surgery for adolescents will increase their life expectancy and decrease their risk of obesity-related comorbidities considerably. Delaying surgery will only lead to prolonged exposure to obesity, increased risk of comorbidities, and a higher weight at the time of surgery and, consequently, after surgery.

Pediatric physicians and surgeons need to monitor long-term compliance with vitamin replacement in light of the large percentage of study participants (57%) with hypoferritinemia and vitamin B12 deficiency on long-term follow-up. This follow-up is significantly less burdensome than monitoring the obese adolescent for diabetes, hypertension, fatty liver, and other complications of obesity. The justification for any surgery, especially in a child or adolescent, depends on balancing risk and benefit.[3] The calculus on the benefit side is clear in light of the marked improvements in weight, obesity-induced comorbidities, and quality of life, not to mention the intractable consequences of lifelong cardio-metabolic disease and early mortality.

Recognizing that children with a BMI greater than 99th percentile are always going to suffer from obesity in adulthood, referring patients to a comprehensive obesity treatment center that also offers weight loss surgery could not only improve the quality of life of these children but also save lives. Early referral and supportive discussion about the dangers of obesity and the benefits of surgical intervention are key. Hopefully, this article provides sufficient evidence to convince pediatric providers of the safety and efficacy of surgery in this unique population.

J. S. Pratt, MD

References

1. Woolford SJ, Clark SJ, Gebremariam A, Davis MM, Freed GL. To cut or not to cut: Physicians' perspectives on referring adolescents for surgery. *Obes Surg.* 2010;20:937-942.
2. Christou NV, Sampalis JS, Liberman M, et al. Surgery decreases long-term mortality, morbidity, and health care use in morbidly obese patients. *Ann Surg.* 2004;240:416-424.
3. Michalsky M, Reichard K, Inge T, Pratt J, Lenders C. American Society for Metabolic and Bariatric Surgery. ASMBS pediatric committee best practice guidelines. *Surg Obes Relat Dis.* 2012;8:1-7.

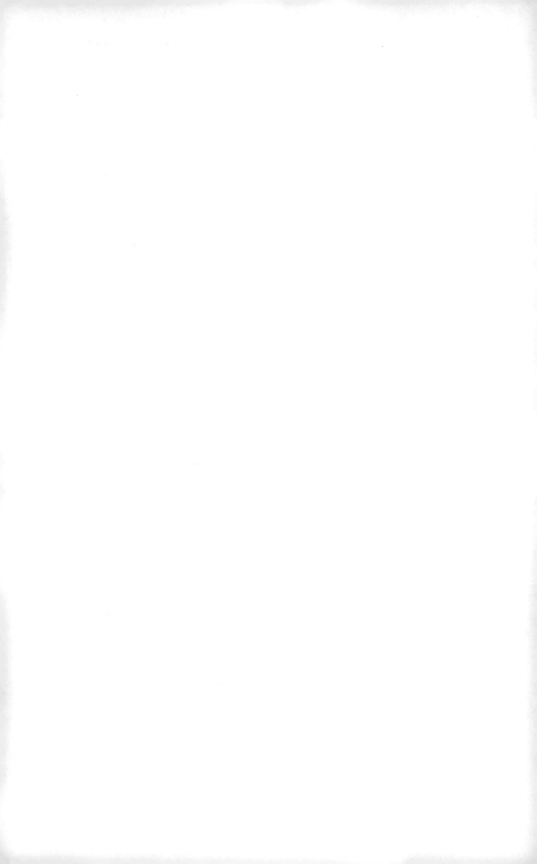

24 Psychiatry

Lithium in the Acute Treatment of Bipolar I Disorder: A Double-Blind, Placebo-Controlled Study

Findling RL, Robb A, McNamara NK, et al (The Johns Hopkins Univ, Baltimore, MD, George Washington Univ, District of Columbia; Case Western Reserve Univ, Cleveland, OH; et al)
Pediatrics 136:885-894, 2015

Background.—Lithium is a benchmark treatment for bipolar disorder in adults. Definitive studies of lithium in pediatric bipolar I disorder (BP-I) are lacking.

Methods.—This multicenter, randomized, double-blind, placebo-controlled study of pediatric participants (ages 7–17 years) with BP-I/manic or mixed episodes compared lithium ($n = 53$) versus placebo ($n = 28$) for up to 8 weeks. The a priori primary efficacy measure was change from baseline to the end of study (week 8/ET) in the Young Mania Rating Scale (YMRS) score, based on last-observation-carried-forward analysis.

Results.—The change in YMRS score was significantly larger in lithium-treated participants (5.51 [95% confidence interval: 0.51 to 10.50]) after adjustment for baseline YMRS score, age group, weight group, gender, and study site ($P = .03$). Overall Clinical Global Impression—Improvement scores favored lithium ($n = 25$; 47% very much/much improved) compared with placebo ($n = 6$; 21% very much/much improved) at week 8/ET ($P = .03$). A statistically significant increase in thyrotropin concentration was seen with lithium (3.0 ± 3.1 mIU/L) compared with placebo (-0.1 ± 0.9 mIU/L; $P < .001$). There was no statistically significant between-group difference with respect to weight gain.

Conclusions.—Lithium was superior to placebo in reducing manic symptoms in pediatric patients treated for BP-I in this clinical trial. Lithium was generally well tolerated in this patient population and was not associated with weight gain, distinguishing it from other agents commonly used to treat youth with bipolar disorder.

▶ Bipolar disorder is a serious condition in childhood that adversely affects the child's social, emotional, and family functioning. Youth with bipolar disorder are at risk of suicide. It is important to identify medications that are effective and safe in treating this disorder in children and adolescents. The atypical antipsychotics have the most evidence of efficacy for treating bipolar disorder in youth; however, there are significant side effects such as weight gain and cardiometabolic syndrome. This article, which demonstrates efficacy of lithium in the treatment of bipolar disorder in children and adolescents, adds to clinicians' evidence-based treatment armamentarium.

This study is important because it is the first double-blind, placebo-controlled study of lithium for the treatment of bipolar I disorder, manic episodes, or mixed episodes in youth. What is unique about this study is that it includes children as young as 7 years old. The studies of atypical antipsychotics for treatment of pediatric bipolar disorder included children aged 10 years and older. Because young children do develop bipolar disorder, this lithium study provides clinicians with reassuring safety and efficacy data for the treatment of young children.

In this 8-week trial, lithium was significantly superior to placebo in the reduction of symptoms of bipolar disorder. It is noteworthy that 47% of the lithium-treated youth were much or very much improved compared to 21% of the placebo-treated youth. The effect size was medium (0.53). Because bipolar disorder in youth tends to be a chronic condition, it would be interesting to know whether a greater percentage of youth would have improved on lithium if the study had been longer than 8 weeks. However, ethical considerations in placebo-controlled treatment trials preclude extended periods of time on placebo.

A strength of the study is the rigorous monitoring of potential adverse events. A suicidal behavior and ideation rating scale, neurological assessments, a structured side effect form, and an open-ended inquiry for treatment-emergent adverse effects were performed at each study visit.

The most common adverse effects found with lithium treatment were vomiting, nausea, and headaches, which are similar to the reports for adults. Vomiting and nausea were managed by dose reduction in some cases, and no youth discontinued the study because of lack of tolerability. Tremor, a common lithium side effect, was reported in 32% of lithium-treated patients compared with 7% of placebo-treated patients. There was a significant increase in thyrotropin concentration in lithium-treated compared to placebo-treated youth. Therefore, it is important to monitor thyroid function when youth are treated with lithium. There was no significant difference between youth treated with lithium and placebo with regard to weight gain (0.9 kg vs 1.2 kg), unlike the case for treatment of youth with atypical antipsychotics. Two lithium-treated and 1 placebo-treated youth discontinued the study because of suicidality; however, these events were viewed as unrelated to the study medication.

A potential limitation of this study is the relative small sample size. However, the recruitment of children with bipolar disorder in clinical trials is challenging. More than 50% of children had comorbid attention deficit hyperactivity disorder (ADHD). It would have been interesting to know whether comorbid ADHD affected lithium treatment response.

Overall, the results of the study support lithium for the treatment of children and adolescents with bipolar I disorder. A medication that does not cause significant weight gain is a welcome addition to medication treatment options for pediatric bipolar I disorder.

K. D. Wagner, MD, PhD

Trends in Pediatric Emergency Department Utilization for Mental Health-Related Visits

Mapelli E, Black T, Doan Q (BC Children's Hosp, Vancouver, Canada)

J Pediatr 167:905-910, 2015

Objective.—To describe trends in utilization of pediatric emergency department (PED) resources by patients with mental health concerns over the past 10 years at a tertiary care hospital.

Study Design.—We conducted a retrospective cohort study of tertiary PED visits from 2003 to 2012. All visits with chief complaint or discharge diagnosis related to mental health were included. Variables analyzed included number and acuity of mental health-related visits, length of stay, waiting time, admission rate, and return visits, relative to all PED visits. Descriptive statistics were used to summarize the results.

Results.—We observed a 47% increase in the number of mental health presentations compared with a 9% increase in the number of total visits to the PED over the study period. Return visits represented a significant proportion of all mental health-related visits (31%-37% yearly). The proportion of mental health visits triaged to a high acuity level has decreased whereas the proportion of visits triaged to the mid-acuity level has increased. Length of stay for psychiatric patients was significantly longer than for visits to the PED in general. We also observed a 23% increase in the number of mental health-related visits resulting in admission.

Conclusion.—Mental health-related visits represent a significant and growing burden for the emergency department at a tertiary care PED. These results highlight the need to reassess the allocation of health resources to optimize acute management, risk assessment, and linkage to mental health services upon disposition from the PED (Figs 1 and 2).

▶ The burden of mental illness is profound and growing. The past 2 decades has seen a marked increase in visits to pediatric emergency departments (ED) for patients with mental health problems in the United States. Lack of access to mental health providers, long waiting times for mental health evaluation for even the highest risk children, inability to pay for care, and insufficient capacity of child and youth mental health providers have all contributed to the burden.

Previous studies have documented increased utilization in all aspects of emergency care including ED length of stay, visit rate, admission rate, ED revisit rates and utilization of consultant services, and laboratory and imaging studies. Coupled with a large gap in the capacity of mental health services, this burden has forced EDs to become the gateway provider of acute mental health care in the United States. In addition, the role of the ED provider has also evolved as health systems take on a more population health-based perspective through the assumption of risk under accountable care structures. Thus, the importance of taking advantage of every health care encounter, maximizing screening, brief interventions, and referrals for a high-risk population and closing the existing gaps of care for children with mental health problems presenting in need is clear.

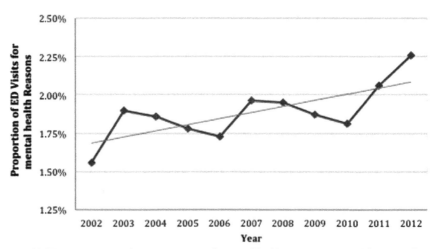

FIGURE 1.—Proportion of PED presentations for mental health reasons. (Reprinted from Mapelli E, Black T, Doan Q. Trends in pediatric emergency department utilization for mental health-related visits. *J Pediatr.* 2015;167:905-910, with permission from Elsevier.)

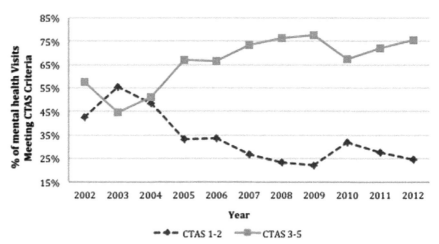

FIGURE 2.—Acuity level distribution for mental health-related visits. (Reprinted from Mapelli E, Black T, Doan Q. Trends in pediatric emergency department utilization for mental health-related visits. *J Pediatr.* 2015;167:905-910, with permission from Elsevier.)

The study by Mapelli et al is a descriptive retrospective examination of the trends of resource use by patients with mental health disorders over an 11-year period to one regional pediatric ED in Canada (Fig 1). Although one might take issue with the lack of generalizability and descriptive simplicity of the study design, one cannot ignore the startling increase in mental health—related visits to this ED over the study period, mirroring increases seen over the same period of time in the United States.

Similar to trends in the United States, this increase in mental health visit burden is way out of proportion compared with visits for non—mental health concerns. Despite a decrease in overall acuity of these mental health visits across the decade studied (Fig 2), the proportion of visits that ended in an admission increased by almost 25% along with a significant increase in ED length of stay, signaling a clear capacity problem with respect to mental health services availability.

The study is another piece of evidence in the mounting armamentarium supporting the call for action to improve the intersection of emergency care and mental health services above and below the US/Canadian border. Feasible and brief ED-based mental health screening, intervention, and referral programs for pediatric patients presenting to EDs are needed. More research is needed to improve the quality of care for patients presenting with mental health complaints. Improving attitudes, knowledge base and management options for general ED providers who provide more than 60% of the care for youth presenting to general EDs is mandatory.

Only then will we be able to ensure the uptake of best practices for the management of patients with mental disorders and psychosocial problems. Most importantly, how these practices integrate with the medical home and the mental health services sector will be a fundamental determinant of long-term success. Studies like this one by Mapelli et al help to bring context to the argument for increasing mental health services capacity in the ED setting.

J. Grupp-Phelan, MD, MPH

Correlates of Body Dissatisfaction in Children
Dion J, Hains J, Vachon P, et al (Université du Québec à Chicoutimi, Saguenay, Canada; et al)
J Pediatr 171:202-207, 2016

Objective.—To assess body dissatisfaction among children between 9 and 14 years of age and to examine factors (age, sex, body mass index, perceived shape, and self-esteem) associated with wanting a thinner or a larger shape.

Study Design.—Through at-school questionnaires, 1515 preadolescent children (51.2% girls) were asked to fill out the Culture Free Self-Esteem Inventory and the Contour Drawing Rating Scale (body dissatisfaction). Trained assessors then weighed and measured the students individually.

Results.—Overall, 50.5% of girls wanted a thinner shape compared with 35.9% of boys. More boys wanted a larger shape compared with girls (21.1% vs 7.2%). Most of the preadolescents who were overweight or obese were unsatisfied whereas 58.0% of girls and 41.6% of boys who were underweight were satisfied with their body. Results of a multinomial logistic regression revealed that age, sex, body mass index, perceived shape, and self-esteem were significant correlates of the 4 body dissatisfaction contrasts (wanting a slightly thinner, much thinner, slightly larger, and much larger shape) and explained 50% of the variance. An interaction between sex and perceived shape was found, revealing that girls who perceived themselves as having a larger shape were more likely to desire a thinner shape than boys.

Conclusions.—The high prevalence rate of body dissatisfaction among children suggests that current approaches in our society to prevent problems related to body image must be improved. The different results between girls and boys highlight the need to take into account sex differences when designing prevention programs that aim to decrease body dissatisfaction.

▶ Body dissatisfaction increases in late childhood and early adolescence as youth struggle to reconcile the changes of impending puberty and become interested in sex and romantic relationships. However, body dissatisfaction has reached epidemic levels in today's youth. This phenomenon is due in part to the increase in obesity over the last several decades, which has put young people at odds with the thin ideal that has endured in the United States and spread worldwide. Although it is a difficult concept to define and study, weight dissatisfaction has been reliably and reproducibly identified in prospective studies as a strong predictor of an eventual eating disorder.[1,2] This study by Dion et al examined correlates of weight dissatisfaction in a large sample of French-speaking children living in Quebec and reported that 57% of boys and girls reported dissatisfaction with their weight or shape. These overall rates are consistent with previous studies in Canada,[3] the United States,[4,5] and internationally.[6]

Children who are dissatisfied with their weight are desperate to lose it by any means. In Project EAT, a large cohort of Midwestern teens averaging 14.9 years old, Neumark-Sztainer et al[4] found that 54.8% of girls and 42.4% of boys were dissatisfied with their weight. Although some of these youth were using healthy weight loss strategies that we suggest in the clinic (eg, decreasing sweets and increasing fruits and vegetables), 56.9% of adolescents were engaging in unhealthy behaviors (eg, skipping meals), and 12.4% reported dangerous practices such as laxative use. These behaviors increased in proportion to degree of overweight, with nearly 18% of very overweight girls engaging in dangerous dieting. These dieting practices are considered a risky health behavior in adolescence[7] because they covary with other health-damaging behaviors such as alcohol and tobacco use,[5] increase risk for eating disorders,[1,2] negatively impact nutritional intake, and predict significant weight gain over time.[8]

Thus, the high rates of weight dissatisfaction reported by Dion et al provide a cautionary reminder for clinicians. In most pediatric clinics, we weigh our patients as soon as they walk through the door. For more than half of the youth seeking our care, this is an inauspicious, often upsetting, starting point to the visit. On a positive note, with proper awareness and sensitivity, weighing at the beginning of the visit may elicit a good discussion of weight dissatisfaction and provide valuable insight into the health risks described above.

This study also reminds us that boys are not immune. Although boys were equally dissatisfied as girls, boys faced the dual dilemma of wanting to be thinner in some cases and larger (more muscular) in others. This bidirectional nature of body dissatisfaction in boys is consistent with that in previous studies[9] and underscores the need to increase skills and sensitivity around working with boys, who are increasingly being diagnosed with eating disorders.[10]

Two unique features of this study population warrant further discussion. First, whereas most studies of weight dissatisfaction focus on adolescents, this study population was children of mean age of 10.4 years. This factor makes the high rates of weight dissatisfaction particularly alarming, given that weight dissatisfaction is known to worsen over time. In the Growing Up Today Study (GUTS), the only study to date that has followed the trajectory of weight dissatisfaction from childhood into adolescence, weight and shape dissatisfaction deteriorated as girls aged from 9 to 18 years.[11] A second unique aspect of this study population is that these were French-speaking children living in Quebec. One shortfall of the Dion et al article is that it did not provide comprehensive descriptive statistics on the study sample so it is difficult to determine whether the sample was representative of the wider population. However, according to a 2015 report by the National Center for Health Statistics,[12] Canadian children age 7 to 11 are far less obese than those in the United States: 11.8 versus 10.1%, respectively. Furthermore, Quebec enjoys the lowest rates of obesity in Canada compared with all territories except for British Columbia. Although the popular press has been busy exploring how French food culture may confer resistance to weight gain,[13] Quebec has taken real and highly progressive stand on obesity prevention. For example, marketing of fast food and soda to children younger than 13 years has been banned in Quebec since 1980.

Unfortunately, the combination of factors that may partially protect children in Quebec from obesity did not serve to protect children in the study by Dion et al from weight dissatisfaction. This finding raises the question, beyond the scope of this study, of how to promote weight satisfaction in youth. One factor that appears to have had a positive effect, paradoxically, is the increase in obesity. Evidence from 24 countries over 9 years shows improved weight satisfaction and decreased dieting behavior among school-age children in association with increasing obesity rates.[6] This finding suggests that as youth are exposed to a wider representation of body types among peers and role models and in the media and their communities, youth are beginning to perceive their higher weights as more acceptable by social comparison.

This finding is not well received by some, who fear that normalizing obesity will act as a disincentive to engage in healthy lifestyle changes. However, readers of this commentary are reminded that this fear is not supported by the evidence. That is, children with weight dissatisfaction are not spurred toward healthy changes. On the contrary, they are practicing dangerous dieting, at risk for eating disorders and overweight, and more likely to be engaging other risky health behaviors. Reduction of these risks through increased weight satisfaction could have tremendous health benefits. Therefore, clinicians, researchers, or parents should take this opportunity to encourage body acceptance at every size and assist this process by shifting the intense focus on weight (which has been roundly unsuccessful) to behavior. In practical terms, this may mean less time plotting body mass index and more time spent discussing reducing soda, avoiding fast food, and limiting screen time and other behaviors that will promote health at every weight.

A. K. Garber, PhD, RD

References

1. Striegel-Moore RH, Bulik CM. Risk factors for eating disorders. *Am Psychol.* 2007;62:181-198.
2. McKnight Investigators. Risk factors for the onset of eating disorders in adolescent girls: results of the McKnight longitudinal risk factor study. *Am J Psychiatry.* 2003;160:248-254.
3. Jones JM, Bennett S, Olmsted MP, Lawson ML, Rodin G. Disordered eating attitudes and behaviours in teenaged girls: a school-based study. *CMAJ.* 2001;165:547-552.
4. Neumark-Sztainer D, Story M, Hannan PJ, Perry CL, Irving LM. Weight-related concerns and behaviors among overweight and nonoverweight adolescents: implications for preventing weight-related disorders. *Arch Pediatr Adolesc Med.* 2002;156:171-178.
5. French SA, Story M, Downes B, Resnick MD, Blum RW. Frequent dieting among adolescents: psychosocial and health behavior correlates. *Am J Public Health.* 1995;85:695-701.
6. Quick V, Nansel TR, Liu D, Lipsky LM, Due P, Iannotti RJ. Body size perception and weight control in youth: 9-year international trends from 24 countries. *Int J Obes (Lond).* 2014;38:988-994.
7. Irwin C, Millstein S. Risk-taking behaviors and biopsychosocial development during adolescence. In: Susman E, Feagans L, Ray W, eds. *Emotion, Cognition, and Development in Children and Adolescents.* Hilisdale, NJ: Edbanm; 1992:75-102.
8. Neumark-Sztainer D, Wall M, Story M, Standish AR. Dieting and unhealthy weight control behaviors during adolescence: associations with 10-year changes in body mass index. *J Adolesc Health.* 2012;50:80-86.
9. Allen KL, Byrne SM, McLean NJ, Davis EA. Overconcern with weight and shape is not the same as body dissatisfaction: evidence from a prospective study of pre-adolescent boys and girls. *Body Image.* 2008;5:261-270.
10. Ornstein RM, Rosen DS, Mammel KA, et al. Distribution of eating disorders in children and adolescents using the proposed DSM-5 criteria for feeding and eating disorders. *J Adolesc Health.* 2013;53:303-305.
11. Calzo JP, Sonneville KR, Haines J, Blood EA, Field AE, Austin SB. The development of associations among body mass index, body dissatisfaction, and weight and shape concern in adolescent boys and girls. *J Adolesc Health.* 2012;51(5):517-523. Epub 2012/10/23.
12. (NCHS) NCfHS. Prevalence of Obesity Among Children and Adolescents in the United States and Canada. 2015. http://www.statcan.gc.ca/daily-quotidien/150826/dq150826a-eng.htm.
13. Guiliano M. *French Women Don't get Fat.* Knopf Books; 2005, French WomenDontGetFat.com.

School-Based Mindfulness Instruction: An RCT

Sibinga EMS, Webb L, Ghazarian SR, et al (Johns Hopkins School of Medicine, Saint Petersburg, FL)
Pediatrics 137:e20152532, 2016

Background and Objective.—Many urban youth experience significant and unremitting negative stressors, including those associated with community violence, multigenerational poverty, failing educational systems, substance use, limited avenues for success, health risks, and trauma. Mindfulness instruction improves psychological functioning in a variety of adult populations; research on mindfulness for youth is promising, but has been conducted in limited populations. Informed by implementation science, we evaluated an adapted mindfulness-based stress reduction (MBSR) program to ameliorate the negative effects of stress and trauma among low-income, minority, middle school public school students.

Methods.—Participants were students at two Baltimore City Public Schools who were randomly assigned by grade to receive adapted MBSR or health education (Healthy Topics [HT]) programs. Self-report survey data were collected at baseline and postprogram. Deidentified data were analyzed in the aggregate, comparing MBSR and HT classes, by using regression modeling.

Results.—Three hundred fifth- to eighth-grade students (mean 12.0 years) were in MBSR and HT classes and provided survey data. Participants were 50.7% female, 99.7% African American, and 99% eligible for free lunch. The groups were comparable at baseline. Postprogram, MBSR students had significantly lower levels of somatization, depression, negative affect, negative coping, rumination, self-hostility, and posttraumatic symptom severity (all $Ps < .05$) than HT.

Conclusions.—These findings support the hypothesis that mindfulness instruction improves psychological functioning and may ameliorate the negative effects of stress and reduce trauma-associated symptoms among vulnerable urban middle school students. Additional research is needed to explore psychological, social, and behavioral outcomes, and mechanisms of mindfulness instruction.

▶ The association between significant adversity and psychological difficulties has been well documented for a long time. Ten years ago, the National Scientific Council on the Developing Child and the FrameWorks Institute coined the term "toxic stress" to describe the underlying physiological disruptions produced by excessive stress system activation that can lead to impairments in learning, behavior, and health.[1] In 2012, the American Academy of Pediatrics issued a technical report[2] and a policy statement[3] that urged pediatricians to support the development of new strategies to address the precipitants of toxic stress in young children and to mitigate their negative effects.

This article presents a rigorously evaluated response to the call for new interventions. The focus on preadolescence as a period of heightened risk is well founded but its characterization by the authors as "primary prevention" is highly problematic because toxic stress can begin to disrupt the developing brain and other biological systems in utero. Some commentators would applaud the study's demonstrated effects on multiple outcomes; others would note the modest magnitude of the reported impacts.

This commentary focuses on a more compelling challenge: how can 21st-century research on the pathophysiology of stress-related impairments in health and development catalyze new, science-based strategies that produce far greater reductions in socioeconomic and racial disparities? Stated bluntly, the biology of adversity is soaring, yet current approaches to protecting the developing brain from the consequences of toxic stress are having marginal impacts. Pediatricians are the logical choice for leadership roles in translating scientific insights into more effective interventions, and the battle against infectious disease presents a promising framework for more creative thinking.

For starters, 1 life-threatening infection was eradicated completely by eliminating the causal agent (think smallpox). The analogous solution for children facing the burdens of poverty, violence, or racial/ethnic discrimination would be to eliminate these pernicious pathogens. Recognizing the complexity of that challenge, the pediatrician's job is to promote more effective strategies for protecting healthy development while others work on eliminating these threats to well-being.

The next category of successful intervention includes preventive approaches that reduce infection by strengthening the body's defenses (think immunization). Science tells us that resilience in the face of adversity can be strengthened by adult caregiving and mentoring that provide buffering protection from stressors and scaffold the development of children's own coping skills, beginning as early as possible.

The third line of defense involves the targeted treatment of infections that have eluded prevention (think specific antibiotics matched to specific bacteria) and alternative measures for those that do not respond to standard therapy (think switching to different medications in the face of drug resistance). For children facing the threat of toxic stress, the question is not "what's the most effective program?" but rather "how can we match specific services to differences in causes, assets, unmet needs, and response to intervention?"

Without overstating the analogy between infectious disease and toxic stress, when the precipitants of significant adversity cannot be prevented or mitigated, targeted intervention from among a suite of options is essential. Mindfulness is one modality that has demonstrated success with some adults and limited but growing evidence of impacts on some children and youth. Although many observers would cite this study as confirmation of the program's evidence-based status for preadolescents, the article's more far-reaching contribution lies in its illustration of how the conventional approach to evaluation research (even when it is done well) does not pave the way for significant impact at scale.

Arguably the most important barrier to breakthrough outcomes that this study demonstrates is its primary focus on mean effects rather than on more important questions about who benefitted most and why (which should trigger targeted replication and scaling) and who benefitted least or not at all and why (which should galvanize the search for new or complementary interventions). Greater attention to response variability would provide a vital source of enhanced theories of change, new hypotheses, and innovative strategies for those who are not well served by existing services. The ultimate value of this segmentation approach is illustrated by how much is learned about the intervention's impact, not by whether sufficient evidence is produced to prove it was effective.

Documenting mean differences on large numbers of outcomes in the absence of an explicit theory of change may generate lots of statistically significant findings but it will not provide a coherent explanation for what caused the effects and how to replicate them. A better understanding of why individual program components produce specific outcomes for different participants can help identify specific effectiveness factors, which can then be integrated selectively into other interventions. When evaluators ask "does it work?" the only pathway to scaling is to replicate every aspect of the program. A modular approach that asks "which features have which impacts for whom and why?" enables a more efficient and cost-effective strategy for selectively scaling the active ingredients of an effective intervention within existing services.

The stresses of poverty and other social adversities are clearly not the same as a serious infection, and the medicalization of socioeconomic disadvantage risks a host of dangerous consequences. That said, a generic, "evidence-based," program recommendation for a child living in poverty is tantamount to prescribing an "effective" antibiotic for a child with an unspecified infection. The evolving principles of precision medicine that focus on underlying causal mechanisms and differential response to treatment for an increasing number of diseases could (and should) be mobilized to drive a comparable transformation in how we address the biological embedding of adversity in the minds and bodies of young children. The study of a mindfulness intervention reported by Sibinga and her colleagues is rigorous and commendable. However, the time has come to move beyond the achievement of statistically significant but small effects and begin to focus more explicitly on what it will take to produce much larger impacts at scale for the remarkably heterogeneous population of children whose physical and mental health is threatened by significant adversity.

J. P. Shonkoff, MD

References

1. National Scientific Council on the Developing Child. (2005/2009/2014). Excessive Stress Disrupts the Architecture of the Developing Brain. Working Paper No. 3. http://www.developingchild.harvard.edu.
2. Shonkoff JP, Garner AS. American Academy of Pediatrics Committee on Psychosocial Aspects of Child and Family Health, Committee on Early Childhood, Adoption, and Dependent Care, Section on Developmental and Behavioral Pediatrics (2012). The lifelong effects of early childhood adversity and toxic stress. *Pediatrics.* 2012;129:e232-e246.
3. Garner AS, Shonkoff JP, American Academy of Pediatrics Committee on Psychosocial Aspects of Child and Family Health, Committee on Early Childhood, Adoption, and Dependent Care, Section on Developmental and Behavioral Pediatrics. Early childhood adversity, toxic stress, and the role of the pediatrician: translating developmental science into lifelong health. *Pediatrics.* 2012;129:e224-e231.

Phenotype and Adverse Quality of Life in Boys with Klinefelter Syndrome

Close S, Fennoy I, Smaldone A, et al (Emory Univ, Atlanta, GA; Columbia Univ School of Medicine, NY; Columbia Univ School of Nursing, NY; et al)

J Pediatr 167:650-657, 2015

Objectives.—To characterize associations among psychosocial well-being, physical phenotype, and sex hormones in a sample of youth with Klinefelter syndrome (KS). We hypothesized that KS physical traits (phenotype) are associated with adverse psychosocial health measures and that testosterone levels are associated with adverse psychosocial health.

Study Design.—Forty-three boys with KS (ages 8-18 years) participated in a cross-sectional study. Participants underwent physical examination, hormone analyses, and psychosocial health questionnaires.

Results.—Using an investigator-developed Klinefelter Phenotype Index Scale, the number of KS physical traits ranged from 1-13 (mean 5.1 ± 1.9). Pubertal boys presented with more KS traits compared with prepubertal boys (5.6 vs 4.2, $P = .01$). Boys diagnosed prenatally had a milder phenotype compared with those diagnosed postnatally. Gonadotropins were elevated without androgen deficiency in 45%. Psychosocial health scores indicated adverse quality of life (QOL) (67%), low self-esteem (38%), poor self-concept (26%), and risk for depression (16%) without a difference between pubertal groups. Linear regression showed that 22% of the variance in QOL ($P = .0001$) was explained by phenotype. Testosterone level was not associated with psychosocial health measures.

Conclusions.—Depending on the degree of phenotypic abnormality, boys with KS may be at risk for impaired QOL. Testosterone levels were not shown to influence psychosocial health. The Klinefelter Phenotype Index Scale may be a useful tool to characterize KS features in boys (Table 2).

▶ Klinefelter syndrome (KS) is a seriously underdiagnosed condition, with only about 10% of the expected number being diagnosed during childhood and adolescent years, and combined only about 25% of the expected number ever receiving a diagnosis. Furthermore, a host of medical conditions with increased morbidity and mortality, as well as social and psychologic challenges, face boys and men with Klinefelter syndrome. Not much is known of interventions that will work in Klinefelter syndrome, and not even testosterone supplementation has been shown to have unequivocal beneficial results when the inevitable hypergonadotropic hypogonadism ensues. The present article shows that prepubertal and pubertal boys with Klinefelter syndrome clearly have a differing phenotype when rigorously examined using a new tool, called the Klinefelter Phenotype Index scale (KSphI; Table 2). In addition, along with low quality of life, poor self-esteem, and poor self-concept, some boys are at risk of depression and even suicidal thoughts.

It is an enigma why boys with KS are not diagnosed during childhood, given the almost pathognomonic usual finding of small testes. This article highlights that boys who were diagnosed both prenatally and postnatally alike have an increased KSphI, indicating that they indeed show a significant number of stigmata related to KS, and to a similar degree independent of ascertainment. Previous studies have suggested that prenatally diagnosed cases might have a milder course, which this study does not support. Included in this index are stigmata such as tall stature, small testes, large waist circumference, increased body mass index (BMI), phallic size, gynecomastia, skeletal abnormalities, high-arched palate, clinodactyly, hand tremor, and hypertelorism. Interestingly, the maximal score on the KSphI is 13, but the sample of children on average

TABLE 2.—KSphI Criteria by Pubertal Group

Physical Characteristic	KSphI Criteria	Presence of the Characteristic			P Value*
		Total Sample, N = 43, n (%)	Prepubertal, N = 16, n (%)	Pubertal, N = 27, n (%)	
Tall stature	0 = <90th percentile; 1 = ≥90th percentile	16 (37.2)	6 (37.5)	10 (37.0)	1.0
Eunuchoid: upper to lower height ratio	0 = non-eunuchoid stature (ratio ≥0.95); 1 = eunuchoid stature (ratio ≤0.94)	22 (51.2)	8 (50.0)	14 (51.9)	1.0
Arm span	0 = ≤4.9 cm of height; 1 = (exceeds height by 5 cm)	10 (23.3)	2 (12.5)	8 (29.6)	.28
WC	0 = <90th percentile; 1 = ≥90th percentile	11 (25.8)	2 (12.5)	9 (33.3)	.17
BMI	0 = ≤85th percentile; 1 = >85th percentile	19 (44.2)	4 (25.0)	15 (55.6)	.06
Testicular volume by TS†	0 = normal volume; 1 = abnormal volume; TS I: 2 mL, TS I: <2 mL; TS II: 3 mL, TS II: <3 mL; TS III: 10 mL, TS III: <10 mL; TS IV: 20 mL, TS IV: <20 mL; TS V: 29 mL, TS V: <29 mL	30 (69.8)	8 (50.0)	22 (81.5)	.04
Phallic length/genital abnormalities for age	0 = normal range; 1 = short (minus 1 SD); 8-12 y ≤4.9 cm; 13 y ≤5.1 cm; 14 y ≤5.6 cm; 15 y ≤9.1 cm; 16 Adult ≤10.8 cm	16 (37.2)	7 (43.8)	9 (33.3)	.53
Gynecomastia	0 = not present; 1 = present	5 (11.6)	0	5 (18.5)	.14
Skeletal abnormalities	0 = not present; 1 = present	4 (9.3)	0	4 (14.8)	.28
High-arched palate	0 = not present; 1 = present	18 (41.9)	3 (18.8)	15 (55.6)	.03
Clinodactyly	0 = not present; 1 = present	23 (53.5)	8 (50.0)	15 (55.6)	.76
Hand tremor	0 = not present; 1 = present	15 (34.9)	4 (25.0)	11 (40.7)	.34
Hypertelorism	0 = not present; 1 = present	0	0	0	N/A
Mean KSphI ± SD		5.1 ± 3.1	4.2 ± 0.98	5.6 ± 2.1	.01

N/A, not applicable.
*Fisher exact test. Significance <.05 shown in boldface.
†TS determined by distribution of pubic hair.
Reprinted from Close S, Fennoy I, Smaldone A, et al. Phenotype and adverse quality of life in boys with Klinefelter syndrome. J Pediatr. 2015;167:650-657, with permission Elsevier.

scored 5, nicely illustrating that any person with Klinefelter syndrome will only present with a limited number of stigmata. This is probably one of the reasons why it is difficult to diagnose cases.

Additionally, the study subjects were examined with the Quality of Life measure, a self-concept scale, a self-esteem scale, and a depression scale. Two-thirds of the sample reported reduced quality of life, a quarter reported poor self-concept and negative self-esteem, and 16% met criteria for depression. And the authors report that 2 individuals actually reported suicidal thoughts. The authors could find no strong relationships between the KSphl (and thus the presence of KS-related stigmata) and any of the psychosocial variables. The authors also found no difference on these measures between prepubertal and pubertal KS boys.

Hormone levels were also examined, and although only a few of the pubertal KS boys had low testosterone levels, as many as 60% has elevated follicle stimulating hormone (FSH) and luteinizing hormone (LH) levels, which could be seen as a sign of relative testosterone insufficiency.

This study illustrates several points. First, typical stigmata are present even in prepubertal KS boys, although each child only presents a limited number of stigmata. Second, boys with KS present with a troublesome psychosocial profile with decreased quality of life, self-concept, self-esteem, and some with outright depression, even in prepuberty. Third, no obvious link between the number of stigmata and the psychosocial traits was present. Although we do not have good and evidence-based treatment for young boys with KS, this study clearly shows the need for the development of psychosocial measures and interventions to improve the lives of KS youth. The study also indicates that relative hypergonadotropic hypogonadism is present in many pubertal KS boys and reinforces the need for randomized controlled trials with early testosterone replacement, perhaps together with psychosocial interventions.

C. H. Gravholt, MD

25 Respiratory Tract

Comparative Effectiveness of Dexamethasone versus Prednisone in Children Hospitalized with Asthma

Parikh K, Hall M, Mittal V, et al (Children's Natl Med Ctr and George Washington School of Medicine, DC; Children's Hosp Association, Overland Park, KS, Children's Med Ctr and Univ of Texas Southwestern Med Ctr, Dallas; et al)

J Pediatr 167:639-041, 2015

Objectives.—To study the comparative effectiveness of dexamethasone vs prednisone/prednisolone in children hospitalized with asthma exacerbation not requiring intensive care.

Study Design.—This multicenter retrospective cohort study, using the Pediatric Health Information System, included children aged 4-17 years who were hospitalized with a principal diagnosis of asthma between January 1, 2007 and December 31, 2012. Children with chronic complex condition and/or initial intensive care unit (ICU) management were excluded. Propensity score matching was used to detect differences in length of stay (LOS), readmissions, ICU transfer, and cost between groups.

Results.—40 257 hospitalizations met inclusion criteria; 1166 (2.9%) received only dexamethasone. In the matched cohort (N = 1284 representing 34 hospitals), the LOS was significantly shorter in the dexamethasone group compared with the prednisone/prednisolone group. The proportion of subjects with a LOS of 3 days or more was 6.7% in the dexamethasone group and 12% in the prednisone/prednisolone group ($P = .002$). Differences in all-cause readmission at 7- and 30 days were not statistically significant. The dexamethasone group had lower costs of index admission ($2621 vs $2838; $P < .001$) and total episode of care (including readmissions) ($2624 vs $2856; $P < .001$) compared with the prednisone/prednisolone group. There were no clinical significant differences in ICU transfer or readmissions between groups.

Conclusions.—Dexamethasone may be considered an alternative to prednisone/prednisolone for children hospitalized with asthma exacerbation not requiring admission to intensive care (Table 1).

▶ Asthma remains a frequently encountered disease among pediatric health care providers, particularly those who work in emergency department (ED) and inpatient hospital settings, where asthma is a leading pediatric diagnosis. And although more than 20 years of asthma guidelines from the National Institutes of Health have directed the use of systemic steroids for children presenting

TABLE 1.—Characteristics of the Study Population by Treatment Group

	Dexamethasone	Prednisolone/Prednisone	P
N	1166 (2.9)	39 091 (97.1)	
Age (y)			<.001
4-6	624 (53.5)	16 492 (42.2)	
7-12	454 (38.9)	17 611 (45.1)	
13-17	88 (7.5)	4988 (12.8)	
Sex			.861
Male	723 (62)	23 945 (61.3)	
Female	443 (38)	15 145 (38.7)	
Race			<.001
Non-Hispanic White	349 (29.9)	10 014 (25.6)	
Non-Hispanic Black	244 (20.9)	19 494 (49.9)	
Hispanic	329 (28.2)	6145 (15.7)	
Asian	78 (6.7)	566 (1.4)	
Other	166 (14.2)	2872 (7.3)	
Payer			<.001
Government	613 (52.6)	22 279 (57)	
Private	477 (40.9)	13 840 (35.4)	
Other	76 (6.5)	2972 (7.6)	
Chest radiography	499 (42.8)	17 822 (45.6)	.059
Antibiotics	225 (19.3)	8463 (21.6)	.054
Magnesium	103 (8.8)	3567 (9.1)	.734
Terbutaline	3 (0.3)	307 (0.8)	.042
Obesity	24 (2.1)	1655 (4.2)	<.001
Atopy	115 (9.9)	7025 (18)	<.001
Median HHI			<.001
Missing	36 (3.1)	493 (1.2)	
<$34 576	230 (19.7)	14 348 (36.7)	
$34 576-$46 100	176 (15.1)	9664 (24.7)	
$46 101-$69 150	373 (32)	7783 (19.9)	
>$69 150	351 (30.1)	6839 (17.5)	

Reprinted from Parikh K, Hall M, Mittal V, et al. Comparative effectiveness of dexamethasone versus prednisone in children hospitalized with asthma. *J Pediatr*. 2015;167:639-644, with permission from Elsevier.

to the ED and hospital settings for asthma care, there have been limitations to the effectiveness of systemic steroids due to patient intolerance (eg, vomiting), patient nonadherence (eg, not filling prescriptions for systemic steroids), and physician nonadherence (eg, not prescribing/administering systemic steroids to patients).

Dexamethasone, particularly when used in the ED, offers a potential solution for the first 2 of these barriers because it is better tolerated and is required for a shorter duration of time compared with traditional steroid preparations (eg, prednisolone). There is strong evidence that dexamethasone is appropriate, and maybe even ideal, for treating children who present to the ED for an asthma exacerbation. The published data goes back 20 years. However, there is a void in the literature as to whether dexamethasone is appropriate and effective for use in hospitalized children, who would presumably be more acutely ill than their counterparts who are discharged to home from the ED. This study is important in attempting to answer the question of whether dexamethasone is as effective as traditional systemic steroids to treat children hospitalized for an asthma exacerbation.

The authors examined electronic medical records of children hospitalized at 42 children's hospitals, who collectively represent 20% of all yearly pediatric hospitalizations for asthma in the United States. The focus of the data was on children 4 to 17 years of age who were being treated exclusively for asthma and who did not have any significant comorbid chronic conditions. The authors then separated the children into 2 groups: (1) those treated exclusively with dexamethasone and (2) those treated with any other systemic steroid preparation. These 2 treatment groups were then compared for a variety of indicators of treatment effectiveness, including total length of hospitalization, readmissions for asthma, hospitalization cost(s), and need for intensive care unit (ICU).

To eliminate other differences between the 2 treatment groups that might affect the treatment effectiveness indicators, the authors made statistical adjustments for a number of sociodemographic and clinical characteristics of the patients, including age, race, payer, income, tests received, treatments received, obesity, and atopy. After those statistical adjustments, the authors observed that patients in receipt of dexamethasone were more likely to have a 1-day hospitalization (vs a 2-day or 3-day or longer hospitalization) and lower hospitalization costs. There were no differences between the treatment groups with regard to readmissions or need for ICU care.

The authors rightly highlight some limitations of their study, including the inability to fully assess clinical severity; lack of information on dosing of any of the steroid preparations, including dexamethasone; and that this was an observational study. Additional limiting considerations not mentioned by the authors include the following: (1) no data were presented on mean length of stay for the treatment groups; rather, data were presented as the percentage of children hospitalized for 1 day, 2 days, or 3 or more days. Although presenting the length of stay data in these categories, being able to see the final average length of stay would be more consistent with the clinical framework in which we view the impact of medications and other interventions on various asthma outcomes. (2) No discussion was presented regarding the representativeness of the studied population to the larger population of children hospitalized for asthma, particularly with regard to the length of stay. Nationally, 2 days is the average duration of hospitalization for pediatric asthma. Therefore, the large percentage of patients who received dexamethasone who had a 1-day hospitalization (71%) were either milder in severity than the typical hospitalized child or there was some truly derived benefit from the use of dexamethasone in reducing length of hospitalization. (3) It is not clear to what extent their statistical adjustments really removed all of the factors that might influence the treatments provided to these patients. In the final analyses, 642 of 1166 in the dexamethasone group were analyzed, whereas 642 of 39 091 children in the "prednisolone/prednisone" group were analyzed. The statistical analyses were required because at first pass, the dexamethasone group was significantly more likely than the prednisolone/prednisone group to be nonblack (79% vs 50%) and to have high household incomes (>$46 101 per year—62% vs 37%; Table 1). The question remains as to whether the apparent subjective nature of how the patients were originally treated was sufficiently eliminated statistically to isolate the clinical effect; this can only be determined with additional and prospective research studies.

Lastly, and most importantly, from a causality framework, the authors with this study have met a number of Sir Bradford Hill's Criteria for Causality (below), but some important gaps in the evidence remain, particularly in terms of consistency, temporal sequence, dose response/biological gradient and experimental evidence (in this case, an experimental design, in which patients are randomly assigned to a treatment, then followed prospectively to measure the outcomes from the treatment).

Sir Bradford Hill Criteria (to establish causality):

1. Strength (effect size): magnitude of the effect of the intervention
2. Consistency (reproducible): similar findings observed by different persons in different places with different samples
3. Specificity: no other factor is a likely explanation of the observed association
4. Temporality: the effect has to occur after the cause (and if there is an expected delay between the cause and expected effect, then the effect must occur after that delay)
5. Biological gradient: more exposure to the intervention/agent results in a larger effect
6. Plausibility: can the observed effect be reasonably explained by known biological mechanisms?
7. Coherence: are epidemiological observations consistent with known scientific/biological/mechanistic findings?
8. Experiment: Findings are consistent with studies with experimental methodologies (eg, random assignment of the treatment has similar results to nonrandomized treatment assignment);
9. Analogy: Is it reasonable or is there evidence that a similar agent (drug) would have the same effect(s)?

This study sheds light on the possibility of using a better tolerated and easier to adhere to medication for the treatment of children admitted to the hospital for asthma. However, the authors statement that "use of dexamethasone for children hospitalized for non-ICU management may be a reasonable practice in the ICU setting" should be taken with caution. We do not know the clinical indications to determine who should receive dexamethasone, the dose to be administered, or even the number of doses to be administered—and what clinical profile is ideal for this formulation. Given the subjective nature with which the medication appears to have already been administered (based on sociodemographics rather than clinical criteria), more evidence to support the use of clinical rather than sociodemographic criteria would provide more equitable inpatient asthma care, regardless of income, race, or other subjective criteria.

S. Okelo, MD, PhD

Disparities in mortality and morbidity in pediatric asthma hospitalizations, 2007 to 2011

Glick AF, Tomopoulos S, Fierman AH, et al (Bellevue Hosp Ctr, NY; et al)
Acad Pediatr 16:430-437, 2016

Objective.—Asthma is a leading cause of pediatric admissions. While several factors including race have been linked to increased overall asthma morbidity and mortality, few studies have explored factors associated with inpatient asthma outcomes. We examined factors associated with mortality and morbidity in children admitted for asthma.

Design/Methods.—Data were obtained from the US Nationwide Inpatient Sample for 2007-2011. Patients 2-18 years old with a primary diagnosis of asthma were included. Predictor variables were sociodemographic and hospital factors and acute/chronic secondary diagnoses. Outcomes were mortality, intubation, length of stay (LOS), and costs. Weighted national estimates were calculated. Multivariable analyses were performed.

Results.—There were 97,379 (478,546 weighted) asthma admissions. Most patients were male (60.6%); 30% were white, 28% black, and 18% Hispanic. Mortality rate was 0.03%. 0.3% were intubated. Median (IQR) LOS was 2 (1-3) days. Median (IQR) costs were $2760 ($1860-4320). Native American race, older age (13-18 years), and West region were significant independent predictors of mortality. Intubation rate was lower in Hispanic compared to white children ($p = 0.028$). LOS was shorter in Asian compared to white children ($p = 0.022$) but longer in children with public insurance and from low income areas ($p < 0.001$). Average costs were higher in black, Hispanic, and Asian compared to white children ($p < 0.05$).

Conclusions.—With the exception of Native Americans, race/ethnicity is not associated with inpatient asthma mortality and has varied effects on morbidity. Recognition of factors associated with increased asthma mortality and morbidity may allow for earlier, more effective treatment and avoidance of complications.

▶ Disparities in asthma hospital admissions have been well documented. African Americans are 2 to 3 times more likely to be admitted to the hospital and at 75% more likely to die from asthma.[1] This study examines what happens after children with asthma are admitted to the hospital. Are there disparities in length of stay (a measure of morbidity) or in deaths?

The authors use the Nationwide Inpatient Sample (NIS), which is an all-payer inpatient data set. The sample represents approximately 20% of the hospital admissions in the United States, and it is publicly available. Given the well-known disparities in asthma hospitalizations among racial/ethnic groups, the primary predictor variable was race/ethnicity.

What isn't easily interpreted from this data set is how sick the children were before they were admitted to the hospital. Asthma outcomes are very much dependent on the local environment, such as poverty rate, overcrowding, access to care, and quality of care. For example, Native Americans were more likely to die, but is that a reflection of the overall system for health care for Native Americans or are there disparities in how they are treated once they are admitted? This issue is difficult to tease out but perhaps an important limitation on analysis of a data set. Native Americans have high prevalence and relatively high asthma morbidity as well as poor access to care, poor self-management skills, and cultural barriers.[2,3] This combination of factors most likely explains the higher mortality found in this study.

However, once these disparities are identified in large data sets, it is our responsibility as health care professionals to look more closely at what is happening. Are there system biases that affect these outcomes, or is it the inequity in the quality of care they receive both in the inpatient and outpatient setting? A recent article found that differences did exist in hospital care across the nation in terms of guideline concordance that directly affected hospital outcomes. The most significant difference was the asthma care plan being given at discharge.[4] In contrast, Krishnan and colleagues reported no racial/ethnic differences in asthma-related deaths among hospitalized patients suggesting that deaths are due to pre-hospitalization factors.[5] In clinical outpatient care, lack of controller medications,[6] asthma care plans,[7] low health literacy,[8] and poor patient-physician communication[9,10] have contributed to disparities in asthma outcomes. Have we made any real progress in changing that on a system-wide basis?

The conclusion in this study that "Black and Hispanic race/ethnicity are not independent predictors of inpatient asthma mortality" is in direct contrast to many previous studies. It is important to understand that in this study, the database only included those who actually came to the hospital for treatment rather than the entire "at-risk" population. As the authors note, this doesn't take into account those who died before getting to the hospital. Akinbami et al recently reported that when one looks at "at-risk" populations, disparities are less apparent in some asthma outcomes; but the disparities between those who die remain.[11]

How do we explain the difference in outcomes found in this article and compared with previous studies? One consideration is that the NIS database doesn't include the "uninsured" and therefore it is not truly representative of the US population where 9.2% of the United States was uninsured in 2015 down from a peak of 18%. In a study done in 2012, uninsured patients were 4 times more likely to die.[12] Also in the current study, Glick and colleagues report that Hispanic children had lower odds of intubation compared with white children, which the authors speculate was due to the increased mortality seen in Hispanic children in the outpatient setting. Another consideration is that undocumented children are less likely to have insurance, which may explain deaths outside of the hospital. Given that the NIS database lacks a substantial number of people who could potentially change the reported disparities in asthma mortality, the findings in this study may not truly reflect asthma mortality outcomes in the United States.

Furthermore, if one doesn't realize that this database is incomplete, one could conclude that there is no need to be concerned about the disparities in asthma mortality that has been shown in previous studies. As the authors duly note, a major weakness of any of the findings in this article is that the study sample is equally proportioned; whites, blacks, and Hispanics each represent 30% of the sample. This distribution isn't a true depiction of the population in the United States. As a result, nothing conclusive can be said about these findings. Even the findings that Hispanics have a longer length of stay and are less likely to be intubated are also potentially suspect.

In the discussion, the authors list the many limitations of this study including "race/ethnicity data missing, lack of all states reporting, and variability in coding." These deficiencies in the dataset are significant and unfortunately limit the ability to generalize or to give credibility to many of the findings regarding disparities in asthma outcomes.

Many studies have reported disparities in asthma mortality and morbidity among racial and ethnic groups.[1,11,13] Rather than repeated descriptions of these disparities, we now need to adopt a "no tolerance" attitude. It is not acceptable for poor children and minority children to have worse asthma outcomes. For there to be virtually no decrease in the large gap that exists between hospitalizations, as well as asthma mortality, for Whites and Blacks is incomprehensible and totally unacceptable. We, as a society and specifically as health care profession, should work together to reduce these inequities. We know that there is a higher poverty rate in the same ethnic groups (blacks, Latinos, Native Americans) that experience poor outcomes. These same groups are more likely to live in substandard housing, experience overcrowding, have more exposure to pollutants, violence,[14,15] and stress,[16,17] all of which are triggers for asthma exacerbations. We must do things differently, such as creating a system-wide intentional and comprehensive multifaceted approach that addresses all of the contributors to asthma disparities.[18] Let's stop describing asthma disparities; rather, let us have a renewed determination to create health equity for all patients with asthma regardless of race and ethnicity.

T. Bryant-Stephens, MD

References

1. Akinbami LJ, Moorman JE, Bailey C, et al. *Trends in asthma prevalence, health care use, and mortality in the United States, 2001–2010.* NCHS Data Brief. NO. Hyattsville, MD: National Center for Health Statistics; 2012.
2. Dixon AE, Yeh F, Welty TK, et al. Asthma in American Indian adults: the Strong Heart Study. *Chest.* 2007;131:1323-1330.
3. Brim SN, Rudd RA, Funk RH, Callahan DB. Asthma prevalence among US children in underrepresented minority populations: American Indian/Alaska Native, Chinese, Filipino, and Asian Indian. *Pediatrics.* 2008;122:e217-e222.
4. Hasegawa K, Tsugawa Y, Clark S, et al. Improving quality of acute asthma care in U.S. hospitals: changes between 1999–2000 and 2012–2013. *Chest.* 2016; 150:112-122.
5. Krishnan V, Diette GB, Rand CS, et al. Mortality in patients hospitalized for asthma exacerbations in the United States. *Am J Respir Crit Care Med.* 2006; 174:633-638.
6. Sarpong E, Miller GE. Racial and ethnic differences in childhood asthma treatment in the United States. *Health Serv Res.* 2013;48:2014-2036.
7. Chandra D, Clark S, Camargo CA Jr. Race/ethnicity differences in the inpatient management of acute asthma in the United States. *Chest.* 2009;135:1527-1534.

8. Harrington KF, Zhang B, Magruder T, Bailey WC, Gerald LB. The impact of parent's health literacy on pediatric asthma outcomes. *Pediatr Allergy Immunol Pulmonol.* 2015;28:20-26.

9. Diette GB, Rand C. The contributing role of health care communication to health disparities for minority patients with asthma. *Chest.* 2007;132:802S-809S.

10. Johnson RL, Roter D, Powe NR, Cooper LA. Patient race/ethnicity and quality of patient-physician communication during medical visits. *Am J Public Health.* 2004;94:2084-2090.

11. Akinbami LJ, Moorman JE, Simon AE, Schoendorf KC. Trends in racial disparities for asthma outcomes among children 0 to 17 years, 2001–2010. *J Allergy Clin Immunol.* 2014;134:547-553.

12. Families USA. Dying for coverage: the deadly consequences of being uninsured. 2012. http://familiesusa.org/sites/default/files/product_documents/Dying-for-Coverage.pdf. Accessed April 27, 2016.

13. Gergen P, Tokias A. Inner city asthma. *Immunol Allergy Clin North Am.* 2015; 35:101-114.

14. Wright RJ, Mitchell H, Visness CM, et al. Community violence and asthma morbidity: the inner-city asthma study. *Am J Public Health.* 2004;94:625-632.

15. Liu SY, Pearlman DN. Hospital readmissions for childhood asthma: the role of individual and neighborhood factors. *Public Health Rep.* 2009;124:65-78.

16. Sandberg S, Paton JY, Ahola S, et al. The role of acute and chronic stress in asthma attacks in children. *Lancet.* 2000;356:982-987.

17. Koinis-Mitchell D, McQuaid EL, Kopel SJ, et al. Cultural-related, contextual, and asthma-specific risks associated with asthma morbidity in urban children. *J Clin Psychol Med Settings.* 2010;17:38-48.

18. Clarke AR, Goddu AP, Nocon RS, et al. Thirty years of disparities intervention research: what are we doing to close racial and ethnic gaps in health care? *Med Care.* 2013;51:1020-1026.

Early Administration of Azithromycin and Prevention of Severe Lower Respiratory Tract Illnesses in Preschool Children With a History of Such Illnesses: A Randomized Clinical Trial

Bacharier LB, for the National Heart, Lung, and Blood Institute's AsthmaNet (Washington Univ in St Louis School of Medicine, St Louis, MO; et al)

JAMA 314:2034-2044, 2015

Importance.—Many preschool children develop recurrent, severe episodes of lower respiratory tract illness (LRTI). Although viral infections are often present, bacteria may also contribute to illness pathogenesis. Strategies that effectively attenuate such episodes are needed.

Objective.—To evaluate if early administration of azithromycin, started prior to the onset of severe LRTI symptoms, in preschool children with recurrent severe LRTIs can prevent the progression of these episodes.

Design, Setting, and Participants.—A randomized, double-blind, placebo-controlled, parallel-group trial conducted across 9 academic US medical centers in the National Heart, Lung, and Blood Institute's AsthmaNet network, with enrollment starting in April 2011 and follow-up complete by December 2014. Participants were 607 children aged 12 through 71 months with histories of recurrent, severe LRTIs and minimal day-to-day impairment.

Intervention.—Participants were randomly assigned to receive azithromycin (12 mg/kg/d for 5 days; n = 307) or matching placebo (n = 300), started early during each predefined RTI (child's signs or symptoms prior to development of LRTI), based on individualized action plans, over a 12- through 18-month period.

Main Outcomes and Measures.—The primary outcome measure was the number of RTIs not progressing to a severe LRTI, measured at the level of the RTI, that would in clinical practice trigger the prescription of oral corticosteroids. Presence of azithromycin-resistant organisms in oropharyngeal samples, along with adverse events, were among the secondary outcome measures.

Results.—A total of 937 treated RTIs (azithromycin group, 473; placebo group, 464) were experienced by 443 children (azithromycin group, 223; placebo group, 220), including 92 severe LRTIs (azithromycin group, 35; placebo group, 57). Azithromycin significantly reduced the risk of progressing to severe LRTI relative to placebo (hazard ratio, 0.64 [95% CI, 0.41-0.98], $P = .04$; absolute risk for first RTI: 0.05 for azithromycin, 0.08 for placebo; risk difference, 0.03 [95% CI, 0.00-0.06]). Induction of azithromycin-resistant organisms and adverse events were infrequently observed.

Conclusions and Relevance.—Among young children with histories of recurrent severe LRTIs, the use of azithromycin early during an apparent RTI compared with placebo reduced the likelihood of severe LRTI. More information is needed on the development of antibiotic-resistant pathogens with this strategy.

Trial Registration.—clinicaltrials.gov Identifier: NCT01272635

► Recurrent episodes of lower respiratory illness (LRTI) in preschool children represent a common yet problematic management conundrum for physicians. It is difficult to manage a condition with uncertain etiology and variable prognosis. Respiratory viruses, including respiratory syncytial virus (RSV) and human rhinovirus (HRV), are frequently detected, while pathogenic bacteria such as *Streptococcus pneumoniae*, *Moraxella catarrhalis*, and *Haemophilus influenzae* are also implicated.[1] Furthermore, the outcome of disease is unpredictable: many episodes are transient with no long-lasting effects, but others may progress to severe LRTI. Recurrent episodes may herald the onset of childhood asthma. Current management is centered around short-acting beta-agonist and corticosteroids (inhaled or systemic), although efficacy is variable. Antibiotic therapy is not recommended given the uncertainty over the role of bacteria.

Reality, however, is quite different. When confronted by an unwell toddler, many physicians will prescribe antibiotics as an adjunct therapy in a bid to minimize symptoms and prevent further deterioration. Anecdotally, this approach appears to show some benefits, although previous trials did not demonstrate conclusive positive outcomes.

However, there has been recent interest in the use of macrolide antibiotics in a broad range of respiratory diseases including cystic fibrosis, non–cystic fibrosis bronchiectasis, asthma, and diffuse panbronchiolitis.[2] In addition to their broad-spectrum antimicrobial properties, macrolide antibiotics such as clarithromycin and azithromycin have immunomodulatory properties and appear to be most effective in conditions where neutrophilic inflammation is dominant.[3] Azithromycin has also been shown to have antiviral effects in in vitro settings.[4] These properties make azithromycin an attractive potential novel therapy for recurrent LRTIs in preschoolers.

In the largest randomized clinical trial on this topic to date, Bacharier and colleagues evaluated the efficacy of azithromycin in preventing progression to severe LRTI in preschoolers with a documented history of recurrent LRTIs. Participants were commenced on a 5-day course of azithromycin (12 mg/kg once daily) or placebo as soon as possible after the onset of LRTI symptoms (as diagnosed by parent or guardian). Compared with placebo, azithromycin therapy led to a significantly lower risk of progression to severe LRTI (hazard ratio: 0.64; 95% confidence interval [CI]: 0.41−0.98, $P = .04$; absolute risk for first RTI: 0.05 for azithromycin, 0.08 for placebo; risk difference: 0.03, 95% CI: 0.00−0.06). The azithromycin group also exhibited fewer symptoms over the duration of RTI, although this is limited to those who eventually progressed to severe LRTI.

Although the overall result of the study seems to be positive, several important questions remain to be addressed. The more severely affected cases (ie, those with chronic unstable asthma needing regular maintenance inhaled corticosteroids and those with more than 4 courses of systemic corticosteroids per year) were excluded from the study. It is likely that this group carries the bulk of morbidity and health care burden, and thus the role of azithromycin in this group cannot be evaluated by the outcomes of the current study. Importantly, the exact mechanism of how azithromycin prevents disease progression remains unclear.

Currently it is not possible to decipher whether it is the antimicrobial, immunomodulatory, or (potential) antiviral aspect that contributes most to azithromycin's positive effect. The authors have endeavored to investigate this issue in the subgroup analyses. Polymorphisms in the interleukin (IL)-8 gene are thought to modulate IL-8 production. By segregating the cohort into the different genotypes (TT, AA/AT), the authors attempted to assess a differential response to azithromycin in "high" and "low" IL-8 producers, but no significant interaction was observed. This lack of effect may reflect the complex immunomodulatory mechanisms of azithromycin. There was also no significant difference in outcomes between those with detectable viral infection and those without it. It is noteworthy that HRV was more commonly detected in subjects who developed severe LRTIs. These subjects were excluded from the study, and thus the effect of azithromycin could not be evaluated. Unfortunately, no bacteriology sample was collected to assess the role of bacteria in the current cohort.

Despite the preceding limitations, there is growing evidence demonstrating the beneficial effects of azithromycin in recurrent LRTIs in preschool children. A recent randomized controlled trial in a Danish cohort of preschool children with recurrent asthma-like symptoms also observed that azithromycin significantly reduced the duration of respiratory symptoms compared with placebo.[5]

Optimism should nonetheless be balanced with caution. Although rare, macrolides do have potential hepatic and cardiac side effects. Given the increasing threat of multidrug-resistant organisms, it is paramount to further examine the role of macrolide antibiotics to prevent widespread inappropriate prescription. Future research should focus on disentangling the etiology of recurrent LRTIs in preschoolers including the role of the airway microbiota. This will not only aid the development of novel biomarkers, but also improve the design of clinical trials that target the patients who are more likely to benefit from macrolide therapy.

E. H. C. Wong, MBBS, MRCP (UK), BSc

S. L. Johnston, MBBS, PhD, FERS, FRCP, FRSB, FMedSci

References

1. Bisgaard H, Hermansen MN, Bonnelykke K, et al. Association of bacteria and viruses with wheezy episodes in young children: prospective birth cohort study. *BMJ.* 2010;341:c4978.
2. Wong EH, Porter JD, Edwards MR, Johnston SL. The role of macrolides in asthma: current evidence and future directions. *Lancet Respir Med.* 2014;2: 657-670.
3. Brusselle GG, Vanderstichele C, Jordens P, et al. Azithromycin for prevention of exacerbations in severe asthma (AZISAST): a multicentre randomised double-blind placebo-controlled trial. *Thorax.* 2013;68:322-329.
4. Gielen V, Johnston SL, Edwards MR. Azithromycin induces anti-viral responses in bronchial epithelial cells. *Eur Respir J.* 2010;36:646-654.
5. Stokholm J, Chawes BL, Vissing NH, et al. Azithromycin for episodes with asthma-like symptoms in young children aged 1–3 years: a randomised, double-blind, placebo-controlled trial. *Lancet Respir Med.* 2016;4:19-26.

Prenatal and infant paracetamol exposure and development of asthma: the Norwegian Mother and Child Cohort Study
Magnus MC, Karlstad Ø, Håberg SE, et al (Norwegian Inst of Public Health, Oslo, Norway; et al)
Int J Epidemiol 45:512-522, 2016

Background.—Paracetamol exposure has been positively associated with asthma development. The relative importance of prenatal vs infant exposure and confounding by indication remains elusive. We examined the association of prenatal and infant (first 6 months) paracetamol exposure with asthma development while addressing confounding by indication.

Methods.—We used information from the Norwegian Mother and Child Cohort Study, including 53 169 children for evaluation of current asthma at 3 years, 25 394 for current asthma at 7 years and 45 607 for dispensed asthma medications at 7 years in the Norwegian Prescription Database. We calculated adjusted relative risks (adj. RR) and 95% confidence intervals (CI) using log-binomial regression.

Results.—There were independent modest associations between asthma at 3 years with prenatal paracetamol exposure (adj. RR 1.13; 95% CI:

1.02–1.25) and use of paracetamol during infancy (adj. RR 1.29; 95% CI: 1.16–1.45). The results were consistent for asthma at 7 years. The associations with prenatal paracetamol exposure were seen for different indications (pain, respiratory tract infections/influenza and fever). Maternal pain during pregnancy was the only indication that showed an association both with and without paracetamol use. Maternal paracetamol use outside pregnancy and paternal paracetamol use were not associated with asthma development. In a secondary analysis, prenatal ibuprofen exposure was positively associated with asthma at 3 years but not asthma at 7 years.

Conclusions.—This study provides evidence that prenatal and infant paracetamol exposure have independent associations with asthma development. Our findings suggest that the associations could not be fully explained by confounding by indication.

▶ In the 1980s, there was a shift from aspirin to acetaminophen use due to the concern of Reye syndrome. This change coincided with the dramatic rise in rates of childhood asthma prevalence over the past few decades. From an epidemiologic standpoint, this begs the question: Is acetaminophen use associated with asthma development? Clearly, asthma development is a multifactorial process without 1 smoking gun; however, the role of acetaminophen needs to be evaluated.

There are plausible mechanisms that could explain this link including acetaminophen decreasing the amount of protective airway glutathione and acetaminophen enhancing T helper cell-2 (Th2) responses. Multiple observational studies have shown an association between acetaminophen use during pregnancy and infancy and the development of asthma later in childhood. Unfortunately, these studies are prone to flaws, most notably the concern of confounding by indication.

The acetaminophen-asthma link is the perfect illustration of confounding by indication. For example, young children with frequent febrile respiratory illnesses are more likely to take acetaminophen to treat the fevers. Additionally, we know that children with frequent respiratory illnesses at a young age are more likely to develop asthma. As such, it is incorrect to blame the acetaminophen use on asthma development without accounting for the indications for the acetaminophen use, especially respiratory illnesses. This issue has been a recurring hurdle for researchers trying to investigate the acetaminophen-asthma link. The authors of this study present some interesting ways to address the confounding by indication dilemma.

This study examined the association of prenatal and early-life acetaminophen exposure with asthma development in the largest cohort to date. The authors found significantly positive associations, as has been described previously. For example, children exposed to acetaminophen in the first 6 months of life had a relative risk of 1.29 of current asthma at 3 years and a relative risk of 1.24 of current asthma at 7 years. Similar significant associations were seen for prenatal exposure to acetaminophen. These results were significant after adjusting for a variety of possible confounders, including maternal respiratory illness during pregnancy and respiratory tract infections in the child during the first 6 months of life.

The uniqueness of this study is that the researchers went further and tried to evaluate possible confounding by indication in a few additional ways. First, they evaluated the reason for acetaminophen use and discovered that prenatal exposure for 3 indications (pain, respiratory infections, and fever) yielded similar associations with asthma development. By contrast, in the absence of prenatal acetaminophen exposure, maternal respiratory infections and fever during pregnancy were not associated with asthma development in the child. These data seem to indicate that it is the actual exposure to acetaminophen that is the driving factor and not the respiratory infections or the fevers alone. Unfortunately, the authors only had data on indications of use for the mother during pregnancy and not for the child during the first 6 months of life. Second, the authors performed sensitivity analyses to understand the possible contribution of background factors such as overall family health behaviors. The authors discovered that maternal acetaminophen intake outside of pregnancy (6 months before pregnancy and 6 months after delivery) and paternal acetaminophen intake were not associated with asthma development in the child. Finally, the authors evaluated the use of ibuprofen during pregnancy, which was rare, as expected. Prenatal exposure to ibuprofen only (no acetaminophen exposure) was associated with current asthma at 3 years (relative risk 1.31; 95% confidence interval: 1.00–1.72), but not with current asthma at 7 years (relative risk 1.16, 95% confidence interval: 0.73–1.83). By contrast, prenatal exposure to acetaminophen was significantly associated with asthma at both ages.

Of course, the ideal way to truly study the acetaminophen-asthma association would not be with an observational study but instead with a randomized controlled trial. Given that acetaminophen is the most commonly used medication in childhood, the results of a randomized controlled trial could have important implications on treatment recommendations. Unfortunately, a randomized controlled trial evaluating the effect of early-life acetaminophen exposure is not an easy task. For one thing, what would be the treatment in the other comparison arm? After acetaminophen, ibuprofen is the second most commonly used medication for fever and pain; however, ibuprofen is generally not recommended during pregnancy, especially in the third trimester. A comparison placebo arm could be considered and may be acceptable in pregnant women; however, treatment of placebo would be unethical in an infant with fever, pain, or discomfort.

These obstacles are the reason that we continue to read reports about observational data and not randomized trials. Although the authors have done an excellent job accounting for possible confounding by indication, they acknowledge in their final sentence that "a randomized controlled trial would be beneficial." Until that trial is done, all articles from observational trials will end with similar wording.

W. J. Sheehan, MD

Childhood Sleepwalking and Sleep Terrors: A Longitudinal Study of Prevalence and Familial Aggregation

Petit D, Pennestri M-H, Paquet J, et al (Hôpital du Sacré-Coeur de Montréal, Quebec, Canada; et al)

JAMA Pediatr 169:653-658, 2015

Importance.—Childhood sleepwalking and sleep terrors are 2 parasomnias with a risk of serious injury for which familial aggregation has been shown.

Objectives.—To assess the prevalence of sleepwalking and sleep terrors during childhood; to investigate the link between early sleep terrors and sleepwalking later in childhood; and to evaluate the degree of association between parental history of sleepwalking and presence of somnambulism and sleep terrors in children.

Design, Setting, and Participants.—Sleep data from a large prospective longitudinal cohort (the Quebec Longitudinal Study of Child Development) of 1940 children born in 1997 and 1998 in the province were studied from March 1999 to March 2011.

Main Outcomes and Measures.—Prevalence of sleep terrors and sleepwalking was assessed yearly from ages 1½ and 2½ years, respectively, to age 13 years through a questionnaire completed by the mother. Parental history of sleepwalking was also queried.

Results.—The peak of prevalence was observed at 1½ years for sleep terrors (34.4% of children; 95% CI, 32.3%-36.5%) and at age 10 years for sleepwalking (13.4%; 95% CI, 11.3%-15.5%). As many as one-third of the children who had early childhood sleep terrors developed sleepwalking later in childhood. The prevalence of childhood sleepwalking increases with the degree of parental history of sleepwalking: 22.5% (95% CI, 19.2%-25.8%) for children without a parental history of sleepwalking, 47.4% (95% CI, 38.9%-55.9%) for children who had 1 parent with a history of sleepwalking, and 61.5% (95% CI, 42.8%-80.2%) for children whose mother and father had a history of sleepwalking. Moreover, parental history of sleepwalking predicted the incidence of sleep terrors in children as well as the persistent nature of sleep terrors.

Conclusions and Relevance.—These findings substantiate the strong familial aggregation for the 2 parasomnias and lend support to the notion that sleepwalking and sleep terrors represent 2 manifestations of the same underlying pathophysiological entity.

▶ If you've practiced in field of pediatrics, dollars to donuts you've seen children with reported non—rapid eye movement (NREM) sleep parasomnias— classically, confusional arousals, sleepwalking, and night terrors, behaviors that are usually initiated during partial arousals from slow-wave sleep, to which the child is fully or substantially amnestic later.[1] Despite the purported common occurrence of this group of disorders, which may start even at very young ages, available studies of the prevalence and course of NREM parasomnias vary in definition, size, and generalizability of the study population, and target age. Further, studies assessing familial aggregation on childhood para-somnia have been typically small, retrospective, and cross-sectional. In the present study, Petit et al have provided a much fuller picture of 2 childhood NREM parasomnias, sleep terrors and sleepwalking, using a prospective, population-derived, longitudinal cohort study design, powerfully adding to our understanding of the prevalence and, importantly, the evolution and familial nature of sleep terrors and sleepwalking in typically developing children.

What they found is of interest both in expanding understanding about what we thought we knew and adding some clinically relevant nuance. First of all, the study indicates that sleep terrors peak prevalence is at 18 months. Take note, though, that the study didn't assess sleep terrors at the 5-month time point, so the first time point at which sleep terrors were assessed had the highest prevalence. That's interesting, because a common belief is that sleep terrors can occur "as early as" 18 months. Based on this data, it's reasonable to surmise that terrors may start even younger than this age. Keep in mind, too, that sleep terrors were assessed by 1 question: "Does your child have night terrors (wakes up suddenly, crying, sometimes drenched in sweat and confused)?" with possible responses of never, sometimes, often, and always. It's possible some behavioral insomnia of childhood was captured by this question, especially if the respondent didn't carefully consider the hallmark confusion and poor responsiveness present with sleep terrors. Grammatically speaking, the question indicates confusion need only be present sometimes. Tricky. At least the study used the same respondent at each time point for all 10 time points, which may increase consistency of interpreting the question across time points.

Second, the study endeavored in earnest to assess familial aggregation of parasomnias in childhood, and it delivered. The authors accomplished this by asking the mother (if she was the biological mother) when the child was 10 years old to report if she or the biological father had a history of sleepwalking in their own childhoods. Big points for going after this important history, but it does leave some room for recall error or just not knowing. It is notable that parental history of sleepwalking was found to predict the emergence of sleep terrors in children, as well as double the likelihood of persistence of sleep terrors into middle childhood (compared with children without a parental history). What's more, the likelihood of child sleepwalking increased with the number of parents with a history of sleepwalking: 2 sleepwalking parents was associated with a 61.5% prevalence of child sleepwalking. It's interesting that neither sex nor age of onset were affected based on family history.

Third, setting family history aside, it is also interesting to know that as many as a third of children who had early childhood sleep terrors went on to develop sleepwalking in later childhood. That's a useful point to keep in mind in clinic.

This study has 2 chief strengths, both related to study design. The first is the strength of the robust study design. The study is nested in the Quebec Longitudinal Study of Child Development, and children were recruited from the Quebec Master Birth Registry, using a randomized, geographically balanced, stratified survey design to study a representative sample of infants born in 1997 and 1998 in Quebec, Canada. Second, the longitudinal nature of the study allowed for analysis of evolution of parasomnias as well as forecasting (ie, the authors were able to assess the probability of developing sleepwalking later in childhood among children who had early sleep terrors). These children were studied at 10 times points from age 1.5 to 13 years for parasomnias—that's a powerful prospective first.

This study has some blind spots. It does not report on concomitant sleep disorders or sleep times, yet links between childhood parasomnias and sleep apnea (which can also be familial) and/or sleep deprivation[2-5] have been reported. Also, although the study population was carefully geographically representative and proportional to births and sex ratio during the enrollment period, due to technical reasons, those in the northern parts of the province as well as Inuit territories and First Nations reserves were excluded. The vast majority of the study population was white (92.8%), and those with known neurological conditions were excluded. Mother was the respondent, a plus that the study surveyed the same individual at each time point but perhaps not inclusive enough of other caregivers who might have information of relevance.

There are 2 take-homes from this work. First: sweet relief! This well-done, large study confirms that night terrors and sleepwalking are very common, although peak ages differ (night terrors: peak prevalence is 34.4% at age 1.5 years; sleepwalking: peak prevalence is 13.4% at 10 years). Perhaps they are more common than previously recognized: the overall prevalence of sleep terrors was 56.2%—that's right, more than half of children studied had sleep terrors reported at some point. That's a sizable leap from previous estimates of 1% to 15%.[6-8] Similarly, the overall prevalence of sleepwalking was also high: 29.1%. In this study, children with sleep terrors were almost twice as likely to also experience sleepwalking.

The second take-home goes beyond the informational. Because family history is elucidated, maybe this study can inform our follow-up questions when encountering parasomnias in clinic: in general, the most useful next question might be, "Who (else) in the family sleepwalks?" That's because the study demonstrates a powerful link between parental history and childhood parasomnia. Furthermore, the perennial challenge of the astute clinician is determining when to dig deeper rather than reassure. This study is helpful in this regard, too: for example, it's useful to know that few new cases of sleep terrors appear for the first time after age 5 (in contrast to new cases of sleepwalking, which keep rising until age 12 years).

Eugene O'Neill wrote, "the past is the present, isn't it? It's the future too."[9] For sleepwalking in particular, this seems to be so. We learn that the key to diagnosis is often a good history. In the case these parasomnias, history may also be key to a good prediction for the future.

S. S. Sullivan, MD

References

1. American Academy of Sleep Medicine. *International classification of sleep disorders*. 3rd edition. Darien, IL: American Academy of Sleep Medicine; 2014.
2. Pilon M, Montplaisir J, Zadra A. Precipitating factors of somnambulism: impact of sleep deprivation and forced arousals. *Neurology*. 2008;70:2284-2290.
3. Espa F, Dauvilliers Y, Ondze B, Billiard M, Besset A. Arousal reactions in sleepwalking and night terrors in adults: the role of respiratory events. *Sleep*. 2002; 25:871-875.

4. Guilleminault C, Palombini L, Pelayo R, Chervin RD. Sleepwalking and sleep terrors in prepubertal children: what triggers them? *Pediatrics.* 2003;111:e17-e25.

5. Carrillo-Solano M, Leu-Semenescu S, Golmard JL, Groos E, Arnulf I. Sleepiness in sleepwalking and sleep terrors: a higher sleep pressure? *Sleep Med.* 2016 [Epub ahead of print].

6. Laberge L, Tremblay RE, Vitaro F, Montplaisir J. Development of parasomnias from childhood to early adolescence. *Pediatrics.* 2000;106:67-74.

7. Simonds JF, Parraga H. Prevalence of sleep disorders and sleep behaviors in children and adolescents. *J Am Acad Child Psychiatry.* 1982;21:383-388.

8. Vela-Bueno A, Bixler EO, Dobladez-Blanco B, Rubio ME, Mattisson RE, Kales A. Prevalence of night terrors and nightmares in elementary school children: a pilot study. *Res Commun Psychol Psychiatr Behav.* 1985;10:177-188.

9. O'Neill E. *Long Day's Journey into Night [reissue edition].* New Haven, CT:: Yale University Press; 1962.

Interventions by Health Care Professionals Who Provide Routine Child Health Care to Reduce Tobacco Smoke Exposure in Children: A Review and Meta-Analysis

Daly JB, Mackenzie LJ, Freund M, et al (Hunter New England Local Health District, Wallsend, Australia; et al)
JAMA Pediatr 170:138-147, 2016

Importance.—Reducing child exposure to tobacco smoke is a public health priority. Guidelines recommend that health care professionals in child health settings should address tobacco smoke exposure (TSE) in children.

Objective.—To determine the effectiveness of interventions delivered by health care professionals who provide routine child health care in reducing TSE in children.

Data Sources.—A secondary analysis of 57 trials included in a 2014 Cochrane review and a subsequent extended search was performed. Controlled trials (published through June 2015) of interventions that focused on reducing child TSE, with no restrictions placed on who delivered the interventions, were identified. Secondary data extraction was performed in August 2015.

Study Selection.—Controlled trials of routine child health care delivered by health care professionals (physicians, nurses, medical assistants, health educators, and dieticians) that addressed the outcomes of interest (TSE reduction in children and parental smoking behaviors) were eligible for inclusion in this review and meta-analysis.

Data Extraction and Synthesis.—Study details and quality characteristics were independently extracted by 2 authors. If outcome measures were sufficiently similar, meta-analysis was performed using the random-effects model by DerSimonian and Laird. Otherwise, the results were described narratively.

Main Outcomes and Measures.—The primary outcome measure was reduction in child TSE. Secondary outcomes of interest were parental smoking cessation, parental smoking reduction, and maternal postpartum smoking relapse prevention.

Results.—Sixteen studies met the selection criteria. Narrative analysis of the 6 trials that measured child TSE indicated no intervention effects relative to comparison groups. Similarly, meta-analysis of 9 trials that measured parental smoking cessation demonstrated no overall intervention effect (n = 6399) (risk ratio 1.05; 95% CI, 0.74-1.50; $P = .78$). Meta-analysis of the 3 trials that measured maternal postpartum smoking relapse prevention demonstrated a significant overall intervention effect (n = 1293) (risk ratio 1.53; 95% CI, 1.10-2.14; $P = .01$). High levels of study heterogeneity likely resulted from variability in outcome measures, length of follow up, intervention strategies, and unknown intervention fidelity.

Conclusions and Relevance.—Interventions delivered by health care professionals who provide routine child health care may be effective in preventing maternal smoking relapse. Further research is required to improve the effectiveness of such interventions in reducing child TSE and increasing parental smoking cessation. The findings of this meta-analysis have policy and practice implications relating to interventions by routine pediatric health care professionals that aim to reduce child exposure to tobacco smoke.

▶ Tobacco smoke exposure (TSE) in children jangles the justice nerve of any pediatrician who cares about health equity. The disproportionate exposure of children living in poverty to second- and third-hand smoke,[1] coupled with the well-documented toxic effects of tobacco smoke,[2] compels us to act to reduce TSE in our pediatric patients. Primary care pediatricians have a unique opportunity to intervene with parents who are smokers: a long-term relationship with parents, access to parents who may not have other sources of health care, and the ability and opportunity to discuss the compelling reasons for parents to quit smoking from the perspective of the child's health. For these and other reasons, national guidelines recommend that pediatricians address TSE in child health settings.[3-5]

Understanding the impact of the clinic-based interventions to reduce TSE is challenging. In this secondary analysis of a 2014 Cochrane review, Daly et al included more recent studies and reexamined the effectiveness of interventions by child health providers to reduce TSE in children. Sixteen studies met their revised selection criteria. Three trials looking at maternal postpartum smoking relapse prevention showed a significant intervention effect. In contrast, 9 trials looking at parental smoking cessation showed no overall intervention effect, and qualitative analysis of 6 trials measuring child TSE showed no intervention effect. The authors report that with the exception of interventions focusing on new mothers, they were unable to find a measurable effect of pediatric interventions on reducing child TSE.

It is heartening to note the evidence supporting the efficacy of interventions with new mothers in reducing child TSE. This underscores the importance of pediatricians counseling postpartum mothers on continued abstinence from smoking. Regarding the other interventions, however, we should exercise caution in interpreting these results and prematurely concluding that they are not worthwhile.

The authors have taken on the admirable but daunting task of evaluating outcomes across a number of different TSE reduction interventions. In the articles reviewed, there was considerable variation in how the interventions were delivered and measured. Some interventions provided behavioral counseling, whereas others used biochemical reports, nicotine therapy (NT), and/or referrals to state quitlines. There was variation even within these types of interventions; in the behavioral counseling interventions, for example, exposure to counseling ranged from 1 to 16 contacts over 6 weeks to 8 years. In addition to variations in intervention content and exposure, there were differences in the types of outcomes measured. Some studies relied on parental self-report, others measured cotinine levels, and still others analyzed parental use of avoidance strategies. The lack of a standard assessment of child TSE across the studies makes it hard to generalize outcomes and conclude that TSE interventions are ineffective.

In addition to variations in outcome measures, there is insufficient information regarding intervention fidelity across the studies. Only 4 of the 16 studies reported adherence to an intervention protocol. Of these, all reported only moderate adherence to the protocol. Variations in trainings for providers and clinic staff, the extent to which clinic practice teams engaged in the intervention and how they championed intervention implementation efforts, the availability and effectiveness of practice change tools, and performance feedback all influence the implementation of clinical interventions.[6] Without more information on these components, it is difficult to draw any conclusions about the efficacy of the TSE reduction interventions.

This meta-analysis, with its great heterogeneity in the types of interventions studied, in the outcomes measured, and limited attention to fidelity, demonstrates primarily that we have not yet been able to systematically implement and effectively evaluate programs to reduce TSE in children. We cannot—and must not—necessarily draw the conclusion that child health centers are not an effective or worthwhile setting in which to deliver such interventions.

To promote implementation of these efforts in busy, often underresourced clinics where low-income children present for care, we must systematically integrate interventions into the clinic workflow. This could include optimizing the electronic health record (EHR) to include diagnosis codes for TSE, adding TSE to the problem lists, including TSE screening questions in intake questionnaires, and building electronic referrals to state quitlines into the EHR to simplify referral processes.[7,8] The authors point out that nicotine replacement therapy (NRT) has been shown to be quite effective in helping smokers quit,[9] but only 2 studies in the meta-analysis provided NRT. Given the efficacy and safety of NRT, pediatricians should be encouraged to take an active role in improving parental access to NRT, either by writing a prescription themselves or by connecting parents to resources like the state quitline, which may be able to provide this medication for free. Only when we have supported the real-world implementation of child TSE reduction efforts and when we have standardized TSE assessment measures can we draw conclusions about the efficacy of such interventions.

Without a doubt, there are tremendous barriers to assisting parents in quitting smoking, including lack of time, pediatric lack of expertise with smoking cessation medications, lack of support resources, and lack of reimbursement for meaningful cessation counseling of the parent. On top of this, tobacco addiction is extraordinarily difficult to address. However, these challenges do not mean we should stop trying. It usually takes a smoker a number of attempts to successfully quit smoking,[10,11] and the pediatrician can play a pivotal role in helping parents take steps toward their final, successful quit attempt. We must continue to develop and study interventions that inform effective delivery of this support, toward the ultimate goal of reducing TSE in our patients and making inroads to health equity for all.

J. Marbin, MD

K. Tebb, PhD

References

1. Mannino DM, Moorman JE, Kingsley B, Rose D, Repace J. Health effects related to environmental tobacco smoke exposure in children in the United States: data from the third national health and nutrition examination survey. *Arch Pediatr Adolesc Med.* 2001;155:36-41.
2. CDC Vital Signs: Secondhand Smoke: An Unequal Danger. 2015. http://www.cdc.gov/vitalsigns/tobacco/.
3. National Center for Chronic Disease Prevention and Health Promotion. *US Office on Smoking and Health. The Health Consequences of Smoking—50 Years of Progress: A Report of the Surgeon General.* Atlanta, GA: Centers for Disease Control and Prevention; 2014.
4. Agency for Healthcare Research and Quality. *Treating Tobacco Use and Dependence.* Rockville, MD: Agency for Healthcare Research and Quality; 2013.
5. Committee on Environmental Health, Committee on Substance Abuse, Committee on Adolescence, Committee on Native American Child. From the American Academy of Pediatrics: policy statement: tobacco use: a pediatric disease. *Pediatrics.* 2009;124:1474-1487.
6. Moulding N, Silagy CA, Weller DP. A framework for effective management of change in clinical practice: dissemination and implementation of clinical practice guidelines. *Quality in Health Care.* 1999;8:177-183.
7. Stead LF, Hartmann-Boyce J, Perera R, Lancaster T. Telephone counselling for smoking cessation. *Cochrane Database Syst Rev.* 2013;(8):CD002850.
8. Sharifi M, Adams WG, Winickoff JP, Guo J, Reid M, Boynton-Jarrett R. Enhancing the electronic health record to increase counseling and quit-line referral for parents who smoke. *Acad Pediatr.* 2014;14:478-484.
9. Lemmens V, Oenema A, Knut IK, Brug J. Effectiveness of smoking cessation interventions among adults: a systematic review of reviews. *Eur J Cancer Prev.* 2008;17:535-544.
10. US Department of Health and Human Services. *How Tobacco Smoke Causes Disease: The Biology and Behavioral Basis for Smoking-Attributable Disease: A Report of the Surgeon General.* Atlanta, GA: U.S. Department of Health and Human Services; Centers for Disease Control and Prevention; National Center for Chronic Disease Prevention and Health Promotion, Office on Smoking and Health; 2010.
11. US Department of Health and Human Services. *Reducing Tobacco Use: A Report of the Surgeon General.* Atlanta, GA: U.S. Department of Health and Human Services; Centers for Disease Control and Prevention, National Center for Chronic Disease Prevention and Health Promotion, Office on Smoking and Health; 2000.

26 Rheumatology

Phenotypic Characterization of Juvenile Idiopathic Arthritis in African American Children

Fitzpatrick L, for the CARRA Registry Investigators (Emory Univ School of Medicine, Atlanta, GA; et al)
J Rheumatol 43:799-803, 2016

Objective.— Juvenile idiopathic arthritis (JIA) affects children of all races. Prior studies suggest that phenotypic features of JIA in African American (AA) children differ from those of non-Hispanic white (NHW) children. We evaluated the phenotypic differences at presentation between AA and NHW children enrolled in the Childhood Arthritis and Rheumatology Research Alliance (CARRA) Registry, and replicated the findings in a JIA cohort from a large center in the southeastern United States.

Methods.—Children with JIA enrolled in the multicenter CARRA Registry and from Emory University formed the study and replication cohorts. Phenotypic data on non-Hispanic AA children were compared with NHW children with JIA using the chi-square test, Fisher's exact test, and the Wilcoxon signed-rank test.

Results.—In all, 4177 NHW and 292 AA JIA cases from the CARRA Registry and 212 NHW and 71 AA cases from Emory were analyzed. AA subjects more often had rheumatoid factor (RF)-positive polyarthritis in both the CARRA (13.4% vs 4.7%, $p = 5.3 \times 10^{-7}$) and the Emory (26.8% vs 6.1%, $p = 1.1 \times 10^{-5}$) cohorts. AA children had positive tests for RF and cyclic citrullinated peptide antibodies (CCP) more frequently, but oligoarticular or early onset antinuclear antibody (ANA)-positive JIA less frequently in both cohorts. AA children were older at onset in both cohorts and this difference persisted after excluding RF-positive polyarthritis in the CARRA Registry (median age 8.5 vs 5.0 yrs, $p = 1.4 \times 10^{-8}$).

Conclusion.—Compared with NHW children, AA children with JIA are more likely to have RF/CCP-positive polyarthritis, are older at disease onset, and less likely to have oligoarticular or ANA-positive, early-onset JIA, suggesting that the JIA phenotype is different in AA children.

▶ Juvenile idiopathic arthritis (JIA) is an umbrella diagnosis encompassing a heterogeneous group of conditions, with the unifying feature of idiopathic inflammation affecting 1 or more joints for at least 6 weeks. Previous studies have reported phenotypic differences in JIA among racial and ethnic groups. This article builds on those studies by describing specific phenotypic

457

characteristics of JIA in African American children, which may have important treatment and prognostic implications. African American children with JIA had a higher prevalence of rheumatoid factor (RF) and anticyclic citrullinated peptide (CCP) antibodies, immunologic markers that predict more destructive arthritis and poorer response to therapy. Patients with these antibodies are considered at higher risk for irreversible joint damage and functional disability and may require more aggressive treatment.

This study introduces a number of recent developments in JIA that are worth reviewing. Phenotypic variation across racial and ethnic groups likely reflects the complex genetic basis of JIA. There is a growing body of literature exploring potential genetic variants associated with JIA. The most well-established genetic associations are between enthesitis-related JIA and human leukocyte antigen (HLA) B27 (also seen in adult spondyloarthritis), and RF-positive polyarticular JIA and HLA DRB1 (also seen in rheumatoid arthritis). In oligoarticular and RF-negative polyarticular JIA, a large number of potentially associated genetic loci have been described, including HLA DRB1, HLA DPB1, PTPN22, and STAT4.[1]

However, most genetic associations show only a modest effect on the risk of developing JIA, suggesting that genetics are only one of multiple factors leading to development of the disease. Given this, increasing attention is also being paid to the impact of environmental exposures on the development of JIA. There is some evidence that implies alteration of the microbiome may affect JIA risk: 2 recent studies report that antibiotic use is associated with increased risk of developing JIA,[2,3] and Stoll et al reported differences in enteric bacteria between patients with enthesitis-related JIA and healthy controls.[4] A number of other environmental factors have been proposed as having a role in the pathogenesis of JIA, including infection, smoking exposure, and lack of breastfeeding, but these have been explored only in small studies with variable results.

The current classification schema for JIA was defined by the International League of Associations for Rheumatology (ILAR) in 2011. The ILAR criteria classify JIA into 7 categories based on clinical and laboratory characteristics: oligoarticular, RF-positive polyarticular, RF-negative polyarticular, systemic-onset, psoriatic, enthesitis-related, and undifferentiated. Increasing recognition of the clinical and genetic heterogeneity described above suggests that revision of the ILAR classification criteria may be appropriate. An interesting recent study by Eng et al proposes an entirely different approach to JIA classification that incorporates immunobiologic data, including genotype and biomarkers such as circulating inflammatory cytokines, in addition to the traditional clinical characteristics and laboratory markers currently used to categorize JIA.[5] The authors applied 2 data modeling techniques, principal components analysis, and cluster analysis, to a cohort of Canadian JIA patients and describe 5 patient clusters that are more homogeneous than the ILAR categories. Because treatment of JIA is in part determined by JIA subtype, improved classification has the potential to better predict optimal therapy for a given patient, ultimately leading to improved outcomes.

K. E. Corbin, MD, MHS
E. Lawson, MD

References

1. Hersh AO, Prahalad S. Immunogenetics of juvenile idiopathic arthritis: a comprehensive review. *J Autoimmun.* 2015;64:113-124.
2. Arvonen M, Virta LJ, Pokka T, Kröger L, Vähäsalo P. Repeated exposure to antibiotics in infancy: a predisposing factor for juvenile idiopathic arthritis or a sign of this group's greater susceptibility to infections? *J Rheumatol.* 2015;42: 521-526.
3. Horton DB, Scott FI, Haynes K, et al. Antibiotic exposure and juvenile idiopathic arthritis: a case-control study. *Pediatrics.* 2015;136:e333-e343.
4. Stoll ML, Kumar R, Morrow CD, et al. Altered microbiota associated with abnormal humoral immune responses to commensal organisms in enthesitis-related arthritis. *Arthritis Res Ther.* 2014;16:486.
5. Eng SW, Duong TT, Rosenberg AM, Morris Q, Yeung RS, on behalf of the REACCH OUT and BBOP Research Consortia. The biologic basis of clinical heterogeneity in juvenile idiopathic arthritis. *Arthritis Rheum.* 2014;66: 3463-3475.

Two-year Efficacy and Safety of Etanercept in Pediatric Patients with Extended Oligoarthritis, Enthesitis-related Arthritis, or Psoriatic Arthritis
Constantin T, for the Paediatric Rheumatology International Trials Organisation (PRINTO) (Istituto G. Gaslini, Genoa, Italy)
J Rheumatol 43:816-824, 2016

Objective.—The main objective was to determine the 2-year clinical benefit and safety of etanercept (ETN) in children with the juvenile idiopathic arthritis (JIA) categories of extended oligoarthritis (eoJIA), enthesitis-related arthritis (ERA), or psoriatic arthritis (PsA).

Methods.—CLIPPER was a 96-week, phase IIIb, open-label, multicenter study. Patients with eoJIA, ERA, or PsA received ETN 0.8 mg/kg once weekly (50 mg max) for up to 96 weeks. The proportions of patients reaching the JIA American College of Rheumatology (ACR) 30/50/70/ 90/100 and inactive disease responses at Week 96 were calculated. Adverse events (AE) were collected throughout the study (intention-to-treat sample).

Results.—There were 127 patients (eoJIA n = 60, ERA n = 38, PsA n = 29) who received ≥ 1 dose of ETN. The mean disease duration was 31.6 (eoJIA), 23.0 (ERA), and 21.8 (PsA) months. At Week 96, JIA ACR 30/50/70/90/100/inactive disease responses (95% CI) were achieved by 84.3% (76.7, 90.1), 83.5% (75.8, 89.5), 78.7% (70.6, 85.5), 55.1% (46.0, 63.9), 45.7% (36.8, 54.7), and 27.6% (20.0, 36.2) of patients, respectively. The most common AE (no. events, events per 100 patient-yrs) overall were headache (23, 10.7), pyrexia (12, 5.6), and diarrhea (10, 4.6). The most common infections were upper respiratory tract infection (83, 38.6), pharyngitis (50, 23.2), gastroenteritis (22, 10.2), bronchitis (19, 8.8), and rhinitis (17, 7.9). No cases of malignancy, active tuberculosis, demyelinating disorders, or death were reported.

Conclusion.—Over 96 weeks of therapy, ETN demonstrated sustained efficacy at treating the clinical symptoms of all 3 JIA categories, with no major safety issues.

▶ Juvenile idiopathic arthritis (JIA), the most common rheumatic disease in childhood, is a chronic disease that if left uncontrolled can be debilitating.[1] JIA has various presentations and is classified into 6 subtypes. Oligoarticular arthritis, affecting 4 or fewer joints, is the most common subtype, generally seen in younger children. Patients with oligoarticular arthritis who have more than 4 affected joints after the first 6 months of diagnosis are classified as having extended oligoarticular JIA, whereas those who continue to have 4 or fewer affected joints throughout their disease course are classified as having persistent oligoarticular JIA. Polyarticular JIA affects 5 or more joints and is separated into 2 subtypes depending on the presence or absence of rheumatoid factor, which confers a higher risk for erosive joint disease. Enthesitis-related arthritis affects primarily axial joints such as hips and the spine as well as entheses, the bony attachment sites of ligaments or tendons. Psoriatic arthritis is characterized by the presence of psoriasis in the patient or a first-degree relative, along with dactylitis and nail changes. Systemic JIA is an autoinflammatory condition in which patients present with arthritis and quotidian fevers along with some combination of characteristic rash, serositis, and generalized lymphadenopathy. Patients who do not meet criteria for any particular subtype or who meet criteria for more than one are characterized as having undifferentiated JIA.

The evolution and availability of biologics has helped make JIA a controllable disease. For pediatric rheumatologists, clinical trial data, practice styles, availability of medications, and insurance approval all play roles in deciding which biologics to choose for patients with JIA. We are also cautious and considerate of the possible adverse events or side effects about which we must give guidance to our patients.

The initial studies of anti–tumor necrosis factor (anti-TNF) agents in children focused on patients with the polyarticular subtype of JIA, despite the fact that polyarticular JIA represents only a small percentage of all JIA patients. Thus, current US Food and Drug Administration–approved indications for anti-TNF medications such as etanercept are only for polyarticular JIA. Pediatric rheumatologists caring for children with other subtypes of JIA have little clinical trial data upon which to base treatment decisions. More recently, studies using anti-TNF agents in other JIA subtypes are being published.

The study by Constantin et al is one of the largest etanercept studies to report prospective long-term efficacy and safety data in patients with the JIA categories of extended oligoarthritis, enthesitis-related arthritis, and psoriatic arthritis. The JIA American College of Rheumatology (ACR) 30/50/70/90/100 criteria is a comprehensive tool used to determine efficacy and clinical response in clinical drug trials based on the percentage of improvement of various core set measures. The ACR Pediatric 30 uses 6 core set variables (physician global assessment of disease activity, patient or parent global assessment of disease impact, number of joints with active arthritis, number of joints with loss of motion, validated measures of physical function, and laboratory measure of acute inflammation). At least 3 of the 6 variables must improve by ≥30% with no more than 1 of the 6 core set variable worsening by less than 30%. The US Food and Drug Administration suggests that 3-month trials using JIA ACR-30 criteria are sufficient to establish efficacy in reduction of signs and symptoms. The authors found that etanercept was not just effective in allowing most patients to reach ACR-30 in the first 12 weeks but also over a 96-week period. Importantly, most patients in all 3 subtypes maintained an ACR 70 response over the 96-week trial. Additionally, approximately 20% of patients in all subtypes achieved completely inactive disease by 96 weeks.

Low patient dropout rates and minimal adverse effects were found throughout all 3 subtypes. Known risks of anti-TNF agents include infections, the development of other autoimmune conditions, and malignancy. Many of the adverse events in this study, including frequent upper respiratory tract infections, are comparable to what is seen in practice. Only a few cases of inflammatory eye disease were reported. Three cases of Crohn disease developed, all in patients with enthesitis-related arthritis. One case was felt to be related to anti-TNF therapy; the other 2 cases were likely part of the patients' underlying disease, as the arthritis seen in enthesitis-related arthritis is on the same spectrum of arthritis seen in inflammatory bowel disease. No cases of malignancy, tuberculosis, demyelinating disease, or death were reported.

It is common to use disease-modifying antirheumatic drugs (DMARDs) like methotrexate in JIA patients before initiating TNF inhibitors and, if adequate response is not seen, to continue a DMARD once a biologic is added. The efficacy of the combination of various DMARDs and anti-TNF therapy is not well studied. In this study, concomitant therapy with one other agent, including methotrexate, hydroxychloroquine, chloroquine, or sulfasalazine, was permitted. It would have been interesting to display particular results for each concomitant therapy with etanercept and its efficacy in each particular JIA subtype. There were likely not enough patients to power any of these analyses. It is also common to switch biologic agents if the initial biologic therapy has failed; these particular patients were not included in the study.

Despite some limitations, this study clearly showed the efficacy and safety of etanercept in certain nonpolyarticular JIA patients, giving pediatric rheumatologists published data to cite when seeking approval for medications. More studies of this sort are needed to support medication management options for the complete spectrum of JIA subtypes.

A. Thakral, MD
M. Curran, MD

Reference

1. Minden K, Niewerth M, Listing J, Biedermann T, Schontube M, Zink A. Burden and cost of illness in patients with juvenile idiopathic arthritis. *Ann Rheum Dis.* 2004;63:836-842.

Prednisone versus prednisone plus ciclosporin versus prednisone plus methotrexate in new-onset juvenile dermatomyositis: a randomised trial

Ruperto N, for the Paediatric Rheumatology International Trials Organisation (PRINTO) (Istituto Giannina Gaslini, Genoa, Italy; et al)
Lancet 387:671-678, 2016

Background.—Most data for treatment of dermatomyositis and juvenile dermatomyositis are from anecdotal, nonrandomised case series. We aimed to compare, in a randomised trial, the efficacy and safety of prednisone alone with that of prednisone plus either methotrexate or ciclosporin in children with new-onset juvenile dermatomyositis.

Methods.—We did a randomised trial at 54 centres in 22 countries. We enrolled patients aged 18 years or younger with new-onset juvenile dermatomyositis who had received no previous treatment and did not have cutaneous or gastrointestinal ulceration. We randomly allocated 139 patients via a computer-based system to prednisone alone or in combination with either ciclosporin or methotrexate. We did not mask patients or investigators to treatment assignments. Our primary outcomes were the proportion of patients achieving a juvenile dermatomyositis PRINTO 20 level of improvement (20% improvement in three of six core set variables at 6 months), time to clinical remission, and time to treatment failure. We compared the three treatment groups with the Kruskal-Wallis test and Friedman's test, and we analysed survival with Kaplan-Meier curves and the log-rank test. Analysis was by intention to treat. Here, we present results after at least 2 years of treatment (induction and maintenance phases). This trial is registered with ClinicalTrials.gov, number NCT00323960.

Findings.—Between May 31, 2006, and Nov 12, 2010, 47 patients were randomly assigned prednisone alone, 46 were allocated prednisone plus ciclosporin, and 46 were randomised prednisone plus methotrexate. Median duration of follow-up was $35 \cdot 5$ months. At month 6, 24 (51%) of 47 patients assigned prednisone, 32 (70%) of 46 allocated prednisone plus ciclosporin, and 33 (72%) of 46 administered prednisone plus methotrexate achieved a juvenile dermatomyositis PRINTO 20 improvement ($p = 0 \cdot 0228$). Median time to clinical remission was $41 \cdot 9$ months in patients assigned prednisone plus methotrexate but was not observable in the other two treatment groups ($2 \cdot 45$ fold [95% CI $1 \cdot 2 - 5 \cdot 0$] increase with prednisone plus methotrexate; $p = 0 \cdot 012$). Median time to treatment failure was $16 \cdot 7$ months in patients allocated prednisone, $53 \cdot 3$ months in those assigned prednisone plus ciclosporin, but was not observable in patients randomised to prednisone plus methotrexate ($1 \cdot 95$ fold [95% CI $1 \cdot 20 - 3 \cdot 15$] increase with prednisone; $p = 0 \cdot 009$). Median time to prednisone discontinuation was $35 \cdot 8$ months with prednisone alone compared with $29 \cdot 4 - 29 \cdot 7$ months in the combination groups ($p = 0 \cdot 002$). A significantly greater proportion of patients assigned prednisone plus ciclosporin had adverse events, affecting the skin and subcutaneous tissues, gastrointestinal system, and general disorders. Infections and infestations were significantly increased in patients assigned prednisone plus ciclosporin and prednisone plus methotrexate. No patients died during the study.

Interpretation.—Combined treatment with prednisone and either ciclosporin or methotrexate was more effective than prednisone alone. The safety profile and steroid-sparing effect favoured the combination of prednisone plus methotrexate.

▶ Juvenile dermatomyositis (JDMS) is an inflammatory myositis that most commonly presents with characteristic inflammation of skin and muscle. Pediatric patients with JDMS can present with a wide spectrum of illness varying from subtle rash and weakness to more profound symptoms including ulcerative skin and gastrointestinal disease as well as severe muscle involvement, resulting in widespread weakness and resulting in difficulty swallowing, talking, breathing, and walking. Fortunately, corticosteroids are an effective therapy for the majority of patients with JDMS. However, the potential for severe short- and long-term side effects of corticosteroids, particularly when given at high doses, has led to a search for steroid-sparing therapies to be used in combination with corticosteroids for both induction and maintenance treatment of JDMS. In some patients with JDMS, it can take months to years to achieve remission, which can lead to significant cumulative exposure to corticosteroids.

Is this article, Ruperto and colleagues report on a sentinel randomized control trial for the treatment of new-onset JDMS.[1] The trial was performed in 54 centers in 22 countries largely across Europe, Latin American, and South America. In this study, 139 pediatric patients (< 18 years of age) with new-onset JDMS were randomized to receive prednisone (corticosteroids) alone, prednisone plus ciclosporin or prednisone plus methotrexate. Methotrexate and ciclosporin are steroid-sparing medications that have been used successfully for the past several decades for the treatment of JDMS and other related autoimmune conditions. A 2010 survey study conducted by the Childhood Arthritis and Rheumatology Research Alliance (CARRA) found that corticosteroids plus methotrexate was the most common combination of medications used for typical cases of JDMS treated by North American rheumatologists.[2] The evolution of this practice has been guided largely by experience and not by data collected in a randomized or prospective fashion.

Fortunately, the results of the study by Ruperto et al reflect what has been observed in clinical practice. Subjects on prednisone alone performed less well on all of the primary outcomes (level of improvement in the Pediatric Rheumatology International Trials Organization (PRINTO) 20 (20% improvement in 3 of 6 core set variables at 6 months), time to clinical remission, and treatment failure) than subjects treated with combination therapy. Subjects on prednisone plus methotrexate had the highest percentage achieving a PRINTO 20. It was the only group with a measurable time to clinical remission (41.9 months) and where a median time to treatment failure was not observed. When comparing the prednisone plus methotrexate to the prednisone plus ciclosporin group, a significantly higher percentage of subjects in the prednisone plus ciclosporin group had adverse events. Infections and infestations were more common in the subjects treated with methotrexate or ciclosporin in addition to prednisone. In all 3 groups, there was a substantial number of treatment failures leading to change in treatments, loss to follow-up, or withdrawal from the study. This observation is not altogether surprising given the potentially unpredictable nature of this condition and how common medication changes are when treating JDMS patients outside of the context of a clinical trial.

Although the results were not unexpected, this trial is important to the field of pediatric rheumatology for several reasons. First, this trial is, to my knowledge, the first randomized control study performed for JDMS. These types of studies are crucial in our field where treatment decisions are often made based on historical practice or personal or expert experience. Second, to conduct a randomized control trial for a disease like JDMS, which is diagnosed with relative infrequency, the authors used PRINTO, an international research network that now includes 550 centers across 60 countries (www.printo.it). By leveraging this network, they were able to achieve enrollment goals over a relatively short recruitment time period of 3.5 years.

Having adequate numbers in each treatment group resulted in the publication of meaningful and interpretable study data without significant limitations. It is the commitment of the international pediatric rheumatology to the development of PRINTO, and similar research networks (eg, the Pediatric Rheumatology Collaborative Study Group [PRCSG] and the Childhood Arthritis and Rheumatology Research Alliance [CARRA]) that has enabled collaborative research in the treatment and outcomes of conditions such as JDMS. Through these networks, new trials and comparative effectiveness studies of other promising treatments for JDMS (eg, intravenous immunoglobulin, rituximab, abatacept) will emerge and will undoubtedly continue to improve health outcomes and quality of life for pediatric patients with rare rheumatic conditions.

A. Hersh, MD

References

1. Ruperto N, Pistorio A, Oliveira S, et al. Prednisone versus prednisone plus ciclosporin versus prednisone plus methotrexate in new-onset juvenile dermatomyositis: a randomised trial. *Lancet.* 2016;387:671-678.
2. Stringer E, Bohnsack J, Bowyer SL, et al. Treatment approaches to juvenile dermatomyositis (JDM) across North America: the childhood arthritis and rheumatology research alliance (CARRA) JDM treatment survey. *J Rheumatol.* 2010;37: 1953-1961.

Efficacy and safety of treatments in Familial Mediterranean fever: a systematic review
Demirkaya E, Erer B, Ozen S, et al (Gülhane Military Med Faculty, Ankara, Turkey; Istanbul Univ, Turkey; Hacettepe Univ, Ankara, Turkey; et al)
Rheumatol Int 36:325-331, 2016

Familial Mediterranean fever (FMF) is an autoinflammatory disease, which can be well controlled with lifelong use of colchicine. Since studies dealing with the efficacy and safety of colchicine were conducted mainly in the sixties and seventies of the previous century, it seems that this topic needs to be updated. Recently, an international expert panel was undertaken for the establishment of recommendations on how to manage FMF. We aimed to summarize the efficacy and safety of the current treatments available to prevent FMF attacks and to avert the appearance of amyloidosis secondary to FMF. A systematic review was performed. Two reviewers and methodologist established the protocol of the review and the epidemiological questions in PICO terms. MEDLINE through PubMed, Embase, and Cochrane Central Trials Register all up to May 31, 2014, were searched, and only randomized controlled trials or quasi-controlled trials were accepted. For each study, a judgment on risk of bias was then rated as high, moderate, or low. Of 1222 initially captured publications, 153 articles were studied in detail. Finally, only seven studies met all criteria and were included. Among these seven studies, four were randomized crossover clinical trials of colchicine including a total of 57 patients, one RCT of *Andrographis paniculata* Herba Nees extract employed in 24 patients, one randomized crossover clinical trial of Rilonacept used in 12 patients, and one RCT of interferon treating 34 acute abdominal attacks in 22 patients. The quality of the colchicine trials was low compared with the other drugs trials. Safety was not clearly mentioned in the trials. Colchicine is an effective treatment in FMF.

▶ Familial Mediterranean fever (FMF) is the archetype and the first discovered (the gene was found in 1997) monogenic autoinflammatory disease. Patients develop, usually during the first decade of life, recurrent and self-limiting episodes of fever, serositis (abdominal, chest, and testicular pain), arthritis, and often erysipelas-like rash in the lower extremity, lasting 1 to 3 days. Untreated patients are at risk of developing amyloidosis, usually with proteinuria as the first manifestation, leading to the nephrotic syndrome and renal failure. It is estimated that there are between 120 000 and 150 000 patients worldwide with FMF (~2000 in the United States), mainly among Sephardic Jews, Turks, Armenians, Arabs, and other Mediterranean populations. This number may be an underestimation based on recent discoveries of FMF in East Asian populations previously not "counted" as those at risk.

There are 3 potential objectives of treating this lifelong disease: (1) aborting, shortening, or easing attacks; (2) preventing attacks; and (3) preventing amyloidosis.

In 1972, Stephen E. Goldfinger, MD, published a Letter to the Editor in the *New England Journal of Medicine*. The letter described the benefit of colchicine in preventing FMF attacks among 5 patients with FMF and this report revolutionized the treatment of FMF.[1] We often tell our students and colleagues that this letter may have saved more lives (and kidneys) than any letter sent to a medical journal in the modern era.

The paper by Demerkaya et al summarizes the strength of the evidence of treating FMF based on the review of 7 controlled studies out of more than 1000 treatment studies. The primary outcome measure in 6 studies was the frequency of attacks. In 1 study, the primary outcome was the abortion of attacks. Multiple outcomes, including quality of life, were examined only in 1 study. Per the criteria employed in the study, only 1 study was considered of Level 1 quality, and all 4 colchicine studies, from the 1970s (!), were of small sample size and poor quality.

However, the strength of the results of the reviewed studies as well as numerous other studies conducted over more than 40 years of follow-up (many were good-quality cohort studies that should not be disregarded even if not controlled), have strongly established colchicine as the cornerstone of FMF therapy. These studies have shown that colchicine not only prevents attacks in most patients (completely in approximately 60% and > 50% decrease in another ∼ 30%) but also prevents amyloidosis, even among nonresponders. Furthermore, prospective studies have established the good long-term safety profile of colchicine, including among children and pregnant women.[2]

Unfortunately, between 5% and 10% of patients are nonresponders, many as a result of noncompliance, and another 5% to 10% are intolerant, mainly due to gastrointestinal adverse effects. Until recently, there were no good alternatives, although numerous medications were tested. Breakthroughs in deciphering the role of pyrin, the mutated protein in FMF, in the regulation of the innate immune system and the inflammsome (a complex of proteins that activates caspases) has led to the understanding that interleukin (IL)-1 plays an important role in the pathogenesis of FMF.

It was since shown, first in case reports/series, then in open-label studies, that led to controlled studies, that IL-1 inhibitors have a remarkable effect (with relative safety) on decreasing the attack frequency and improving the quality of life of the vast majority (there are rare nonresponders) of patients with severe disease not responsive or intolerant to colchicine. There are few case reports showing that IL-1 inhibition was even able to reverse the effects of amyloidosis on the kidney. Demerkaya et al reported only on the controlled study of rilonacept but the results of controlled studies on the other IL-1 inhibitors are expected shortly. IL-1 inhibition has already become standard of care for these patients.[3] There are currently 3 IL-1 inhibitors on the market: (1) anakinra, an IL-1 receptor antagonist, with a very short half-life, given by daily subcutaneous (SC) injection; (2) rilonacept, a soluble IL-1 receptor, which "traps" IL-1, given by weekly SC injection; and (3) canakinumab, a humanized Il-1β antibody, with a very long half-life, given by SC injection every 4 weeks.

It does appear, however, that all FMF medications (including colchicine, with the exception of the small study quoted in this review; interferon-α; and even IL-1 inhibitors) are not effective in shortening attacks once these are established, although attacks are often milder with therapy. Thus, we again emphasize the role of colchicine in FMF as a "prophylactic" medication, preventing both attacks and amyloidosis. The use of intermittent colchicine only during attacks is not the standard of care.

Despite the remarkable efficacy of IL-1 inhibitors it is still necessary to continue treatment with colchicine, still the only agent proven to prevent amyloidosis. However likely, it may take many years of long-term follow-up to assess whether IL-1 inhibitors are independently able to prevent amyloidosis.

One important point made by the authors that is crucial in assessing the efficacy of future biologic/advanced therapies is to achieve consensus on defining those patients needing these therapies (ie, stratifying patients by severity of their disease, defining nonresponse to colchicine, and agreeing on clear and meaningful outcome measures).

From the study of Demerkaya et al, it is clear that despite our excitement on being able to help the most severe FMF patients with biologic modifiers the cornerstone of FMF therapy for the vast majority of patients will remain the "old" medicine, colchicine.

M. Heshin-Bekenstein, MD

P. J. Hashkes, MD, MSc, RhMSUS

References

1. Goldfinger SE. Colchicine for familial Mediterranean fever. *N Engl J Med.* 1972; 287:1302.
2. Padeh S, Gerstein M, Berkun Y. Colchicine is a safe drug in children with familial Mediterranean fever. *J Pediatr.* 2012;161:1142-1146.
3. Hentgen V, Grateau G, Kone-Paut I, et al. Evidence-based recommendations for the practical management of familial Mediterranean fever. *Semin Arthritis Rheum.* 2013;43:387-391.

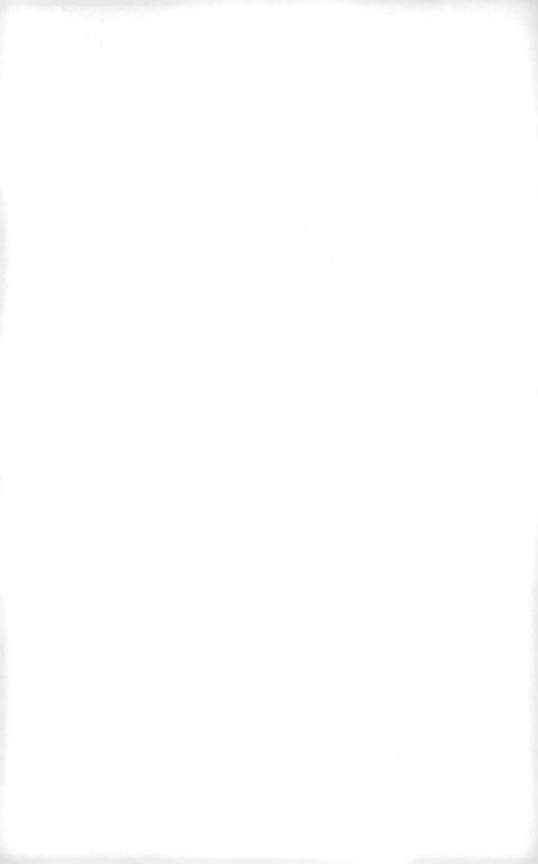

27 Therapeutics and Toxicology

Elevated Blood Lead Levels in Children Associated With the Flint Drinking Water Crisis: A Spatial Analysis of Risk and Public Health Response
Hanna-Attisha M, LaChance J, Sadler RC, et al (Hurley Children's Hosp/ Michigan State Univ College of Human Medicine, Flint; Hurley Med Ctr Res, Flint, MI; Michigan State Univ College of Human Medicine, Flint)
Am J Public Health 106:283-290, 2016

Objectives.—We analyzed differences in pediatric elevated blood lead level incidence before and after Flint, Michigan, introduced a more corrosive water source into an aging water system without adequate corrosion control.

Methods.—We reviewed blood lead levels for children younger than 5 years before (2013) and after (2015) water source change in Greater Flint, Michigan. We assessed the percentage of elevated blood lead levels in both time periods, and identified geographical locations through spatial analysis.

Results.—Incidence of elevated blood lead levels increased from 2.4% to 4.9% ($P < .05$) after water source change, and neighborhoods with the highest water lead levels experienced a 6.6% increase. No significant change was seen outside the city. Geospatial analysis identified disadvantaged neighborhoods as having the greatest elevated blood lead level increases and informed response prioritization during the now-declared public health emergency.

Conclusions.—The percentage of children with elevated blood lead levels increased after water source change, particularly in socioeconomically disadvantaged neighborhoods. Water is a growing source of childhood lead exposure because of aging infrastructure.

▶ It is unfortunate that it takes a public health emergency to call attention to critical public health issues. Dr. Hanna-Attisha and coauthors highlight the narrative of hundreds of young children in Flint, Michigan, who were exposed to lead following the corrosion of the metal from water pipes due to a shift in the water supply from Lake Huron to the Flint River. Exposure to lead, a known neurotoxin, can adversely affect the behavioral and developmental health of young children. This timely study from Flint has underscored the importance of lead in drinking water.

In the recent past, the majority of lead exposure was from lead in paint or gasoline. Fortunately, bans on lead-based paint and leaded gasoline have led to reductions in the numbers of children in the United States with elevated blood lead levels. As this article points out, however, an aging drinking water infrastructure calls pediatricians and public health officials to consider drinking water as a possible exposure to lead. Although lead was banned from many drinking water plumbing materials starting in1986, it was not completely banned from lead in brass until 2014.

The American Academy of Pediatrics recommends serum-based lead screening for at-risk children at 1 and 2 years of age, a time when children are more mobile and capable of putting lead-containing paint chips, dust, soil, toys, or candies in their mouths. Screening at this older age will miss a critical timeframe of exposure for young infants who may be drinking formula constituted from lead-contaminated tap water. Indeed, because young infants are consuming so much water in formula relative to their body size, they are at greatest risk for lead-related health impacts. The Centers for the Disease Control and Prevention simply assumes that the Environmental Protection Agency (EPA) Lead and Copper Rule is protecting these children—an assumption that has proven to be without basis in Flint and many other US cities.

So what guidance can clinicians provide to families of young children who are concerned about exposure to lead in drinking water after hearing about the case in Flint?

In the majority of US homes water is supplied through public water suppliers. The first recommended step in identifying exposure to lead in drinking water is to examine the public water supplier report for elevated lead levels, but unfortunately these reports may not be accurate because utilities like those in Flint, Michigan, are sampling in ways that miss lead in water risks. It is also important to know if the home has a lead service line connection, or has leaded materials—but unfortunately city records on service line materials are often in error.

Families may want to consider testing drinking water for lead using a laboratory that is certified by the Environmental Protection Agency, particularly if homes are old, have lead pipes, or show signs of decay.[1] Unfortunately, we now know that a single measurement of low lead is not conclusive proof that water is safe. Clearly, there is a lot to be concerned about given the uncertainty regarding identification of lead in drinking water, which is why lead in water is in the news.

Many families may forgo testing and implement mitigation strategies instead. If there is a high risk of lead service lines or exposure to lead in drinking water, pediatric providers should recommend the following: (1) flushing or running water lines prior to use (especially after periods of not using water) and (2) using NSF-certified lead filters to reduce lead exposure.[2] This is certainly the case for all families preparing infant formula in homes that might have lead service pipes. Of course, the EPA also recommends that hot tap water should not be used to make infant formula.

As many infants and children spend substantial time in child care facilities and schools, it is important to also consider exposure to lead in these settings. Currently no federal laws require testing of drinking water sources for lead in schools or child care. Pediatric providers can help decrease lead exposure among children by advocating for changes in these laws and by providing families with resources to ensure the accessibility of safe drinking water in these settings.[3]

A. I. Patel, MD, MSPH, MSHS

M. A. Edwards, PhD, MS

References

1. United States Environmental Protection Agency. Contact Information for Certification Programs and Certified Laboratories for Drinking Water. https://www.epa.gov/dwlabcert/contact-information-certification-programs-and-certified-laboratories-drinking-water. Accessed March 20, 2016.
2. NSF International. Search for NSF Certified Drinking Water Treatment Units, Water Filters. http://info.nsf.org/Certified/DWTU/. Accessed March 20, 2016.
3. California Food Policy Advocates. Parents Making Waves. A Toolkit for Promoting Drinking Water in Schools. http://waterinschools.org/parents-making-waves/. Accessed March 20, 2016.

Exposure to select phthalates and phenols through use of personal care products among Californian adults and their children

Philippat C, Bennett D, Calafat AM, et al (Univ of California, Davis; Ctrs for Disease Control and Prevention, Atlanta, GA)

Environ Res 140:369-376, 2015

Introduction.—Certain phenols and phthalates are used in many consumer products including personal care products (PCPs).

Aims.—We aimed to study the associations between the use of PCPs and urinary concentrations of biomarkers of select phenols and phthalates among Californian adults and their children. As an additional aim we compared phenols and phthalate metabolites concentrations measured in adults and children urine samples collected the same day.

Method.—Our study relied on a subsample of 90 adult–child pairs participating in the Study of Use of Products and Exposure Related Behavior (SUPERB). Each adult and child provided one to two urine samples in which we measured concentrations of selected phenols and phthalate metabolites. We computed Spearman correlation coefficients to compare concentrations measured in adults and children urine samples collected the same day. We used adjusted linear and Tobit regression models to study the associations between the use of PCPs in the past 24 h and biomarker concentrations.

Results.—Benzophenone-3 and parabens concentrations were higher in adults compared to their children. Conversely children had higher mono-*n*-butyl phthalate and mono-isobutyl phthalate concentrations. No significant difference was observed for the other compounds. The total number of different PCPs used was positively associated with urinary concentrations of methyl, propyl and butyl parabens and the main metabolite of diethyl phthalate in adults. Among children, the use of a few specific products including liquid soap, haircare products and sunscreen was positively associated with urinary concentrations of some phenols or phthalate metabolites.

Discussion.—These results strengthen the body of evidence suggesting that use of PCPs is an important source of exposure to parabens and diethyl phthalate in adults and provide data on exposure to selected phenols and phthalates through use of PCPs in children (Table 3).

▶ Phenols and phthalates are classes of synthetic chemicals that are found in many consumer products including personal care products (PCPs). This use results in a high potential for widespread exposure. The primary roles of these chemicals in PCPs are antibacterial agents, preservatives, plasticizers, and fixatives. Evidence is emerging from human and animal studies that these chemicals are associated with significant health outcomes including neurodevelopmental disorders, endocrine disruption, reproductive health, and respiratory health.

If these associations are confirmed, it will be important to understand how to avoid or minimize exposure. Therefore, a better understanding of effects of exposure to different sources will help investigators develop interventions. In this study, the investigators aimed to evaluate the relationship between self-reported, recent PCP use (previous 24 hours) and urinary concentrations (biologic markers of exposure) of phthalate and phenol metabolites in children and their parents. The investigators also explored within-subject correlation between samples collected 1 year apart.

The investigators reported that the adults in this California sample were primarily female (90%) and well educated (72% associates degree or higher). The children were on average 5.6 years old and evenly split by sex (49% female). The most frequently used PCPs in adults were toothpaste (100%), liquid soap (88%), and deodorant (74%-76%) compared with toothpaste (98%), liquid soap (86-88%), and shampoo (34-37%) in children. Urinary concentrations were greater than the limit of detection in greater than 90% of samples for all metabolites other than triclosan and butylparaben, confirming extensive measureable levels of exposure. The concentrations were not normally distributed, so the investigators log transformed the markers. The investigators reported correlations of the different metabolites and evaluated adjusted associations between reported number of PCPs used and biomarker concentrations for children and adults, presented in extensive tables in the article (Table 3). The comparison of levels between children and adults showed potential differences in exposure (ie, different PCPs used by adults compared with children) based on difference in biomarker concentrations. They also found that several of the metabolites were associated with increased total reported numbers of PCPs used. Temporal variability (>1 year) for adults was low for a few of the metabolites but higher for others. The correlations were lower in children showing more temporal variability.

There were many limitations to this study. Primary limitations include small sample size, nonrepresentative sample, no dose response information collected (only reported use of a product, not the amount used or amount of chemical in the products), not much variation in the reported use of some products

TABLE 3.—Adjusted Associations Between the Use of Specific PCPs and Phenol and Phthalate Metabolite Urinary Concentrations Among Children (n = 83, SUPERB Study, 1st and 2nd Study Visit, 2007–2009)

	Benzophenone-3		Triclosan		Methyl Paraben		Propyl Paraben		Butyl Paraben		Monoethyl Phthalate		Mono-n-Butylphthalate		Mono-Isobutyl Phthalate	
	Ratio	95% IC	Ratio	95% IC	Ratio	95% IC	Ratio	95% IC	Ratio	95% IC	Ratio	95% IC	Ratio	95% IC	Ratio	95% IC
Number of PCPs used																
≤ 3[a]																
3–5	1.13	[0.75; 1.70]	0.95	[0.61; 1.47]	0.85	[0.58; 1.26]	1.07	[0.73; 1.56]	1.27	[0.78; 2.06]	0.80	[0.55; 1.16]	0.81	[0.58; 1.13]	0.79	[0.56; 1.12]
5–10	1.22	[0.75; 1.98]	0.97	[0.57; 1.65]	1.19	[0.76; 1.88]	1.36	[0.88; 2.12]	1.34	[0.77; 2.32]	1.07	[0.69; 1.67]	0.72	[0.50; 1.06]	0.86	[0.57; 1.29]
Number of scented PCPs used																
≤ 2[a]																
2–3	0.82	[0.53; 1.26]	1.45	[0.90; 2.34]	0.75	[0.49; 1.14]	0.67	[0.45; 0.99]	0.71	[0.42; 1.18]	1.40	[0.94; 2.09]	0.74	[0.52; 1.06]	0.89	[0.61; 1.28]
3–8	1.10	[0.72; 1.69]	1.23	[0.78; 1.95]	1.10	[0.73; 1.63]	1.28	[0.87; 1.87]	1.19	[0.74; 1.92]	1.35	[0.92; 1.99]	0.96	[0.69; 1.35]	1.28	[0.90; 1.83]
Shampoo	1.26	[0.86; 1.85]	0.86	[0.56; 1.32]	0.80	[0.56; 1.15]	1.17	[0.82; 1.67]	0.97	[0.63; 1.51]	1.04	[0.73; 1.50]	0.98	[0.73; 1.33]	1.21	[0.87; 1.67]
Other haircare products[b]	0.94	[0.61; 1.43]	1.15	[0.72; 1.83]	0.86	[0.58; 1.27]	1.02	[0.69; 1.51]	1.74	[1.09; 2.76]	0.93	[0.63; 1.38]	0.93	[0.67; 1.29]	1.30	[0.91; 1.85]
Bar soap	0.61	[0.41; 0.90]	0.87	[0.56; 1.37]	0.65	[0.45; 0.94]	0.79	[0.55; 1.15]	0.49	[0.32; 0.77]	0.93	[0.64; 1.35]	1.09	[0.79; 1.51]	0.93	[0.66; 1.31]
Liquid soap	1.47	[0.91; 2.37]	1.23	[0.72; 2.08]	0.94	[0.59; 1.49]	0.76	[0.49; 1.18]	1.46	[0.82; 2.59]	1.65	[1.07; 2.56]	0.99	[0.67; 1.46]	1.13	[0.75; 1.71]
Hand sanitizer	0.71	[0.48; 1.06]	0.98	[0.64; 1.51]	1.30	[0.89; 1.90]	1.01	[0.70; 1.47]	1.21	[0.75; 1.95]	0.83	[0.57; 1.19]	0.78	[0.56; 1.08]	0.66	[0.47; 0.93]
Hand/body lotion	1.05	[0.62; 1.76]	0.92	[0.53; 1.60]	1.11	[0.68; 1.82]	0.97	[0.60; 1.57]	0.74	[0.40; 1.37]	0.66	[0.41; 1.06]	0.78	[0.51; 1.19]	1.01	[0.65; 1.58]
Chapstick/lipbalm	0.90	[0.56; 1.44]	1.11	[0.67; 1.85]	1.25	[0.79; 1.96]	1.10	[0.71; 1.71]	0.91	[0.52; 1.60]	0.98	[0.64; 1.52]	0.91	[0.62; 1.35]	0.93	[0.62; 1.40]
Suntan lotion	3.10	[1.83; 5.25]	1.24	[0.68; 2.26]	1.91	[1.14; 3.18]	1.39	[0.84; 2.30]	1.68	[0.89; 3.18]	0.77	[0.47; 1.26]	1.63	[1.05; 2.54]	1.40	[0.88; 2.22]

We reported the adjusted ratio of the bionmarker concentrations in exposed and unexposed subjects (exponential of the beta coefficient). Our models were adjusted for participant sex, age, education level and race of the adult, creatinine concentration and the total number of other personal care products used, not counting the one being examined. Analysis restricted to PCPs used by at least 5 subjects.

[a]Reference category.

[b]Includes hair conditioner, gel, spray and mouse.

Reprinted from Philippat C, Bennett D, Calafat AM, et al. Exposure to select phthalates and phenols through use of personal care products among Californian adults and their children. *Environ Res.* 2015;140:369-376, with permission from Elsevier.

(toothpaste, 100%), no collection of brand information for PCPs, potential exposure misclassification due to report of exposure, and limitations of short half-life of the metabolites affecting levels that were collected, among others.

Despite the limitations, this study has several important findings. First, investigators found that their questionnaire data may be a broad surrogate indicator of exposures in adults, but they were not as useful in children. Possible reasons for poor performance in children are the differences and types of PCPs used, although it could also have been weaknesses in their survey. A second key finding is that PCPs are possibly a significant contributor of exposure to some phenols, parabens, and phthalates in both adults and children, but additional research is needed to clarify the relationships. A third key finding is that there was weak correlation of the metabolites over repeated measures (1 year apart) suggesting variability in exposures over time.

Although this study did not evaluate health effects, the findings have some clinical implications. It found widespread measurable levels of exposure, suggesting most of the study population was being exposed, and PCP use was associated with many of the phthalate and phenol metabolites. If studies continue to show health effects of exposure to phthalates and phenols, reduction in use of PCPs containing these chemicals, improved labeling of PCPs to increase consumer awareness, or policy changes to remove of these chemicals from PCPs could be feasible ways to minimize exposure.

R. Gilden, PhD, RN
A. Spanier, MD, PhD, MPH, FAAP

Serial Free Bisphenol A and Bisphenol A Glucuronide Concentrations in Neonates

Nachman RM, Fox SD, Golden WC, et al (Johns Hopkins Bloomberg School of Public Health, Baltimore, MD; Frederick Natl Laboratory for Cancer Res, MD; Johns Hopkins Univ School of Medicine, Baltimore, MD)
J Pediatr 167:64-69, 2015

Objective.—To determine the balance of metabolism of free bisphenol A (BPA) to the inactive conjugate, BPA glucuronide (BPAG), in neonates.

Study Design.—Free BPA and BPAG concentrations were measured in 78 urine samples collected between December 2012 and August 2013 from a cohort of 44 healthy full term ($\geq$37 weeks' gestation) neonates at 2 intervals (3-6 days and 7-27 days of age). A questionnaire was administered at the time of sample collection. Neonates recruited into the study were born in an urban, tertiary care hospital.

Results.—Only BPAG was detected in the urine samples; concentrations ranged from <0.1 μg/L to 11.21 μg/L (median: 0.27 μg/L). Free BPA concentrations were below the limit of quantification of 0.1 μg/L. Age, but not sex or type of diet, was significantly associated with urinary BPAG concentration ($P = .002$).

Conclusions.—Our results illustrate widespread BPA exposure in healthy full-term neonates and efficient conjugation of BPA to its readily excretable and biologically inactive form (BPAG) as early as 3 days of age. Factors other than type of diet may be important contributors to BPA exposure in neonates.

▶ Bisphenol A (BPA) was synthesized by the Russian chemist Aleksandr Dianin in 1891. Many years later, it was identified as the basis for a polymer that made plastics hard. Given the ever accelerating American lifestyle, polycarbonate plastics came into use in water bottles, aluminum cans, as well as thermal paper (where BPA is used as a developer to facilitate printing receipts). Of note, when diethylstilbestrol (DES) was being developed as a pharmaceutical estrogen to treat pregnant women and prevent miscarriage, BPA was considered but was not sufficiently potent.

It would take many years after that initial warning before the US Food and Drug Administration (FDA) would ban BPA from baby bottles and sippy cups, but indeed it is still used in aluminum cans. That said, as increasing concerns arise about a diverse array of health effects, including on neurodevelopment, asthma and obesity in children, many manufacturers are shifting to an alphabet soup of bisphenols: F, S, Z, and SIP, among other alternatives. Unfortunately, because of the flawed Toxic Substances Control Act (TSCA) of 1976, toxicity testing data was not required to prove safety for these newer alternatives, and early data suggest that these alternatives are as estrogenic and toxic to embryos as BPA.

The present study examined only BPA and measured urinary BPA, identifying that the liver develops a capacity to detoxify BPA by glucuronidating it. Does that mean BPA in newborns is not a problem? Not at all. Although BPA is thought to have a half-life of 1 to 2 days, it is lipid soluble, and BPA levels in urine do not decline with fasting in the expected time line, suggesting that other compartments such as fat can store BPA and prolong half-life. Indeed, BPA can cause oxidant stress, make fat cells bigger, and, as an estrogen, even short-term exposures can be problematic at important developmental windows of vulnerability. There is novelty in BPA-glucuronide (BPA-G) measurement, and most studies have chosen not to measure free BPA and BPA-G separately because of contamination concerns.

The study by Nachman and colleagues is limited to a single center, and genetic variability may contribute to differential glucuronidation. Arbuckle and colleagues[1] were among the first to document BPA-G and free BPA in pregnancy, when the effects on developmental programming may be more substantial. Could measurement of total as opposed to free BPA have confounded the findings of some studies in pregnancy that have not documented the effects on body mass in humans as consistently as those identified in animals and tissues? Possibly. However, there is substantial evidence that BPA should be removed from food uses, with 1 naturally derived alternative (oleoresin) costing $0.022 per can. Substitution with an alternative free of health effects has been found to produce $1.7 billion/year in annual benefits, which is comparable to the costs of replacement with oleoresin ($2.2 billion/year).[2]

Future studies should measure the bisphenol alphabet soup (especially S) and examine exposure at more than 2 time points given the short half-life and windows of susceptibility. No studies have examined impacts of bisphenols and trajectories of fetal growth in humans, which are increasingly straightforward to study. Yet further research is not needed to realize the needed real reform of the TSCA, including proactive testing of new chemicals for endocrine disrupting effects, lest we repeat the DES story. Although Europe is actively developing criteria for endocrine disruption that could limit dangerous and unnatural experiments, bans in Europe do not necessarily preclude the United States and other manufacturers worldwide from using it in products that end up being sold in the United States. The US FDA more generally should take a more proactive approach to requiring testing of chemicals that are inadvertently or intentionally added to food.

L. Trasande, MD, MPP

References

1. Arbuckle TE, Marro L, Davis K, et al. Exposure to free and conjugated forms of bisphenol A and triclosan among pregnant women in the MIREC cohort. *Environ Health Perspect.* 2015;123:277-284.
2. Trasande L. Further limiting bisphenol A in food uses could provide health and economic benefits. *Health Aff.* 2014;33:316-323.

Pollution, Poverty, and Potentially Preventable Childhood Morbidity in Central California

Lessard LN, Alcala E, Capitman JA (California State Univ-Fresno)
*J Pediatr.*168:98-204, 2016

Objective.—To measure ecological relationships between neighborhood pollution burden, poverty, race/ethnicity, and pediatric preventable disease hospitalization rates.

Study Design.—Preventable disease hospitalization rates were obtained from the 2012 California Office of Statewide Health Planning and Development database, for 8 Central Valley counties. US Census Data was used to incorporate zip code level factors including racial diversity and poverty rates. The pollution burden score was calculated by the California Office of Environmental Health Hazard Assessment using 11 indicators. Poisson-based negative binomial regression was used for final analysis. Stratification of sample by age, race/ethnicity, and insurance coverage was also incorporated.

Results.—Children experiencing potentially preventable hospitalizations are disproportionately low income and under the age of 4 years. With every unit increase in pollution burden, preventable disease hospitalizations rates increase between 21% and 32%, depending on racial and age subgroups. Although living in a poor neighborhood was not associated with potentially avoidable hospitalizations, children enrolled in Medi-Cal who live in neighborhoods with lower pollution burden and lower levels of poverty, face 32% lower risk for ambulatory care sensitive condition hospitalization. Children living in primary care shortage areas are at increased risk of preventable hospitalizations. Preventable disease hospitalizations increase for all subgroups, except white/non-Hispanic children, as neighborhoods became more racially diverse.

Conclusions.—Understanding the geographic distribution of disease and impact of individual and community level factors is essential to expanding access to care and preventive resources to improve the health of children in California's most polluted and underserved region (Fig 1).

▶ The concept that social, societal, and individual factors interact with environmental ones is not a new idea. Pediatricians are well aware that children are vulnerable to lead poisoning in part because they have increased absorption relative to adults and developing, susceptible brains. But clinicians also understand that poor children are more likely to live in old houses that are in disrepair

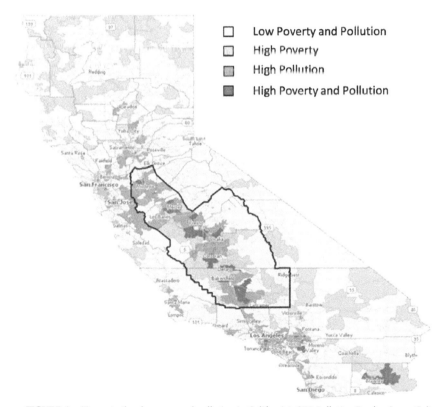

☐ Low Poverty and Pollution

☐ High Poverty

▨ High Pollution

■ High Poverty and Pollution

FIGURE 1.—Top quintile of poverty and pollution in California's SJV. Pollution Burden Score, California Office of Environmental Health Hazard Assessment (OEHHA) CalEnviroScreen version 1.0 and Individuals Living in Poverty, American Community Survey, 2012. (Reprinted from Lessard LN, Alcala E, Capitman JA. Pollution, poverty, and potentially preventable childhood morbidity in central California. *J Pediatr.* 2016;168:198-204, with permission from Elsevier.)

and in neighborhoods with greater contamination from traffic and industry and have nutritional deficiencies that increase absorption of lead. Poor children are also least likely to have the advantages of excellent preventive health care or educational opportunities that may mitigate the neurocognitive effects of lead. The current crisis in Flint, Michigan has brought these issues front and center.

Studies of childhood asthma risk have found an increased risk when there is concurrent exposure to air pollution and a stressful home or community environment.[1,2] Similarly, increased effects of exposure to tobacco smoke, lead, and polychlorinated biphenyls have been noted in less-optimal home environments.[3-5]

Many studies showed the importance of the early social, family, and economic environment not only on childhood health and development but also on lifelong health and risk for disease. It now is evident that the chemical environment has similar effects and can work through identical mechanistic pathways.

This study by Lessard et al is unique in that it uses a measure of cumulative burdens of environmental hazards combined with economic status to analyze the incidence of preventable hospitalizations in children.[6] The metric for cumulative environmental burden was adapted from the CalEnviroScreen, a quantitative method for evaluating multiple pollution levels and sources in a community while also accounting for the community's vulnerability to pollution.[7] This assessment combines both measures of exposure to pollutants (eg, air pollution, factory emissions) and personal and community/social factors of vulnerability (eg, income, community violence, non—English-speaking family).

The CalEnviroScreen (and the similar Environmental Justice Screen, at the US Environmental Protection Agency) resulted from the recognition that health and disease are the result of many factors, both social and environmental.[8] These burdens have been distributed unevenly in the population and are the basis of the Environmental Justice movement. Children of color in California (as in many places) are more likely to live in communities with higher pollution burdens and poverty. Lessard et al found that living in a community with either a high pollution burden or a shortage of primary care physicians was associated with increased risk for preventable hospitalizations (Fig). Simply living in a low-poverty area was not associated with a decreased risk of preventable hospitalization. However, for those with public health insurance (a measure of low income), residing in a community with lower pollution burden and low rates of poverty reduced the risk of preventable hospitalization by 32%.

A commentary published with this article concludes that we do not know enough to formulate a plan of action to reduce the effects of these hazards on children.[9] Although their evaluation of the limitations of this study is accurate, the authors of the commentary miss the key messages for a clinical audience. A strong body of toxicologic and epidemiologic evidence is developing that supports the impact of cumulative exposures on children's health. While Lessard et al are limited in the endpoints examined and used ecologic exposure measures, it provides real world evidence for these cumulative effects on children's health. The authors deserve credit for thinking big, and it is appropriate that this article has been chosen as a cutting-edge attempt to document the multifactorial origins of disease. As methodology improves, this approach of integrating data from multiple large data sets offers the possibility to identify community and subgroup risk factors for disease that have been previously unexaminable.

Ultimately, understanding the cumulative effects of social, societal, and chemical environments should point to effective intervention strategies. The CalEnviroScreen is being used to direct a portion of the funds generated by legislation from the Regulation for the California Cap on Greenhouse Gas Emissions and Market-Based Compliance Mechanisms (ie, California's Carbon Cap and Trade Program) to disadvantaged communities. These investments are aimed at improving public health, quality of life, and economic opportunity in California's most burdened communities while reducing pollution that causes climate change. Rosalind Wright, MD, MPH, a pioneer in the study of how the social environment can modify the effects of chemical exposures, has said "It is likely that only by addressing the multiple factors, both social and environmental, contributing to the development of disease, will we be able to see a noticeable improvement in health as a result of interventions."[9]

M. D. Miller, MD, MPH

References

1. Clougherty JE, Levy JI, Kubzansky LD, et al. Synergistic effects of traffic-related air pollution and exposure to violence on urban asthma etiology. *Environ Health Perspect.* 2007;115:1140-1146.
2. Shankardass K, McConnell R, Jerrett M, et al. Parental stress increases the effect of traffic-related air pollution on childhood asthma incidence. *Proc Natl Acad Sci U S A.* 2009;106:12406-12411.
3. Rauh VA, Whyatt RM, Garfinkel R, et al. Developmental effects of exposure to environmental tobacco smoke and material hardship among inner-city children. *Neurotoxicol Teratol.* 2004;26:373-385.
4. Bellinger D, Leviton A, Sloman J. Antecedents and correlates of improved cognitive performance in children exposed in utero to low levels of lead. *Environ Health Perspect.* 1990;89:5-11.
5. Vreugdenhil HJ, Lanting CI, Mulder PG, et al. Effects of prenatal PCB and dioxin background exposure on cognitive and motor abilities in Dutch children at school age. *J Pediatr.* 2002;140:48-56.
6. California Environmental Protection Agency. California communities' environmental health screening tool, version 2.0 (CALENVIROSCREEN 2.0): guidance and screening tool. http://oehha.ca.gov/ej/ces2.html. Accessed March 25, 2016.
7. US Environmental Protection Agency. EJ Screen, Environmental Justice Screening and Mapping Tool. https://www.epa.gov/ejscreen. Accessed March 25, 2016.
8. Sacks JD, Nichols JL. A need for better studies to identify those populations at greatest risk of a pollutant-related health effect. *J Pediatr.* 2016;168:11-13.
9. Wright R. Presentation at 2013 Symposium on Cumulative Impacts on Children's Health and the Environment at California Environmental Protection Agency". Sacramento, CA. January 16, 2013.

28 Training and Professionalism

Perceptions and Expectations of Host Country Preceptors of Short-Term Learners at Four Clinical Sites in Sub-Saharan Africa
Lukolyo H, Rees CA, Keating EM, et al (Baylor College of Medicine, Houston, TX)
Acad Pediatr 16:387-393, 2016

Objective.—The demand for global health electives among medical students and residents has grown substantially, yet perspectives of international hosts are not well documented. This study aimed to assess how host country supervising clinical preceptors perceive learners on short-term global health electives of up to 6 weeks.

Methods.—This study used a cross-sectional survey design and assessed international clinical preceptors' perceptions of short-term learners' (STLs) professional behaviors, medical knowledge, competency in systems-based care, as well as the benefits and burdens of hosting STLs. Surveys were sent to all clinical preceptors (n = 47) at 4 clinical sites in sub-Saharan Africa in 2015.

Results.—Thirty-two preceptors (68%) responded to the survey. Most respondents (97%) were satisfied in their role hosting STLs and reported that STLs enhanced patient care and the professional image of the clinical site. Nearly half of respondents (45%) reported decreased self-perceived efficiency in clinical care tasks. Qualitative data identified concerns related to STLs' professionalism and teamwork. Respondents also identified knowledge gaps in understanding differences in health systems and epidemiology in host country settings. Respondents preferred that rotations last at least 4 weeks and that STLs complete predeparture training.

Conclusions.—STLs were largely positively regarded by international host clinical preceptors. To improve mutuality of benefits, sending institutions should ensure learners understand host country expectations of professionalism and that learners are well prepared for medical, ethical, and cultural challenges through participation in predeparture curricula that prepare them clinically and emotionally for these international experiences. Rotations of at least 4 weeks may enhance benefits to learners and hosts (Fig 1).

▶ Medical students and residents have long been transformed by international health experiences. Several studies (many of them cited by the authors of this article) support the idea that such international rotations lead trainees to more likely work with underserved populations at home or abroad in the future as well as other potential benefits of such exposures. Over the last few decades, the term *international health* has matured into *global health*, which has developed into a possible career track for those in the health care field.

The demand for global health experiences has meant most major medical schools offer some kind of elective or rotation abroad. In the past, more often than not, international health experiences and rotations were not properly prepared for, were not suitably supervised, and were not appropriately debriefed. More recently, there have been attempts to develop best practices for such experiences and to develop global health competencies that every trainee should be expected to achieve, which has led to more robust research and higher standards in global health education and experience.

One of the literature gaps regarding such international experiences, Global Health Electives (GHEs), as the article terms them, has been evaluations of these GHEs from the host country's perspective. This study adds to the limited data on this topic, and it is important because this should be the ethical focus of evaluation of the electives that are sending those from rich countries to have experiences in resource-scarce settings. The authors used a survey they developed through and iterative process that thankfully included input from those on the ground in clinics in the countries they were evaluating. This survey was administered to both US, foreign, and local preceptors at 4 clinical sites operated by Baylor focused on pediatric human immunodeficiency virus.

The authors found some things that are no surprise to those that work in global health and have been involved with trainees—short-term learners (STLs)—taking part in GHEs. Among other things, the GHE preceptor respondents said that they liked precepting, that they liked having the STLs, but that the STLs made them less efficient in their work (Fig). In the open-ended qualitative data collected, the preceptors discussed several themes in which they were less positive about the STLs: professionalism issues; trainee motivation issues; the fact that longer rotations are preferable and a learning curve means STLs are of little use early on; the need for prerotation training, which respondents thought needed to be better defined and implemented; and the desire for some cultural background training for the STLs.

Some limitations are outlined by the authors. Their results focused on Baylor clinical sites, which are well resourced and specialty focused and not especially generalizable to other sites and institutions. As more evaluations of the impact of such income-rich trainees' learning in income-scarce host countries are done, surveys of others beside the preceptors would be more informative. Preceptors are likely biased, as they are likely invested in, and often have secondary gain (financial, social, professional) from the GHE programs. Surveying patients, all health care workers, and people who the STLs interact with

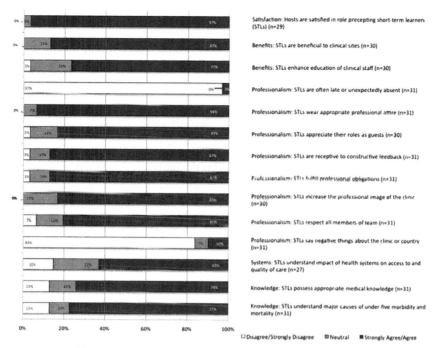

FIGURE 1.—Host preceptor responses from Baylor International Pediatric AIDS Initiative clinics in sub-Saharan Africa in 2015 (n = 32). (Reprinted from Lukolyo H, Rees CA, Keating EM, et al. Perceptions and expectations of host country preceptors of short-term learners at four clinical sites in Sub-Saharan Africa. *Acad Pediatr* 2016;16:387-393, with permission from Academic Pediatric Association.)

would give more information on how such rotations and electives can be ethically sound.

However, this article reinforces important components of global health electives that most working in global health understand to be best practices. Predeparture training is important, and most programs don't do enough of it, or don't do it as thoroughly and well as they could. Professionalism and cultural humility should be part of this predeparture training and should be part of a trainee's evaluation on the rotation. Rotations should be at least 4 weeks if the trainee is likely to be helpful rather than a drain on efficiency of those at the site.

This article is most helpful as a draft template for the type of questions and evaluation that every institution should be doing of their international elective offerings. To truly understand the impact of these rotations, we need more information from the host site perspectives. Building on the spirit of this article, it would be wonderful to see even more introspection around global health elective experiences, so we can really "first do no harm" as we send trainees to do work abroad.

C. C. Stewart, MD

Prevalence of Depression and Depressive Symptoms Among Resident Physicians: A Systematic Review and Meta-analysis

Mata DA, Ramos MA, Bansal N, et al (Harvard Med School, Boston, MA; Yale Univ, New Haven, CT; Univ of Cambridge, UK; et al)
JAMA 314:2373-2383, 2015

Importance.—Physicians in training are at high risk for depression. However, the estimated prevalence of this disorder varies substantially between studies.

Objective.—To provide a summary estimate of depression or depressive symptom prevalence among resident physicians.

Data Sources and Study Selection.—Systematic search of EMBASE, ERIC, MEDLINE, and PsycINFO for studies with information on the prevalence of depression or depressive symptoms among resident physicians published between January 1963 and September 2015. Studies were eligible for inclusion if they were published in the peer-reviewed literature and used a validated method to assess for depression or depressive symptoms.

Data Extraction and Synthesis.—Information on study characteristics and depression or depressive symptom prevalence was extracted independently by 2 trained investigators. Estimates were pooled using random-effects meta-analysis. Differences by study-level characteristics were estimated using meta-regression.

Main Outcomes and Measures.—Point or period prevalence of depression or depressive symptoms as assessed by structured interview or validated questionnaire.

Results.—Data were extracted from 31 cross-sectional studies (9447 individuals) and 23 longitudinal studies (8113 individuals). Three studies used clinical interviews and 51 used self-report instruments. The overall pooled prevalence of depression or depressive symptoms was 28.8% (4969/17 560 individuals, 95% CI, 25.3%-32.5%), with high between-study heterogeneity ($Q = 1247$, $\tau^2 = 0.39$, $I^2 = 95.8\%$, $P < .001$). Prevalence estimates ranged from 20.9% for the 9-item Patient Health Questionnaire with a cutoff of 10 or more (741/3577 individuals, 95% CI, 17.5%-24.7%, $Q = 14.4$, $\tau^2 = 0.04$, $I^2 = 79.2\%$) to 43.2% for the 2-item PRIME-MD (1349/2891 individuals, 95% CI, 37.6%-49.0%, $Q = 45.6$, $\tau^2 = 0.09$, $I^2 = 84.6\%$). There was an increased prevalence with increasing calendar year (slope = 0.5% increase per year, adjusted for assessment modality; 95% CI, 0.03%-0.9%, $P = .04$). In a secondary analysis of 7 longitudinal studies, the median absolute increase in depressive symptoms with the onset of residency training was 15.8% (range, 0.3%-26.3%; relative risk, 4.5). No statistically significant differences were observed between cross-sectional vs longitudinal studies, studies of only interns vs only upper-level residents, or studies of nonsurgical vs both nonsurgical and surgical residents.

Conclusions and Relevance.—In this systematic review, the summary estimate of the prevalence of depression or depressive symptoms among resident physicians was 28.8%, ranging from 20.9% to 43.2% depending on the instrument used, and increased with calendar year. Further research is needed to identify effective strategies for preventing and treating depression among physicians in training (Fig 2).

▶ Depression causes major morbidity and mortality in young adults, including many resident physicians. With increasing system changes and stressors in the medical field, several articles in the popular press report high rates of burnout, depression, and even suicide among physicians. Beyond compelling individual physician stories, there is a need to understand the full scope, prevalence, and multiple factors involved in depression. We must appreciate how depressive symptoms can affect resident physicians to plan training curricula, refine regulatory policies, and improve systems of care. Residency is a key period in a career continuum of provider health and wellness.

One strength of this study is the long-term view of publications from the period of 1963 to 2016. Older generations of physicians who trained in a different era before the Accreditation Council for Graduate Medical Education (ACGME) duty-hour regulations might ask, "Didn't depression go away with q2 call?" However, many studies included in this analysis were after 2003 when the ACGME instituted additional duty hour restrictions. Even among recent studies, there is still a high rate of depression (Fig 2). In addition, statistical analysis did not demonstrate a significant effect by the year of study. Residency remains stressful with different stressors of electronic medical records, medical consumerism, and other demands that are not related to the number of hours, night calls, or length of shifts.[1,2]

Another key distinction the reader must appreciate is the difference in key terms "depressive symptoms" and "depression" and the level of scores on the various scales. There is great heterogeneity in this body of literature, and readers must understand how the 2-item Primary Care Evaluation of Mental Disorders questionnaire (PRIME-MD) could vary as a proxy for depression versus other scales and structured interviews. We must be careful to distinguish more general concepts of "depressive symptoms" from externally verified "depression" and the different diagnostic subtypes. Only 3 of the 54 included studies had results based on structured interviews. The issue of self-report versus external diagnosis and review is key in our attempts to understand depression among physicians. The longitudinal nature of depressive symptoms is also critical to understand because depression is generally a longer term disorder with variable waxing and waning of symptom levels. It is not a transient or acute phenomenon. Thus, a snapshot of one point of time, or even scales that ask about the last 2 weeks, may give a limited glimpse into this chronic condition. However, the pooled results are fairly consistent even for different scales and methods.

One may debate nuances in different screening measures, self-report validity, and scales, yet a subset of the 7 longitudinal studies provides evidence that the prevalence of depression seems to increase during graduate medical education training. Residency is a stressful time for young adults, many of whom start with a high level of depressive symptoms. In fact, studies of medical students show high levels of depressive symptoms even before starting residency.[3]

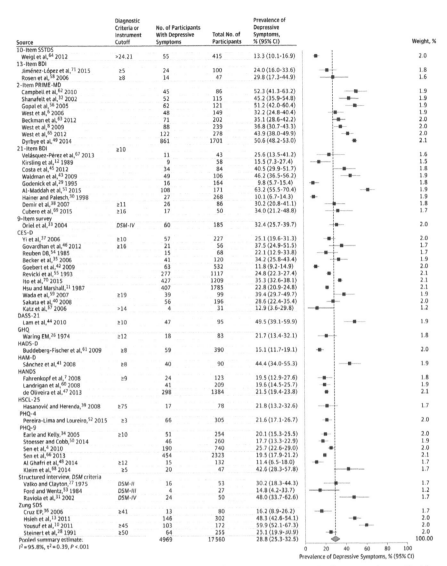

Source	Diagnostic Criteria or Instrument Cutoff	No. of Participants With Depressive Symptoms	Total No. of Participants	Prevalence of Depressive Symptoms, % (95% CI)	Weight, %
10-Item SSTDS					
Weigl et al,[64] 2012	>24.21	55	415	13.3 (10.1-16.9)	2.0
13-Item BDI					
Jiménez-López et al,[71] 2015	≥5	24	100	24.0 (16.0-33.6)	1.8
Rosen et al,[58] 2006	≥8	14	47	29.8 (17.3-44.9)	1.6
2-Item PRIME-MD					
Campbell et al,[62] 2010		45	86	52.3 (41.3-63.2)	1.9
Shanafelt et al,[32] 2002		52	115	45.2 (35.9-54.8)	1.9
Gopal et al,[56] 2005		62	121	51.2 (42.0-60.4)	1.9
West et al,[6] 2006		48	149	32.2 (24.8-40.4)	1.9
Beckman et al,[63] 2012		71	202	35.1 (28.6-42.2)	2.0
West et al,[8] 2009		88	239	36.8 (30.7-43.3)	2.0
West et al,[65] 2012		122	278	43.9 (38.0-49.9)	2.0
Dyrbye et al,[49] 2014		861	1701	50.6 (48.2-53.0)	2.1
21-Item BDI	≥10				
Velásquez-Pérez et al,[67] 2013		11	43	25.6 (13.5-41.2)	1.6
Kirsling et al,[12] 1989		9	58	15.5 (7.3-27.4)	1.5
Costa et al,[45] 2012		34	84	40.5 (29.9-51.7)	1.8
Waldman et al,[43] 2009		49	106	46.2 (36.5-56.2)	1.9
Godenick et al,[29] 1995		16	164	9.8 (5.7-15.4)	1.8
Al-Maddah et al,[51] 2015		108	171	63.2 (55.5-70.4)	1.9
Hainer and Palesch,[30] 1998		27	268	10.1 (6.7-14.3)	1.9
Demir et al,[38] 2007	≥11	26	86	30.2 (20.8-41.1)	1.8
Cubero et al,[69] 2015	≥16	17	50	34.0 (21.2-48.8)	1.7
9-Item survey					
Oriel et al,[33] 2004	DSM-IV	60	185	32.4 (25.7-39.7)	2.0
CES-D					
Yi et al,[37] 2006	≥10	57	227	25.1 (19.6-31.3)	2.0
Govardhan et al,[46] 2012	≥16	21	56	37.5 (24.9-51.5)	1.7
Reuben DB,[54] 1985		15	68	22.1 (12.9-33.8)	1.7
Becker et al,[35] 2006		41	120	34.2 (25.8-43.4)	1.9
Goebert et al,[42] 2009		63	532	11.8 (9.2-14.9)	2.0
Revicki et al,[55] 1993		277	1117	24.8 (22.3-27.4)	2.1
Ito et al,[70] 2015		427	1209	35.3 (32.6-38.1)	2.1
Hsu and Marshall,[11] 1987		407	1785	22.8 (30.9-24.8)	2.1
Wada et al,[59] 2007	≥19	39	99	39.4 (29.7-49.7)	1.9
Sakata et al,[60] 2008		56	196	28.6 (22.4-35.4)	2.0
Katz et al,[57] 2006	>14	4	31	12.9 (3.6-29.8)	1.2
DASS-21					
Lam et al,[44] 2010	≥10	47	95	49.5 (39.1-59.9)	1.9
GHQ					
Waring EM,[26] 1974	≥12	18	83	21.7 (13.4-32.1)	1.8
HADS-D					
Buddeberg-Fischer et al,[61] 2009	≥8	59	390	15.1 (11.7-19.1)	2.0
HAM-D					
Sánchez et al,[41] 2008	≥8	40	90	44.4 (34.0-55.3)	1.9
HANDS					
Fahrenkopf et al,[7] 2008	≥9	24	123	19.5 (12.9-27.6)	1.8
Landrigan et al,[60] 2008		41	209	19.6 (14.5-25.7)	1.9
de Oliveira et al,[47] 2013		298	1384	21.5 (19.4-23.8)	2.1
HSCL-25					
Hasanović and Herenda,[39] 2008	≥75	17	78	21.8 (13.2-32.6)	1.7
PHQ-4					
Pereira-Lima and Loureiro,[52] 2015	≥3	66	305	21.6 (17.1-26.7)	2.0
PHQ-9					
Earle and Kelly,[34] 2005	≥10	51	254	20.1 (15.3-25.5)	2.0
Stoesser and Cobb,[50] 2014		46	260	17.7 (13.3-22.9)	1.9
Sen et al,[4] 2010		190	740	25.7 (22.6-29.0)	2.0
Sen et al,[66] 2013		454	2323	19.5 (17.9-21.2)	2.1
Al Ghafri et al,[48] 2014	≥12	15	132	11.4 (6.5-18.0)	1.7
Kleim et al,[68] 2014	≥5	20	47	42.6 (28.3-57.8)	1.7
Structured interview, DSM criteria					
Valko and Clayton,[27] 1975	DSM-II	16	53	30.2 (18.3-44.3)	1.7
Ford and Wentz,[53] 1984	DSM-III	4	27	14.8 (4.2-33.7)	1.2
Raviola et al,[31] 2002	DSM-IV	24	50	48.0 (33.7-62.6)	1.7
Zung SDS					
Cruz EP,[36] 2006	≥41	13	80	16.2 (8.9-26.2)	1.7
Hsieh et al,[13] 2011		146	302	48.3 (42.6-54.1)	2.0
Yousuf et al,[10] 2011	≥45	103	172	59.9 (52.1-67.3)	2.0
Steinert et al,[28] 1991	≥50	64	255	25.1 (19.9-30.9)	2.0
Pooled summary estimate.		4969	17 560	28.8 (25.3-32.5)	100.00

$I^2 = 95.8\%, \tau^2 = 0.39, P < .001$

Prevalence of Depressive Symptoms, % (95% CI)

FIGURE 2.—Meta-analysis of the Prevalence of Depression or Depressive Symptoms Among Resident Physicians Contributing studies are stratified by screening modality and ordered by increasing sample size. The area of each square is proportional to the inverse variance of the estimate. The dotted line marks the overall summary estimate for all studies, 28.8% (4969/17 560 individuals, 95% CI, 25.3%-32.5%, $Q = 1247.11$, $\tau^2 = 0.39$, $I^2 = 95.8\%$ [95% CI, 95.0%-96.4%], $P < .001$). (Refer to footnotes of Table 1 and Table 2 for expanded names of diagnostic instruments.) *Editor's Note:* Please refer to original journal article for full references. (Reprinted from Mata DA, Ramos MA, Bansal N, et al. Prevalence of depression and depressive symptoms among resident physicians: a systematic review and meta-analysis. *JAMA.* 2015;314:2373-2383, with permission from American Medical Association.)

In addition to overall prevalence, the comparison of different subgroups is very interesting. This article challenges some of the commonly held beliefs that depression is presumed to be higher among different specialties, United States versus international residents, by different age, or by gender. These factors were not significant in this systematic review. This is important because many proposed strategies for detection and early intervention attempt to focus on "high-risk" groups. Simply being a resident seems to be high risk alone, and graduate medical education leaders and organizations need to continue to address these needs in a more comprehensive versus targeted approach. The article does not speculate on the reasons for depressive symptoms, but long hours, debt and financial stress, and other more subtle individual factors of personality may be involved.

Although it is beyond the scope of this review to address how many residents seek assistance or treatment, it is known to be well below the 28% prevalence rate of depressive symptoms cited. General stigma of mental illness is an issue for all patients. It is likely an even greater factor among resident physicians who are evaluated, scrutinized, and competing for top fellowship and practice positions, when the stakes and potential professional stigma are even higher. We must consider how disclosure of depressed mood to evaluators and superiors in residency is managed, and how these factors influence answers to scales in these studies, even those which promise anonymity. Issues of confidentiality and potential concerns of disclosure to future employers, credentialing agencies, and licensing boards is a real fear and an issue to scrutinize given the magnitude of depressive symptoms.[4]

Of note, this article does not address suicidality and its relationship with depression; however, there are many reports that suggest physician suicide is also greater than the general population rate. Depression is one important part of a much larger issue of mental health issues facing resident physicians. Despite some limitations, it is quite clear that depressive symptoms are common in resident physicians. Among a relatively healthy young cohort of physicians, we must focus on mental health morbidity and mortality moving forward to ensure that healers are healed.

J. L. Rushton, MD, MPH

References

1. Institute of Medicine (US) Committee on Optimizing Graduate Medical Trainee (Resident) Hours and Work Schedule to Improve Patient Safety, Ulmer C. In: Miller Wolman D, Johns MME, eds. *Resident Duty Hours: Enhancing Sleep, Supervision, and Safety.* Washington, DC: National Academies Press (US); 2009. Impact of Duty Hours on Resident Well-Being:5.
2. Sen S, Kranzler HR, Didwania AK, et al. Effects of the 2011 duty hour reforms on interns and their patients: a prospective longitudinal cohort study. *JAMA Intern Med.* 2013;173:657-663.
3. Schwenk TL, Davis L, Wimsatt LA. Depression, stigma, and suicidal ideation in medical students. *JAMA.* 2010;304:1181-1190.
4. Center C, Davis M, Detre T, et al. Confronting depression and suicide in physicians: a consensus statement. *JAMA.* 2003;289:3161-3166.

Training Physicians to Provide High-Value, Cost-Conscious Care: A Systematic Review

Stammen LA, Stalmeijer RE, Paternotte E, et al (Maastricht Univ, the Netherlands; OLVG Hosp, Amsterdam, the Netherlands; et al)

JAMA 314:2384-2400, 2015

Importance.—Increasing health care expenditures are taxing the sustainability of the health care system. Physicians should be prepared to deliver high-value, cost-conscious care.

Objective.—To understand the circumstances in which the delivery of high-value, cost-conscious care is learned, with a goal of informing development of effective educational interventions.

Data Sources.—PubMed, EMBASE, ERIC, and Cochrane databases were searched from inception until September 5, 2015, to identify learners and cost-related topics.

Study Selection.—Studies were included on the basis of topic relevance, implementation of intervention, evaluation of intervention, educational components in intervention, and appropriate target group. There was no restriction on study design.

Data Extraction and Synthesis.—Data extraction was guided by a merged and modified version of a Best Evidence in Medical Education abstraction form and a Cochrane data coding sheet. Articles were analyzed using the realist review method, a narrative review technique that focuses on understanding the underlying mechanisms in interventions. Recurrent patterns were identified in the data through thematic analyses. Resulting themes were discussed within the research team until consensus was reached.

Main Outcomes and Measures.—Main outcomes were factors that promote education in delivering high-value, cost-conscious care.

Findings.—The initial search identified 2650 articles; 79 met the inclusion criteria, of which 14 were randomized clinical trials. The majority of the studies were conducted in North America (78.5%) using a pre-post interventional design (58.2%; at least 1619 participants); they focused on practicing physicians (36.7%; at least 3448 participants), resident physicians (6.3%; n = 516), and medical students (15.2%; n = 275). Among the 14 randomized clinical trials, 12 addressed knowledge transmission, 7 reflective practice, and 1 supportive environment; 10 (71%) concluded that the intervention was effective. The data analysis suggested that 3 factors aid successful learning: (1) effective transmission of knowledge, related, for example, to general health economics and prices of health services, to scientific evidence regarding guidelines and the benefits and harms of health care, and to patient preferences and personal values (67 articles); (2) facilitation of reflective practice, such as providing feedback or asking reflective questions regarding decisions related to laboratory ordering or prescribing to give trainees insight into their past and current behavior (56 articles); and (3) creation of a supportive environment in which the organization of the health care system, the presence of role models of delivering high-value, cost-conscious care, and a culture of high-value, cost-conscious care reinforce the desired training goals (27 articles).

Conclusions and Relevance.—Research on educating physicians to deliver high-value, cost-conscious care suggests that learning by practicing physicians, resident physicians, and medical students is promoted by combining specific knowledge transmission, reflective practice, and a supportive environment. These factors should be considered when educational interventions are being developed.

▶ The low value—defined as the quality for cost—of much of American health care is an outrage and threatens patients' well-being physically and financially. Medical error is among the top 3 causes of death in the United States based on available estimates, and the rising costs of care have not only suppressed wages for the average family over the past 2 decades but now crowd out needed investments in education, infrastructure, and public programs. Yet despite the national spotlight on high costs and inconsistent quality found throughout much of the health care system, most medical educators have until recently preferred to bury their heads in the sand rather than prepare the next generation of clinicians to deliver high value care.

But gatekeepers of medical training won't be able to ignore the burning issues of costs and quality much longer, especially as their academic medical centers, bastions of Flexnerian orthodoxy and "cost is no issue" naïveté, are forced either to adapt to regulatory and public demands for high value care or face extinction. Lucky for them, the Stammen article provides a roadmap for preparing physicians to practice in the fast-approaching, value-based future.

The article is the most rigorous published review to date of the growing literature on training in value-based care. Looking back over 30 years, the authors find a remarkably promising proportion of positive studies showing improved quality and reduced costs associated with value-based educational interventions for medical trainees and practicing physicians.

The limitations of the studies reviewed are predictable and commonplace in evaluations of educational interventions. To counterbalance the preponderance of pre—post study designs in the review, the authors make an effort to highlight results from the minority of studies with more rigorous methodologies, which also demonstrate an eyebrow-raising high success rate. They acknowledge that only an eighth of the studies included had samples of more than 100 participants, with another third of the studies forgoing any description of the sample size at all.

Many of the articles evaluate change in knowledge but not clinical behavior change, although the authors try to focus on studies with meaningful outcomes for patient care. Of the studies they find that do track clinical outcomes and costs, few measured whether the improvements were sustained well beyond the conclusion of the intervention. The authors rightly point out that the high rate of positive trials found indicates a high likelihood of publication bias.

Despite these caveats, in their review, the authors find that content knowledge transmission, reflective practice, and a supportive culture toward high-value care emerge as the building blocks of successful value-based training, a conclusion sufficiently generic to be both nonthreatening to the medical education neophyte just beginning to conceive a value-based curriculum and practically useless to the educator who will eventually implement it.

In other words, the article perfectly encapsulates the opportunity medical education has at this moment: a nearly blank slate opportunity to define the strategy, create and iterate new curricula, build the evidence, and reform from top to bottom to prepare future physicians to deliver high-value care. It's precisely because we know so little about how to teach value well that makes this moment so exciting and full of possibility, especially in pediatrics.

For the minority of children who are medically complex or who find themselves in the emergency department or hospital, pediatrics faces the same challenges of low quality and high cost rampant throughout the rest of American medicine. The available evidence would suggest that many of these children would be better off if pediatricians were better trained to safely do less—less continuous pulse oximetry monitoring for the bronchiolitic, less computed tomography for minor head trauma, less harm from unnecessary phlebotomy and polypharmacy. In just the past year, academic pediatricians have seen a host of educational tools emerge to address this need, from value-based pediatric case modules (http://hvc.acponline.org/pedcases) to full high-value pediatric curricula (https://www.mededportal.org/publication/10146). As these resources are increasingly adopted, pediatrics can hopefully reduce overuse of low-value care.

In terms of underuse of high-value care, however, there is a strong case to be made that we pediatricians have greater opportunity to improve value than any other field of medicine. Why? Because primary prevention is our core strength and the benefits to our patients accrue for decades. Consider this: the highest-value care is not switching to a generic or reducing hospital length of stay but preventing the need for the medication or the hospitalization in the first place. So while the internists work to marginally reduce the costs of their multicomorbid high utilizers in intensive care, pediatricians have the opportunity to reshape children's health today to eliminate the chance of them ever becoming tomorrow's high cost patients. This puts the long-standing pediatric emphasis on prevention in a new, high-value light. As counterintuitive as it may be, substantially increasing our investment in upstream pediatric primary prevention efforts that work may deliver the largest savings in health care costs over the long run. This uniquely pediatric approach to increasing value over the life course flips the typical approach to cost containment on its head.

So although we can learn quite a bit from the value training conversation taking place in other fields of medicine, let's not forget that health care for kids really is different in important ways and the keys to improving value in pediatrics will be similarly unique. We have an opportunity in pediatrics to take value-based training in a new direction by teaching trainees what works to keep kids (and the adults they will become) healthy, to focus on the problem of underuse of high-value pediatric services (ie, vaccination, developmental screening, home nurse visitation for at-risk infants) that represents the greatest threat to quality care for the nation's kids, and to emphasize how the field of pediatrics is perfectly positioned to deliver high-value care in the most critical time of life to ensure lifelong health.

A. Schickedanz, MD

Work—Life Balance Burnout, and Satisfaction of Early Career Pediatricians
Starmer AJ, Frintner MP, Freed GL (Boston Children's Hosp, MA; American Academy of Pediatrics, Elk Grove Village, IL; Univ of Michigan, Ann Arbor)
Pediatrics 137:e20153183, 2016

Background and Objective.—Data describing factors associated with work—life balance, burnout, and career and life satisfaction for early career pediatricians are limited. We sought to identify personal and work factors related to these outcomes.

Methods.—We analyzed 2013 survey data of pediatricians who graduated residency between 2002 and 2004. Dependent variables included: (1) balance between personal and professional commitments, (2) current burnout in work, (3) career satisfaction, and (4) life satisfaction. Multivariable logistic regression examined associations of personal and work characteristics with each of the 4 dependent variables.

Results.—A total of 93% of participants completed the survey (n = 840). A majority reported career (83%) and life (71%) satisfaction. Fewer reported current appropriate work—life balance (43%) or burnout (30%). In multivariable modeling, excellent/very good health, having support from physician colleagues, and adequate resources for patient care were all found to be associated with a lower prevalence of burnout and a higher likelihood of work—life balance and career and life satisfaction. Having children, race, and clinical specialty were not found to be significantly associated with any of the 4 outcome measures. Female gender was associated with a lower likelihood of balance and career satisfaction but did not have an association with burnout or life satisfaction.

Conclusions.—Burnout and struggles with work—life balance are common; dissatisfaction with life and career are a concern for some early career pediatricians. Efforts to minimize these outcomes should focus on encouragement of modifiable factors, including health supervision, peer support, and ensuring sufficient patient care resources.

▶ Although there is a growing body of literature looking at personal and career satisfaction, burnout, and work—life balance for physicians, there remains a paucity of data looking at these factors among pediatricians. Previous studies make it clear that no specialty is immune to burnout, imbalance, or dissatisfaction. In previous studies, pediatrics has had one of the lowest rates of burnout, yet still has more than a third of its workforce experiencing it.[1] This fact underscores that action is not optional, especially given the potential impact of burnout on quality of patient care and on the primary care workforce shortage.[2]

It is imprudent to draw actionable conclusions from multispecialty studies that do not account for unique demographic and practice issues facing pediatricians.

This study focuses on wellness in early career physicians (≤10 years of practice), who often experience additional stressors such as simultaneously starting a career and a family, needing rapid knowledge and skills attainment, and building a patient panel or meeting productivity goals. This study approximates others in that nearly a third of respondents are experiencing burnout. The most striking finding of this study, however, is that 3 of the independent variables positively influenced all four of the dependent variables (work—life balance, burnout, personal and career satisfaction). These variables were excellent or very good self-reported health, personal support from physician colleagues, and adequate resources for patient care. Surprisingly, they are all potentially modifiable factors. This fact validates the use of resources to promote them in an attempt to reduce burnout, dissatisfaction, and imbalance. Depression and inadequate sleep were modifiable variables that negatively affected at least 2 of the dependent variables. Furthermore, having a negative life event in the previous 12 months decreased life satisfaction and increased burnout. These are also targetable factors for additional screening and support.

This study can be applauded for identifying preventable factors affecting the well-being of pediatricians. It also confirmed that the nonmodifiable factors of race or having children do not negatively affect wellness measures. This is an especially important finding given that most early-career pediatricians are women with young children. One factor that potentially weakens the findings is that burnout was measured with a single survey item: "I am currently experiencing burnout in my work." Because burnout encompasses symptoms of emotional exhaustion, depersonalization, and a lack of sense of personal accomplishment,[3] it is less likely that a single item, without a shared definition, accurately captures it.

The study also uses cross-sectional data from 1 survey of pediatricians 9 to 11 years out of residency. Although these data cannot be generalized to pediatricians at other points in their careers, interventions based on screening for wellness indicators across career stages hardly seem ill advised. Future longitudinal analysis using additional surveys through the PLACES study will help guide burnout prevention and wellness promotion across the pediatric career spectrum. Further data will also help determine whether the factors making the most impact on wellness in each career phase change over time. Certainly, more detailed studies are needed because this survey did not go into potential causative factors such as time spent on the electronic health record (EHR), which patient care resources were lacking, and the contributors to hectic work environments.

The relative dearth of data on burnout in pediatricians has made it difficult to advocate for action. Like most health issues, increased awareness, surveillance, and prevention are the key to reducing the magnitude of the problem. These initial data support advocating for options such as peer support programs and health coaches and provide direction to pediatric departments for gathering more detailed information. We cannot wait until this problem reaches crisis proportions before we take action.

S. Colianni, MD, FAAP

References

1. Shanafelt TD, Boone S, Tan L, et al. Burnout and satisfaction with work-life balance among US physicians relative to the general US population. *Arch Intern Med.* 2012;172:1377-1385.
2. Song Z, Chopra V, McMahon L. Addressing the primary care workforce crisis. *Am J Manag Care.* 2015;21:e452-e454.
3. Linzer M, Levine R, Meltzer D, Poplau S, Warde C, West CP. 10 bold steps to prevent burnout in general internal medicine. *J Gen Intern Med.* 2014;29:18-20.

Pediatricians Working Part-Time Has Plateaued

Cull WL, Frintner MP, O'Connor KG, et al (American Academy of Pediatrics, Elk Grove Village, IL)

J Pediatr 171:294-299, 2016

Objective.—To examine trends in pediatricians working part-time and residents seeking part-time work and to examine associated characteristics.

Study Design.—The American Academy of Pediatrics (AAP) Periodic Survey of Fellows and the AAP Annual Survey of Graduating Residents were used to examine part-time employment. Fourteen periodic surveys were combined with an overall response rate of 57%. Part-time percentages were compared for surveys conducted from 2006-2009 and 2010-2013. The AAP Annual Surveys of Graduating Residents (combined response rate = 60%) from 2006-2009 were compared with 2010-2013 surveys for residents seeking and obtaining part-time positions following training. Multivariable logistic regression models identified characteristics associated with part-time work.

Results.—Comparable percentages of pediatricians worked part-time in 2006-2009 (23%) and 2010-2013 (23%). There was similarly no statistically significant difference in residents seeking part-time work (30%-28%), and there was a slight decline in residents accepting part-time work (16%-13%, aOR .75, 95% CI .56-.96). Increases in working part-time were not found for any subgroups examined. Women consistently were more likely than men to work part-time (35% vs 9%), but they showed different patterns of part-time work across age. Women in their 40s (40%) were more likely than other women (33%) and men in their 60s (20%) were more likely than other men (5%) to work part-time.

Conclusions.—There has been a levelling off in the number of pediatricians working part-time and residents seeking part-time work. Overall, women remain more likely to work part-time, although 1 in 5 men over 60 work part-time (Fig 1, Table 1).

▶ The issue of part-time employment has been a frequent topic of the Women in Medicine Special Interest Group of the Academic Pediatric Association as

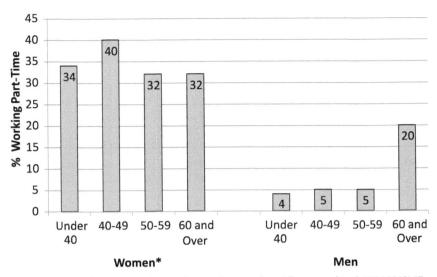

FIGURE 1.—Pediatrician part-time employment by age and sex (all years combined, 2006-2013).*For all age groups, women were statistically significantly more likely than men to work part-time. (Reprinted from Cull WL, Frintner MP, O'Connor KG, et al. Pediatricians working part-time has plateaued. *J Pediatr.* 2016;171:294-299, with permission from Elsevier.)

well as other women-physician focused groups. The assumption has always been that women, especially during their childbearing years, preferred to work part-time at least until their children had achieved some level of independence. Men, on the other hand, may select part-time employment later in life, often after they retire (Fig 1).

The concerns facing these women and men are often different. For younger individuals the questions are as follows: Do you take night call or weekend coverage? Who covers your malpractice, and can it be prorated? Do you get benefits such as health insurance and retirement? If you are a woman, are you covered by your husband's benefits?

How acceptable is working part-time? Traditionally, the quality of one's work as a physician has been measured by the quantity of one's work, especially in academia. But times have changed as duty hours altered the expectations of newly trained physicians, and more companies and groups have accepted the request for part-time employment, with the expectation on the part of the employee of at least some benefits. The medical community started to look at other industries and rather than the potentially pejorative term of "women-friendly" or "family-friendly," Fortune 500 companies prided themselves on being "employee friendly." And rather than talking about "part-time" began using the phrase "flexible schedules."

The American Academy of Pediatrics (AAP), through its various resident and physician survey instruments, has been monitoring both the interest in as well as the experience with part-time employment for pediatricians. The interest in part-time employment had continued to increase over a number of years but in this most recent report has seemed to level off (Table 1). It remains to be

TABLE 1.—The Percentage of Pediatricians Working Part-Time From 2006-2013 by Subgroups (n = 10 268)

	2006-2009 % Part-Time	2010-2013 % Part-Time	Δ (Time 2-Time 1)*
Total	23	23	0
Sex			
Female (n = 5675)	36	34	−2
Male (n = 4593)	8	9	1
Age			
Less than 40 y (n = 2771)	27	24	−3
40-49 y (n = 3003)	26	26	0
50-59 y (n = 2870)	18	18	0
60 y and older (n = 1562)	22	24	2
Specialty			
Pediatric primary care (n = 7290)	27	26	−1
Pediatric subspecialist (n = 2872)	15	15	0
Primary practice location			
Suburban (n = 4257)	27	27	0
Rural (n = 1126)	22	23	1
Urban, not inner city (n = 2761)	21	21	0
Urban, inner city (n = 1962)	19	18	−1

*None of the differences were significant at $P \leq .05$.
Reprinted from Cull WL, Frintner MP, O'Connor KG, et al. Pediatricians working part-time has plateaued. *J Pediatr.* 2016;171:294-299, with permission from Elsevier.

seen whether the current rate continues to stay level, to increase, or to decrease over the next few years.

So why is part-time employment of interest? And what are the factors that have lead to the increase in part-time employment over the past decade? In the days when part-time employment opportunities were less available, data and workshops equipped physicians interested in part-time employment with tools and information to assist in their negotiations. And perhaps gave some individuals the courage or network to attempt to obtain such a position. Careers in academia often seemed to be problematic because scholarly productivity was felt to be incompatible with part-time work. But it would be inaccurate to suggest that these sorts of discussions or workshops are a thing of the past. At the 2016 Pediatric Societies Meeting, the Women in Medicine Special Interest Group held a session titled "Strategies to Navigate and Support a Part-Time Faculty Career Path."

In the early 1990s, more than 20 years ago, there was concern about the "Feminization of Pediatrics." This term referred to the "worrisome" trend in which more pediatricians were women and their commitment to advance research as related to child health was deemed suboptimal. What greater evidence of this substandard commitment was there than a request for part-time work? It was bad enough that women would be late in the morning (hard to get to those 7:00 AM meetings when you couldn't drop you children off at preschool before 7:30 AM) or leave by 5:00 PM (extended care ended at 5:30 PM). In the late 1990s, I had the opportunity to present the notion of part-time employment to the Association of Medical School Pediatric Department Chairs, and there was the uniform sentiment that having part-time academicians was not in the best interest of the department or children.

In addition to the fear that child health research would be negatively affected by women (and part-time employment), another issue of concern was related to the integrity of the pediatric workforce. Children were potentially in danger because of the lack of sufficient pediatricians to meet their needs.

But how to calculate the need and the resources? Some say that 2 part-time employees give you more than one full-time employee. But this may be the rhetoric of those promoting part-time opportunities or may reflect a varying definition of part time. At my institution, anything less than 32 hours qualifies as part time, and there are no health benefits with such a position. It would be of interest if the AAP continues to survey its members and better define what the actual hours are, what the call is, what happens with malpractice insurance, and what the benefits are. It is possible that although the trend has leveled off, the nature of part-time positions has changed significantly since 2006, and, as the authors note, this has not been addressed in the present report.

C. D. Berkowitz, MD

Pediatricians' Experience with Clinical Ethics Consultation: A National Survey

Morrison W, Womer J, Nathanson P, et al (The Children's Hosp of Philadelphia, PA; Perelman School of Medicine at the Univ of Pennsylvania, Philadelphia; et al)
J Pediatr 167:919-924, 2015

Objective.—To conduct a national survey of pediatricians' access to and experience with clinical ethics consultation.

Study Design.—We surveyed a randomly selected sample of 3687 physician members of the American Academy of Pediatrics. We asked about their experiences with ethics consultation, the helpfulness of and barriers to consultation, and ethics education. Using a discrete choice experiment with maximum difference scaling, we evaluated which traits of ethics consultants were most valuable.

Results.—Of the total sample of 3687 physicians, 659 (18%) responded to the survey. One-third of the respondents had no experience with clinical ethics consultation, and 16% reported no access to consultation. General pediatricians were less likely to have access. The vast majority (90%) who had experience with consultation had found it helpful. Those with fewer years in practice were more likely to have training in ethics. The most frequently reported issues leading to consultation concerned end-of-life care and conflicts with patients/families or among the team. Intensive care unit physicians were more likely to have requested consultation. Mediation skills and ethics knowledge were the most highly valued consultant characteristics, and representing the official position of the hospital was the least-valued characteristic.

Conclusion.—There is variability in pediatricians' access to ethics consultation. Most respondents reported that consultation had been helpful in the past. Determining ethically appropriate end-of-life care and mediation of disagreements are common reasons that pediatricians request consultation.

▶ Pediatricians and other child health professionals deal with complicated ethical issues every day. In primary care, they often have to deal with parents whose values and preferences clash with those of the pediatrician.[1] Sometimes, this can undermine the trust that is an essential component of a therapeutic doctor-patient-parent relationship.[2] In subspecialties like neonatology, oncology, and neurology, pediatricians must care for children with complex chronic conditions. Sometimes, they must help families make end-of-life decisions. Clinicians who participate in research must balance their obligations as doctors with the rigorous demands of science. It is not surprising, given the ubiquity of ethical conundrums, that pediatricians sometimes feel the need for guidance from ethics consultants or ethics committees. What is perhaps surprising is how seldom they feel that need.

Kesselheim and colleagues showed that, at 46 freestanding children's hospitals, ethics consultants were consulted less than 1 time per month.[3] Thomas and colleagues found a similar paucity of ethics consults.[4] Now, Morrison and colleagues show that most pediatricians have not asked for an ethics consult in the last year and that, of those who did, most had only asked for a very few. They also show that when people did consult an ethicist, they generally found the response to be helpful.

There is a mystery wrapped up in these statistics. Ethical dilemmas are common. Ethics consultations are infrequent. When they occur, they are helpful. Why don't more occur?

Ethics consultation is designed "to help patients, staff, and others to resolve ethical concerns."[3,5] In actuality, it is more often a mechanism to arbitrate or mediate intractable disputes that have resisted resolution by other means.[6] The relatively low rate of ethics consultation suggests that most ethical concerns are resolved before they become intractable. To put it another way, ethicists' expertise is not really in ethics. It is in mediation and arbitration.

Streuli and colleagues suggest another role for such consults. They note that, in their children's hospital, ethics consultation works only when there is "an underlying institutional clinical ethics framework embodying a comprehensive set of transparently articulated values and opinions."[7] To put this another way, ethics is less about individual values and more about institutional values. In hospitals, the relevant institution is the hospital itself. Hospitals develop policies and practices that define the moral climate of the institution. Outside of hospitals, the institution is the profession of pediatrics itself. Pediatricians need to know whether their own practices are in sync with professional norms. Generally, this is something that they can learn by talking to other pediatricians. After all, the norms of a profession are the norms of the practitioners of that profession. The dilemmas for which an outside opinion is necessary, then, are those in which there is either intraprofessional disagreement or a challenge to the profession from somebody who is outside of it. The most common outside challenge comes from patients (or, in pediatrics, parents). This explains why the most common reasons for ethics consultation are to resolve disagreements among professionals or between professionals and the patient or family.

What, then, do ethics consultants do? The process of discussing and resolving ethical issues begins with consideration of the ethical beliefs of the individuals involved, including patients, families and professionals. The process must also honor the institutional ethos or the ethical norms of the profession. But different doctors and different hospitals may have slightly different missions. Some are religious institutions, some are secular. Some are private, some public. Some doctors are religious, others not. Doctors and hospitals in different communities serve different subcultures of patients. All of these factors may lead different doctors to develop different policies and practices about issues like prenatal counseling, medical futility, or the provision of innovative treatment. Societal norms related to these issues put constraints on both hospitals and individuals, creating a need for ethical discussion and processes.

The mediating and arbitrating role of the ethics consultant is a way of defining the limits of acceptable practice in a multicultural society that values pluralism and individuality but is not completely morally relativistic. The ethics consultant teases out the core beliefs that must be upheld in every case, regardless of the personal beliefs of the individuals involved. At the same time, the consultant tries to find the compromises that will best preserve the prerogative of individuals to preserve their own moral integrity. The most valuable skill for such a task is the delicate skill of mediating between disagreeing parties whose disagreements are often about deeply held values. The next decade will likely see more emphasis on mediation skills in the training of clinical ethicists.

J. D. Lantos, MD

References

1. Leask J, Kinnersley P. Physician communication with vaccine-hesitant parents: the start, not the end, of the story. *Pediatrics*. 2015;136:180-182.
2. Kluger J. Health. Vaccinate or leave. More pediatricians are firing families for not giving their kids shots. *Time*. 2011;178:57.
3. Kesselheim JC, Johnson J, Joffe S. Ethics consultations in children's hospitals: results from a survey of pediatric clinical ethicists. *Pediatrics*. 2010;125:742-746.
4. Thomas SM, Ford PJ, Weise KL, Worley S, Kodish E. Not just little adults: a review of 102 paediatric ethics consultations. *Acta Paediatr*. 2015;104:529-534.
5. Fox E, Berkowitz KA, Chanko BL et al. Integrated Ethics: Improving Ethics Quality in Health Care. http://www.ethics.va.gov/ECprimer.pdf. Accessed February 9, 2016.
6. Fiester A. Bioethics mediation & the end of clinical ethics as we know it. *Cardozo J Conflict Resol*. 2014;15:501-513.
7. Streuli JC, Staubli G, Pfändler-Poletti M, Baumann-Hölzle R, Ersch J. Five-year experience of clinical ethics consultations in a pediatric teaching hospital. *Eur J Pediatr*. 2014;173:629-636.

Sex Differences in Academic Rank in US Medical Schools in 2014

Jena AB, Khullar D, Ho O, et al (Harvard Med School, Boston, MA; Massachusetts General Hosp, Boston; et al)
JAMA 314:1149-1158, 2015

Importance.—The proportion of women at the rank of full professor in US medical schools has not increased since 1980 and remains below that of men. Whether differences in age, experience, specialty, and research productivity between sexes explain persistent disparities in faculty rank has not been studied.

Objective.—To analyze sex differences in faculty rank among US academic physicians.

Design, Setting, and Participants.—We analyzed sex differences in faculty rank using a cross-sectional comprehensive database of US physicians with medical school faculty appointments in 2014 (91 073 physicians; 9.1% of all US physicians), linked to information on physician sex, age, years since residency, specialty, authored publications, National Institutes of Health (NIH) funding, and clinical trial investigation. We estimated sex differences in full professorship, as well as a combined outcome of associate or full professorship, adjusting for these factors in a multilevel (hierarchical) model. We also analyzed how sex differences varied with specialty and whether differences were more prevalent at schools ranked highly in research.

Exposures.—Physician sex.

Main Outcomes and Measures.—Academic faculty rank.

Results.—In all, there were 30 464 women who were medical faculty vs 60 609 men. Of those, 3623 women (11.9%) vs 17 354 men (28.6%) had full-professor appointments, for an absolute difference of -16.7% (95% CI, -17.3% to -16.2%).Women faculty were younger and disproportionately represented in internal medicine and pediatrics. The mean total number of publications for women was 11.6 vs 24.8 for men, for a difference of -13.2 (95% CI, -13.6 to -12.7); the mean first- or last-author publications for women was 5.9 vs 13.7 for men, for a difference of -7.8 (95% CI, -8.1 to -7.5). Among 9.1% of medical faculty with an NIH grant, 6.8% (2059 of 30 464) were women and 10.3% (6237 of 60 609) were men, for a difference of -3.5% (95% CI, -3.9% to -3.1%). In all, 6.4% of women vs 8.8% of men had a trial registered on ClinicalTrials.gov, for a difference of -2.4% (95% CI, -2.8% to -2.0%). After multivariable adjustment, women were less likely than men to have achieved full-professor status (absolute adjusted difference in proportion, -3.8%; 95% CI, -4.4% to -3.3%). Sex-differences in full professorship were present across all specialties and did not vary according to whether a physician's medical school was ranked highly in terms of research funding.

Conclusions and Relevance.—Among physicians with faculty appointments at US medical schools, there were sex differences in academic faculty rank, with women substantially less likely than men to be full professors, after accounting for age, experience, specialty, and measures of research productivity.

▶ Jena et al report on a comprehensive cross-sectional dataset of US physicians with medical school faculty appointments. The study focused on sex differences at the full professor level and the combined associate and full professor levels. This analysis is particularly robust because of the ability to control for a variety of potential confounding factors including age, years since residency, specialty, authored publications, National Institutes of Health funding, clinical trial investigations, and research ranking of the faculty member's institution. Despite controlling for all of these predictors of academic rank, significant sex differences were still identified across nearly all specialties, including pediatrics, suggesting that female sex is an independent predictor of the decreased numbers of women at higher academic levels.

Given the specific context of pediatrics, in which women make up 52% of faculty across ranks, the end result that sex differences persist in the field is disheartening and suggests that sex equity challenges could be even more significant in specialties with less female faculty representation. Prior research has documented sex-specific national discrepancies in leadership positions in medical schools, including pediatrics, with the percentage of women chairs hovering at 20%.[1] However, at the same time, women make up 75% of all active pediatric residents from US and Canadian medical schools. We are left to wonder what, then, occurs between a recent graduate's first entry into the ranks of academic medicine from residency to a faculty career to account for this large discrepancy?

Studies have documented institutional and environmental factors that serve to impede women's advancement through the faculty ranks including institutional barriers,, unsupportive work environments, personal choice, and unconscious sex biases. In addition, women faculty members face an entire social context of preconceived notions. In a study of respondents across the general population using the publicly availability Implicit Association Test (available through Project Implicit), robust preferences in the general population for the concepts of male paired with science and female paired with liberal arts have been demonstrated, along with equally strong preferences for the concepts of male paired with career and female paired with home. In a study of 4 large public accounting firms, men were favored over women in being given important career-advancing projects by their supervisor. The supervisors' biases that women were less likely to have a successful outcome in a challenging assignment (and potentially reflect negatively on the supervisor) appeared to drive this outcome. While in a different industry, this observation underscores the importance of the critical role of the faculty's supervisor in guiding and mentoring faculty in their career development.

Given these prior research findings, it is perhaps not surprising that Jena et al find this result of continued sex differences despite controlling for traditional variables associated with academic rank. There are, however, limitations to their study that provide avenues for future research and possible interventions. First, the authors mention that they do not have information on faculty line or track, (ie, primary clinician-educator roles, in which many women faculty find themselves). If biases did not exist, however, we would expect high proportions of women as full professors in these tracks. In practice, this does not appear to be the case, although analysis by faculty line could identify tracks in which less sex bias could potentially exist.

Second, it is true that women professionals are more likely than men to experience career interruptions because of their children, which may adversely affect career progression. Additionally, research finds that faculty compensation packages differ significantly between men and women faculty from the very beginning of their careers despite controlling for generally agreed upon predictors of compensation. These differences in career experiences as well as the provision of institutional resources may have an outsized contributing role in sex differences at the highest ranks.

Finally, the greatest limitation of the study is the assumption that the authors are able to control for a variety of predictor factors, without taking into account the inability to control for other potentially more significant predictors. As such, the model inevitably suffers from omitted variable bias. It can be argued, for example, that unconscious biases and institutional barriers in the work environment, especially in leadership and mentors, although difficult to quantify, likely have a major impact on both the predictor variables and the dependent variable. This finding makes model estimation difficult, as the predictors themselves are subject to biases.

These limitations, however, do not discount the major finding of this study, which is the persistence of the sex gap in academic leadership. It is important for the academic medicine community to understand that despite objective metrics for advancement, sex biases still persist within the field. This systemic bias has negative consequences for the quality of academic medicine by limiting the numbers of excellent academic physicians who also happen to be women. Research shows that diversity is valuable for corporate and academic teams alike. For example, a McKinsey analysis found that sex-diverse and ethnically diverse companies have higher financial performance than their more homogenous counterparts. In the academic world, mixed sex teams and teams with higher ethnic diversity are found to produce higher-impact research articles than single-sex and single-ethnicity teams, respectively.,

In the field of pediatrics, sex diversity in leadership is especially important. Pediatrics draws a high number of women to the field in the earlier career stages; however, if women faculty members in the field continue to suffer from stymied advancement opportunities, sex equality at senior ranks will face significant obstacles. We must identify and mitigate such obstacles if we anticipate that contributions fueled by sex equity can be achieved in academic medicine.

M. Fassiotto, PhD
Y. Maldonado, MD
C. Sandborg, MD

Article Index

Chapter 1: Adolescent Medicine

Chapter 2: Allergy

Chapter 3: Anesthesia Pain

Chapter 4: Blood

Chapter 12: Health Policy and Economics

Chapter 13: Heart and Blood Vessels

Chapter 14: Hospital Critical Care

Chapter 15: Infectious Diseases

Chapter 16: Musculoskeletal

Chapter 17: Neonatology

Chapter 21: Oncology

Chapter 22: Ophthalmology

Chapter 23: Pediatric Surgery

Chapter 24: Psychiatry

Chapter 25: Respiratory Tract

Chapter 26: Rheumatology

Chapter 27: Therapeutics and Toxicology

Chapter 28: Training and Professionalism

Author Index

Edwards Brothers Malloy
Ann Arbor MI. USA
December 13, 2016